Medical-Surgical Nursing

SIXTH EDITION

Lippincott Certification Review

Medical-Surgical Nursing

SIXTH EDITION

Clinical Editor

LAURA M. WILLIS, DNP, APRN, FNP-C, CMSRN

Family Nurse Practitioner
Springfield Regional Medical Group
Urbana Family Medicine and Pediatrics
Urbana, Ohio

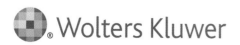

Philadelphia • Baltimore • New York • London
Buenos Aires • Hong Kong • Sydney • Tokyo

Acquisitions Editor: Nicole Dernoski
Editorial Coordinator: Lindsay Ries
Clinical Editor: Laura Willis
Art Director: Elaine Kasmer
Manufacturing Coordinator: Kathy Brown
Production Project Manager: Marian Bellus
Prepress Vendor: SPi Global

Sixth Edition

9 8 7 6 5 4 3 2 1

Printed in China

Library of Congress Cataloging-in-Publication Data
Names: Willis, Laura M., 1969- author.
Title: Lippincott certification review. Medical-surgical nursing / Laura M. Willis.
Other titles: Lippincott's review for medical-surgical nursing certification | Medical-surgical nursing
Description: Sixth edition. | Philadelphia : Wolters Kluwer, [2018] | Preceded by: Lippincott's review for medical-surgical nursing certification. 5th ed. c2012 | Includes bibliographical references and index.
Identifiers: LCCN 2017053869 | ISBN 9781496387332
Subjects: | MESH: Medical-Surgical Nursing | Certification | Examination Questions | Outlines
Classification: LCC RD99.25 | NLM WY 18.2 | DDC 617.0231076—dc23 LC record available at https://lccn.loc.gov/2017053869

LWW.com

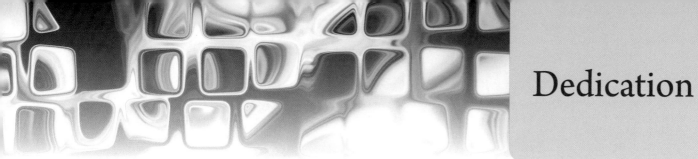

Dedication

It is with appreciation that I dedicate this book to:

The leaders and mentors who have shaped and molded me over the past two decades. I am humbled to have each of your influence in my life and my career.

To my family. I love you all so much.

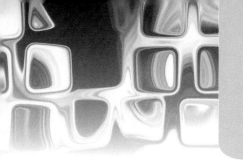

Contributors and Consultants

Diego Acero, MSN, FNP-C
Transplant Coordinator
Northwell Health
Manhasset, NY

Kaye L. Claytor, PhD, CMSRN, ACNS-BC
Education Specialist
Clarian Health
Indianapolis, Indiana

Keelin C. Cromar, MSN, RN
Adjunct Faculty
Mississippi Gulf Coast Community College
Perkinson, MS

Phyllis Magaletto, MS, RN, BC
Instructor, Medical-Surgical Nursing
Cochran School of Nursing
Yonkers, New York

Katrin Moskowitz, DNP, FNP
Nurse Practitioner
Midstate Medical Center
Meriden, CT
and
Charlotte Hungerford Hospital
Torrington, CT

Joyce W. Pompey, DNP, APRN-BC, RNC
Assistant Professor
School of Nursing
University of South Carolina Aiken
Aiken, South Carolina

Cherie Rebar, PhD, MBA, RN, COI
Professor of Nursing
Wittenberg University
Springfield, OH

Amy Slusher, MSN, APRN, FNP-C
Nurse Practitioner
Optum
Blue Ash, OH

Estella J. Wetzel, MSN, APRN, FNP-C
Family Nurse Practitioner
Springboro Family Medicine
Springboro, OH

Fawn Workman, MSN, APRN, FNP-C
Nurse Practitioner
Bon Secours Depaul Medical Center
Chesapeake, VA

Medical-surgical nursing is alive and well! Once considered a basic skill required of all nurses, medical-surgical nursing has become increasingly complex, evolving into a vital specialty nursing practice. Medical-surgical nurses must care for a growing number of health care consumers with complex medical needs as well as keep current with continuing developments in health care science, technology, and economics. They must overcome the challenges these developments can bring to providing patient care while continuing to provide high-quality nursing care to diverse patient populations in all stages of life—from adolescents to the elderly.

Specialty certification is the most important step a registered nurse can take in his or her career. It signifies a nurse's commitment to professional growth and development and, most importantly, to provide safe, effective, timely, and high-quality patient care. Research by the American Board of Nursing Specialties confirms that certification validates specialized knowledge, enhances professional credibility and autonomy, indicates professional growth, and provides evidence of professional commitment.

Lippincott's Review for Medical-Surgical Nursing Certification will certainly help you in your pursuit of certification as a medical-surgical nurse. This thoroughly updated review book offers the most current content typically included in medical-surgical nursing certification tests by both the Medical-Surgical Nursing Certification Board (MSNCB) of the Academy of Medical Surgical Nurses (AMSN) and the American Nurses Credentialing Center (ANCC).

The core content of this new edition has been attentively revised to reflect the best available practices that influence medical-surgical nursing. It includes review topics on the foundations of nursing, legal and ethical aspects of nursing, principles of medical-surgical nursing and wound care, and disruptions in homeostasis. It also reviews the different body systems and associated diseases that certification exams frequently cover and that medical-surgical nurses commonly encounter.

The content includes cultural and ethnic beliefs and practices, evidence-based practice, safety issues, health maintenance and wellness, and lifestyle management. Covered are collaboration, patient's bill of rights and self-determination, the developmental theories of Jean Piaget and Abraham Maslow, nutrition, substance abuse, abuse and neglect, complementary therapies, obesity, herbal remedies, adult immunizations, and laboratory values.

The post test practice questions have been completely revised along with revisions to many of the questions at the end of each chapter.

Whether you're a newly graduated nurse exploring the specialty of medical-surgical nursing, a displaced nurse reentering the nursing profession, or a seasoned nurse wanting to update your skills and knowledge in medical-surgical nursing or become certified in this prestigious specialty, I know you'll find this book a valuable addition to your library. More importantly, this book will give you the knowledge and confidence you need to ace the medical-surgical nursing certification exam.

I wish you well as you move forward in this major endeavor—becoming certified as a medical-surgical nurse.

Laura M. Willis, DNP, APRN, FNP-C, CMSRN
Family Nurse Practitioner
Springfield Regional Medical Group
Urbana Family Medicine and Pediatrics
Urbana, Ohio

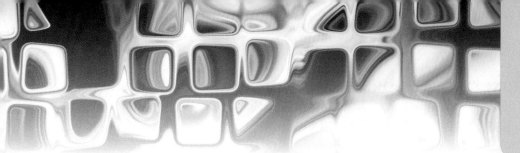

Contents

Chapter 1

Medical-Surgical Nursing Certification

Medical-surgical nurses are the backbone of health and wellness care in the United States. Indeed, new nursing graduates are strongly encouraged to work in a hospital as a medical-surgical nurse for 1 to 2 years to hone their skills before branching out into other areas of nursing. In 1972, the American Nurses Association (ANA) recognized this valuable specialty by certifying medical-surgical nurses through the American Nurses Credentialing Center (ANCC). Almost 151,000 nurses have been certified to date in more than 30 specialty and advanced practice areas of nursing. Further, as of 1990, a new medical-surgical nursing organization, the Academy of Medical-Surgical Nurses (AMSN), was founded to serve the specific educational needs of this group of nurses. The AMSN has also developed a certification examination to recognize the knowledge base of the practicing medical-surgical nurse.

The ANCC Certification Examination

The ANA offers two examinations for medical-surgical nursing certification: a basic medical-surgical nurse examination and a clinical specialist examination in adult health (formerly medical-surgical nursing). The ANCC administers the computer-based examinations in cities throughout the United States and its territories. The tests last about 4 hours.

Eligibility and Application

The ANCC establishes criteria for eligibility to take the examination. Requirements for the basic examination differ from those of the clinical specialist examination. The criteria discussed in this book were in effect as of the 2010 examination. Because requirements can change, candidates should obtain the latest criteria before applying for certification. (See *ANCC Certification Eligibility Requirements*, page 2.) The medical-surgical nursing examination is available to nurses with an associate's degree or diploma, thus establishing two levels of credentialing. Nurses certified at the baccalaureate level are designated as Board Certified, or "RN-BC"; nurses certified at the associate or diploma level are designated as Certified, or "RN-C." The credential approved for clinical nurse specialists is "APRN-BC."

After you have decided to prepare for the examination, obtain the certification catalog by writing to the American Nurses Credentialing Center, 8515 Georgia Ave., Suite 400, Silver Spring, MD 20910-3492, or by calling toll-free 1-800-284-2378 or accessing online. This catalog provides all the information you'll need to apply. Examination information, catalogs, and applications may also be obtained through the ANCC Web site at www.nursecredentialing.org.

Pay careful attention to all steps in the application process. Failure to complete any step correctly may make you ineligible to take the examination on the date you had planned. All applicants must pay a nonrefundable application fee and an examination fee set each year by the credentialing center.

Box 1-1: ANCC Certification Eligibility Requirements

The American Nurses Credentialing Center's (ANCC) eligibility criteria for certification in medical-surgical nursing, as of 2017, are listed below. Note that the requirements for the basic nursing examination differ from those of the specialist examination.

Criteria for a medical-surgical nurse (RN-BC [Registered Nurse–Board Certified])

By the time of application, you must:

1. hold a current, active unrestricted professional registered nurse (RN) license in the United States or its territories or the professional, legally recognized equivalent in another country
2. have practiced the equivalent of 2 years full-time as an RN
3. have practiced as a licensed RN in medical-surgical nursing for a minimum of 2,000 hours within the past 3 years
4. have received 30 contact hours within the last 3 years in medical-surgical nursing.

Criteria for a clinical nurse specialist in adult health (ACNS-BC [Adult Health Clinical Nurse Specialist–Board Certified])

By the time of application, you must:

1. hold a current, active RN license in the United States or its territories or the professional, legally recognized equivalent in another country
2. hold a master's degree or higher in nursing
3. have been prepared in medical-surgical nursing through a master's degree program or a formal postgraduate master's program in nursing
4. have graduated from an accredited institution granting graduate-level academic credit for all of the course work (including advanced health assessment, advanced pharmacology, and advanced pathophysiology) that includes both didactic and clinical components, and a minimum of 500 hours of supervised clinical practice in medical-surgical nursing.

Source: American Nurses Credentialing Center. Silver Spring, MD. Retrieved from www.nursecredentialing.org.

Certification Test Plan

After establishing your eligibility, the credentialing center will mail or e-mail you a link to the handbook that contains the current examination blueprint, or test plan. The test plan outlines the test content and the ratio (weighting) of each content area. Information about the test plan, especially its content, can provide considerable guidance in helping you organize your study plan.

In the ANCC catalog for 2017, medical-surgical examination topics included biophysical and psychosocial concepts, pathophysiology of body systems, patient care, health promotion and wellness, management and leadership, and legal and ethical issues and trends. Examination topics for the clinical specialist in medical-surgical nursing included clinical practice, consultation, management, education, research, and issues and trends.

The Board on Certification for Medical-Surgical Nursing Practice, one of the many ANCC certification boards, develops the certification examination. The test objectively evaluates knowledge, comprehension, and application of medical-surgical nursing theory and practice to patient care. The test development committee defines the content areas covered in each test and the emphasis placed on each area.

Certified medical-surgical nurses from around the country contribute questions for each examination. The committee reviews each test item for accuracy, readability, and relevance to the test plan. Sample questions approved by the committee are compiled into an examination that will be used on the next test date. All computer-based examinations offer on-site testing results. The certificate and ANCC pin are mailed about 8 weeks after successful completion of the examination.

Each test contains 175 multiple-choice questions. Of those questions, 150 are scored questions and 25 are unscored, pretest questions. The pretest questions aren't distinguishable from the scored questions. A candidate's score is based solely on the 150 scored questions. Candidates have 4 hours to complete the test. A break usually is provided.

If the candidate takes a paper-and-pencil exam instead of a computer exam, test results are mailed about 6 to 8 weeks after the examination. No results are released early or over the telephone to protect the privacy of candidates.

The AMSN Certification Examination

The AMSN is a professional organization for nurses who practice medical-surgical/adult health care. The organization developed the Scope and Standards of Medical-Surgical Nursing Practice; it builds on the ANA's Standards of Clinical Practice and helps to establish the responsibilities of medical-surgical nurses in all types of health care settings.

The AMSN founded the Medical-Surgical Nursing Certification Board (MSNCB) to promote and implement a certification examination for medical-surgical nurses. The tests are offered as computer-based exams, available throughout the year, or as paper-and-pencil exams, administered four times a year. The test lasts 4 hours.

Eligibility and Application

The MSNCB establishes criteria for eligibility to take the examination. However, because requirements can change, candidates should obtain the latest criteria before applying for certification. (See *AMSN Certification Eligibility Criteria*) The medical-surgical certification examination does not require a BSN degree. Nurses who are certified through this examination are designated as "RN-CMSRN."

MSNCB works with a testing center, the Center for Nursing Education. The certification catalog and examination application may be obtained by writing to MSNCB, East Holly Avenue, Box 56, Pitman, NJ 08071. Or download an application from the Web site www.amsn.org.

Again, be sure to read all directions, and pay careful attention to all steps in the application process. Failure to complete the application properly may lead to ineligibility to take the examination.

Certification Test Plan

If the application is completed properly, an examination permit is mailed approximately 2 weeks before the test. The permit will include the test center address and the time you should report to the center. You must have the examination permit to be admitted to take the exam.

The paper-and-pencil exam contains 175 questions, including 25 unscored, pretest questions. The exam must be completed in 4 hours, and results are mailed approximately 8 weeks after the exam.

The computer-based exam contains 150 scored questions, with no pretest questions. The test must be completed in 3 hours, and the results are available immediately after the exam is completed.

Strategies for a Successful Certification Examination

When you're ready to take a medical-surgical nursing certification examination, you'll need to learn about the certification process. Certification is a way to validate your knowledge, skills, and abilities as a medical-surgical nurse. The certification test is based on predetermined standards, so you should become certified in your area of clinical expertise.

Start by selecting the organization you want certification from. Next, research the requirements for certification. You can begin your research by typing "medical-surgical certification" into a search engine. Some Web sites you might want to look more closely at include www.msncb.org and www.nursecredentialing.org. Certifying organizations provide a test content outline, test reference list, and sample tests with practice questions. They typically list review courses with locations and dates as well as test-taking strategy courses. If you must choose only one course, select the review course. You can learn about successful test-taking strategies by reading further.

Box 1-2: AMSN Certification Eligibility Criteria

The Academy of Medical-Surgical Nurses (AMSN) eligibility criteria, as of 2017, are listed below.

By the time of application you must:
- hold a current and unrestricted license as a registered nurse (RN) in the United States or any of its territories

OR

- hold a current, full, unrestricted license to practice as a first-level nurse in the country in which one's nursing education was completed, and meet the eligibility criteria for licensure as an RN in accordance with requirements of the Commission of Graduates of Foreign Nursing Schools (CGFNS)
- have practiced a minimum of 2 full years as an RN in an adult medical-surgical clinical setting
- have accrued a minimum of 2,000 hours within the past 3 years of clinical practice in an adult medical-surgical setting.

Source: Academy of Medical-Surgical Nurses. Pitman, NJ. Retrieved from www.amsn.org.

Three essential components lead to successful certification: following a well-thought-out study plan and reviewing diligently, preparing carefully for examination day to avoid unexpected surprises, and learning successful test-taking strategies. Each component calls for a closer look.

Following a Study Plan

Successful test preparation calls for a well-thought-out study plan. This book provides you with an organized source for that review; you can also use the test center content outline to help guide your study plan. It is also helpful to determine what type of learner you are such as visual, auditory, etc. Then, identify the concepts you find most difficult and content where you have a knowledge gap, and place those topics first on your study outline. Next, divide the study plan into weeks and then subdivide that into days. Divide the topics into study sessions for each day.

To help organize your thoughts, make note cards that concisely cover major topics. Be creative with the note cards. Use mnemonic devices to help you recall information you otherwise can't easily remember. Try some brightly colored pens or pencils to help make the cards decorative and visually memorable.

Make sure you allow at least a week for each of the major content areas. Then, divide each week into a pattern of study by days. Study a topic thoroughly on its assigned day of the week, and then reserve a day to take practice exams, using good test-taking strategies. Mark off each topic as you complete it.

Use 2 of the last 3 days before the exam to review topics you're still weak on and to take practice exams. When you take practice exams, also practice pacing yourself so that you'll be able to complete the exam. Give yourself about a minute to answer each question; use a stopwatch if necessary. Finally, reserve the day before the exam for rest and relaxation.

You may want to try combining study with exercise. For instance, walking while studying can help you to relieve stress, relax, and maintain your physical health. Just remember, if you walk and study, be safe; don't walk on busy streets or use equipment that could lead to an accident.

Some certification centers offer the choice of taking the test using either paper and pencil or a computer. Make sure you take practice tests using the appropriate method. If you plan to take the test on a computer—the most popular method—then take online practice tests. If you plan to take a paper-and-pencil version of the test, take practice exams using that method.

Most medical-surgical certification exams range from 3½ to 4 hours. The week before the exam, take a practice test that's the same length as the actual exam and spend the full 3½ to 4 hours taking the exam. Think of this as pre-examination calisthenics. If you have time, take a full-length exam twice, on separate days. However, *don't* attempt a practice exam the day before the real exam; you'll tire yourself out unnecessarily.

After you've completed the study plan, use the last day for rest, relaxation, and final last-minute preparation for the test. Eat nutritiously, participate in light exercise, and get plenty of sleep the night before the exam.

Preparing for Examination Day

Careful planning can help you avoid unexpected surprises on test day. Make sure you know the *exact* location of the test center. Drive to the center a few days before the actual test at about the time the test is scheduled. Time the drive so you know how long it will take to arrive.

Collect the required identification. Most test centers will accept a driver's license, passport, or US military identification. Make sure your identification is current (not expired) and that your name and address are correct. Test centers may not allow books, calculators, food, drinks, notes, cell phones, or personal electronics; check the test center's rules before you arrive. Also, check to see what *is* allowed. If the center allows pencils and paper, make sure you bring them with you.

The evening before the exam, fill your car's gas tank, lay out your clothes, pack a small bag of peanut-covered chocolate (or another high-energy snack if you're allergic to peanuts) and a bottle of water, and gather together your note cards. Plan to wear layered clothing, shoes with covered toes to prevent cold feet, and generally comfortable attire.

On day of the test, arrive 30 minutes ahead of time. Before entering the test site, eat your snack; the peanuts will provide long-term energy, the sugar will give you quick energy, and the chocolate will make the neurons in your brain fire faster. Then drink enough water to quench your thirst. Next, pull out your note cards one last time and look at them. Don't analyze them or attempt to learn anything in the last minute; just try to see what each card looks like.

When you arrive at the center, you'll be checked in to the test site and then admitted to the examination room. Before you enter, take one last bathroom stop. Once you're in the examination room, at the start of the test write, down everything you can still "see" from your note cards (if you're allowed to have paper and pencil in the examination room). Write down everything you can visualize, but don't spend more than 10 minutes transcribing note cards from memory.

Finally, remember that you've studied hard, learned extensively from clinical practice, and prepared well to take the medical-surgical nursing certification examination. Have confidence in yourself; you're ready for the test!

Learning Test-Taking Strategies

You can improve your chances of passing any standardized multiple-choice examination by using proven test-taking techniques. These include knowing how timed examinations are administered, understanding all the parts of a test question, and taking specific steps to help make sure that you've selected the correct answer. And if you come across a question you absolutely don't know the answer to, you need to know how to make a good guess!

Because you aren't penalized for guessing, you should try to respond to every question. Answering other questions may stimulate your recall of the correct answer for a question you've left unanswered. If you still have no idea of a correct answer, certain tricks can give you a greater than 50% chance of guessing accurately.

Keep in mind that the people writing questions for certification exams are experts in the content area and know test-taking strategies thoroughly, so the following tricks may not always work for you. But generally, you're more likely to guess correctly if you select option B or C. Also, longer answers tend to be correct, and if you come across two similar answers, one of those answers is probably correct. Eliminating at least one answer that you're sure is incorrect will also improve your chances of guessing correctly. And if all other strategies fail, you still have a one in four chance of guessing correctly.

To try out your test-taking strategies, you can take online tests from other disciplines that you know nothing about. In such cases, all you have to rely on are good test-taking strategies. If you score at least 60% on such tests, you've mastered those strategies.

All questions on a certification examination are carefully crafted and pretested to ensure readability and uniformity. Understanding the components of a question can help you analyze what it's asking, increasing the likelihood that you'll respond correctly. (See *Parts of a Test Question*, page 6.)

Time management is crucial when taking a standardized test because you receive no credit for unanswered questions. Because of that, you should try to pace yourself to finish the test on time. Remember, you'll have about a minute to answer each question. Don't spend too much time on any one question. If you're taking a paper-and-pencil exam, place a light pencil mark next to a question you're unsure of and come back later, if time is available.

Computer-based exams also allow you to mark questions you're unsure about to return to later if time permits. Make sure you know how to mark questions before starting the test; the proctor can help you if you need assistance.

For both computer and paper-and-pencil tests, read every question carefully. If a clinical situation precedes the question, study the information given. Watch for key words (such as *most, first, best,* and *except*); they're important guides to which option you should select. For example, if a question reads, "Which of the following nursing actions should the nurse perform first?" you may find that all the options are appropriate for the patient's condition but only one clearly takes precedence over the others.

As you read the stem, cover up the answers on a paper test or ignore the computer screen with the answers and try to answer the question without regard to the answer options. Then look at the options to see if your answer is listed. If so, it's probably correct. By knowing the answer, you save time and have avoided second-guessing yourself.

If you're not sure of the answer, read all the choices. If you select an option before reading every choice, you'll deny yourself the chance to evaluate them all. Try to find an option that most closely resembles the one you thought would be correct and to eliminate at least two answers. Then, choose your best selection. If you don't find a best selection, look for the best option available. Remember, you're looking for the best answer among those choices given. It may not be what *you* think is the best response, but it's all you have to work with. Mark that question to return to later if time permits.

For some questions, you may see two options that seem correct and have trouble deciding between them. Look at them again, knowing that there must be a difference. Read the stem again; you may discover something

Box 1-3: **Parts of a Test Question**

Multiple-choice questions on certification examinations are constructed according to strict psychometric standards. As shown here, each question has a stem and four options, including a key (correct answer) and three distractors (incorrect answers). A brief clinical situation or case study commonly precedes each question. Note how clearly the question is written, with no unnecessary words in the stem. Each option should be relatively uniform in length.

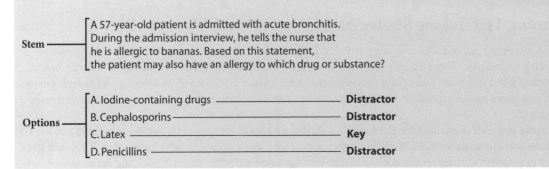

Stem —
A 57-year-old patient is admitted with acute bronchitis. During the admission interview, he tells the nurse that he is allergic to bananas. Based on this statement, the patient may also have an allergy to which drug or substance?

Options —
A. Iodine-containing drugs —— **Distractor**
B. Cephalosporins —— **Distractor**
C. Latex —— **Key**
D. Penicillins —— **Distractor**

you didn't see before that will help you make a selection. If not and you still can't choose, make an educated guess using good test-taking strategies. As a last resort, select B or C. Again, mark that question to return to later.

Despite thorough preparation, you may not know the answer to some questions. Relax. Remember that you're an expert practitioner and possess a wealth of information. Think of patient cases you've had, and recall information about them that you can apply to the question. Mentally review your note cards, or look at your scratch paper if that's allowed. Remind yourself of the principle involved, and recall what you know about applying that principle to practice situations. Don't spend too long on the question, though; mark the question and move on. As you look at other questions, you may find information that helps you make an accurate selection for the question you had trouble with.

After you've answered the last question, take a deep breath. Take a brief moment to reflect on how many test questions you knew the correct answer to. Remember that you planned and studied and are now well prepared to discriminate between the choices for test items you were uncertain about. Return to the questions you didn't answer or those you marked for later review, and then answer those questions or review your answers for possible changes. Don't be afraid to change a selection if you later think of a better choice.

Finally, complete the exam and submit it. For a paper-and-pencil exam, be sure to erase any stray pencil marks before turning in the exam. If you're taking a paper-and-pencil exam, you'll be notified of your results in a few weeks. If you're taking a computerized exam, you'll find out the results right away—which can be frightening. Take another deep breath, and view your results. Whether you scored high enough to pass the certification exam or not, you should feel good that you created a study plan, worked on a timeline, and prepared to take the test. If you weren't successful, as soon as you leave the test center, write down the test items you were uncertain about. Then, go back and alter your study plan to include the items you listed.

Taking the certification examination shows confidence in your knowledge of medical-surgical nursing. An organized study program, good test-taking strategies, and last-minute review of test items can lead to successful certification as a medical-surgical nurse.

Selected References

American Nurses Credentialing Center. (2017). Silver Spring, MD. Retrieved from www.nursecredentialing.org.

Academy of Medical-Surgical Nurses. (2017). Pitman, NJ. Retrieved from www.amsn.org.

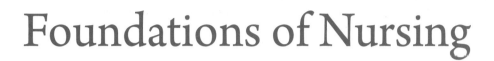

Chapter 2

Foundations of Nursing

Nursing Process

History of the Nursing Process

- In the 1970s, the American Nurses Association (ANA) mandated that the nursing process be part of nursing practice and instituted a five-step process (assessment, diagnosis, planning, implementation, and evaluation)
- In 1982, the North American Nursing Diagnosis Association, now known as NANDA International (NANDA-I), was established to develop, review, and update nursing diagnoses; this organization meets every 2 years

Purpose of the Nursing Process

- The nursing process provides the core for problem solving, clinical decisions, and patient-focused care
- It uses the scientific method of observation, measurement, data collection, and data analysis to evaluate the needs of individuals, families, or communities
- The nursing process provides an organized and universal method of communication for nurses in education, practice, and research
- Through the nursing process, nurses have adopted a body of knowledge that's unique to nursing; this knowledge encompasses illness, illness prevention, and health maintenance

Standards of Practice

- The Standards of Clinical Nursing Practice are directly related to the nursing process
  - Standard I ("The nurse collects patient health data") relates to step 1 of the nursing process (assessment)
  - Standard II ("The nurse analyzes the assessment data in determining diagnosis") relates to step 2 of the nursing process (diagnosis)
  - Standard III ("The nurse identifies expected outcomes individualized to the patient") and Standard IV ("The nurse develops a care plan that prescribes interventions to attain expected outcomes") relate to step 3 of the nursing process (planning)
  - Standard V ("The nurse implements the interventions in the care plan") relates to step 4 of the nursing process (implementation)
  - Standard VI ("The nurse evaluates the patient's progress toward outcomes") relates to step 5 of the nursing process (evaluation)
- These clinical standards use the steps of the nursing process to help achieve the standards of practice that have been set forth by state nurse practice acts and the ANA standards of professional performance as well as the Academy of Medical-Surgical Nurses Scope and Standards of Nursing Practice
- These varying standards help assure quality nursing care and provide the gauge by which to measure quality

Steps of the Nursing Process

- Assessment
  - Assessment is the collection and organization of data
  - Data collection involves the formation of a database from the patient interview, patient history, subjective data (what the patient says or believes), objective data (vital signs, laboratory results), and physical assessment (inspection, palpation, percussion, and auscultation)
  - Assessment also includes psychological, sociocultural, spiritual, economic, and lifestyle factors
  - Data organization and documentation involves clustering and recording related findings, reviewing the amount and completeness of data, and evaluating it through comparison with normal or baseline data
- Diagnosis
  - Diagnosis is the identification of actual or potential health conditions or needs as indicated by the assessment data; it is also defined as the responses to actual or potential health problems
  - The diagnostic statement consists of three parts: identifying the problem or need, identifying the cause of the problem or need ("related to"), and identifying related signs and symptoms ("as evidenced by")
  - A sample diagnostic statement is "ineffective breathing pattern related to fatigue, as evidenced by shortness of breath, shallow respirations, and tachycardia"
  - Nursing diagnoses are organized in a taxonomy based on human response patterns (see *NANDA-I Taxonomy II by Domain*, page 323); they also may be grouped by functional health patterns (health maintenance, nutritional-metabolic, elimination, activity-exercise, altered sleep, cognitive-perceptual, self-perception-self-concept, role-relationship, sexuality-reproductive, coping-stress tolerance, and value-belief)
- Planning
  - Planning involves determining achievable outcomes, setting priorities, establishing goals, selecting appropriate interventions, and documenting care
  - Priorities can be based on Maslow's hierarchy of needs (in which physical needs, such as oxygen and safety, take priority over psychosocial needs, such as self-esteem and self-actualization) or other factors
  - Goals are established by identifying the desired outcomes; short-term and long-term goals can be defined and are measurable and time-specific
  - Specific nursing interventions are selected to develop an individualized care plan; interventions should specify times, frequencies, and amounts
  - The care plan is documented so that all health care team members know the patient's individualized plan
- Implementation
  - Implementation involves providing actual care to the patient according to the care plan
  - Data collection, documentation, and assessment continue during this step
- Evaluation
  - To provide effective care, the goals, outcomes, and appropriateness of interventions must be continuously evaluated and modified in relation to the care plan

---

Box 2-1: Practice Roles of the Nurse

No matter what the practice setting, the medical-surgical nurse assumes various roles.

Caregiver

- As a caregiver, the nurse assesses the patient, analyzes his needs, develops nursing diagnoses, and plans, delivers, and evaluates nursing interventions and patient outcomes.

Advocate

- As an advocate, the nurse helps the patient and his family members interpret information from other health care providers and make decisions about health-related needs.
- The nurse ensures the health, welfare, and safety of the patient.
- The nurse makes every attempt to respect the patient's decisions and to communicate those wishes to other members of the health care team.
- The nurse accepts the patient's decisions, even if they differ from the decisions the nurse would make.

(continued)

Box 2-1: Practice Roles of the Nurse (continued)

Educator

- With a greater emphasis on health promotion and illness prevention, the nurse's role as an educator becomes increasingly important.
- As an educator, the nurse assesses learning needs, plans and implements teaching strategies to meet those needs, and evaluates the effectiveness of the teaching.
- The nurse employs interpersonal communication skills and principles of adult learning to provide patient teaching.
- The nurse considers the educational, cultural, and socioeconomic background of the patient when planning and providing patient teaching.

Coordinator

- As a coordinator, the nurse practices leadership and manages time, people, resources, and the environment in which the nurse provides care.
- The nurse carries out these tasks by directing, delegating, and coordinating activities.
- The nurse plays an important role in coordinating the efforts of all team members to meet the patient's goals and may conduct team conferences to facilitate communication among team members.

Discharge planner

- As a discharge planner, the nurse assesses the patient's needs for discharge starting at the time of admission, including the patient's support systems and living situation.
- The nurse links the patient with available community resources.

Change agent

- As a change agent, the nurse works with the patient to address his health concerns and with staff members to address organizational and community concerns.
- The nurse employs a knowledge of change theory, which provides a framework for understanding the dynamics of change, human responses to change, and strategies for effecting change.
- The nurse serves as a role model in the community, assisting consumers in bringing about change to improve the environment, work conditions, or other factors that affect health.
- The nurse works to bring about change through legislation by helping to shape and support the laws that mandate the use of safety seats and motorcycle helmets.

Researcher

- As a researcher, the nurse takes part in nursing research, which promotes growth in the science of nursing and develops a scientific basis for nursing practice, and applies research findings to nursing practice.
- Even if not trained in nursing research methods, the nurse participates by remaining alert for nursing problems and asking questions about care practices.
- The nurse improves nursing care by incorporating research findings into nursing practice and by communicating research to others.

Roles of the Nurse

General Information

- Nursing's goal is to protect, promote, restore, and maintain the health of people as well as prevent illness and injury, facilitate healing, and alleviate suffering of individuals, families, and communities
- Although the expectations for providing nursing care have expanded and increased, this goal has remained constant

Roles

- In adapting to changing health care needs, nurses assume various roles in health care settings
- Each role has specific responsibilities, but some facets of these roles are common to all nursing positions
- Medical-surgical nurses are not only caregivers but also educators, advocates, coordinators, agents of change, discharge planners, and researchers (see *Practice Roles of the Nurse*, pages 8–9)
- Medical-surgical nurses as caregivers conduct independent assessments and implement patient care based on knowledge and skills and collaborate with other members of the health care team to implement and evaluate that care

Collaborative Practice

General Information

- Successful collaboration requires respect for the unique contribution of each member of the health care team
- An interdisciplinary approach to care serves the patient's needs best

Nurse-Physician Collaboration

- Collaboration is facilitated when nurses and physicians work together regularly and can contribute to improved patient outcomes and lower health care costs
- Methods of encouraging nurse-physician collaboration include scheduling times to develop and sustain working partnerships, communicating openly and directly, and agreeing to discuss conflicts when they arise

Collaboration with Other Members of the Health Care Team

- Collaboration with other health care providers, such as social workers, nutritionists, and physical, occupational, and respiratory therapists, improves the quality of health care services
- Interdisciplinary care conferences allow team members to learn about other health professionals' contributions to patient care; such conferences reflect a facility's commitment to collaborative practice

Case Management

General Information

- Case management is a system of patient care delivery that focuses on achieving outcomes within specific time frames and using resources appropriately
- It includes the entire episode of illness, crossing all settings in which the patient receives care
- Research shows that nursing case management improves quality of care, achieves better outcomes, and reduces health care costs

Case Management Versus Managed Care

- Case management differs from managed care, although both systems are designed to reduce costs and achieve quality outcomes
- Case management provides continuity of the care provided by linking people across clinical settings
- Managed care provides continuity of the care plan by linking tasks, shifts, and departments within the organization

Goals of Case Management

- The goals of case management are the same regardless of setting: increased positive outcomes
- An organization may designate individual case managers or group practice case managers; the latter can represent practitioner or clinical nurse specialist practices

Role of Case Managers

- Case managers are accountable for patient and cost outcomes and may provide administrative, educational, and research services
- They collaborate with the attending physician, patient, family members, and other service providers
- They evaluate the patient's physical and mental health, functional capability, support systems, and financial resources
  - Interdisciplinary teams or individual providers perform the assessments, with the case manager coordinating the process
  - Standardized instruments for collecting data are key to coordinating care

- With the patient and family, case managers formulate a care plan that includes mutually agreed-on goals with measurable objectives so that outcomes can be evaluated (critical pathways)
- They help provide the patient with appropriate resources to fulfill the care plan; case managers troubleshoot for the patient when barriers are identified
- They use performance improvement (PI) to evaluate the quality and cost-effectiveness of patient care

Characteristics of Case Managers

- The ANA recommends that nurse case managers hold a baccalaureate degree in nursing and have 3 years of clinical experience; however, many organizations prefer nurses with master's degrees who are clinical specialists in the areas related to the patient's condition
- Successful case managers possess expert clinical knowledge and skills, can set realistic goals and outcomes, and clearly understand the financial aspects of health care systems and strategies for quality improvement
- They skillfully communicate, negotiate, and collaborate with other health care providers and know what resources are available in health care institutions and the community

Nursing Research

General Information

- For nursing research to achieve full impact, its findings must be applied in practice; nurses in administration, research, and practice must collaborate to create an environment in which nurses raise questions about policies, look for solutions to problems, and develop protocols for testing innovations in nursing care
- The level of participation in research varies with the nurse's educational background
- An associate degree or diploma in nursing qualifies the nurse to assist in identifying clinical problems in nursing practice, to collect data in a structured format, and to work with advanced practice nurses in applying research findings
- A baccalaureate degree in nursing allows the nurse to identify clinical problems that need further research, to critique research findings for use in practice, to collect data, and to implement research findings
- A master's degree in nursing permits the nurse to act as clinical expert in collaborating with an experienced researcher and to provide leadership for integrating findings in clinical nursing practice
- A doctoral degree allows the nurse to formulate nursing knowledge through research and theory development and to conduct funded independent research projects

Types of Research

- *Quantitative research* is a deductive process that aims to describe, explain, and test hypotheses and examine cause-and-effect relationships that apply to a wider universe; this type of research emphasizes facts and data to validate or extend existing knowledge
- Specific terms are associated with quantitative research
  - *Control* involves the use of design techniques to decrease the possibility of error, thereby increasing the potential for findings that accurately reflect reality
  - *Hypothesis* is a formal statement of the expected relationships between two or more variables
  - *Sampling* is the selecting of subjects that are representative of the population being studied
  - *Randomization* is a sampling procedure used to provide each member of the study population with an equal chance of being selected for an intervention
  - *Independent* variable describes the treatment or experimental variable that's manipulated or varied by the researcher to create an effect on the dependent variable
  - *Dependent variable* is the response, behavior, or outcome that the researcher hopes to predict or explain; changes in the dependent variable are presumed to be caused by the independent variable
- *Qualitative research* is an inductive process that aims to understand, describe, and identify the meaning of phenomena for a particular context; this type of research emphasizes the development of new insights, theory, and knowledge in the form of words rather than numbers
- Specific terms are associated with qualitative research
  - *Bracketing* requires the researcher to lay aside what's known about the experience being studied and be open to new insights

- *Intuiting and reflecting* refer to focused awareness on the phenomena under study
- *Theoretical sampling* is the selecting of subjects on the basis of concepts that have theoretical relevance to an evolving theory
- *Saturation* describes the point at which data collection is ended because continuing would result in "more of the same"

Research Process

- The quantitative research process consists of 10 steps: formulating the problem, reviewing related literature, developing a theoretical framework, identifying research variables, formulating research questions or hypotheses, selecting the research design, defining the population and sampling procedures, developing a plan for data collection and analysis, implementing the research plan, and communicating findings
- The qualitative research process follows different steps
  - The initial literature review is less exhaustive to avoid over sensitizing the researcher to the subject matter; after key concepts emerge, a more extensive literature review is conducted, and its insights are woven into the analysis
  - A theoretical framework is seldom used because the goal of qualitative research is to develop concepts, constructs, models, or theories based on the data; a theoretical framework can result from data analysis
  - Variables aren't preselected for study; they become evident as data collection proceeds
  - Research questions are broad at first and then become more focused as data are collected; hypotheses aren't formulated
  - Guidelines for data collection exist, but the direction of the research can change as dictated by the data

Evidence-Based Nursing Practice

General Information

- Evidence-based nursing practice (EBNP) is the foundation of our practice and is essential in guiding our practice
- It differs from research utilization, which starts with a research-based innovation that's evaluated for possible use in practice; it instead uses the best clinical evidence from research in making patient care decisions and informing nursing practice
- It differs from evidence-based medicine because it doesn't rely solely on randomized control trials
- In general, rigorous studies are the best type of evidence for informing a nurse's actions, decisions, and interactions with patients
- Research-based evidence may come from both nursing studies and a broad array of other disciplines
- Sources for EBNP include quantitative and qualitative research, Eastern and Western therapies, patient advocacy, tradition, assumptions, and clinical practice guidelines
- EBNP also includes holistic forms of medicine, clinician expertise, and patient values, preference, and beliefs
- Nurses who incorporate high-quality research evidence in their practice are demonstrating professional accountability to their patients and those they mentor
- Several current trends shape the need for nursing research in nursing practice:
  - A heightened focus on evidence-based practice
  - A stronger knowledge base resulting from multiple confirmatory strategies
  - Greater stress on integrative reviews
  - Increased emphasis on multidisciplinary collaboration
  - Expanded dissemination of research findings
  - Increased interest in outcomes research
  - Emphasis on the visibility of nursing research

Benefits of EBNP

- EBNP often results in streamlined care that saves time and leads to desired outcomes
- It eliminates useless, outdated practices and rituals and decisions based on ritual, opinion, custom, and authority
- It eliminates nurses' stress and frustration in applying basic education to patient care problems and new technology
- It can decrease nursing care costs by avoiding repetitious, undesirable, and expensive alternative outcomes

Implementation

- EBNP's emphasis is on identifying the best available evidence and integrating it with clinical expertise, patient input, and existing resources
- It can be implemented in the form of procedures, protocols, guidelines, standards of care, and clinical pathways
- The first step in implementing EBNP is formulating a clinical question
- The nurse should next search for peer-reviewed articles on that clinical question
- Critically evaluating and comparing the articles for quality and usefulness is the third step
- After that, the nurse implements the information from the articles into practice
- Finally, the nurse evaluates the process and outcome of the changes made in local practice

Quality Assurance

- A peer review of a research article provides an objective assessment of its quality, which depends on its validity and reliability
  - The validity of research refers to its ability to measure what it claims to measure
  - The reliability of a research refers to its ability to be repeated using a different design or setting but providing the same results
- Using randomization, double-blinding, and control groups or large populations helps ensure research quality
- Not all research studies can use these methods; they may require alternatives that call for training and experience
- Randomization requires randomly assigning people to different groups, making it a hallmark of high-quality research
- When evaluating outcomes from applying EBNP, nurses should determine and document patient responses

Barriers to EBNP

- *Research-related barriers* include flaws in research design and method, lack of research reliability, and inaccessibility of findings
- *Nurse-related barriers* include lack of skills in evaluating a study, poor attitudes and lack of motivation to engage in EBNP, and resistance to change
- *Organizational barriers* include resistance to change, lack of intellectual curiosity and openness, lack of time and support for EBNP, and reluctance to expend resources
- *Profession-related barriers* include lack of interaction among nurses, lack of role models, and lack of independence in practice

Improving EBNP

- It is important to value research as a way of knowing and as the foundation for informing and basing practice
- Nurses can take several steps to improve their use and application of research evidence:
  - Read widely and critically
  - Attend professional conferences
  - Learn to expect evidence that a procedure is effective
  - Become involved in a journal club and national or state nursing organizations
  - Pursue and participate in EBNP projects
- Administrators can also take steps to promote the use of research evidence:
  - Foster a climate of intellectual curiosity
  - Offer emotional and moral support
  - Provide financial or resource support for using research evidence
  - Reward and acknowledge efforts for using research evidence
  - Seek opportunities for institutional research utilization or EBNP projects
- Successfully implementing EBNP requires the support of management, administration, and physicians

Performance Improvement and Benefits

Performance Improvement

- PI ensures a specified degree of excellence in patient care and related processes through continuous measurement and evaluation; it is used to implement change, not to identify problems or solutions
- It is a continuous three-stage cycle: measurement of observed nursing practice, comparison of observed practice with expectations (standards of practice), and implementation of change to reconcile discrepancies between observations and expectations
- Three approaches are used to evaluate the quality of care:
  - *Structure evaluation* examines the components of services, such as the setting and environment, which affect quality of care
  - *Process evaluation* examines the activities and behaviors of the health care provider such as the nurse
  - *Outcome evaluation* measures demonstrative changes in the patients' behaviors and attitudes
- Two types of review are used to evaluate the quality of care:
  - *Retrospective review* is a critical examination of past or completed health care delivery to a specified patient population; chart audits, postcare conferences, interviews, and questionnaires are used for this type of review
  - *Concurrent review* is a critical examination of a patient's movement toward desired alterations in health status (outcomes) and patient care management (process) while patient care and treatment are in progress; chart audits, interviews, observation, and inspection of the patient are the usual sources of data
- Before a PI program is implemented, written descriptions are needed of the scope of services provided to patients, the structure of the PI committee and its relation to other committees, the person responsible for PI activities, the procedures to be followed, the methods by which assessments are made, and the type of documentation necessary

Benefits

- PI programs benefit nurses and patients with ongoing goal of improving quality of care
- They help describe the scope of nursing practice and the effectiveness of nursing interventions in improving and maintaining patient health
- They give patients an opportunity to critique the care received, which helps ensure accountability for the care provided

Risk Management and Related Reports

Risk Management

- Risk management seeks to prevent accidents and injuries and control liability
- It has three main goals:
  - Decrease the number of claims by promptly identifying and following up on adverse events
  - Reduce the frequency of preventable injuries and accidents leading to lawsuits by maintaining or improving the quality of care
  - Control costs related to claims by pinpointing trouble spots early and working with the patient and his family
- Risk managers identify, analyze, and evaluate risks within their facility and formulate plans to decrease the frequency and severity of accidents and injuries

Occurrence Reports

- An occurrence, or incident, report is filled out when an event occurs that's inconsistent with a health care facility's ordinary routine, regardless of whether an injury occurs
- Examples of events that require an incident report to be filed include medication errors, injuries from medical equipment (such as a burn), falls (even if the patient wasn't injured), and accidents and injuries involving family members, visitors, or staff members

- An occurrence report has two functions:
  - It informs the administration of the incident, so the risk manager can work to prevent similar incidents
  - It alerts the administration and the facility's insurance company to a potential claim and the need for further investigation
- An occurrence report should be objective and include the names of the persons involved and any witnesses, the patient's account of what happened, factual information about the event, the consequences to the patient, who discovered the patient, your immediate action, who was notified and at what time, and the patient's response to the event
- An occurrence report shouldn't include your assumptions, opinions, suggestions, or accusations

Consultation

General Information

- In a consultation, the nurse draws on internal and external resources to identify and resolve a patient problem; the nurse consultant must build a relationship while maintaining objectivity
- *Formal consultation* uses a written agreement that follows specific steps, whereas *informal consultation* relies on a verbal agreement between colleagues or other staff members
- As health care organizations decentralize, staff nurses will become more involved in consultations

Models of Consultation

- *Patient-centered case consultation* provides expert advice on handling a particular patient or group of patients
- *Consultee-centered case consultation* focuses on work difficulties with patients, which are used as a learning opportunity
- *Program-centered administrative consultation* provides expert advice on developing new programs or improving existing ones
- *Consultee-centered administrative consultation* considers work problems in the areas of program development and organization

Formal Consultation Process

- The process begins with the initial contact, in which clear communication and an understanding of the consultation's goal are particularly important
- The second step is to formulate a contract, with a mutually agreed-upon detailed scope of work, which helps minimize misunderstandings
- The negotiating process is followed by problem identification and diagnostic analysis, which results in a plan of action
- The plan of action is implemented, and feedback is obtained
- Finally, the consultant provides findings and recommendations

Informal Consultation

- Informal consultation occurs among colleagues and requires the same principles and skills as those of formal consultation
- Increased specialization in nursing has resulted in more nurse clinicians tapping the expertise of other nurses to improve patient care
- The decision whether to implement the recommendations of the consultant rests with the individual or group who sought the consultation

Patient Teaching

General Information

- The educational process uses a problem-solving approach similar to that of the nursing process
- Assessment and evaluation are continuous, so that planning and teaching strategies can be adapted to fit the situation

Educational Process

- The educational process involves the development of a teaching plan based on a patient's and family's needs
- The patient's educational needs and type of teaching plan depend on the patient's current knowledge and perceived need, education and reading ability, environment (including culture and support systems), readiness to learn, and learning style
- The teaching plan outlines the learning objectives, content, and teaching methods to be used
- During implementation, the nurse must document activities and monitor progress so that changes can be made quickly if needed
- The effects of teaching can be evaluated by testing skills with return demonstrations, creating hypothetical situations and testing the patient's response, and letting the patient explain his understanding of a topic
- If further education is needed, the nurse can refer a patient to other resources in the community

Documentation

- The nurse documents all teaching activities
- The nurse also documents when the patient isn't ready to learn because of difficulty coping with an illness, uncontrolled pain, or other factors
- The nurse documents the data on which patient assessment is based and includes the action taken

Practical Aspects of Teaching

- Teaching by nurses may be informal and may occur while the nurse performs other activities
- Accurate assessment of a patient and caregiver's needs are the key to effective and efficient use of nursing time
- Empowering patients and caregivers with information, education, and encouragement to participate in identifying their needs facilitates long-term success
- To meet patient and family learning needs, the nurse can use creative methods, such as waiting-room teaching sessions and printed materials and other media
- Before patients are discharged, the nurse must ensure that they're aware of the critical information pertaining to their condition and document this in the medical record

Health and Wellness Promotion

Health

- The World Health Organization describes health as a "state of complete physical, mental, and social well-being and not merely the absence of disease or infirmity"
- Sociologists view health as a condition that allows for the pursuit and enjoyment of desired cultural values, including the ability to carry out activities of daily living, such as working and performing household chores
- Others take a more holistic and subjective view of health and describe it as a level of wellness in which a person is striving to attain his full potential
- One of the nurse's primary functions is to help patients reach an optimal level of wellness
- Multiple factors can affect a patient's health status; the nurse must be aware of these factors when assessing the patient and plan to tailor interventions accordingly
  - Genetics—a person's biological and genetic makeup—can cause illness and lead to chronic conditions
  - Cognitive abilities affect a person's view of health and his ability to seek out and use resources
  - Demographics, such as age and sex, can determine the prevalence of certain diseases in particular groups
  - Culture helps determine a person's perception of health, motivations to seek care, and the types of health practices performed
  - Lifestyle choices and environment such as diet, level of activity, and exposure to toxins can influence a patient's health
  - Health beliefs and practices can affect health positively or negatively
  - Previous health experiences can influence a patient's reaction to illness and the decision to seek care
  - Spirituality affects a person's view of illness and health care
  - Support systems affect the degree to which a person adapts and copes with a situation

Illness

- Illness can be defined as a sickness or deviation from a healthy state; it is considered a broader concept than disease
- Illness occurs when a person is no longer in a state of perceived "normal" health
- Illness also encompasses how a patient interprets a disease's source and importance, how that disease affects his behavior and relationships with others, and how the patient tries to remedy the problem
- The nurse must understand the meaning a person attaches to the experience of being ill
- Disease commonly refers to a specific biological or psychological problem that's supported by clinical manifestations and results in body system changes, organ malfunction, or psychological symptoms that deviate from the patient's baseline
- A disease is detected when it causes a change in metabolism or cell division that produces signs and symptoms
- In the absence of intervention, resolution of the disease depends on many factors functioning over a period of time, such as the extent of the disease and the presence of other diseases
- Manifestations of disease may include hypofunction, hyperfunction, or changes in mechanical function
- Disease occurs or progresses through stages
  - In *exposure* or *injury*, target tissue is exposed to a causative agent or injury
  - During the *latency* or *incubation period*, no evident signs or symptoms occur
  - In the *prodromal period*, the patient generally has mild, nonspecific signs and symptoms
  - During the *acute* phase, the disease is at its full intensity, possibly with complications; this is called the *subclinical acute* phase if the patient still functions as though the disease weren't present
  - *Remission* is a secondary latency phase that occurs in some diseases and is commonly followed by another acute phase
  - During *convalescence*, the patient progresses toward recovery
  - During *recovery*, the patient returns to health or normal functioning, with no remaining signs or symptoms of disease
- Illness can be acute or chronic
  - *Acute illness* refers to a disease or condition that has a relatively abrupt onset, high intensity, and short duration; if no complications occur, most acute illnesses end in full recovery, with a patient returning to his previous or similar level of functioning
  - *Chronic illness* refers to a noncommunicable disease that typically has a slower onset, less intensity, and a longer duration than acute illness, with a patient typically experiencing periods of exacerbation; the nurse's goal is to help the patient regain and maintain the highest possible level of health, although a patient may fail to return to his previous level of functioning

Health and Wellness Promotion

- Good health practices have the benefit of fewer illnesses, a longer life span, and lower health care costs
- Health promotion involves addressing and preventing causes of illness and finding ways to help them correct poor health practices
- *Healthy People 2020* sets forth major comprehensive health goals for the United States, with the aim of reducing mortality and morbidity across the life span
  - Increase the quality and years of life
  - Eliminate health disparities among segments of the population, such as those that occur by gender, race, education, disabilities, geographic location, and sexual orientation
- Health indicators used to measure the health of the nation are physical activity, tobacco use, responsible sexual behavior, mental health, obesity, substance abuse, injury and violence, environmental quality, immunization, and access to health care
- The components of health promotion are self-responsibility, stress reduction and management, physical fitness, and nutritional awareness
  - Self-responsibility is based on the theory that the individual has a responsibility to control his life and can make choices to live a healthy lifestyle or not
  - Stress reduction and management recognizes the role stress can play in disease and focuses on the importance of managing stress
  - Physical fitness has become increasingly important as the nation struggles with obesity
  - Nutritional awareness involves understanding the importance of a healthy diet and recognizing the role diet can play in disease or wellness

Patient Safety

General Information

- Patient safety is such an integral part of nursing that the Joint Commission has developed National Patient Safety Goals to protect patients
- The purpose of National Patient Safety Goals is to improve patient safety by focusing on problems in health care safety and how to solve them

Patient Identification

- Nurses should follow certain procedures to ensure correctly identifying each patient
  - Use at least two patient identifiers according to the facility's policy to identify the patient
  - Don't use the patient's room number as a patient identifier
  - Use two patient identifiers when administering medications and blood products, taking blood samples and other specimens for testing, providing treatment, and performing procedures
  - Label containers used for blood and other specimens in front of the patient

Caregiver Communication

- Nurses should maintain clear, effective, and timely communication among caregivers
  - When verbal or telephone orders are necessary, write down the order for the medication or treatment prescribed and read the complete order back to the person who prescribed it to verify its accuracy
  - When reading the order back to the person who prescribed it, receive confirmation from the person who gave the order
  - For critical test results reported over the telephone, follow specific guidelines:
    - Write down the test result or enter it into a computer
    - Verify the critical test results by reading them back to the person giving the results
    - Receive confirmation from the person who gave the test result
    - Make sure that test results are given only to the patient's licensed, responsible caregiver
    - Measure and assess the timeliness of reporting and the timeliness of receipt by the licensed responsible caregiver
    - If appropriate, take action if critical test results aren't reported or received in a timely manner

Medication Safety

- Look-alike and soundalike drugs used in the facility should be identified and reviewed at least annually and measures should be taken to prevent errors caused by interchanging these drugs
- Medications, medication containers (syringes, medicine cups, and basins), or other solutions used on and off the sterile field in perioperative and other procedural settings must be clearly labeled
- Specified measures must be taken to reduce the likelihood of harm to patients on anticoagulation therapy

Infection Protection

- Health care–associated infections are a leading cause of sickness and death in health care facilities, prolong stays in facilities, and increase health care costs
- Handwashing is one of the most effective techniques for reducing the risk of health care–associated infections
- The Joint Commission mandates following the current hand hygiene guidelines of the World Health Organization or Centers for Disease Control and Prevention:
  - Wash your hands with soap and water when visibly soiled, before eating, and after going to the bathroom
  - Use an alcohol-based hand rub or soap and water when decontaminating hands that aren't visibly soiled
  - Perform hand hygiene before putting on gloves
  - Perform hand hygiene before and after each patient contact
  - Perform hand hygiene before handling an invasive device for patient care
  - Perform hand hygiene after contact with inanimate objects in close proximity to the patient
  - Perform hand hygiene after contact with bodily fluids or excretions, wound dressings, nonintact skin, or mucous membranes

- Health care facilities must implement evidence-based practices to prevent health care–associated infections from multiresistant organisms in acute care health care facilities, central line–associated bloodstream infections, and surgical site infections

Patient Safety Risks

- According to the Joint Commission, health care facilities should identify safety risks inherent in their patient populations
  - Identify patients who may be at risk for suicide
  - Identify specific factors that may increase or decrease risk for suicide
  - Address immediate patient safety needs
  - Ensure that the setting for treatment is appropriate
  - Give patients and their family members information, such as crisis hotline numbers, for crisis situations

Delegation

General Information

- Delegation occurs when a nurse assigns tasks and the authority to complete those tasks to other personnel, such as unlicensed assistive personnel (UAP)
- The ANA defines a *UAP* as an individual trained to function in an assistive role to the registered professional nurse in the provision of patient care activities, as delegated by and under the supervision of that nurse
- Further definition and clarification regarding delegation of nursing tasks may be defined by Nurse Practice Acts in individual states

Delegation Process

- The nurse should know facility policy regarding delegation and only delegate tasks (but not the nursing process) that the UAP is competent to perform
- UAPs make observations, collect clinical data, and report findings to the nurse in a timely manner
- Responsibility for the task is delegated but not the accountability, so the nurse should receive regular updates from the UAP, ask specific questions, and make frequent rounds of patients
- The nurse must evaluate the task and the outcome and ensure that they're accurately documented in the medical record

Review Questions

Question 1. The registered nurse has an unlicensed assistant working with her for the shift. When delegating tasks, the nurse understands that the unlicensed assistant:

A. interprets clinical data.
B. collects clinical data.
C. is trained in the nursing process.
D. can function independently.

Correct answer: B Unlicensed personnel make observations, collect clinical data, and report findings to the nurse. Option A is incorrect because the registered nurse, who has learned critical thinking skills, interprets the data. Option C is incorrect because although unlicensed assistants are trained to perform skills, they don't learn the nursing process. Option D is incorrect because unlicensed assistants don't function independently; they're assigned tasks by a registered nurse who retains overall responsibility for the patient.

Question 2. When performing an assessment, the nurse identifies the following signs and symptoms: impaired coordination, decreased muscle strength, limited range of motion, and reluctance to move. These signs and symptoms indicate which nursing diagnosis?

A. Health-seeking behaviors
B. Impaired physical mobility
C. Disturbed sensory perception
D. Deficient knowledge

Correct answer: B Impaired physical mobility is a limitation of physical movement and is defined by the patient's signs and symptoms. Options A, C, and D are nursing diagnoses with different defining signs and symptoms.

Question 3. When prioritizing a patient's care plan based on Maslow's hierarchy of needs, the nurse's first priority would be:

A. allowing the family to see a newly admitted patient.
B. ambulating the patient in the hallway.
C. administering pain medication.
D. using two nurses to transfer the patient.

Correct answer: C In Maslow's hierarchy of needs, pain relief is on the first layer. Activity (option B) is on the second layer. Safety (option D) is on the third layer. Love and belonging (option A) are on the fourth layer.

Question 4. When a nurse asks another nurse for advice on handling a particular patient problem, she's seeking what type of consultation?

A. Patient-centered case consultation
B. Consultee-centered case consultation
C. Program-centered administrative consultation
D. Consultee-centered administrative consultation

Correct answer: A Patient-centered case consultation (option A) provides expert advice on handling a particular patient or group of patients. Consultee-centered case consultation (option B) focuses on work difficulties with patients, which are used as a learning opportunity. Program-centered administrative consultation (option C) provides expert advice on developing new programs or improving existing ones. Consultee-centered administrative consultation (option D) considers work problems in the areas of program development and organization.

Question 5. When implementing an evidence-based nursing program to decrease the incidence of pressure ulcers on a medical-surgical unit, which of the following is the most important to ensure its success?

A. Obtaining support from management, administration, and physicians
B. Determining and documenting patient outcomes
C. Identifying a significant problem that needs to be addressed
D. Evaluating research based on its validity and reliability

Correct answer: A To successfully implement an evidence-based nursing program, it is important to obtain the support of management, administration, and

physicians. Option B is part of evaluating evidence-based nursing program implementation. Option C is part of the first step of the evidence-based nursing program process. Option D is part of the critical evaluation of resources.

Question 6. When planning the implementation of evidence-based practices to prevent falls, which of the following steps should the nurse take first?

A. Identify the common causes of falls.
B. Gather and review currently existing literature and guidelines for the prevention of falls.
C. Identify fall prevention practices that are applicable to the patient care setting.
D. Gather data to identify the effectiveness of the new practice guidelines.

Correct answer: B Options A, B, and C are correct steps in planning for the implementation of evidence-based practices; however, option B would be the initial step, followed by options A and C. Option D is part of the evaluation phase of evidence-based practice implementation.

Question 7. Which measure most effectively reduces the risk of health care–associated infections?

A. Keeping employee health records up-to-date
B. Performing hand hygiene
C. Providing annual influenza vaccinations
D. Always wearing a mask when caring for patients

Correct answer: B Performing hand hygiene in compliance with the World Health Organization or Centers for Disease Control and Prevention guidelines is the most effective in reducing the risk of health care–associated infections. Keeping employee health records up-to-date (option A), providing annual influenza vaccinations (option C), and always wearing a mask when caring for patients (option D) aren't the most effective ways to reduce the risk of health care–associated infections.

Question 8. Which action should the nurse take when receiving a telephone order from a physician?

A. Inform the physician that telephone orders are not permitted.
B. Write the order in the patient's medical record immediately.
C. Write down the order and then read back the complete order to the physician.
D. Immediately carry out the order.

Correct answer: C When receiving a telephone or other verbal order, the nurse should write down the order and then read back the complete order to the physician to verify its accuracy. Options A, B, and D aren't appropriate actions for the nurse to take when receiving a telephone order from a physician.

Question 9. A secondary latency phase that occurs in some diseases that is commonly followed by another acute phase is referred to as:

A. remission.
B. convalescence.
C. the acute phase.
D. the subclinical acute phase.

Correct answer: A A secondary latency phase that occurs in some diseases that is commonly followed by another acute phase is referred to as remission. Convalescence (option B) is progression toward recovery. The acute phase (option C) refers to the disease at its full intensity, possibly with complications. The subclinical acute phase (option D) occurs when the patient is in the acute phase but still functions as if the disease weren't present.

Question 10. Qualitative research emphasizes developing new insights, theories, and knowledge. Which term in qualitative research describes the researcher laying aside what is known about the experience being studied?

A. Bracketing
B. Saturation
C. Intuiting
D. Theoretical sampling

Correct answer: A Bracketing requires the researcher to lay aside what's known about the experience being studied and be open to new insights. Saturation (option B) describes the point at which data collection is ended because continuing would result in acquiring more of the same information or data. Intuiting (option C) refers to the focused awareness on the phenomena being studied. Theoretical sampling (option D) is the selecting of subjects on the basis of concepts that have theoretical relevance to an evolving theory.

Selected References

Academy of Medical-Surgical Nurses. (n.d.). Retrieved from www.amsn.org.

Anderson, T. (2009). *Nursing consultation: Honoring the privilege.* Retrieved from www.Medscape.com.

Brant, J. M. (2015, November). Bridging the research-to-practice gap: The role of the nurse scientist. *Seminars in Oncology Nursing, 31,* 298–305. Retrieved from http://dx.doi.org/10.1016/j.sonen.2015.08.006.

Campbell, E. J., & Richter, J. M. (2017, April). Performance improvement: Quality is in the cards. *Digestive Diseases and Sciences, 62,* 821–822. Retrieved from http://dx.doi.org/10.1007/S10620-017-4480-7.

Daly, P. (2017, February). An integral approach to health science and healthcare. *Theoretical Medicine and Bioethics, 38*(1), 15–40. Retrieved from http://dx.doi.org/10.1007/S11017-017-9396-X.

Elsous, A., Radwan, M., & Mohsen, S. (2017). Nurses and physicians attitudes toward nurse-physician collaboration: A survey from Gaza Strip, Palestine. *Nursing Research and Practice,* 1–7. Retrieved from http://dx.doi.org/10.1155/2017/7406278.

Emiliana, M. D., Lindolpho, M. D., Valente, G. S., Chrizostimo, M. M., Chaves Sa, S. P., & Da Rocha, I. D. (2017, May). Perception of nursing consultation by elderly people and their caregivers. *Journal of Nursing UFPE, 11,* 1791–1797. Retrieved from http://dx.doi.org/10.5205/reoul.11077-98857-1-SM.1105201706.

Finnell, D. S., Thomas, E. L., Nehring, W. M., McLaughlin, K. A., & Bickford, C. J. (2015, May). Best practices for developing specialty nursing scope and standards of practice. *Online Journal of Issues in Nursing, 20*(2). Retrieved from http://dx.doi.org/10.3912/OJIN.Vol20No02Man01.

Friesen-Storms, J., Loo, A. V., Beurskens, A., & Bours, G. (2014). Systemic implementation of evidence-based practice in a clinical nursing setting: A participatory action research project. *Journal of Clinical Nursing, 24,* 57–68. Retrieved from http://dx.doi.org/10.1111/jocn.12697.

Healthy People 2020. (n.d.). Retrieved from www.HealthyPeople.gov.

Hoarle, K. (2015, November/December). Risk management poised to grow as healthcare evolves. *Biomedical Instrumentation and Technology, 49,* 433–435. Retrieved from http://dx.doi.org/10.2345/0899-8205-49.

Hudon, C., Chouinard, M., Bouliane, D., Diadiou, F., & Lambert, M. (2015, November/December). Case management in primary care for frequent users of health care services with chronic diseases: A qualitative study of patient and family experience. *Annals of Family Medicine, 13,* 523–528. Retrieved from www.annfammed.org.

Karnick, P. M. (2016). Evidence-based practice and nursing theory. *Nursing Science Quarterly, 29,* 283–284. Retrieved from http://dx.doi.org/10.1177/0894318416661107.

Knier, S., Stitcher, J. F., Ferber, L., & Catterall, K. (2015, January/February). Patients' perceptions of the quality of discharge teaching and readiness for discharge. *Rehabilitation Nursing, 40*(1), 30–39. Retrieved from http://dx.doi.org/10.1002/RNJ.164.

Maijala, V., Tossavainen, K., & Turunen, H. (2015). Identifying nurse practitioners' required case management competencies in health promotion practice in municipal public primary healthcare. A two-stage modified Delphi study. *Journal of Clinical Nursing, 24*(17–18), 2554-2561. Retrieved from http://dx.doi.org/10.1111/jocn.12855.

McCusker, K., & Gunaydin, S. (2015). Research using qualitative, quantitative or mixed methods and choice based on the research. *Perfusion, 30,* 537–542. Retrieved from http://dx.doi.org/10.1177/0267659114559116.

NANDA Nursing Diagnosis List. (n.d.). Retrieved from www.nandanursingdiagnosislist.org.

Pagura, I. (2016, Spring). Work health and safety: Risk management. *Journal of the Australian Traditional-Medicine Society, 22,* 164–166.

Park, J., & Lee, K. (2014). The association between managed care enrollments and potentially preventable hospitalization among adult Medicaid recipients in Florida. *BMC Health Services Research, 14*(247), 2–12. Retrieved from www.biomedcentral.com.

Pidgeon, K. (2015, November/December). The genesis of a trauma performance improvement plan. *Journal of Trauma Nursing, 22,* 315–320. Retrieved from http://dx.doi.org/10.1097/JTN.0000000000000166.

Rivas, F. J., Martin-Iglesias, S., Pacheco del Cerro, J. L., Arenas, C. M., Lopez, M. G., & Lagos, M. B. (2016, January). Effectiveness of nursing process use in primary care. *International Journal of Nursing Knowledge, 27*(1), 43–48. Retrieved from http://dx.doi.org/10.1111/2047-3095.12073.

Roche, M. A., Friedman, S., Duffield, C., & Twigg, D. E. (2017, June). A comparison of nursing tasks undertaken by regulated nurses and nursing support workers: A work sampling study. *Journal of Advanced Nursing, 73,* 1421–1432. Retrieved from http://dx.doi.org/10.1111/JAN.13224.

Ryan, E. J. (2016). Undergraduate nursing students' attitudes and use of research and evidence-based practice—An integrative literature review. *Journal of Clinical Nursing, 25,* 1548–1556. Retrieved from http://dx.doi.org/10.1111/jocn.13229.

The Joint Commission. (n.d.). Retrieved from www.jointcommission.org.

The Nursing Process. (n.d.). Retrieved from www.nursingworld.org.

Walton, B. G. (2016, September/October). Developing a nursing IQ-Part II: The expertise of nursing process. *Ohio Nurses Review, 91*(5), 24–34.

Weiss, M. E., Sawin, K. J., Gralton, K., Johnson, N., Klingbeil, C., Lerret, S., …, Schiffman, R. (2017, May/June). Dish charge teaching, readiness for discharge, and post-discharge outcomes in parents of hospitalized children. *Journal of Pediatric Nursing, 34,* 58–64. Retrieved from http://dx.doi.org/10.1016/J.PEDN.2016.12.021.

World Health Organization. (n.d.). Retrieved from www.who.int.

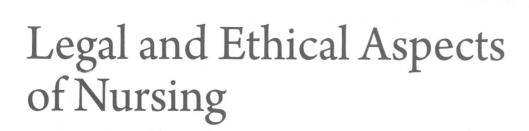

Chapter 3

Legal and Ethical Aspects of Nursing

Nurse Practice Acts

- State statutes
  - Each state has statutes, or nurse practice act (NPA), that define the levels of nursing (e.g., advanced practice nurse [nurse practitioner, clinical nurse specialist, certified nurse-midwife, certified nurse-anesthetist], registered nurse, licensed practical nurse, and nursing assistant); they're the most important laws governing nurses and nursing practice
    - Most statutes set licensure requirements for each level of nursing
    - They may prescribe minimum educational qualifications for licensure
  - Regulatory boards created by the NPA govern nursing practice in the state
  - The NPA may provide for a board of nursing accreditation and approval of educational programs within the state
- Disciplinary actions
  - The state board of nursing may take action against a nurse who violates the NPA or the licensing board's regulations (see *Common Legal Concerns for Nurses*, page 24)
    - A nurse can be disciplined for habitual substance abuse that affects the ability to practice, fraud or deceit in obtaining a nursing license, incompetence, criminal felony conviction, and unprofessional conduct
    - Other actions or conditions that would inhibit the nurse's safe and effective nursing practice are also grounds for discipline
  - A licensed nurse has a limited property right to the license
    - The state must follow specific procedures to determine if a nurse's license should be revoked to protect public safety
    - The licensee must be notified of the complaint, must have an opportunity to respond to the complaint and present evidence, and must be allowed to have a hearing before an impartial panel and to appeal the panel's decision
- Possible sanctions
  - The nurse's license may be revoked
  - The license may be suspended for a predetermined time
  - The license may be suspended for an undetermined time, and the nurse may reapply after completing a course of study or treatment
  - Conditions may be placed on the license to limit the nurse's practice
  - The nurse may voluntarily surrender the license or enter into a consensual agreement with the nursing board, agreeing to limitations on the license or supervision of practice for a time
  - The nurse may receive a disciplinary warning or reprimand

Box 3-1: Common Legal Concerns for Nurses

Three areas commonly cause legal problems for nurses: confidentiality, consent to treatment, and the right to refuse treatment.

Confidentiality

Confidential information is any information that the patient communicates to the nurse or practitioner for diagnosis or treatment with the expectation that it won't be disclosed. Nurses have an ethical and legal duty to avoid disclosing such confidential information to unauthorized people who aren't involved in the patient's care and treatment.

A nurse who discloses confidential information without the patient's permission may be subject to a lawsuit or disciplinary action for unprofessional conduct. The nurse can be liable for invasion of privacy, defamation, intentional or negligent infliction of emotional distress, or breach of an implied contract of secrecy. Some states provide a statutory penalty against health care providers who violate the patient's right to confidentiality.

However, confidential information can be disclosed under certain circumstances. For example, the nurse must disclose such information when authorized by a patient (but only to the extent authorized), when a patient is a danger to himself or others, or when required by law for a reportable communicable disease or suspected abuse. In some cases, the court may order disclosure of confidential patient information.

Consent to treatment

The law presumes that adults are legally capable of consenting to treatment. To provide a valid consent, a patient must be mentally capable of understanding the nature and consequences of treatment. Expressed consent is obtained orally or in writing; implied consent is obtained by the patient's voluntarily submitting to treatment. Medical treatment performed without a patient's expressed or implied consent may result in legal claims of battery or negligence.

Therefore, informed consent should be obtained before a patient undergoes an invasive procedure, receives anesthesia or blood, or undergoes procedures that carry a significant risk of harm. Informed consent requires the health care provider (physician, nurse practitioner, physician assistant, nurse-midwife) to provide appropriate information including risks, benefits, and potential outcomes. The adequacy of this information is evaluated by two questions: Did the health care provider provide information that a reasonably competent health care provider in the same situation would provide? Did the patient receive sufficient information such that a reasonable person in the same circumstances could make an informed decision? If a patient receives appropriate information and refuses care or treatment against medical advice, the physician or health care provider is responsible for documenting that the informed consent conversation took place, the general facts discussed, and the patient's decision.

Exceptions to informed consent

Informed consent isn't required if a delay to obtain consent for emergency treatment would cause imminent harm that outweighs the risk of treatment, if the patient would be substantially harmed by disclosing the risks of treatment, if the patient waives the right to consent and asks not to be informed, or if compulsory treatment is mandated by law or a court order.

Right to refuse treatment

Adults are presumed to be legally capable of refusing treatment. In fact, mentally competent patients with terminal conditions can refuse life-sustaining treatment without creating legal liability for their health care providers.

The Patient Self-Determination Act of 1990 encourages persons to express their wishes about life-sustaining treatment should they become legally incapacitated. The act requires health care facilities that participate in Medicare and Medicaid to develop programs to inform patients about advance directives, such as living wills and durable powers of attorney and do-not-resuscitate (DNR) orders. Under this act, the health care facility must provide patients with written materials explaining their rights under their state laws to make decisions concerning medical care, including the right to accept or refuse treatment and the right to execute an advance directive. A living will expresses a patient's wishes about withholding or withdrawing life-sustaining treatment. A durable power of attorney designates a person to make health care decisions, including termination of life support, for a patient who can no longer do so. A DNR order authorizes health care personnel not to initiate resuscitative measures. The Patient Self-Determination Act specifically prohibits covered health care facilities from conditioning the provision of care or discriminating against an individual based on whether the individual has executed an advance directive.

When a patient is no longer mentally capable of making health care decisions, a court order, statute, or law may authorize a surrogate decision-maker to accept or refuse medical treatment for the patient based on the patient's prior documentation or expressed wishes.

Legal Concepts of Responsibility

- Individuals
  - In the absence of mental or legal incapacity, a person is responsible for his/her own actions; a nurse, as a professional, is legally accountable for providing a nursing assessment and care
  - Although the nurse may be individually accountable, other people or entities may also be legally responsible for a nurse's negligence
- Employers and supervisors
  - An employer is automatically liable for its employees' actions within the scope of their employment; the employer is thereby encouraged to hire competent employees
  - A nurse in a management or supervisory position may be liable for the actions of a negligent nurse under their supervision; liability can result if the supervisor didn't adequately assess the nurse's competence or the assignment's requirements, didn't adequately supervise the nurse's performance, or knew the nurse's limitations and didn't provide adequate training or staffing
- Independent contractors
  - An independent contractor is one who contracts with another to do a specific job; in nursing, the private duty nurse who is employed by an agency but hired on a per diem basis by a health care facility is the most common example of an independent contractor
  - The independent contractor's actions aren't directly controlled by the employer; the contractor has independent discretion in performing the job
  - The employer may not be liable for the negligent actions of an independent contractor unless the employer knew or should have known of the independent contractor's incompetence
- Corporations
  - A health care facility is obligated to carefully monitor the credentials and competence of employees and independent contractors
  - A health care facility that doesn't ensure its workers' competence may be liable for injuries caused by the workers' negligence

Possible Civil Actions

- Torts
  - A tort is a civil action for damages for injury to a person, property, or reputation
  - Torts are classified as unintentional or intentional
- Unintentional torts
  - *Professional negligence* and *professional malpractice* are the most common legal claims against nurses
    - Negligence is the failure to exercise the degree of care that a person of ordinary prudence would exercise under the same circumstances; for example, if a nurse notices water on the floor of a room and doesn't wipe it up, and the water causes a patient to fall and injure himself, this constitutes negligence
    - The plaintiff in a negligence suit must prove that the nurse's actions caused harm
    - Professional malpractice or professional negligence requires a plaintiff to introduce proof of duty, breach of duty, proximate cause, and damages or harm; proof of the nurse's standard of care is critical to establishing the first three elements
    - Unlike negligence cases, professional negligence cases require expert testimony as to the duty of care, its breach, and its causal relationship to the injury
  - A nurse also can be sued for *negligent infliction of emotional distress*
    - In many states, a plaintiff can be awarded damages for severe emotional distress resulting from a nurse's negligent actions
    - Some states require that the plaintiff have physical manifestations of the emotional distress, such as palpitations, gastric discomfort, or insomnia
- Intentional torts
  - *Assault* is an act that places a patient in fear of harmful or offensive touching
  - *Battery* is touching a patient without justification or permission

- *Defamation* results when a nurse communicates false information verbally (slander) or in writing (libel) about a patient that damages the patient's reputation or causes the patient to be shunned or avoided by the community
- *Invasion of privacy* occurs when a nurse gives unauthorized access to the patient or information about the patient; taking photographs of a patient without permission is an invasion of privacy
- *Fraud* and *misrepresentation* are false or misleading statements by the nurse that the patient relies on to his detriment
- *False imprisonment* is unjustifiable restriction of patient movement
- *Intentional infliction of emotional distress* results when a nurse's actions produce distress so severe that no reasonable person could be expected to endure it
- Contract actions
  - Contract actions are determined by whether the parties performed obligations agreed to in a contract
  - A breach of contract results when one party fails to perform as required by the contract
  - Nurses are most commonly involved in employment contracts and malpractice insurance contracts

Possible Defenses to a Health Care Negligence Suit

- Comparative and contributory negligence
  - With comparative negligence (the more common defense), the jury compares the degree of negligence of the parties or of various defendants and apportions damages (i.e., compensation or indemnification) accordingly
  - With contributory negligence, because the plaintiff's conduct contributes to the cause of the injury and falls below the standard by which individuals are expected to conform, the plaintiff can't recover damages, even though the defendant violated a duty of care to the plaintiff and would be liable
- Statutes of limitation
  - A statute of limitation sets a time limit within which the legal action must be brought; a nurse can't be sued for negligence if the claim is made after the time limit expires
  - Statutes of limitation for health care negligence are established by the state legislature
  - These statutes may not apply in some cases, such as those involving fraudulent concealment of negligence or later discovery of negligence
- Good Samaritan laws
  - All states have Good Samaritan laws to protect people who render assistance at the scene of an emergency
  - Some statutes protect all citizens; others cover only specified health care providers
  - Those protected under Good Samaritan laws are liable only for grossly negligent acts
- Statutory defenses
  - Many states have statutes that prescribe special procedures for health care negligence cases
  - A suit may be dismissed if the statutory requirements aren't met

Professional Liability Insurance for Nurses

- Types of policies
  - A *claims-made* policy provides coverage for claims made during the policy period
  - An *occurrence policy* provides coverage for negligence that occurs during the policy period
- Obligations of the insurer and the insured
  - Insurers must provide and pay for legal counsel to defend the nurse in the lawsuit and must pay damages (within coverage limits) for which the nurse is judged liable
  - The nurse must notify the insurer that a claim has been made and must assist as needed in preparing the defense (see *Reducing Nursing Liability*, page 28)

Patient's Bill of Rights

- Self-determination
  - Self-determination is often used synonymously with autonomy
  - It means having a form of personal liberty to choose and implement one's own decisions, free from deceit, duress, constraint, or coercion
  - It involves the right of patients to decide what will or will not happen to their bodies
  - Basic elements of self-determination include the patient's ability to decide, the power to act upon his own decision, and respect for the individual autonomy of others
  - Although self-determination is often addressed in relation to death and dying, it concerns all aspects of consent and its refusal
  - To practice this right, the individual must be competent to make his own decisions about accepting or refusing treatment
  - Some states uphold the patients in orally expressed desires, provided they're documented, including the patient's awareness of consequences of his actions
  - The Patient Self-Determination Act has three basic premises:
    - Patients who are informed of their rights are more likely to take advantage of them
    - If patients are more actively involved in decisions about their medical care, then that care will more closely respond to their needs
    - Patients may choose care that is less costly
- Informed consent
  - Informed consent is the voluntary authorization by a patient to a care provider to do something to the patient
  - Some states accept oral forms of consent as being equally as valid as written consent
  - Contents of an informed consent include the procedural information, associated risks and benefits, alternatives to the procedure, and the name of the person who will perform the procedure
  - Generally, physicians have the responsibility to obtain informed consents
  - Nurses can witness and have the responsibility to advocate for the patient to ensure that all criteria for autonomous decision-making are met
  - Four exceptions to consents are emergency situations, therapeutic privilege, patient waiver, and prior patient knowledge
- Living wills
  - Living wills, or health care directives, are directives from competent individuals to medical personnel regarding treatment they wish to receive
  - A living will takes effect when the previously competent person becomes sick and can no longer make decisions for himself
  - It typically contains information about the conservator or health care agent, the patient's code status, and the patient's desire for organ donation; it may also contain other information
  - Because living wills aren't typically legally enforced, medical practitioners may choose to abide by them or to ignore them as they see fit
  - There's no protection for the practitioner against criminal or civil liabilities for proceeding under a living will's directions
- Durable power of attorney
  - Durable (or medical) power of attorney for health care allows competent patients to appoint a surrogate to make decisions for them in the event that they lose competence
  - The power includes the right to ask questions, select and remove physicians from the patient's care, assess risks and complications, and select treatments

Ethical Aspects of Nursing

- General information
  - Ethics is a branch of philosophy that examines values, actions, and choices to determine right and wrong
    - Nursing ethics is part of normative ethics, a type of ethics that's based on the criteria by which people make moral judgments
    - As the basis for professional codes of ethics, ethical theories attempt to provide a system of principles and rules for resolving ethical dilemmas
    - The American Nurses Association's "Code of Ethics for Nurses" provides guidance for carrying out nursing responsibilities consistent with the ethical obligations of the profession

Box 3-2: Reducing Nursing Liability

The nurse can take measures to reduce liability in several areas.

Liability Area	Prevention Measures
Competent practice	• Know your practice area, and stay current in the field. • Recognize your strengths and limitations. • Be familiar with the American Nurses Association's Standards of Practice and the standards of practice of appropriate specialty groups. • Build a good relationship with your patients. • Review and follow your facility's nursing policies and procedures.
Charting	• Record information accurately, promptly, and legibly. • Use only approved abbreviations. • Record the assessment of the patient completely. • Record all nursing actions and the patient's responses to them. • Correct mistaken entries by drawing a single line through them and initialing the line; don't obliterate the mistaken entry. • Correct errors in computer documentation as directed by the computer program used. • Never falsify, alter, or destroy a patient's record.
Access to medical records	• Follow Health Insurance Portability and Accountability Act guidelines as developed by the health care facility. • Release copies of medical records to the patient on proper request and to others authorized by the patient. • Release human immunodeficiency virus or acquired immunodeficiency syndrome test results as required by state law. • Don't release alcohol or other substance abuse counseling records unless explicitly authorized; a general authorization is insufficient. • Don't release protected documents to the patient, such as incident reports and peer-review materials.
Common sources of injuries **Falls**	• Know the facility's fall-risk policies and procedures. • Assess every patient's risk of falling based on the facility's protocol. • Monitor all patients identified as at risk, and document accordingly.
Medications	• Know the facility's protocols and procedures regarding specific drugs, such as insulin and anticoagulants. • Keep current about commonly used drugs in your practice. • Review package insert information before administering drugs. • Be vigilant when preparing and administering drugs. • Question all unusual orders. • Recheck orders questioned by the patient.
Restraints	• Follow institutional policy regarding restraints. • Exhaust all alternative methods of care before considering restraints. • Monitor restrained patients according to the facility's policies and standards.
Inadequate patient education	• Assess the patients' cognitive ability and willingness to learn, and document accordingly. • Assess the patient's knowledge before and after teaching. • Use written, verbal, and audiovisual teaching methods. • Use return demonstration of physical skills. • Document the patient's response to teaching.
Abandonment	• Don't leave a patient without arranging for continuing care. • Give a complete report when transferring care, and reconcile the patient's drugs across the continuum. • Document the completion of treatment.
Malfunctioning equipment	• Check equipment according to the manufacturer's recommendation and the facility's protocol. • Have malfunctioning equipment fixed or replaced immediately. • Notify appropriate authorities of the problem and the action taken.

- Morality involves rules of conduct about right and wrong
  - It's based on norms of conduct determined by society
  - Society's moral codes guide what people ought to do; professional codes, such as the code of ethics for nurses, communicate the goals and ideals of a profession
- Although *ethics* and *morals* are theoretically distinct terms, they're used interchangeably to describe right and wrong actions
- Professional code of ethics for nurses
  - Nurses have a contract with society to behave in accordance with rules dictated by society and the nursing profession
  - Whereas NPAs set the legal standards for safe nursing practice, the code for nurses delineates nursing's moral ideals, provides guidelines for ethically principled behavior, and holds nurses morally accountable for their actions (see *Code of Ethics for Nurses*, page 31)
- Ethical theories
  - *Deontology* holds that an act's moral rightness is determined by the inherent duty one has to act in accordance with rules and principles
    - It presumes that the rightness of an act is determined by the intent to conform with a moral rule, not by the consequences of the act
    - Immanuel Kant is a principal deontologic theorist
  - *Utilitarianism* holds that an act's moral rightness is determined by its ability to produce good consequences and to avoid harmful ones
    - It presumes that the rightness of an act is determined by its consequences, not by the person's intent
    - John Stuart Mill and Jeremy Bentham are utilitarian theorists
- Ethical principles
  - *Autonomy* is a state of being self-regulating, self-defining, and self-reliant
    - Immanuel Kant believed that all people are worthy of unconditional positive regard (Kantian principle of "respect for persons"); he also introduced the concept of freedom of will
    - John Stuart Mill believed that a person should be respected for his freedom of thought and action
    - The principle of autonomy that actions and choices shouldn't be restricted by others has many clinical applications
      - A patient's right to informed consent derives from the principle of autonomy
      - The principle of "respect for persons" dictates that a patient has a right to treatment and a right to refuse treatment
      - Advance directives, such as living wills and durable powers of attorney for health care, maintain a patient's autonomy
  - *Beneficence* is a moral principle that holds that individuals should promote good
    - Based on the duty to help, beneficence requires nurses to act in their patients' best interests
    - This principle may create a duty when the law doesn't
    - This principle often conflicts with the principle of autonomy—for example, a nurse may violate the autonomy principle by preventing a patient from acting on suicidal impulses (a beneficent act)
  - *Nonmaleficence* mandates that a nurse doesn't harm others or put them at risk for harm; this principle causes many debates about euthanasia, withholding and withdrawing treatment, and the use of artificial hydration and nutrition
  - *Justice* is a moral concept that maintains equals should be treated equally and those who aren't equal should be treated according to their differences; it is used when there are scarcities or competition for resources or benefits
  - *Veracity* obligates the nurse to be truthful with patients
  - *Privacy* requires the nurse to restrict access to the patient appropriately; *confidentiality* requires the nurse to deny access to information about the patient
  - *Fidelity* refers to a nurse's faithfulness in keeping a promise; in practice, the nurse makes an implied promise to care for a patient
- Ethical dilemmas
  - An ethical dilemma arises when a nurse must choose between competing claims or select from equally undesirable alternatives
  - When faced with an ethical dilemma, the nurse should apply a rational decision-making process by gathering all the facts, identifying the problem or dilemma, listing possible actions, choosing the most appropriate action, and evaluating the results of the action

Cultural and Ethnic Beliefs and Practices

- Definitions
  - Madeleine Leininger, a nurse anthropologist and theorist, has defined culture as the learned and shared values, beliefs, norms, and practices of a particular group that guide thinking, decision-making, and actions in a patterned way
  - *Cultural sensitivity* is the understanding of the diverse needs, characteristics, and values of individuals, families, and groups
  - *Cultural competency* is the ability to work and interact effectively with people of other cultures
  - Culture is not limited to a specific ethnic background or racial heritage but rather is an adapted way of life that is learned from families and other social interactions
  - Culture includes several elements
    - Patterns of behavior
    - Acquired and transmitted symbols
    - Assigned values
    - Selected ideals
    - Language
    - Religious practices and beliefs
- Cultural diversity
  - *Cultural diversity* describes the diverse groups in society, which have varying races and national origins, religious affiliations, languages, physical size, gender, sexual orientation, age, disabilities, socioeconomic status, occupational status, and geographic location
  - Differences are based on ideology and values
    - *Ideology* refers to a group's opinions or ways of thinking
    - *Values* refers to a group's norms, customs, ideas, and behaviors
  - The nurse brings personal cultural heritage along with cultural and philosophical views into the clinical setting
  - The nurse-patient encounter includes the interaction of three cultural systems: the cultural systems of the nurse, of the patient and family, and of the setting
- Sensitivity to cultures
  - Several factors may affect sensitivity to other cultures
  - Stereotyping occurs when an individual assumes that all members of a culture or ethnic group act alike
  - Stereotyping may be positive or negative
    - Negative stereotyping includes racism, ageism, and sexism—beliefs that a certain race, age group, or gender is inherently superior to others—leading to discrimination against those considered inferior
    - Positive stereotyping can be just as harmful as negative stereotyping; it can include such statements as "Asians are good at math," "Italians are great cooks," or "Native Americans are spiritual"
- Cultural sensitivity in nursing care
  - To be able to provide culturally competent care to people from diverse backgrounds, the nurse must be sensitive to culturally diverse needs, characteristics, and values of individuals, families, and groups
  - To provide effective nursing care, the nurse should deliver care with respect for any and all cultural beliefs and practices of the patient and family
  - The incorporation of the nurse's own cultural diversity experiences and awareness brings competency to everyday practice
  - Culturally sensitive care acknowledges the impact that a patient's cultural norms or beliefs may have on wellness, treatment of illnesses, causes of disease, and definitions of health and wellness
  - Ethnocentrism, or the belief that one's own cultural values and beliefs are superior or the only correct values and beliefs, can interfere with the delivery of effective nursing care
  - The nurse must at all times be sensitive to the beliefs and values of those being cared for and understand how beliefs and values influence healing and health care practices
  - The broad range of cultural diversity requires the nurse to be sensitive to and have a willingness to learn about the values and norms of those being cared for
  - Inquiry and active listening can help both the nurse and the patient and family meet expectations

Code of Ethics for Nurses

The American Nurses Association's "Code of Ethics for Nurses" provides ethical standards of conduct and guidelines for all aspects of nursing practice.

1. The nurse, in all professional relationships, practices with compassion and respect for the inherent dignity, worth, and uniqueness of every individual, unrestricted by considerations of social or economic status, personal attributes, or the nature of health problems.

2. The nurse's primary commitment is to the patient, whether an individual, family, group, or community.

3. The nurse promotes, advocates for, and strives to project the health, safety, and rights of the patient.

4. The nurse is responsible and accountable for individual nursing practice and determines the appropriate delegation of tasks consistent with the nurse's obligation to provide optimum patient care.

5. The nurse owes the same duties to self as to others, including the responsibility to preserve integrity and safety, to maintain competence, and to continue personal and professional growth.

6. The nurse participates in establishing, maintaining, and improving health care environments and conditions of employment conducive to the provision of quality health care and consistent with the values of the profession through individual and collective action.

7. The nurse participates in the advancement of the profession through contributions to practice, education, administration, and knowledge development.

8. The nurse collaborates with other health professionals and the public in promoting community, national, and international efforts to meet health needs.

9. The profession of nursing, as represented by associations and their members, is responsible for articulating nursing values, for maintaining the integrity of the profession and its practice, and for shaping social policy.

Reprinted from American Nurses Association. (2008). *Guide to the code of ethics for nurses: Interpretation and application.* Washington, DC: American Nurses Association, with permission.

Organ Donation

- Uniform Anatomical Gift Act
  - This legislation was approved in 1968 by the National Conference of Commissioners on Uniform State Laws
  - It allows people to control the disposition of their organs after death
- United Network for Organ Sharing (UNOS)
  - UNOS maintains the nation's organ transplant waiting list under contract with the Health Resources and Services Administration of the U.S. Department of Health and Human Services (DHHS)
  - UNOS's organ-sharing policy, Required Request, increases the probability of a successful transplant
    - Legalized in 1987, this initiative requires that the family of every potential organ and tissue donor be asked about donating their family member's organs
    - Its purpose is to ensure that no potential donor is missed and that the family of every potential donor understands the option to donate
- Centers for Medicare and Medicaid Services (CMS) (formerly the Health Care Financing Administration)
  - CMS requires health care facilities to report all deaths to the regional organ procurement organization (OPO)
  - The OPO then enters donor information into the UNOS computer
- Organ collection
  - For most organs—such as the heart, liver, kidney, and pancreas—the patient must be pronounced brain dead and kept physically alive until the organs are harvested
  - Such tissue as the eyes, skin, bone, and heart valves may be taken after death
- Nursing interventions
  - Follow your facility's policy for identifying and reporting a potential organ donor
  - Contact your local regional OPO when a potential donor is identified
    - Typically, a specially trained person from your facility along with someone from your regional OPO will speak with the family about organ donation
    - The OPO coordinates the donation process after a family consents to donation

Health Care Regulation and Policies

- Agency for Healthcare Research and Quality (AHRQ) (formerly the Agency for Health Care Policy and Research)
  - AHRQ works collaboratively with the public and private sectors to improve quality and safety of patient care
  - As part of the DHHS, AHRQ supports research designed to improve the quality of health care, advance the use of information systems, reduce health care costs, improve patient safety, decrease medical errors, and broaden access to essential services
  - AHRQ supports the development of evidence reports through its 12 evidence-based practice centers and the dissemination of evidence-based guidelines through the AHRQ's National Guideline Clearinghouse
- Reimbursement
  - Reimbursement for health care services involves numerous plans (private and governmental), methods of coverage, and options depending on an individual's income, employment status, and age
  - Each type of plan differs in coverage, payment terms, medical treatment procedures, and choice of health care providers
  - Common types of private plans include indemnity plans, preferred provider organizations (PPOs), health maintenance organizations (HMOs), and point-of-service (POS) plans
    - An indemnity, or fee-for-service, plan allows the individual to use any health care facility or practitioner
      - The individual submits a claim, and the insurance company reimburses the individual or the health care provider
      - Indemnity plans are flexible but carry higher premiums than other types of health coverage
      - Typically, the individual must meet a deductible before reimbursement begins
    - A PPO provides a network of hospitals, practitioners, and clinics that discount their fees to insurance companies in exchange for being part of a network
      - If an individual chooses to use a provider outside the network, he'll most likely pay a higher deductible
      - This type of plan is typically less expensive but doesn't offer the flexibility of an indemnity plan
    - An HMO is a network of providers that deliver all the medical services an individual requires
      - Except in emergencies, any use of health care providers outside the HMO must be authorized by the HMO, or services may not be reimbursed
      - HMOs don't require the individual to pay a deductible, but most do require a small co-payment
      - POS is an HMO option whereby the primary health care provider may refer an individual to a health care provider outside the HMO network with minimal or no additional cost
  - Government reimbursement programs include Medicare and Medicaid
    - The CMS is the federal agency that provides health insurance through Medicare and Medicaid
    - Medicare, authorized by Congress in 1965, is a federal health insurance plan for people age 65 or older, some disabled people younger than age 65, and people with end-stage renal disease
      - Part A of Medicare pays for hospital care, skilled nursing facility care, hospice care, and some skilled nursing home care for most people when they turn age 65; it is funded by Medicare taxes
      - Part B pays for practitioners, services, outpatient hospital care, and some other medical services not covered in part A, such as physical and occupational therapy, and some home health care and supplies; part B requires most enrollees to apply monthly
      - Part C—In 1997, Congress created Medicare Advantage (Part C), formerly known as Medicare + Choice. Individuals with Medicare Parts A and B can choose to receive all of their health care through one of these provider organizations such as HMOs, PPOs, POS, or private fee-for-service plans
      - Part D—Individuals with Medicare, regardless of income, health status, or prescription drug usage, have access to prescription drug coverage
    - Medicaid became a law in 1965 under Title XIX of the Social Security Act to provide medical care to eligible needy individuals
      - Medicaid is jointly funded by the federal and state governments to assist states in the provision of adequate medical care to needy individuals
      - The Medicaid program varies considerably state to state and within each state over time

- Occupational Safety and Health Administration (OSHA)
  - In 1970, Congress approved the Occupational Safety and Health Act that placed safety and health enforcement under the federal agency called OSHA
  - OSHA ensures compliance of standards through an inspection program, with penalties for violations
  - OSHA established the National Institute for Occupational Safety and Health to conduct research and training in occupational safety and health in workplaces covered by OSHA
- The Joint Commission
  - The Joint Commission is an independent, nonprofit organization
  - It sets standards in areas such as patient rights, patient safety, health care provider credentialing, management of human resources, management of information, leadership and management, performance improvement, utilization management, emergency care, and environmental protection
  - It also evaluates health care organizations—such as hospitals (including general, psychiatric, pediatric, and rehabilitation), health care networks, home care agencies, long-term care facilities, assisted living residences, behavioral health care organizations, ambulatory care providers, and clinical laboratories—in those areas and then grants or denies accreditation
  - Health care organizations that don't receive Joint Commission accreditation don't receive reimbursement from insurance companies and Medicare
- Health Insurance Portability and Accountability Act (HIPAA)
  - In 1996, Congress approved HIPAA, which is intended to limit the ability of employers to deny employees with pre-existing medical conditions health insurance coverage
  - In 2009, the American Recovery and Reinvestment Act (ARRA) included new changes to HIPAA standards; the changes expand HIPAA's coverage and strengthen its protection
  - For a health care provider or health care organization, covered entities include all employees, including clinical staff members—such as physicians, nurses, and technicians—as well as nonclinical staff members, such as employees working in registration, billing, housekeeping, and food services; ARRA updates may also include nonemployees (such as volunteers) in this definition
- Privacy rules
  - The DHHS has developed privacy rules that include, but are not limited to, electronic medical records (EMRs); these privacy rules apply to all health care providers who transmit information electronically and prohibit the release of personal health information (PHI) without permission
  - PHI is any information that can be used to identify an individual patient; examples of PHI include a patient's name, date of birth, social security number, medical record number, address, diagnosis, license numbers, photographs, and other specific account numbers
  - Volunteers of a health care facility as well as business associates—such as contracted staff members—are expected to protect the privacy and security of health information as if they were employees
  - The National Alliance for Healthcare Information Technology defines an EMR as the health-related information of an individual that is created, gathered, managed, and consulted by licensed clinicians and staff members from a single organization who are involved in that individual's health and care
    ○ The EMR can be created in both ambulatory services (offices and off-site facilities) and health care facilities
  - The electronic heath record is a combined electronic record of health-related information on an individual that's created and gathered cumulatively across more than one health care organization and is managed and consulted by licensed clinicians and staff members involved in the individual's health and care
  - Deidentified information refers to any health or health care information that doesn't reveal a patient's commonly identifiable information (including information that could identify the patient through relatives, household members, and employers), such as a case study presented at a conference that uses a fictitious name in place of the patient's real name; this information isn't protected by privacy rules, so there are no limits on the use of this type of information
  - Disclosure is the act of sharing information; HIPAA defines disclosure as "the release, transfer, provision of access to, or divulging in any other manner of information outside the entity holding the information"
  - There are two types of disclosure
    ○ In *authorized disclosure*, the patient gives written permission to disclose information for uses outside of treatment, payment, and operations
    ○ In *unauthorized disclosure*, no written authorization is received
  - Protecting the privacy of PHI and following privacy rules is the responsibility of everyone at a health care facility, regardless of an individual's role; it's not intended to get in the way of providing quality care to patients or meeting patients' other needs

- To ensure following privacy rules while working, the nurse should ask herself three questions:
  - ○ Do I need this information to treat this patient?
  - ○ Do I need this information to bill this patient?
  - ○ Do I need this information to do other hospital-related business?
- If the answer to all three questions is "no," then the nurse doesn't need the information and shouldn't be accessing or asking for it
- Exceptions to disclosing PHI include required public health reporting; disasters or situations of imminent danger; reporting abuse of children, the elderly, or protected populations; and other state-specific required reporting, such as knife or gunshot wounds
- EMRs pose special challenges and require safeguards to ensure that information remains private
  - ○ The health care facility should ensure that each employee's computer password allows access to only the information needed to do one's job
  - ○ Employees should position computer screens away from visitors and use privacy screens whenever possible
  - ○ Employees shouldn't share or post passwords
  - ○ Employees should log out of computers immediately after each use
  - ○ Health care facilities should make sure all computers automatically log users out after a set period of inactivity
  - ○ Health care facilities should limit fax machine access to only those who need the information being faxed and should use preprogrammed numbers whenever possible to reduce the risk of incorrect dialing

Review Questions

Question 1. The nurse leaves a patient who is elderly and confused to find someone to assist with transferring the patient to bed. While the nurse is gone, the patient falls and is hurt. The nurse is at fault because the nurse hasn't:

A. properly educated the patient about safety measures.
B. restrained the patient.
C. documented that the patient was left in the room.
D. arranged for continual care of the patient.

Correct answer: D By leaving the patient, the nurse is at fault for abandonment. The better courses of action are to turn on the call bell or elicit help on the way to the patient's room. Options A and C are incorrect because neither excuses the nurse from responsibility for ensuring the patient's safety. Option B is incorrect because restraints are only to be used as a last resort, when all other alternatives for ensuring patient safety have been tried and have failed; moreover, restraints won't ensure the patient's safety.

Question 2. The nurse is caring for a patient admitted to the emergency department after a motor vehicle accident. Under the law, the nurse must obtain informed consent before treatment unless the patient:

A. is mentally ill.
B. refuses to give informed consent.
C. is in an emergency situation.
D. asks the nurse to give substituted consent.

Correct answer: C The law doesn't require informed consent in an emergency situation when the patient can't give consent and no next of kin is available. Option A is incorrect because even though a patient who is declared mentally incompetent can't give informed consent, mental illness doesn't by itself indicate that the patient is incompetent to give such consent. Option B is incorrect because a mentally competent patient may refuse or revoke consent at any time. Option D is incorrect because although the nurse may act as a patient advocate, the nurse can never give substituted consent.

Question 3. Which of the following acts committed by a nurse is an intentional tort?

A. Battery
B. Breach of confidentiality
C. Negligence
D. Abandonment

Correct answer: A Battery, touching a patient without justification or permission, is an intentional tort. Option B is incorrect because although a nurse who breaches a patient's confidentiality can be subject to a lawsuit or disciplinary action, the act isn't an intentional tort. Option C is incorrect because negligence, the failure to exercise the degree of care that a person of ordinary prudence would exercise under the same circumstances, is an unintentional tort. Option D is incorrect because although abandonment is a liability for nurses, the act isn't an intentional tort.

Question 4. OSHA is responsible for:

A. compensating workers injured in the workplace.
B. providing rehabilitation for workers injured in the workplace.
C. inspecting high-hazard workplaces for compliance with protective standards.
D. disciplining workers injured in the workplace.

Correct answer: C OSHA is responsible for preventing work-related injuries, illnesses, and deaths. Options A and B are incorrect because it's the responsibility of workers' compensation to compensate workers for injuries occurring in the workplace and to provide rehabilitative services. Option D is incorrect because it's the employer's responsibility to improve the safety and health of employees. Employers who violate OSHA standards are subject to fines and penalties.

Question 5. A patient became seriously ill after a nurse gave the patient the wrong medication. After recovery, the patient filed a lawsuit. Who is most likely to be held liable?

A. No one because it was an accident
B. The hospital
C. The nurse
D. The nurse and the hospital

Correct answer: D Nurses are always responsible for their actions. The hospital is liable for negligent conduct of its employees within the scope of employment. Consequently, the nurse and the hospital are liable. Therefore, options B and C are incorrect. Option A is incorrect because although the mistake wasn't intentional, standard procedure wasn't followed.

Question 6. Which of the following is incorrect about informed consent?

A. It can be revoked by the state, especially when the benefits outweigh the risks.
B. A person has to be mentally competent to sign an informed consent.
C. Physicians can waive informed consents in emergency situations.
D. The name of the procedure, its risks and benefits, and other alternative procedures make up all the essential elements of informed consent.

Correct answer: D An informed consent should also contain the name of the health care professional who will be performing the procedure. The other options are correct statements about informed consent.

Question 7. Which of the following is considered identifiable health information?

A. A photograph of a patient's leg showing a unique tattoo
B. A patient's chart listing his history of a stroke last year
C. A blank menu for a regular diet on the patient's overbed table
D. A laboratory report with the patient's name, address, Social Security number, date of birth, and room number deleted

Correct answer: A Any information that can identify the person or that relates to a past, present, or future physical or mental condition is considered identifiable health information. Options B, C, and D don't contain information that can identify the patient.

Question 8. In a negligence suit against a nurse, what must the plaintiff prove?

A. The nurse intended to cause harm.
B. The nurse's actions caused harm.
C. The nurse knew they caused harm.
D. The nurse was sorry for causing harm.

Correct answer: B In a negligence suit, the plaintiff must prove that the nurse's actions caused harm to the patient. The plaintiff doesn't need to prove that the nurse intended to cause harm (option A), knew they caused harm (option C), or was sorry they caused harm (option D).

Question 9. A nurse failed to administer a medication to a patient according to accepted standards. Consequently, the patient suffered adverse effects. Failure to provide patient care and to follow appropriate standards is called:

A. breach of duty.
B. breach of contract.
C. battery.
D. tort.

Correct answer: A Breach of duty means that the nurse provided care that didn't meet the accepted standard. When investigating breach of duty, the court asks: How would a reasonable, prudent nurse with comparable training and experience have acted in comparable circumstances? A breach of contract (option B) results when one party fails to perform as required by a contract. Battery (option C) is touching a patient without justification or permission. A tort (option D) is a civil action for damages for injury to a person, property, or reputation.

Question 10. The belief that one's own cultural values and beliefs are superior or the only correct values and beliefs is:

A. cultural competency.
B. cultural diversity.
C. ethnocentrism.
D. cultural sensitivity.

Correct answer: C Ethnocentrism is the belief that one's own cultural values and beliefs are superior or the only correct values and beliefs. Cultural competency (option A) is the ability to work and interact effectively with people of other cultures. Cultural diversity (option B) describes the diverse groups in society, which have varying races and national origins, religious affiliations, languages, physical size, gender, sexual orientation, age, disabilities, socioeconomic status, occupational status, and geographic location. Cultural sensitivity (option D) is the understanding of the diverse needs, characteristics, and values of individuals, families, and groups.

Selected References

Agency for Healthcare Research and Quality. Rockland, MD. Available at www.ahrq.gov.

American Nurses Association. (2008). *Guide to the code of ethics for nurses: Interpretation and application*. Washington, DC: American Nurses Association.

Occupational Safety and Health Administration. Washington, DC. Available at www.osha.gov.

United Network for Organ Sharing. Richmond, VA. Available at www.unos.org.

Chapter 4

Principles of Medical-Surgical Nursing

Adult Growth and Development

- General information
  - Growth refers to the increase in physical size and changes in physical appearance and body function that occur with aging
  - Development refers to changes in a person's psychological, intellectual, and social functioning
- Principles of growth and development
  - Growth and development occur from conception until death
  - These processes are influenced by heredity and environment
  - These processes are continuous and orderly, yet each person experiences them in a unique way
- Theories of growth and development
  - Psychosocial, behavioral, social-learning, cognitive, and humanist theories describe human growth and development
  - In Erik Erikson's psychosocial theory, each person goes through predictable, age-related stages
    - Each stage involves a key conflict or core problem that may be completely, partially, or unsuccessfully resolved
    - Healthy personality development is associated with positive resolution of key conflicts (see *Stages of adult development*, pages 38–39)

Human Behavior

- General information
  - Several theorists aim to explain or predict human behavior
  - Two theorists of human behavior typically referred to in nursing practice are Jean Piaget and Abraham Maslow
- Jean Piaget
  - Piaget's theory of human behavior suggests that individuals reach cognitive maturity by middle to late adolescence
  - During his life, Piaget explored how intelligence and cognitive functioning develop in children
  - He believed that human intelligence progresses through a series of stages based on age, with the child at each successive stage demonstrating a higher level of functioning than at previous stages
  - He strongly believed that biological changes and maturation were responsible for cognitive development, and he divided cognitive development into four stages
    - The *sensorimotor stage* lasts from birth to age 2 years
      - The child develops a sense of self as separate from the environment and develops the concept of object permanence—that is, the child realizes that tangible objects don't cease to exist just because they are out of sight
      - The child begins to form mental images

Box 4-1: Stages of Adult Development

As adults age, they enter different stages of physical, cognitive, and psychosocial development and face various challenges and health problems and concerns.

Development	Challenges	Health Problems and Concerns
Young adulthood (ages 18 to 35) **Physical** • By the mid-20s, a person reaches adult height, and body systems are fully developed. • Young adults are at peak physical strength, maximum physiologic reserve, and prime reproductive capability. **Cognitive** • With stimulation, young adults continue to develop their intellectual abilities. **Psychosocial** • The key conflict is "intimacy versus isolation." • Young adults struggle to form commitments without losing their identity. • With positive resolution, the young adult develops satisfying, intimate relationships. • With negative resolution, the young adult becomes self-absorbed and focuses only on his or her own needs.	• Selecting and preparing for a vocation • Becoming financially independent • Establishing a new living arrangement • Managing a home • Selecting a marriage partner • Choosing an alternative lifestyle such as homosexuality • Developing a satisfactory sex life • Becoming a parent and raising children • Finding a congenial social group • Assuming civic responsibilities	*Health problems* • Childbirth or infertility • Substance abuse • Stress and stress-related illnesses such as peptic ulcer disease • Sexually transmitted diseases • Accidents and injuries *Health concerns (when illness occurs)* • Loss of independence and disruption of lifestyle • Disruption of employment and loss of employment benefits such as health insurance • Decreased self-esteem
Middle adulthood (ages 36 to 65) **Physical** • Middle-aged adults experience a slow decline in body functions. The rate of decline varies greatly and is affected by heredity, diet, exercise, rest, and stress. • Typical physical changes include hair thinning and graying, skin wrinkling, diminished eyesight and hearing, menopause, decreased metabolism, weight gain, decreased strength and endurance, loss of bone mass and density, muscle and joint stiffness, and decreased libido. **Cognitive** • Intellectual performance remains relatively stable. **Psychosocial** • The key conflict in middle age is "generativity versus stagnation." • Middle-aged adults need to be productive and accept responsibility for their family, work, and community. • With positive resolution, the middle-aged adult is productive and satisfied with life. • With negative resolution, the middle-aged adult becomes egocentric, stagnant, and dissatisfied.	• Maintaining satisfactory employment • Preparing for retirement • Adjusting to the physical changes of middle age • Developing satisfying relationships with grown children, friends, and other adults • Helping children become responsible, happy adults • Resolving the empty-nest crisis as children leave home • Becoming a grandparent • Relating to aging parents • Developing leisure activities • Maintaining social and civic responsibilities	*Health problems* • Chronic diseases (such as arthritis, hypertension, coronary artery disease, osteoporosis, diabetes, and lung disease) and depression, anxiety, or other emotional problems • Cancer, particularly of the lung, breast, colon, rectum, and prostate • Substance abuse • Accidents and injuries *Health concerns* • Loss of job and employment benefits such as health insurance • Awareness of mortality and fear of early death • Ability to meet commitments to children, aging parents, and community • Concerns about retirement and retirement benefits

(continued)

Box 4-1: Stages of Adult Development (continued)

Development	Challenges	Health Problems and Concerns
Older adulthood (age 66 and older) **Physical** • The maximum life span is typically age 110; the average is age 80. • The body systems of older adults function adequately unless stressed, which taxes their decreased physiologic reserves. • Older adults experience decreased strength, endurance, cardiac output, vital capacity, GI motility, and skin elasticity and secretions; weakened muscles and joints; bone and muscle loss; diminished eyesight and hearing; and altered renal function. **Cognitive** • Intellectual abilities generally remain stable. • Normal changes include increased response time and minor short-term memory loss; other cognitive changes warrant investigation. **Psychosocial** • The key conflict in older adulthood is "integrity versus despair." • Older adults focus on a life review and acceptance of the worth of their life. • With positive resolution, the older adults are satisfied with their accomplishments. • With negative resolution, the older adult has feelings of hopelessness, regret, and despair.	• Adjusting to retirement and an altered financial situation • Maintaining satisfactory housing arrangements • Adjusting to the death of a spouse, family members, and friends • Adjusting to decreased physical strength • Adjusting to declining health • Adjusting to mental changes and short-term memory loss • Maintaining social relationships • Finding leisure activities	*Health problems* • Chronic diseases (especially arthritis, cardiovascular disease, cerebrovascular disease, cancer, diabetes, osteoporosis, Alzheimer's disease, glaucoma, benign prostatic hyperplasia, pneumonia, and other respiratory disease), fractures, and cataracts • Greater susceptibility to adverse drug reactions • Longer recovery from illness • Vague or atypical symptoms of illness *Health concerns* • Loss of functional abilities • Disruption of current lifestyle and living arrangements

- ○ The *preoperational stage* lasts from ages 2 to 7 years
  - ○ The child develops the ability to express self with language, understands the meaning of symbolic gestures, and begins to classify objects
  - ○ The child has difficulty taking the viewpoint of others
  - ○ The child classifies objects by a single feature
- ○ The *concrete operational stage* lasts from ages 7 to 11 years
  - ○ The child begins to apply logic to thinking, understands spatiality and reversibility, can classify objects according to several features, and can place them in a series based on a single dimension, such as size
  - ○ The child is increasingly social and able to apply rules
  - ○ The child's thinking remains concrete
- ○ The *formal operational stage* begins at age 11 years and continues through adulthood
  - ○ The child can think logically about abstract positions and test hypotheses
  - ○ The child further develops logical thinking and reasoning
  - ○ The child achieves cognitive maturity
- ● Abraham Maslow
  - ● Maslow described a hierarchy of needs based on the basic drives or needs that motivate people; he posited that an individual must meet each level before he or she can move on to the next level
  - ● Maslow's hierarchy consists of five basic levels
    - ○ *Physiological needs* are a person's most basic needs and must be met; these biological needs include oxygen, food, water, shelter, and freedom from pain
    - ○ At the next level, a person needs *safety and security*, including protection and freedom from harm or threatened deprivation

- ○ The next level of need is *love, affection, and belonging,* when a person seeks to overcome feelings of loneliness and alienation; this stage carries the need for enduring intimacy, friendship, and acceptance and includes both giving and receiving of love and affection
  - ○ At the next level, the person tries to meet *esteem needs* and self-respect
    - ○ When a person successfully meets these needs, he or she feels self-confident and valuable as a person
    - ○ When a person doesn't meet these needs, he or she feels inferior, helpless, and worthless
  - ○ At the top level of *self-actualization,* the person meets the need of doing what the person was "born to do"; this level includes the need for beauty, truth, and justice
- Traumatic life circumstances or compromised health can cause a person to regress to a lower level of motivation

Death and Dying

- General information
  - There are multiple definitions of death. According to the Uniform Determination of Death Act (1981), death is defined as the irreversible cessation of circulatory and respiratory functions. Dying is a process that ends with death
  - Several categories of death include cell death, brain death, cardiac death, spiritual death, and functional death (Rubel, 2016)
  - Many factors influence an adult's views of death: ethnic, social, and cultural background; religious beliefs; personal values; previous experiences with death; and developmental stage
  - Young and middle-aged adults usually spend little time considering the possibility of their own death; they view it as an intrusion or an injustice and are most concerned with who will take care of their family if they should die
  - Older adults begin to consider the possibility of death and tend to view it as a phase of life; although some older adults welcome death as freedom from pain, others fear dying alone or suffering needlessly
- Responses to death
  - Each person responds to death in his or her own way which can range from fear of death to acceptance of death; there are no right or wrong responses
  - Current research supports that an individual's personal experiences with death can have a positive impact on the attitudes toward death and can decrease death anxiety.
  - The circumstances of a death can influence a person's response
    - ○ Sudden, unexpected deaths such as accidental deaths or suicide may be harder to accept than those that have been anticipated for some time
    - ○ Other influences on the response to death include age, kinship or relationship status, previous losses, and the survivor's own personality and coping style
    - ○ A premature death, such as that of a child, is harder to accept than that of an elderly person
  - Elisabeth Kübler-Ross described a typical pattern of response to death (see *Dealing with death and dying,* page 41)
  - Other more recent models also describe responses to death
    - ○ Pattison (1970) developed a living-dying interval theory. This theory begins when a patient learns that death is imminent and ends at the actual time of death. The person may go between denial and acceptance of the prognosis
    - ○ Corr (1992) created a task-based model in response to death and dying. This focused on how people cope with dying by completing physical, psychological, social, and spiritual tasks
    - ○ Doka (1996) described a phase-based model for coping with dying. The phases include prediagnostic, acute, chronic, terminal, and recovery phases of life-threatening illnesses
    - ○ Life review and spiritually based approaches to death and dying are other models (Rubel, 2016)

Assessment

- General information
  - A nursing assessment includes a comprehensive health history, thorough physical examination, and (when applicable) review of diagnostic test results
  - A thorough, accurate nursing assessment is critical in determining appropriate nursing diagnoses

Box 4-2: Dealing with Death and Dying

Elisabeth Kübler-Ross discovered that most people pass through five stages in response to death and dying. Although some individuals experience the stages in a different order and others revisit some stages, knowledge of these stages can help the nurse evaluate—and deal with—a patient's responses to death and dying.

Stages of death and dying

1. *Denial and isolation:* the initial response characterized by shock and disbelief
2. *Anger:* expressions of rage and resentment
3. *Bargaining:* attempts to strike a bargain, typically with God, in exchange for prolonged life
4. *Depression:* feelings of loss, grief, and intense sadness
5. *Acceptance:* a quiet stage characterized by a gradual, peaceful withdrawal from life

Nursing implications

For a Dying Patient's Psychosocial and Spiritual Needs	For a Dying Patient's Physical Needs	For Family Members' Psychosocial and Spiritual Needs
• Help the patient make final plans. • Help the patient control personal routines and affairs as long as possible. • Provide opportunities for reminiscence and validation of self-worth. • Support the patient's expression of difficult feelings. • Use touch as a communication tool, if acceptable to the patient. • Provide for formal spiritual support, such as clergy visits or last rites.	• Regularly perform routine personal care measures, such as turning, positioning, bathing, and grooming. • Be alert for constipation, a common problem. • Anticipate bowel and bladder incontinence as death nears. • Be sensitive to individual preferences for lighting and noise control. • Use pain medications and comfort measures as needed to maintain patient comfort. • Offer favorite liquids and soft foods; appetite wanes as death nears. • Remember that hearing is the last sense to be lost.	• Allow flexible visitations. • Encourage family members to participate in patient care. • Recommend rest breaks for family members. • Visit the patient regularly, and perform routine personal care activities while family members are present. • Encourage the family to personalize the patient's room. • Provide for bereavement follow-up. • Recognize the need for formal counseling in difficult situations. • Encourage the use of support groups when available.

- Health history
    - Excellent communication techniques and interviewing skills are the key to obtaining a good health history
    - The nurse begins the history by obtaining *biographic data:* name, address, age, date of birth, sex, race, marital status, education, occupation, and financial status
    - The nurse then determines the patient's *chief complaint* or reason for seeking health care
    - Next, the nurse obtains a *history of current illness*, including a description of the symptom's location, duration, frequency, intensity, precipitating factors, and relieving factors
    - The nurse continues by ascertaining a *personal history*
        - The personal history includes childhood illnesses and childhood and recent immunizations
        - It also includes questions about disorders, such as allergies, heart disease, and diabetes; accidents; and emotional problems or mental illness
        - It investigates prior hospitalizations, surgery, and transfusions
        - It assesses work history, including occupational exposure to toxins or other harmful substances
        - If the patient is female, it addresses age at menarche, age at menopause, and pregnancy history
        - The personal history evaluates lifestyle and health habits, including sexual orientation and activity; alcohol and tobacco use; diet; over-the-counter, herbal, and recreational drug use; and sleeping patterns
        - It explores prescription medication use
    - Then the nurse obtains a *family history*
        - It ascertains the ages of the patient's parents and the number, sex, and age of siblings
        - It also inquires about a family history of various diseases and emotional problems or mental illness
    - The nurse concludes the history with a *review of physical status*
        - *General:* Assess overall health status, malaise, fatigue, chills and fever, night sweats, recent weight gain or loss, and increased sensitivity to heat or cold

- *Skin, hair, and nails:* Ask about skin disease or rash, urticaria, acne, psoriasis, alopecia, hirsutism, pigmentation changes, jaundice, and increased skin dryness or moisture
- *Head:* Inquire about trauma, headache, vertigo, syncope, and change in level of consciousness (LOC)
- *Eyes:* Investigate visual acuity, use of glasses or contact lenses, photophobia, diplopia, night blindness, nystagmus, eye infections, eye pain, and halos around lights
- *Ears:* Assess tinnitus, ear infections, ear pain, ear discharge, loss of hearing, use of hearing aids, and occupational or lifestyle exposure to damaging sounds
- *Nose:* Ask about problems with smell, frequent colds, sinus infections or pain, and epistaxis
- *Mouth:* Have the patient discuss condition of the teeth, use of dentures or partial plates, bleeding or swollen gums, frequent sore throats, hoarseness, and difficulty swallowing
- *Neck:* Evaluate for pain, tenderness, and swelling
- *Cardiovascular:* Inquire about edema, dyspnea, orthopnea, number of pillows needed when supine, cough, chest pain, intermittent claudication, hypertension, palpitations, anemia, varicosities, and results of the last electrocardiogram and blood cholesterol levels
- *Respiratory:* Learn about any dry or productive cough, color of sputum, hemoptysis, dyspnea, wheezing, and last chest X-ray
- *GI:* Discuss dietary intake, polyphagia, polydipsia, anorexia, nausea, vomiting, heartburn, bowel habits, diarrhea, constipation, change in stool color, blood or mucus in stool, flatulence, hemorrhoids, location and intensity of abdominal pain, jaundice, and ascites
- *Genitourinary:* Check into nocturia, frequency, burning, decreased urinary stream, hesitancy, pain, dribbling, polyuria, and incontinence
- *Musculoskeletal:* Assess for joint pain or stiffness, decreased mobility, edema, and heat or tenderness
- *Neurologic:* Ask about seizures, headaches, fainting spells, decreased LOC, paresis or paralysis, paresthesia, aphasia, tremor, head injuries, and loss of memory
- *Mental status:* Inquire about mood swings, anxiety, depression, insomnia, and suicidal ideation
- *Reproductive*
  - *Male*: Ask about testicular self-examination, penile discharge, sexually transmitted diseases, sexual activity, safer sex practices (such as the use of latex condoms with spermicide and having one known partner), impotence, and infertility
  - *Female*: Inquire about age of menarche; date, duration, and flow of last menses; vaginal discharge; sexually transmitted diseases; sexual activity; use of birth control; safer sex practices; age of menopause; last Papanicolaou test; breast tenderness or discharge; breast self-examination; and last mammogram
- Physical examination
  - To perform an effective physical examination, the nurse must be proficient in the following techniques
    - *Inspection* uses the senses of sight and smell to observe the patient, such as when the nurse observes a patient's gait or smells a fruity odor on the patient's breath
    - *Palpation* uses the sense of touch to gather data, such as when the nurse takes a radial pulse or feels the breasts for lumps
    - *Percussion* involves striking one object against another to generate a vibration that produces an audible sound wave, such as when the nurse taps over clear lung fields (resonance), a body organ (dullness), or an air-filled stomach (tympany)
    - *Auscultation* uses the sense of hearing to listen for sounds, usually with a stethoscope, produced by body organs, such as when the nurse takes an apical pulse or listens over the carotid artery for a bruit
  - The nurse usually conducts the physical examination from head to toe and from least to most sensitive areas
    - The nurse begins with a *general assessment*
      - Check height, weight, and vital signs
      - Observe general appearance and grooming, breath and body odor, overall mental state, posture, and ability to move
    - Next, the nurse examines the *head*
      - Note condition of scalp and hair and distribution of hair
      - Note head size and contour and facial symmetry
    - Then the nurse checks the *eyes*
      - Check visual acuity, visual fields, and extraocular movements
      - Note condition of conjunctivae, sclerae, and eyebrows
      - Check pupil size and reaction to light and corneal reflex
      - Examine the retinas using an ophthalmoscope

- ○ The nurse continues by assessing the *ears*
  - ○ Observe ear size, shape, and position
  - ○ Examine the tympanic membrane with an otoscope, noting color, landmarks, external canal condition, and any wax or foreign bodies
  - ○ Conduct hearing screening tests
    - ○ For the *Weber test*, hold a vibrating tuning fork at the middle of the patient's forehead and check for equal distribution of sound; the sound should be equal on both sides; lateralization indicates abnormality
    - ○ For the *Rinne test*, hold a vibrating tuning fork over the mastoid process; when the vibration stops, place the tuning fork near the external ear; the patient should still be able to hear the vibration
- ○ Then the nurse assesses the *nose*
  - ○ Observe nares for patency, appearance, and septal deviation
  - ○ Test for sinus tenderness and the ability to discriminate smells
- ○ The nurse examines the *mouth and throat* next
  - ○ Note condition of the teeth and use of dentures or partial plates
  - ○ Observe mucous membranes, tongue, tonsils, and pharynx
  - ○ Determine the patient's ability to discriminate different tastes
  - ○ Test for the gag reflex and ability to move the uvula
  - ○ Palpate the lymph nodes
- ○ The nurse evaluates the *neck*
  - ○ Observe for mobility
  - ○ Palpate thyroid for size and shape
  - ○ Palpate trachea for midline placement
  - ○ Auscultate for carotid bruits
- ○ The nurse assesses the *heart*
  - ○ Inspect for visible pulsations and jugular vein distention
  - ○ Palpate for point of maximal impulse at the fifth intercostal space, at the midclavicular line
  - ○ Palpate for thrills or ventricular heave
  - ○ Auscultate heart sounds and assess apical pulse for rate, rhythm, and quality
- ○ The nurse also assesses the *lungs*
  - ○ Inspect chest for size, shape, and symmetrical excursion
  - ○ Note use of accessory muscles
  - ○ Palpate for symmetrical excursion and tactile fremitus
  - ○ Auscultate for breath sounds
- ○ Next, the nurse checks the *breasts*
  - ○ Observe for symmetry, dimpling, or retraction
  - ○ Palpate for masses and palpable lymph nodes
- ○ Then the nurse evaluates the *abdomen*
  - ○ Inspect for size, contour, and scars
  - ○ Auscultate all quadrants for bowel sounds
  - ○ Percuss for tympany and area of dullness at liver margin
  - ○ Palpate for tenderness or masses; the liver, spleen, and kidneys normally aren't palpable
- ○ The nurse assesses the *musculoskeletal system*
  - ○ Note symmetry, alignment, and joint range of motion
  - ○ Palpate for tenderness, muscle tone, and crepitus in joints
- ○ The nurse also assesses the *nervous system*
  - ○ Note LOC, orientation, speech, and gait
  - ○ Check deep tendon and plantar reflexes
  - ○ Check sensory perceptions of pain, touch, position, vibration, and temperature
  - ○ Test cranial nerve function
  - ○ Test motor system for muscle tone and strength
- ○ The nurse then examines the *genitalia*
  - ○ For a male patient, inspect general appearance, circumcision (if any), pubic hair distribution, urethral opening, scars, swelling, and discharge; also palpate for tenderness, descended testicles, masses, swelling, and palpable inguinal lymph nodes
  - ○ For a female patient, inspect external genitalia and pubic hair distribution, check vaginal mucosa and cervix with a speculum, and perform bimanual examination of uterus and ovaries

○ Finally, the nurse assesses the *rectum*
  ○ Inspect for hemorrhoids and fissures
  ○ Note stool color
  ○ Palpate rectum for shape, tenderness, and internal hemorrhoids; for male patient, palpate posterior prostate for symmetry and tenderness

Therapeutic Communication

- General information
  - Therapeutic communication is as important for a medical-surgical nurse as for a psychiatric and mental health nurse
  - A therapeutic relationship facilitates application of the nursing process and is based on the patient's needs
    ○ It focuses on the patient; personal issues that interfere with a nurse's ability to relate to a patient must be resolved through peer supervision or counseling
    ○ It's influenced by the nurse's style of interaction (see *Interaction styles affecting therapeutic communication*, page 45)
- Uses of therapeutic communication
  - Therapeutic communication enhances the patient's coping skills by helping the patient become an integral part of the treatment plan, actively participate in recovery, and try new health-promoting behaviors
  - It decreases patient defensiveness by building a trusting nurse-patient relationship; it also helps the nurse identify health problems, such as substance abuse, and promotes cooperation with nursing interventions
  - It can clarify issues, which reduces misunderstandings and facilitates the design of an individualized care plan
  - It can promote healing (see *Therapeutic communication techniques for medical-surgical nursing*, page 46)
- Types of messages
  - *Constructive messages* confirm the patient's importance, keep the lines of communication open, and allow for further data collection; examples include "What would you like from me?" "What do you think about … ?" and "I can see you're in pain; let's talk about your options for managing it"
  - *Destructive messages* negate the patient's importance, close the lines of communication, and put all parties on the defensive; examples include "The doctor ordered this," "There are other patients on this floor besides you," and "We're doing the best we can"
- Patient perceptions
  - Patients are affected not only by what they know about their situation but also by how they perceive it
  - Therapeutic communication allows the nurse to assess the patient's knowledge of their condition; examples include "What's your understanding of your condition?" "What have you been told about your condition?" and "What questions do you have about your condition?"
  - Therapeutic communication allows the nurse to assess how the patient perceives their condition; examples include "What are your thoughts about what's happening to you?" "How does this illness affect your life?" and "Based on your condition, what do you anticipate happening?"
  - Therapeutic communication lets the nurse assess how the patient feels about his or her health; examples include "How do you feel about your condition?" and "On a scale of 1 to 5, how comfortable are you with knowing that you have … ?"
- Steps to therapeutic communication
  - Respect privacy
  - Convey unconditional positive regard; patients need to feel valued no matter how they look or act
  - Choose words carefully; the use of *why* can sound accusatory, and other words can hinder self-disclosure
  - Use an appropriate sequence of questions
    ○ First, ask for descriptions; for example, "Tell me about the pain"
    ○ Second, ask what the patient thinks about the situation; for example, "What do you think this pain is all about?"
    ○ Third, ask the patients how they feel about the situation; for example, "How do you feel about having this pain?"
  - Use the nursing process in a culturally relevant way
    ○ Assess the patient's health beliefs and practices to avoid misunderstandings and noncompliance
    ○ Formulate a culturally relevant etiology statement in the nursing diagnosis to allow development of individualized care plans
    ○ Devise plans or goals that are compatible with the patient's values; incompatible plans will frustrate the patient and the nurse

○ Use culturally relevant interventions; whenever possible, interweave the patient's usual health practices with scientific health practices

○ Evaluate outcomes within the context of the patient's background

● Establish a therapeutic environment

○ Address the reality of the patient's experience

○ If a patient asks, "Am I going to die?" an appropriate nursing response is "Tell me why you're asking that question"

○ Avoid responses that close off exploration, such as "You'll have to ask your doctor" or "Yes, you know your illness is terminal"

○ Provide patients with the information that they need about their condition and the health care system

○ Tell patients what to expect from the system and the nurse, and explain what's expected of them

○ Tell them who has access to information about their condition

○ Inform them of the unit rules

○ Explain procedures and medications

○ Provide the names of personnel associated with their care

○ Empower patients

○ Include them in care conferences

○ Ask them what they think of the care plan, what they want the nurse to know about them, and what they expect from the nurse

○ Anticipate patients' needs

○ Begin discharge planning when a patient enters care, and include significant others in the planning

○ Provide written materials; most patients are moderately anxious and comprehend only fragments of information at a time

○ Allow for privacy and space needs

○ Conserve patients' energy for healing; don't expect or require them to do more than is realistic

○ Don't wait for patients to tell you of their needs such as a need for pain medication; ask about their needs regularly

○ Arrange for diversionary activities as patients recover

○ Be accountable to patients

○ Keep patients informed of care plans

○ Ask them about care, and determine if they would like to change anything

---

Box 4-3: Interaction Styles Affecting Therapeutic Communication

Interaction styles range from defensive to sympathetic to holistic. To enhance therapeutic communication, the nurse should strive to achieve a holistic style.

Defensive style

Nurses who interact defensively have an intense need to be perfect and feel a need to justify everything. They're closed, they withhold information, and they don't risk exposing personal vulnerabilities. They tend to blame their patients and feel frustrated when the patients don't "measure up."

This interaction style can produce anxiety, defensiveness, fatigue, guilt, frustration, and burnout.

Sympathetic style

Nurses who interact sympathetically have poor boundaries and can't clearly separate their own emotional responses from the patient's needs and wants. Sympathizers tend to project their own feelings onto others. They take on others' burdens as their own and feel a need to make everything turn out right. They experience a sense of personal failure if the patient's problem isn't resolved.

This interaction style can cause an emotional outflow of energy, emotional exhaustion, and a sense of futility.

Holistic style

Nurses who interact holistically have healthy ego boundaries: They understand what belongs to their patients and what belongs to them. Holistic nurses provide an atmosphere for patient growth and allow it to happen in whatever manner is meaningful to their patients.

This interaction style can lead to self-awareness, centeredness, differentiation of nurse and patient needs, controlled energy outflow, vitality, tranquility, and satisfaction.

Box 4-4: Therapeutic Communication Techniques for Medical-Surgical Nursing

The medical-surgical nurse can use various techniques to achieve therapeutic communication.

Technique	Description	Example
Broad opening	General statement or question designed to encourage the patient to talk about whatever is most important at the moment	Patient (in bed): "Hello." Nurse: "How are you doing?" or "How is it going?"
Clarification	Seeking validation for what was said	Nurse: "What do you mean when you say…?" or "You're awfully quiet today. What's going on?"
Concreteness	Seeking further information by asking how, what, where, when, and who, which helps the nurse gather more information and helps the patient become more objective about a situation	Patient: "They said…" Nurse: "Who said…?" Patient: "I feel so bad." Nurse: "Tell me how you feel bad."
Confrontation	Calling the patients' attention to discrepancies in their communication patterns or discrepancies between what they say and do	Patient: "I don't have any concerns about…" Nurse: "You say you aren't concerned, but I notice your muscles are tense" or "You say you don't have any concerns, yet you've asked me the same question four times."
Empathy	Putting yourself temporarily in another's position	Patient: "I should never have agreed to this surgery." Nurse: "Sounds like you're having second thoughts."
Focusing	Helping the patient direct attention to something specific	Patient: "This is so complicated, I don't know where to begin. How will I ever learn how to take care of…" Nurse: "For now, I want you to concentrate on…"
Reflection	Paraphrasing what the patient has said	Patient: "I'm useless. I can't even scratch my own nose." Nurse: "You're convinced you'll never be able to do anything for yourself."
Silence	Refraining from speech to gather information, collect personal thoughts, or give the patient an opportunity to speak when ready	Patient: "It's so awful to lose your husband" (weeps vigorously). Nurse: remains quietly with the patient but doesn't try to take away the patient's pain.

Review Questions

Question 1. The nurse is assessing pain in a patient with appendicitis. Which initial statement or question will be most effective in eliciting information?

A. "Tell me how you feel."
B. "Point to where you're feeling pain."
C. "Does your pain medication relieve your pain?"
D. "Coughing makes your pain worse, doesn't it?"

Correct answer: A Asking the patient to describe how he or she is feeling is an open-ended question, allowing for the widest range of responses. Asking the patient to point to the pain (Option B) may be an important follow-up question but is too limiting to be the nurse's first question. Asking if pain medication relieves their pain (Option C) is a closed question requiring only a yes-or-no response and should be avoided. Option D is leading as well as closed. It suggests to the patient that coughing should make the pain worse.

Question 2. When performing an abdominal assessment, the nurse should follow which examination sequence?

A. Auscultation, inspection, percussion, palpation
B. Inspection, auscultation, percussion, palpation
C. Palpation, auscultation, percussion, inspection
D. Percussion, palpation, auscultation, inspection

Correct answer: B The correct sequence for abdominal assessment is inspection, auscultation, percussion, and palpation because this sequence prevents altering bowel sounds with palpation before auscultation. The correct sequence for all other assessments is inspection, palpation, percussion, and auscultation.

Question 3. To maintain a therapeutic environment with a patient and their family, the nurse can use communication techniques such as clarification. An example of clarification is:

A. "How is it going?"
B. "You say you aren't concerned, but you've asked me many questions on this same subject."
C. "What do you mean when you say…?"
D. "For now, I would like to concentrate on…"

Correct answer: C Option C is an example of clarification or seeking validation. Option A isn't an example of clarification but is instead an example of a broad-opening technique. Option B is an example of confrontation, which calls attention to discrepancies in what the patient is saying. Option D is an example of focusing or helping the patient direct his or her thoughts.

Question 4. In the stages of death and dying as defined by Elisabeth Kübler-Ross, loss, grief, and intense sadness are symptoms of:

A. depression.
B. denial.
C. anger.
D. acceptance.

Correct answer: A Loss, grief, and intense sadness indicate depression. Denial (Option B) is indicated by the refusal to admit the truth or reality. Anger (Option C) is manifested by rage and resentment. Acceptance (Option D) is evidenced by a gradual, peaceful withdrawal from life.

Question 5. In the levels of basic human needs as defined by Abraham Maslow, which of the following levels is most basic?

A. Physiologic
B. Safety and security
C. Love, affection, and belonging
D. Esteem

Correct answer: A Physiologic needs (Option A) are the most basic needs and essential for sustaining life. Once physiologic needs are met, needs for safety and security (Option B) can be met, followed by love, affection, and belonging (Option C), and esteem (Option D).

Question 6. According to the stages of development, what conflict does the older adult experience?

A. Intimacy versus isolation
B. Generativity versus stagnation
C. Identity versus role confusion
D. Integrity versus despair

Correct answer: D The key conflict the older adult (age 66 and older) faces is integrity versus despair. Intimacy versus isolation (Option A) is the key conflict in young adulthood; generativity versus stagnation (Option B) is the key conflict in middle adulthood; and identity versus role confusion (Option C) is the key conflict of adolescence.

Question 7. The nurse is caring for a patient who has just been diagnosed with a terminal illness. The patient says to the nurse, "I can't believe this! I feel…" and pauses. The nurse allows the patient time to gather his or her thoughts. What type of therapeutic communication is this?

A. Clarification
B. Empathy
C. Reflection
D. Silence

Correct answer: D The nurse allows the patient time to gather his or her thoughts by using silence. Clarification (Option A) would be seeking validation for what the patient said. Empathy (Option B) would be the nurse placing self temporarily in the patient's position. Reflection (Option C) would be paraphrasing what the patient said.

Question 8. A patient becomes angry attending a treatment group and complains about it to the nurse. Which response could the nurse give that would best demonstrate clarification?

A. "Can you tell me what about the treatment group made you angry?"
B. "Why are you upset? Attending the treatment group will help you get well."
C. "It sounds like group today was pretty upsetting."
D. "Treatment groups have been carefully planned by the staff to help patients."

Correct answer: A Option A uses clarification to seek validation of what the patient said. Using "why," as in Option B, is accusatory and can hinder self-disclosure. Option C is an example of empathy, and Option D is a destructive sentence that negates the patient's importance.

Question 9. Which of Piaget's cognitive developmental stages takes place from ages 7 to 11?

A. Formal operational
B. Concrete operational
C. Preoperational
D. Sensorimotor

Correct answer: B The concrete operational stage takes place between ages 7 and 11. The formal operational stage (Option A) occurs at age 11 and above. The preoperational stage (Option C) takes place between ages 2 to 7, and the sensorimotor stage (Option D) occurs from birth to age 2 years.

Question 10. Which interaction style describes nurses who cannot clearly separate their own emotional responses from the patient's needs and wants?

A. Holistic
B. Defensive
C. Sympathetic
D. Silence

Correct answer: C A sympathetic interaction style occurs when the nurse can't clearly separate his or her own emotional responses from the patient's needs and wants. Nurses who use a holistic interaction style (Option A) have healthy ego boundaries and provide an atmosphere that promotes patient growth. Nurses who tend to blame their patients and feel frustrated when they do not "measure up" have a defensive interaction style (Option B). Silence (Option D) is a type of therapeutic communication technique, not an interaction style.

Selected References

Corr, C. A., & Corr, D. M. (2013). *Death & dying, life & living* (7th ed.). Belmont, CA: Wadsworth.

Doka, K. J. (1996). Coping with life-threatening illness: A task model. *OMEGA—Journal of Death and Dying, 32*(2), 111–122. Retrieved from http://journals.sagepub.com/doi/pdf/10.2190/0WEH-QUBG-67VG-YKJK

Pattison, E. M. (1977). *The experience of dying.* Englewood Cliffs, NJ: Prentice Hall.

Rubel, B. (2016). *Death, dying, and bereavement: Providing compassion during a time of need* (3rd ed.). Brockton, MA: Western

Schools. Retrieved from https://www.westernschools.com/ce-course/nursing-ce-course/death-dying-and-bereavement-providing-compassion-during-a-time-of-need-3rd-edition-3890.aspx

Sumegi, A. (2014). *Understanding death: An introduction of ideas of self and afterlife in world religions.* Malden, MA: Wiley-Blackwell.

The uniform determination of death act: An effective solution to the problem of defining death. (1982). *Washington and Lee Review, 39*(4). Retrieved from http://scholarlycommons.law.wlu.edu/wlulr/vol39/iss4/14

Chapter 5

Principles of Wound Care

Introduction

- Skin, the body's largest organ and the outer covering of the body, serves as a protective barrier against microorganisms
- The skin is subject to injury from various external and internal factors
  - *External factors* include extremes of heat and cold (burns or frostbite), mechanical forces such as pressure and shearing, allergens, chemicals, radiation, and excretions and secretions (for instance, from an ostomy or draining wound)
  - *Internal factors* include emaciation, drugs, altered circulation and impaired oxygen transport, altered metabolic state, and infections

Definitions

- *Angiogenesis* is a physiological process in which the formation of new granulation vessels forms from preexisting vessels
- *Cellulitis* is the inflammation of cellular or connective tissue
- *Colonization* refers to the presence of bacteria that cause no local or systemic indications of infection
- *Dehiscence* is the separation of the layers of a surgical wound (may be serious surgical complication)
- *Eschar* is thick, leathery, necrotic, devitalized tissue
- *Friction* is the mechanical force exerted when skin rubs against a coarse surface such as bed linens
- *Full thickness* describes a wound that involves skin loss with extensive destruction, tissue necrosis, or damage to muscle, bone, or supporting structures
- *Infection* is the invasion and multiplication of microorganisms in body tissue in a sufficient quantity (greater than 1 million organisms per gram of tissue) to overwhelm tissue defenses; an infection can produce purulent exudate, odor, erythema, warmth, tenderness, edema, pain, fever, and an elevated white blood cell (WBC) count
- *Maceration* is the softening of tissue by wetting or soaking; it can produce skin degeneration and disintegration if left uncontrolled
- *Partial thickness* describes a wound that involves damage to epidermal and, possibly, dermal skin layers
- *Sloughing* is the separation of necrotic tissue from viable tissue
- *Shearing* is trauma caused by tissue layers sliding against one another; it results in disruption or strangulation of blood vessels and can result in skin tear injuries
- A *wound* is any disruption to the anatomic or physiologic function of tissue

Types of Wounds

- An *acute* wound heals uneventfully within an expected time frame unless underlying systemic conditions interrupt the process; examples include surgical incisions, trauma wounds, skin tears, and lacerations.
- A wound is *chronic* when underlying pathophysiology causes the wound or interferes with the course of healing; several types exist (see *Characteristics of acute and chronic wounds*, pages 50–51)

Wound Healing Process

- A dynamic process that restores anatomic and functional integrity, wound healing works on a continuum from injury to healing
  - In *healing by primary intention*, the wound is surgically closed (such as with sutures, staples, glue, or Steri-Strips), and healing occurs by fibrous adhesion; granulation tissue isn't apparent, and there's little or no scar tissue; examples include surgical wounds and superficial traumatic wounds
  - In *healing by secondary intention*, the wound's edges are too far apart to be surgically closed, and there's marked tissue loss; the wound is instead closed naturally by the formation and adhesion of granulation tissue and epithelialization; examples include pressure ulcers, dehisced surgical wounds, and traumatic injuries
  - In *healing by tertiary intention*, also known as *delayed primary closure*, there's a delay in wound closure, resulting in granulation of the wound edges; later surgical closure results in more scar formation; these wounds are sometimes left open for several days to allow edema or infection to resolve or exudate to drain
- Wound healing consists of several phases
  - The *injury* is a break in the skin's integrity

Box 5-1: Characteristics of Acute and Chronic Wounds

The following chart summarizes the type and cause, location, related signs and symptoms, and appearance of acute and chronic wounds. Specific nursing measures vary with the type of wound.

Type and Cause	Location	Related Signs and Symptoms	Appearance
Surgical wound			
• Sterile incision, which is then closed with glue, staples, sutures, or Steri-Strips • Heals by first intention	• Anywhere on body • Usually follows integumentary cleavage line, which enhances healing	• Vary with type of surgery	• Even, sharp wound margins • Clean, with no drainage or scab formation
Arterial ulcer (ischemic ulcer)			
• Insufficient arterial perfusion to an extremity • Risk increases with history of peripheral vascular disease, diabetes mellitus, or advanced age.	• Between toes (web space) or on tips of toes • Over phalangeal heads • Around lateral malleolus • On areas subjected to trauma or rubbing from shoes	• Thin, shiny, dry skin • Thickened nails • Pallor in affected limb on elevation and dependent rubor • Cyanosis • Decreased temperature in affected limb • Absent or diminished pulses in affected limb • Severe pain	• Punched-out appearance of wound edges • Gangrene or necrosis • Deep, pale wound bed • Blanched, purpuric • Signs of cellulitis • Minimal exudate
Diabetic ulcer			
• Peripheral neuropathy • Risk increases with history of diabetes mellitus or arterial insufficiency	• On plantar aspect of foot • Over metatarsal heads • Under heels	• Diminished or absent sensation in foot • Foot deformities • Increased temperature in foot without sweating • Atrophy of subcutaneous fat • Altered gait • Signs of peripheral vascular disease	• Even, well-defined wound margins • Depth of wound bed variable, possibly with undermining • Signs of cellulitis or underlying osteomyelitis • Variable amounts of exudate • Possible necrosis • Possible granulation tissue

(continued)

Box 5-1: Characteristics of Acute and Chronic Wounds (continued)

Type and Cause	Location	Related Signs and Symptoms	Appearance
Venous ulcer			
• Disturbance in return blood flow from legs • Risk increases with history of valve incompetence, perforating veins, deep vein thrombophlebitis or thrombosis, previous ulcers, obesity, or advanced age	• On medial lower leg and ankle • Above medial malleolus	• Edema • Possible dilated superficial veins • Dry, thin skin • Evidence of previously healed ulcer • Lack of pain sensation at wound site • Possible dermatitis	• Irregular wound margins • Superficial wound bed • Ruddy, granular tissue • Moderate to heavy exudate
Pressure ulcer			
• Excessive pressure (either high pressure over a short time or low pressure over a longer time) that causes localized tissue damage	• On bony prominences, especially sacrum and heels	• Possible local pain	• **Suspected deep tissue injury**: purple or maroon localized area of discolored intact skin or blood-filled blister resulting from damage of underlying soft tissue from pressure, shear, or both; may be preceded by tissue that's painful, firm, mushy, boggy, and warmer or cooler than adjacent tissue • **Stage I:** intact skin with localized nonblanchable redness, usually over a bony prominence; possibly no visible blanching on darkly pigmented skin, although color may differ from surrounding area
• Risk increases with history of advanced age, inadequate tissue perfusion, incontinence, or prolonged immobility	• On areas where friction and shear can damage tissue	• Foul-smelling odor	• **Stage II:** partial-thickness tissue loss presenting as a shallow, open ulcer with a red-pink wound bed without slough; may also present as an intact or open and ruptured serum-filled blister. May involve epidermis, dermis, or both. • **Stage III:** full-thickness tissue loss, possibly with visible subcutaneous fat but with no exposed bone, tendon, or muscle; slough may be present but doesn't obscure depth of tissue loss; involves the subcutaneous tissue. • **Stage IV:** full-thickness tissue loss with exposed bone, tendon, or muscle; slough or eschar may be present on some parts of wound bed; often includes undermining and tunneling • **Unstageable:** full-thickness tissue loss in which the base of the ulcer is covered by slough (yellow, tan, gray, green, or brown) or eschar (tan, brown, or black) or both in the wound bed

- *Hemostasis* is a brief period of vasoconstriction at the site of injury as the body attempts to prevent excessive bleeding
- The *inflammatory phase* starts right after the injury and lasts from 2 to 6 days; this defensive reaction to tissue injury involves increased blood flow and capillary permeability and aids in phagocytosis or autolytic debridement; it's marked by increased heat, redness, swelling, and pain in the affected area
- During the *proliferative phase*, granulation tissue forms and epithelialization begins
  - Granulation tissue is a pink-to-red, moist tissue that contains new blood vessels, collagen, fibroblasts, and inflammatory cells; the tissue fills the open deep wound and acts as a kind of scaffolding for the eventual migration of epithelial cells
  - During epithelialization, epithelial cells migrate across the wound's surface, forming a layer of new tissue; these cells look silvery and form a perimeter around the granulation tissue
- As *epithelial closure* occurs, the wound contracts and begins to close
- During the final *maturation phase*, collagen reorganizes and strengthens, a process that continues for months and sometimes years; chronic wounds may regain 50% of their original tensile strength after 2 to 3 weeks, but they'll ultimately regain only 70% to 75% of their original strength

Factors That Affect Wound Healing

- Local factors
  - Moisture—for instance, from incontinence—leads to skin maceration and edema, making the epidermis more susceptible to abrasion; the chemicals and bacteria in urine and stool also cause tissue breakdown
  - Necrotic debris and other foreign material in a wound interfere with optimal healing and must be removed; by increasing the bacterial count, dead tissue increases the risk of infection. Debridement of necrotic tissue is essential to decrease the risk for infection
  - Infection at a level of more than 1 million organisms per gram of tissue inhibits granulation and epithelialization
- Systemic factors
  - Aging has a profound impact on all body systems; it affects wound healing by decreasing the inflammatory response, delaying angiogenesis, decreasing collagen synthesis and degradation, slowing epithelialization (resulting in a thinner epidermal layer), decreasing cohesion between the epidermal and dermal layers, decreasing the function of sebaceous glands (resulting in dryness), and altering the function of melanocytes (resulting in skin discoloration)
  - Malnutrition delays or prevents healing by depriving the body of the nutrients it needs to combat the physiologic stress of infection and to meet the increased metabolic demands of tissue repair; patients with chronic or difficult-to-heal wounds have special dietary needs (see *The role of nutrition in wound healing*, page 54)
  - Dehydration can hasten debilitation and death; a patient with a large wound can lose far more than 1 L of water per day, the water loss of a healthy adult. Optimal hydration is a vital part of a patient's plan of care, especially those patients with large wounds or burns
  - Vascular insufficiency can lead to poor healing and the development of leg ulcers
    - Arterial insufficiency results in an inadequate blood supply, often in the patient's extremities, and may lead to tissue hypoxia, infection, and death.
    - Cardiovascular insufficiency leads to systemic hypoxemia, which impedes wound healing
    - Venous insufficiency—impaired flow toward the heart and elevated pressure in the venous system— leads to the leakage of fibrinogen around capillaries into the dermis; this results in formation of a fibrin layer that blocks tissue oxygenation, nutrient exchange, and waste removal
- Metabolic factors
  - A patient with diabetes mellitus requires strict maintenance of normal blood glucose levels for proper wound healing, particularly for the acute phase of tissue repair, during periods of stress, after surgery, and for combating sepsis; poorly controlled diabetes results in notoriously slow and complicated wound healing for several reasons. Diabetes also puts the patient at higher risk of infection
    - Impaired circulation caused by thickening of the capillary basement membrane results in reduced local blood flow, which often leads to ischemia and pain

- ○ Reduced sensation from diabetic neuropathy significantly reduces sensation in the lower extremities, making patients less aware of injuries and serious infections
- ○ Hyperglycemia impairs the inflammatory response and collagen synthesis and produces leukocyte dysfunction, which increases the risk of infection
- Renal failure or insufficiency increases the risk of infection and wound dehiscence and delays granulation
- A newly recognized disorder, reperfusion injury is thought to result from the uncontrolled release of free radicals (superoxide anion, hydroxyl radicals, and hydrogen peroxide) when ischemic tissue is reperfused or reoxygenated; oxygen-free radicals can cause damage to cell membranes, lipids, proteins, blood vessels, and deoxyribonucleic acid and can trigger the inflammatory process
- Neurologic factors
  - The absence of pain sensation can lead to significant tissue damage from pressure or trauma; a patient who doesn't feel pain can't respond to alleviate the pain
  - Immobility and impaired sensory perception contribute to pressure ulcer development and delayed healing (see table *Characteristics of acute and chronic wounds for pressure ulcer staging*, pages 50–51)
- Psychological factors
  - Stress, depression, and sleep disorders can alter the immune response
  - A stressed, depressed, or sleep-deprived patient is less likely to participate in self-care, including wound care
  - The sleep deprivation that can result from many psychological disorders interferes with the restorative properties of rest and sleep
  - Some patients with severe psychiatric disorders may deliberately injure themselves or interfere with wound care measures
- Immunologic deficiencies
  - Immunologic deficiencies impair many aspects of the inflammatory phase of healing
  - Such deficiencies also predispose patients to infection
- Clotting disorders
  - Clotting disorders interfere with the coagulation cascade critical in wound healing
  - Platelet aggregation normally initiates hemostasis and the release of chemotactic and growth-promoting substances, but clotting factor deficiencies (for instance, from hemophilia, malnutrition, or hepatic disease), thrombocytopenia, and anticoagulation therapy can prolong bleeding into a wound and delay healing
- Other factors
  - Glucocorticoid therapy (for instance, with prednisone or hydrocortisone) can interfere with healing by suppressing the inflammatory response, preventing macrophages from migrating into the wound, reducing fibroblast and endothelial cell activity, and delaying contraction and epithelialization
  - Medications, including anti-inflammatory drugs, cancer-fighting agents, anticoagulants, and antiprostaglandins, interfere with the normal healing process

Nursing Assessment

- General assessment
  - Determine the patient's age
  - Ask about allergies to drugs, dressings, and local anesthetics
  - Ask about urinary and fecal incontinence
  - Note any chronic illnesses that can interfere with wound healing, including diabetes mellitus, chronic obstructive pulmonary disease, and arteriosclerotic heart disease
  - Assess the patient's nutritional status, including general appearance and skin turgor, and hydration status; look for signs of weight loss
  - Make sure the patient's laboratory values fall within the normal range: serum albumin level, 3.5 to 5 g/dL; serum transferrin level, 200 to 400 mg/dL; total lymphocyte count, 1,800 to 3,000 µL; and thyroxine-binding prealbumin level, 15.7 to 29.6 mg/dL
  - Assess the patient's oxygenation and circulation status, noting indications of respiratory and circulatory impairment and peripheral vascular disease; ask if the patient smokes

Box 5-2: The Role of Nutrition in Wound Healing

The following chart outlines the role protein, calories, vitamins, and minerals play in wound healing.

Nutrient	RDA/Healthy Adults	Effects of Deficiency	Effects on Healing
Protein	0.8/kg	Impairs all aspects of healing and host defenses	Improves tissue integrity; increase to 1.5 to 2 g/kg needed for healing
Calories	• Resting: 1,500 • Sedentary: 2,000 • Very active: 3,500	Muscle wasting	May need to increase fivefold for positive nitrogen balance to promote healing
Vitamin C	60 mg	Collagen instability; decreased tensile strength	Necessary for collagen synthesis; not stored in body so deficiency occurs quickly
Vitamin A	1,000 mcg	Decreased epithelialization, collagen synthesis, resistance to infection by way of decreased macrophage production	Supplementation reverses effects of glucocorticoids
Vitamin B_6	2 mcg	Decreased protein synthesis	Needed for protein metabolism
Vitamin B_{12}	2 mcg	Decreased protein synthesis	Needed for cell proliferation and tissue synthesis
Folate	200 mcg	Decreased protein synthesis	Enables transport of oxygen; decreased absorption in elderly patients so supplementation may be necessary
Zinc	15 mg	Decreased immunity, collagen synthesis	Enables protein synthesis and tissue repair; healing improves after supplementation in true deficiency

- Assess the patient's immune status; ask about corticosteroid use, and ask if the patient has been diagnosed with cancer and is undergoing chemotherapy; determine whether the patient tests positive for the human immunodeficiency virus
- Ask about use of medications, including steroids, nonsteroidal anti-inflammatories, immunosuppressants, antineoplastics, anticoagulants, and antiprostaglandins
- Determine the patient's stress level, asking about family support and community resources
- Wound assessment
  - Determine the wound's cause. Ask patient explicitly to describe how it occurred
  - Note the wound's location
  - Measure the wound's length, width, and depth in centimeters
  - Determine the wound's stage
  - Observe the wound margins, looking for undermining, tunneling, and sinus tracts
  - Look for exudate in the wound, observing the amount and type (serous, serosanguineous, sanguineous, or purulent); note any odor
  - Assess circulation, sensation, and movement distal to wound
  - Assess ROM and strength against resistance of all body parts surrounding wound site
  - Assess the tissue in the wound bed
    - Granulation tissue will look beefy red
    - Epithelial tissue will look pearly pink
    - Sloughing necrotic or devitalized tissue will look soft and yellow-gray; eschar necrotic tissue will look thick and black
  - Note signs of infection, including induration, fever, erythema, edema, an elevated WBC count, and purulent drainage

Management

- Prevention of pressure ulcers
  - Identify patients at risk, including bedridden and chairbound patients and patients who have difficulty repositioning themselves
  - Using a valid risk assessment tool, assess at-risk patients for pressure ulcers on admission and at regular intervals; document your assessment on the Braden or Norton scale
  - Identify risk factors that contribute to skin breakdown, including immobility, incontinence, nutritional deficiencies, and an altered level of consciousness
- Prevention of vascular ulcers
  - Identify patients at risk, including those with chronic diseases such as diabetes mellitus and cardiovascular, renal, and neurologic disease
  - Identify risk factors that can contribute to vascular ulcers, including aging, malnutrition, and therapy with such drugs as glucocorticoids, anti-inflammatories, antineoplastics, anticoagulants, and antiprostaglandins
- Prevention of skin tear injuries
  - Identify patients at risk, especially elderly patients and those with a history of skin tears
  - Use a valid skin integrity risk assessment tool and a classification system such as Payne-Martin (see *Payne-Martin classification system for skin tears*, page 57)
- Early intervention
  - Treat the underlying disorder—for example, monitor blood glucose levels, administer insulin or an oral antidiabetic, and teach proper nutrition to the patient with diabetes
  - Minimize skin exposure to moisture from incontinence, perspiration, or wound drainage
  - Clean skin as soon as it becomes wet, and bathe the patient regularly
    - Avoid soap that dries the skin
    - Use warm, not hot, water
    - Use cream on dry, scaly skin
    - Don't rub reddened areas over bony prominences
  - Use topical moisture barriers to protect skin from urine and feces
  - Make sure the patient receives adequate protein, calories, vitamins, and minerals
  - Encourage daily activity and, if possible, exercise
  - If the patient is bedridden, take steps to minimize pressure on vulnerable skin areas
    - Reposition the patient—from back to side, to opposite side, to back—at least every 2 hours
    - When the patient is on the side, make sure the patient isn't lying directly on the trochanter
    - Use pillows or foam wedges to keep bony prominences from direct contact with the bed
    - Avoid massaging the skin over bony prominences
    - Take steps to reduce shearing and friction
      - Use the sheet to lift or reposition the patient in bed; don't drag the patient up in bed
      - Have an overhead trapeze bar installed for a patient who has enough strength in the upper extremities to reposition independently
      - Use a slide board for transferring the patient from a bed to a stretcher
      - Place sheepskin directly under the patient (unless he's incontinent)
      - Elevate the head of the bed to no more than 30 degrees, unless contraindicated
    - Lift the patient's heels off the bed, or use a device that totally relieves pressure on the heels
    - Consider using a pressure-reducing or pressure-relieving mattress for a patient who is at high risk for developing pressure ulcers
  - If the patient is chairbound, take steps to minimize pressure on vulnerable skin areas
    - Make sure the patient shifts weight frequently
    - Seat the patient on a 4″ pressure-reducing, high-density foam pad—not a doughnut-type device
    - Consider postural alignment, distribution of weight, balance and stability, and pressure relief when positioning a patient in a chair or wheelchair
    - Use elbow and heel pads to protect skin and minimize friction
- Treatment
  - Protect the wound from further trauma
    - Use pressure-reducing devices
    - Reduce friction and shear

- ○ Elevate the head of the bed no more than 30 degrees
- ○ Use a sheet to reposition the patient in bed
- ○ Remove dressings gently.
- ○ Use nonadhering dressings or those with minimal adherent
- ○ Use wraps, such as a stockinette or soft gauze, to protect areas at high risk of skin tearing
- ● Prevent infection and promote a clean wound base
  - ○ Cover the wound to protect it from infection
  - ○ Remove or debride any necrotic tissue
    - ○ *Mechanical debridement* is the manual removal of devitalized tissue using physical forces, such as whirlpooling, wet-to-dry gauze dressings, and wound irrigation
    - ○ *Sharp debridement* is the removal of foreign material or devitalized tissue with a sharp instrument, such as a scalpel or scissors
    - ○ *Autolytic debridement* uses synthetic dressings to cover the wound; this allows the enzymes naturally present in the wound fluid to digest devitalized tissue
    - ○ *Chemical* or *enzymatic debridement* involves the topical application of a proteolytic substance (such as enzymes) to break down devitalized tissue
  - ○ Use pressurized irrigation (a 35-mL syringe with a #18 needle or angiocatheter) to clean the wound surface or cavity; use a noncytotoxic agent such as normal saline solution
  - ○ Absorb excess exudate with collagen or calcium alginates or absorbent powders, beads, or paste
  - ○ Pack dead space with collagen or calcium alginates or moistened saline nonwoven gauze dressings
- ● Use a moisture-retentive dressing that keeps the wound bed moist but leaves the surrounding skin dry
  - ○ Use one of the following dressings for a wound with light to moderate exudate
    - ○ A *transparent film* is a clear, adherent, nonabsorptive, polymer-based dressing that is permeable to oxygen and water vapor but not to water; it's used to treat partial-thickness wounds and wounds with eschar (to promote autolysis)
    - ○ A *hydrogel* is a nonadherent dressing composed of water and a polymer that has some absorptive properties; it's used to treat partial- to full-thickness wounds, dry wounds, wounds with minimal drainage, wounds with necrosis or slough, and infected wounds
    - ○ A *foam dressing* is made up of a spongelike polymer; it can be adherent and has some absorptive properties and is used to treat partial- to full-thickness wounds and wounds with minimal to heavy drainage (including around tubes)
    - ○ A *hydrocolloid* is an adhesive, moldable wafer made of a carbohydrate-based material, usually with a backing that's impermeable to oxygen, water, and water vapor; the thin version has some absorptive properties; it's used to treat partial- to full-thickness wounds, wounds with minimal to moderate drainage, and wounds with necrosis or slough
  - ○ For a wound with moderate to heavy exudate, use a foam dressing, a collagen or calcium alginate dressing (a nonwoven, absorptive dressing made from seaweed), or a hydrocolloid dressing, which is more absorbent than the thin dressing
- ● Take steps to improve the patient's overall condition
  - ○ Provide nutritional support
    - ○ Arrange for a nutritional consultation
    - ○ Provide nutritional supplements as needed
    - ○ Make sure the patient is hydrated
  - ○ Maintain the patient's oxygenation and circulation
    - ○ If the patient experiences venous insufficiency, use compression to optimize venous return
    - ○ If the patient is diabetic, take steps to control blood glucose level
    - ○ Institute measures to optimize the patient's arterial blood supply and avoid circulatory impairment
  - ○ Help the patient reduce their stress level by involving the patient and family in care; contact the appropriate community resources
- ● Minimize the patient's pain
  - ○ Provide sufficient analgesia before, during, and after dressing changes
  - ○ Choose dressings that maximize the time between dressing changes and that cause minimal tissue trauma
  - ○ Teach the patient relaxation techniques and guided imagery to help control pain and maximize the effects of pain medication

Box 5-3: Payne-Martin Classification System for Skin Tears

This classification system improves documentation and allows for better tracking of outcomes of care for patients with skin tears.

Category I: Skin tear without tissue loss

A: Linear type—Epidermis and dermis pulled apart as if an incision has been made

B: Flap type—Epidermal flap completely covers the dermis to within 1 mm of the wound margin

Category II: Skin tears with partial tissue loss

A: Scant tissue loss type—25% or less of the epidermal flap lost

B: Moderate to large tissue type—More than 25% of the epidermal flap lost

Category III: Skin tears with complete tissue loss

Adapted from Payne, R. L., & Martin, M. L. (1993). Defining and classifying skin tears: Need for a common language. *Ostomy & Wound Management, 39*(5), 16–20, 22–24, 26, with permission.

Review Questions

Question 1. Which of the following includes all sites that are at high risk and likelihood for external pressure–related pressure ulcers?

A. Sacrum, trochanter, calcaneus, coccyx
B. Ribs, coccyx, occiput
C. Sacrum, coccyx, tibia, and patellar
D. Coccyx, sternum, patellar, sacrum

Correct answer: A High-risk areas for the development of pressure ulcers include pressure points at the occipital part of the head, elbows, sacrum, coccyx, and calcaneus (heels). The only choice that includes all of these choices is option A. The ribs, tibia, sternum, and patellar are not high-risk pressure points.

Question 2. A client has been having an allergic rash to new detergent. The client has been scratching frequently and presents with large areas of skin excoriation. What is the most appropriate nursing diagnosis for this client?

A. Risk for impaired skin integrity
B. Impaired skin integrity
C. Impaired tissue integrity
D. Risk for infection

Correct answer: B Impaired skin integrity is the best answer because the client has actual impairment due to the scratching from the rash, so the patient is no longer at risk. Since the damage is at the skin level and it does not involve deeper tissues, choice C is incorrect. Even though the patient is at risk for infection, surface excoriation is not at a high risk for infection. The best answer would be B.

Question 3. The nurse is assessing the laboratory values of a patient with a large hip wound healing by secondary intention. Which of the following laboratory values indicates that the patient is receiving adequate nutrition?

A. Serum albumin level of 4 g/dL
B. Thyroxine-binding prealbumin level of 12 mg/dL
C. Transferrin level of 100 mg/dL
D. Total lymphocyte count of 1,100 μL

Correct answer: A A serum albumin level of 4 g/dL indicates adequate nutrition. Options B, C, and D are incorrect because these laboratory values indicate poor nutrition.

Question 4. Which of the following puts a client a risk for developing pressure ulcers?

A. Advanced age
B. Prolonged immobility
C. Incontinence
D. All of the above

Correct answer: D All of these three choices puts a client at risk for the development of pressure ulcers.

Question 5. A home nurse visits a client who sprained their ankle while going for a run this morning. The client has an ice bag on the ankle. Which of the following conditions puts the patient at risk of using ice on the ankle?

A. Herpes zoster
B. Athlete's foot
C. Diabetes
D. Osteopenia

Correct answer: C Reduced sensation from diabetic neuropathy significantly reduces sensation in the lower extremities, making patients less aware of injuries and serious infections. Clients with neurological or circulatory impairment are at risk for injury with ice use.

Question 6. Which of the following information collected by the nurse BEST reflects a systemic response to a wound infection?

A. Pain
B. Exudate
C. Edema
D. Hyperthermia

Correct answer: D Hyperthermia is a common systemic response to infection. With hyperthermia, microorganisms and endotoxins stimulate phagocytotic cells that release pyrogens, which stimulate the hypothalamic thermoregulatory center, resulting in fever. The other three choices are considered local responses to infection or injury.

Question 7. When working with the elderly population, a nurse would know that aging affects wound healing by all of the following EXCEPT:

A. decreasing the inflammatory response.
B. delaying angiogenesis.
C. increasing collagen synthesis and degradation.
D. slowing epithelialization (thinning the epidermal layer).

Correct answer: C Aging does not increase but instead decreases collagen synthesis and degradation. Advanced age does have the impact on the other three choices.

Question 8. You are assessing a client's wound and notice a superficial pressure ulcer on the client's sacrum that appears as a shallow crater involving the epidermis and the dermis. Which of the following stages would the nurse BEST describe this pressure ulcer?

A. Stage I
B. Stage II
C. Stage III
D. Unstageable

Correct answer: B Stage II ulcers involve a partial-thickness skin loss, which involves the epidermis, dermis, or both. Stage I involved a nonblanchable erythema of intact skin. Stage III ulcers are full-thickness tissue loss with possibly visible subcutaneous fat. Unstageable ulcers are full-thickness tissue loss in which the base of the ulcer is covered by slough or eschar.

Question 9. One of your family members comes to you and explains that the doctor has just diagnosed them with a diabetic ulcer. As a nurse, you know that the most common location of this type of wound would be:

A. on plantar aspect of foot.
B. on the occipital lobe.
C. on the medial lower leg.
D. on bony prominences.

Correct answer: A Diabetic ulcers are most often found on the plantar aspect of the foot, over metatarsal heads or under the heels. Pressure ulcers are often found on bony prominences and may be found on the occipital lobe. Venous ulcers are often found on the medial lower leg.

Question 10. Which substance enables protein synthesis and tissue repair during wound healing?

A. Zinc
B. Vitamin B_6
C. Folate
D. Vitamin C

Correct answer: A Zinc enables protein synthesis and tissue repair. Folate enables the transport of oxygen during wound healing. Vitamin B_6 decreases collagen and protein synthesis, and vitamin C is needed for collagen synthesis.

Selected References

Dynamed. (2017, Mar 6). *Pressure ulcers.* Ipswich, MA: EBSCO Information Services. Retrieved from http://www.dynamed.com.frontier.idm.oclc.org/topics/dmp~AN~T116231/Pressure-ulcer on May 1, 2017

Dynamed. (2017, Apr 11). *Zinc.* Ipswich, MA: EBSCO Information Services. Retrieved from http://www.dynamed.com.frontier.idm.oclc.org/topics/dmp~AN~T908294/Zinc on May 1, 2017

Ousey, K. (2016). The importance of hydration in wound healing: Reinvigorating the clinical perspective. *Journal of Wound Care,* 25(3), 122–130.

Palese, A. (2017). Prevalence and incidence density of unavoidable pressure ulcers in elderly patients admitted to medical units. *Journal of Tissue Viability,* 26(2), 85–88.

Chapter 6

Disruptions in Homeostasis

Stress

- General information
  - Stress is the body's response to stressors or stimuli that are perceived as threatening
  - Stressors can be *biophysical* (such as disease, trauma, and overexertion), *chemical* (such as pollution, drugs, and alcohol), *psychosocial* (such as job loss, divorce, and bankruptcy), or *cultural* (such as traveling, being separated from family members during hospitalization, and delegating decision-making to health care providers)
  - The body responds to stress physiologically and psychologically
- Selye's stress theory
  - Hans Selye's theory describes a general adaptation syndrome that consists of three stages of a hormonally controlled stress response
    - The first stage is the alarm reaction, in which the person is alerted to the presence of a stressor and the need to act
    - The second stage is resistance
      - In this stage, the pituitary gland secretes corticotropin
      - Corticotropin stimulates the production of glucocorticoids and mineralocorticoids, which promote and inhibit inflammation, allowing the body to protect or surrender tissue
    - If resistance continues and the body doesn't adapt, the third stage is exhaustion, which can lead to disease or death
  - According to Selye, stress can result from positive or negative events
- Physiologic stress responses
  - Physiologic responses to stress involve the central nervous system, hypothalamus, sympathetic nervous system, anterior and posterior pituitary gland, adrenal medulla, and adrenal cortex
    - Hormones and catecholamines are secreted or stimulated by these organs in response to a stressor
    - Their release results in the body's fight or flight response to stress
  - The initial reaction to stress is increased alertness in preparation for fight or flight
  - Blood vessels dilate, heart rate increases, the rate and depth of respirations increase, and bronchodilation occurs; these reactions increase the oxygen supply to organs and muscles
  - The arterioles in the skin, kidneys, and abdominal viscera constrict; blood is shunted from the GI tract and periphery to the brain, heart, and major muscles
  - Gluconeogenesis increases; decreased insulin secretion and increased fatty acid metabolism increase the amount of glucose available for energy
  - Localized sweat production increases, and muscles become tense
  - Pain tolerance increases as endorphins (endogenous opiates) are released
  - Repeated physiologic stress responses can damage the body, resulting in problems such as kidney failure, gastric ulcers, and exacerbation of an existing disorder
  - The body's level of physiologic response to stress varies according to the stimuli; most physiologic stress responses aren't helpful in coping with the daily stresses of life
- Psychological stress responses
  - Psychological stress responses result when the body's ability to adapt to change is exceeded; a person adapts to psychological stress through coping strategies, such as problem solving, reappraising stressors, and rehearsing responses to stress

- The body's psychological response to stress varies according to the stressor's intensity and duration and the perceived control over the stressor
  - Psychological stress can cause physical manifestations, such as hypertension and digestive disorders, and psychological manifestations, such as anxiety attacks and eating disorders
  - When psychological stress exceeds a person's coping abilities, crisis (extreme psychological disequilibrium) may occur
- Nursing assessment of stress
  - The nurse should identify the source and duration of the stress, the patient's resources and coping strategies, and the effects of the stress on the patient and family members
  - Sources of stress include illness and hospitalization
    - Stressors related to illness include pain, fear of loss of a body part or function, fear of prognosis, and fear of disfigurement
    - Stressors related to hospitalization or treatment include perceived loss of control, increased dependence, change in environment, loss of roles as worker and provider for family, change in routine, and lack of trust in the caregivers
  - The duration of the stress depends on the stressor, which can be acute or chronic, intermittent or continuous
  - External resources include family members and significant others; internal resources include past experiences with illness or hospitalization, education, and spirituality
  - Coping strategies consist of past methods that have been effective for the patient, such as information seeking, relaxation techniques, prayer, counseling, physical or mental activity, meditation, discussion of options, and review of events or event rehearsal
  - Repeated stress responses can have physical effects
    - Immediate responses include rapid speech, restlessness, rapid heart rate, light-headedness, and palpitations
    - Long-term responses include headaches, neck and stomach aches, muscle cramps, and changes in eating, elimination, and sleep patterns
  - Repeated stress responses can cause psychosocial symptoms, including changes in family or working relationships, denial or anger, hopelessness, silence, or the inability to make decisions
  - The nurse can use life-event questionnaires to measure stressors in a patient's life and hardiness scales to determine a patient's ability to cope with or adapt to stress
- Nursing interventions
  - Physical interventions reduce tension and support organ function
  - Massage, heat application, warm baths, stretching exercises, and physical activity can reduce muscle tension, serve as distractions, and increase the ability to put stressors in perspective
    - Activities to protect organ function include monitoring for complications such as ileus and GI bleeding, checking urine output, and assessing glucose levels
  - Educational interventions include teaching the patient or family about stress and the body's response to it and rehearsing events to prepare the patient for stress-producing events
    - Teaching plans should include what to expect from the stress-producing situation
    - Event rehearsal helps the patient to review an expected sequence of events and deal with anxiety-producing situations in a controlled environment before the actual event occurs
  - Emotional support can be given through counseling, encouraging discussions, sharing feelings, verbalizing difficulties, and supporting family problem solving; helping patients to separate themselves from the issue can help maintain their self-esteem
  - Social support activities include evaluating financial status, assisting with insurance forms, providing referrals for home health care assistance, and evaluating spirituality needs (with appropriate referrals to clergy)

Shock

- General information
  - Shock is an acute state of reduced perfusion of all body tissues
  - Inadequate circulating blood volume results in decreased delivery of oxygen to tissues and decreased gas exchange in the capillaries
  - Inadequate oxygenation leads to impaired cellular metabolism and an inability to excrete metabolic waste products

- Pathogenesis of shock
  - Initial stage
    - Decrease in cardiac output leads to decrease in mean arterial pressure
    - Sympathetic nervous system is stimulated, leading to initiation of stress response
    - Signs and symptoms include normal to slightly increased heart rate, normal to slightly decreased blood pressure, thirst, and pale, cool, moist skin over the face
  - Compensatory stage
    - Decrease in mean arterial pressure stimulates the sympathetic nervous system to release epinephrine and norepinephrine to try to achieve homeostasis
    - Stimulation of alpha$_1$-adrenergic fibers causes vasoconstriction of vessels in the skin, GI organs, kidneys, muscles, and lungs, shunting blood to the heart and brain
    - Stimulation of beta-adrenergic fibers causes vasodilation of coronary and cerebral arteries, increases heart rate, and increases force of myocardial contractions, resulting in increased cardiac output
    - Reduced renal blood flow leads to release of renin and production of angiotensin, resulting in vasoconstriction and stimulation of the adrenal cortex to release aldosterone, increasing renal sodium reabsorption
    - Increased serum osmolarity stimulates the release of antidiuretic hormone (ADH), resulting in increased water reabsorption by the kidneys and increased venous blood return to the heart and, ultimately, increased cardiac output
    - Signs and symptoms include restlessness, normal or decreasing blood pressure, bounding or thready pulse, tachycardia, tachypnea, normal or hypoactive bowel sounds, slightly decreased urine output, and pale, cool skin (flushed and warm in septic shock)
  - Progressive stage
    - Compensatory mechanisms become ineffective and possibly even counterproductive
    - Falling cardiac output and vasoconstriction cause cellular hypoxia and anaerobic metabolism; metabolic acidosis occurs as lactic acid levels rise
    - Renal ischemia stimulates the renin-angiotensin-aldosterone system, causing further vasoconstriction
    - Fluid shifts from intravascular to interstitial space
    - Signs and symptoms include falling blood pressure; narrowed pulse pressure; cold, clammy skin; rapid, shallow respirations; tachycardia; weak, thready, or absent pulses; arrhythmias; absent bowel sounds; anuria; and subnormal body temperature (subnormal or elevated in septic shock)
  - Irreversible stage
    - Compensatory mechanisms are ineffective
    - Lactic acid continues to accumulate, and capillary permeability dilation increases, resulting in loss of intravascular volume and tachycardia; this further aggravates falling blood pressure and cardiac output
    - Coronary and cerebral perfusion decline, and organ systems fail
    - Signs and symptoms include unresponsiveness; areflexia; severe hypotension; slow, irregular heart rate; absent pulses; slow, shallow, irregular respirations; Cheyne-Stokes respirations; and respiratory and cardiac arrest
- Types of shock (see *Comparing types of shock*, pages 63–64)
  - *Cardiogenic shock* results from an inadequate pumping function that causes decreased cardiac output and stroke volume, leading to inadequate tissue perfusion and a precipitous drop in blood pressure and urine output; it results from such occurrences as acute myocardial infarction (MI), acute mitral insufficiency, right ventricular infarction, arrhythmias, heart failure, myocarditis, cardiac tamponade, and cardiac surgery
  - *Hypovolemic shock* results from decreased intravascular volume in relation to the vascular bed's size; loss of blood plasma into the tissues leads to decreased circulating blood volume and venous return, reduced cardiac output, and inadequate tissue perfusion
    - This type of shock is classified by the amount of blood loss: class I is an acute loss of up to 15% of blood volume; class II, 16% to 30%; class III, 31% to 40%; and class IV, more than 40%
    - Absolute, or measurable, external fluid losses can be caused by hemorrhage, burns, trauma, surgery, dehydration, intestinal obstruction, diabetes mellitus, diabetes insipidus, diuretic therapy, peritonitis, pancreatitis, cirrhosis, hemothorax, and hemoperitoneum
    - Relative, or immeasurable, internal fluid losses in the intravascular space can be caused by venous or arterial pooling and in the extravascular space, by capillary leakage

- *Distributive shock* results from poor distribution of blood to the tissues, which is caused by acute vasodilation without simultaneous expansion of the intravascular volume; anaphylactic, neurogenic, and septic shock are types of distributive shock
    - *Anaphylactic shock* results from an antigen-antibody reaction that releases histamine into the bloodstream, which causes widespread dilation of arterioles and capillary beds and bronchial hypersensitivity; it can be caused by allergic reactions to contrast media used in diagnostic tests, drugs, foods, animal and insect bites, and blood
    - *Neurogenic shock* results from decreased vasomotor tone with generalized vasodilation; it can result from general or spinal anesthesia, epidural block, spinal cord injury, vasovagal syncope, barbiturate or phenothiazine ingestion, and insulin shock
    - *Septic shock* results from a systemic response to microorganisms in the blood, causing vasodilation with selective vasoconstriction and poor distribution of blood; it commonly stems from overt infection, localized infection that spreads to the systemic circulation, urinary tract infection, postabortion or postpartal infection, or immunosuppressant therapy
  - *Obstructive shock* results from a physical obstruction that reduces cardiac output despite normal contractility and intravascular volume; it's caused by pulmonary embolism, dissecting aortic aneurysm, atrial myxoma, cardiac tamponade, and tension pneumothorax
- Complications of shock
  - Myocardial depression may be caused by decreased coronary blood flow and acidosis and can lead to arrhythmias, MI, and cardiac failure
  - Acute respiratory distress syndrome, also known as shock lung, may result from decreased perfusion to pulmonary capillaries
  - Renal failure may occur when prolonged renal hypoperfusion causes acute tubular necrosis
  - Hepatic insufficiency may stem from poor perfusion to the liver and can lead to recirculation of bacteria and cellular debris
  - Disseminated intravascular coagulation may occur because shock causes excessive consumption of clotting factors
  - GI ulcerations may occur when reduced blood flow increases acid production
- Nursing interventions
  - Ensure an adequate airway
    - Encourage coughing and deep breathing; administer medications for pain as needed to ensure deep breathing; suction as needed; and position the patient to maintain a patent airway and maximum ventilation
    - Turn the patient frequently, and elevate the head of the bed, unless contraindicated
    - Administer oxygen as prescribed
    - Perform postural drainage and chest physiotherapy to mobilize secretions
    - Evaluate breath sounds for crackles and wheezes
  - Maintain hemodynamic stability
    - Assess pulse rate and rhythm
    - Assess blood pressure for changes, using a Doppler ultrasound transducer if a sphygmomanometer doesn't provide an audible blood pressure
  - Maintain a normal temperature
    - Prevent hypothermia (core temperature less than 95°F [35°C]) by setting the room thermostat higher, warming the room with infrared lights, covering the patient with warmed blankets, using a warming mat as prescribed, warming lavage solutions, and using a fluid warmer when infusing I.V. solutions or blood
    - Prevent hyperthermia (increase in body temperature and metabolic rate) by removing excess blankets, administering medications as prescribed to decrease temperature, giving a tepid sponge bath, and using a cooling mat as prescribed
  - Maintain normal volume status to prevent fluid imbalance
    - Assess skin turgor for signs and symptoms of dehydration
    - Note signs of extreme thirst
    - Monitor urine output (amount, color, and specific gravity)
    - Monitor drainage (wound, gastric, and chest tube drainage)
    - Check for abnormal breath sounds
    - Assess the patient for weight gain or loss

  ○ Infuse fluids as prescribed
  ○ Assess blood loss, if possible
- Prevent complications of shock
  ○ Assess nutritional status to ensure adequate caloric intake to meet metabolic demands
  ○ Watch for signs of decreased tissue perfusion, such as changes in skin color and temperature, level of consciousness (LOC), peripheral pulses, and urine output
  ○ Prepare for transfer to the critical care unit if the patient's status deteriorates
- Reduce patient and family anxiety
  ○ Explain all procedures in understandable terms
  ○ Medicate the patient for pain to ensure patient comfort
  ○ Teach the patient relaxation techniques used to reduce anxiety
  ○ Give family members time to ask questions and express concerns
- Follow infection control policies

Box 6-1: Comparing Types of Shock

Some assessment findings and treatments are common to all types of shock. Others are specific to the type of shock.

Assessment Findings	Treatment
All types of shock	
• Acid-base imbalance, such as metabolic acidosis and respiratory alkalosis	• Increase perfusion to vital organs.
• Anuria or oliguria	• Increase peripheral perfusion.
• Anxiety and restlessness	• Decrease myocardial oxygen demand and workload.
• Changes in respiratory rate such as tachypnea	• Relieve pulmonary congestion.
• Confusion, lethargy, and coma	• Correct acid-base imbalances.
• Cool, clammy skin	• Ensure adequate oxygenation.
• Decreased pulse pressure and tachycardia	
• Decreased urine creatinine clearance and elevated urine specific gravity	
• Elevated blood urea nitrogen and serum creatinine, potassium, and lactate levels	
• Elevated hematocrit (with volume depletion)	
• Extreme thirst	
• Hypotension	
• Hypothermia (except in septic shock)	
Cardiogenic shock	
• Ashen or cyanotic skin	• Administer an inotropic medication, such as dobutamine, dopamine, milrinone (Primacor), or inamrinone
• Decreased level of consciousness	• Administer a vasopressor, such as dopamine, norepinephrine, or phenylephrine (Levophed)
• Decreased sensorium	
• Gallop rhythm, faint heart sounds, and, possibly, a holosystolic murmur	• Administer a vasodilator, such as nitroglycerin or nitroprusside (Nitropress)
• Jugular vein distention	• Administer morphine to reduce preload and afterload.
• Mean arterial pressure <60 mm Hg in adults	• Maintain normal pH and partial pressure of oxygen in blood.
• Pale, cold, clammy skin	• Intubate the patient and administer oxygen as needed.
• Pulmonary crackles	• If the patient has no signs of pulmonary edema, infuse fluid; if the patient has signs of pulmonary edema, administer a diuretic such as furosemide (Lasix)
• Rapid, irregular, thready pulse	
• Rapid, shallow respirations	
• Severe anxiety	• Ensure adequate relief of pain and anxiety.
• Urine output <20 mL/hour	• Correct electrolyte imbalances.
	• Control arrhythmias.
	• Use intra-aortic balloon pump therapy to reduce left ventricle's workload.
	• Place patient on ventricular-assist device if needed.

(continued)

Box 6-1: Comparing Types of Shock (continued)

Assessment Findings	Treatment
Hypovolemic shock	
• Decreased sensorium	• Increase intravascular volume with the appropriate solution, such as blood or a blood product, a colloid preparation, a plasma expander, or a crystalloid solution.
• Mean arterial pressure <60 mm Hg in adults (in chronic hypotension, mean pressure may fall below 50 mm Hg before signs of shock)	
	• Administer a vasopressor, such as norepinephrine, epinephrine, or dopamine.
• Pale, cool, clammy skin	
• Rapid, irregular, thready pulse	• Administer an inotropic medication, such as dobutamine, dopamine, milrinone (Primacor), or inamrinone (Levophed)
• Rapid, shallow respirations	
• Urine output usually <20 mL/hour	• Maintain a patent airway, and supply oxygen as needed.
Distributive shock: septic shock	For both phases:
Hyperdynamic phase (warm shock)	• Initiate antibiotic therapy.
• Adequate urine output	• Initiate vasopressor therapy, such as dopamine or norepinephrine.
• Chills and temperature above 100°F (37.8°C)	
• Normal or decreased blood pressure	• Initiate inotropic therapy such as dobutamine.
• Rapid heart rate	• Control hypothermia and hyperthermia.
• Signs of high cardiac output	• If patient develops disseminated intravascular coagulation, initiate heparin therapy.
• Warm, pink extremities	
• Widening pulse pressure	• Administer colloids or crystalloid infusions.
Hypodynamic phase (cold shock)	
• Abnormal prothrombin time, blood culture positive for infectious organisms, leukocytosis, and thrombocytopenia	
• Cold extremities	
• Narrowing pulse pressure	
• Oliguria	
• Signs of intense arterial vasoconstriction	
• Signs of low cardiac output	
Distributive shock: anaphylactic shock	
• Abdominal pain, diarrhea, nausea, and vomiting	• Administer adrenalin and an antihistamine.
• Feelings of impending doom	• Administer a vasopressor, such as norepinephrine or dopamine.
• Flushing, pruritus, and urticaria	
• Hoarseness, inspiratory stridor, and wheezing or respiratory distress	• Administer a steroid.
	• Administer a bronchodilator if needed.
• Seizures or unresponsiveness	
Distributive shock: neurogenic shock	
• Bradycardia	• Administer a vasopressor, such as dopamine and epinephrine.
• Hypotension	• Use a plasma expander to ensure adequate volume.
• Hypothermia	• If bradycardia develops, administer atropine.

Inflammation and Infection

- Inflammation
  - The inflammatory process is a defense mechanism that's activated in response to localized injury or infection; also called the local adaptation syndrome, this process acts to limit the spread of infection and promote wound healing
  - The inflammatory process occurs in three phases
    - In the first phase, blood vessels at the injury site constrict to control bleeding; vasoconstriction is followed by the release of histamines and increased capillary permeability to encourage blood flow and attract white blood cells (WBCs) to the area
    - In the second phase, exudate is produced, the amount of which depends on the wound's size, location, and severity; exudate is composed of cells and fluid that have escaped from blood vessels and may be serous, sanguineous, purulent, or a combination of the three
    - In the final stage, damaged cells are repaired by regeneration or formation of scar tissue

- Infection
  - The infectious process results from a combination of several factors
    - A causative agent (pathogen) must be present
    - A reservoir must be available for the pathogen
    - The reservoir must have a means of exit, such as the nares, feces, or wound drainage
    - The pathogen must be transmitted directly or indirectly to the new host; direct transmission requires contact between the reservoir and the new host, whereas indirect transmission usually occurs when an inanimate object carries the pathogen
    - The pathogen must enter the host through a portal of entry, such as the GI tract, respiratory tract, or a wound
    - The pathogen's virulence and the host's susceptibility also affect the infection process
  - Signs and symptoms of systemic and localized infections
    - *Systemic infections* are generalized and produce symptoms in multiple body systems
      - Prodromal symptoms, which may be vague, include malaise, weakness, fatigue, aches, and anorexia
      - Progression of infection is evidenced by symptoms such as fever, tachycardia, leukocytosis with a shift in differential, and lymphadenopathy
      - Severe untreated systemic infections can produce altered mental status, seizures, and shock
    - *Localized infections* are limited to a specific body region and produce symptoms in only one or two body systems
      - Presenting signs and symptoms include pain, warmth, swelling, erythema, and itching at the affected site
      - Progression of infection is evidenced by increasing redness and induration and the development of exudate
  - Diagnostic findings for both types of infection include elevated WBC counts and positive aerobic or anaerobic cultures
  - Medical treatments for infections include antibiotic therapy, surgery to remove an infected body part, dead tissue debridement, and abscess drainage; these procedures remove the infection or reduce the number of organisms to be eliminated
  - Nursing interventions for a patient with an infection consist primarily of monitoring and teaching
    - Monitor the progression of infection
      - Take the patient's vital signs
      - Measure the extent of induration or visible erythema
      - Assess the patient's LOC
      - Administer oral, parenteral, or topical antibiotics
      - Apply heat to localized infections
      - Apply sterile dressings to draining or open wounds
      - Monitor drainage for amount, color, and odor
      - Maintain standard precautions
      - Document infection progression, treatments performed, and patient response
      - Encourage adequate nutrition for wound healing
    - Teach the patient to prevent future infections
      - Instruct the patient to protect intact skin and mucous membranes by using precautions to prevent breakdown
      - Stress the importance of handwashing
      - Encourage nutritional maintenance of immune system responses
      - Discuss avoidance of pathogens transmitted by way of the respiratory or GI tract
      - Promote good hygiene
      - Teach about wound care and antibiotic therapy

Fluid Imbalances

- General information
  - Water accounts for 60% of the total body weight in adults and 80% in infants; the leaner the person, the greater the proportion of water to total body weight
  - The *intracellular fluid (ICF) compartment* includes water in the cells; this compartment accounts for 70% of total body water, or about 25 L of fluid in an adult
  - The *extracellular fluid (ECF) compartment* includes water outside the cells; this compartment accounts for 30% of total body water, or about 15 L of fluid (including 5 L of blood)

- Additional fluids are contained in other body compartments
  - Interstitial fluid is found in the spaces between cells
  - Plasma, an intravascular fluid, is found within arteries, veins, and capillaries
  - Cerebrospinal fluid and intraocular fluid are found in the spinal cord and eyes, respectively
- Alterations in the amount or composition of body fluids can cause complications; a 10% fluid loss (4 L) is serious, and a 20% loss (8 L) is fatal
- Body fluids transport nutrients to and remove wastes from cells
- Fluid movement
  - Body compartments are separated by semipermeable membranes that control fluid movement through filtration, hydrostatic pressure, and osmosis
    - Filtration is the passage of water and solutes across a semipermeable membrane
    - Hydrostatic pressure is pressure caused by a fluid column in an enclosed area such as a blood vessel wall
    - Osmosis is the passage of water through a semipermeable membrane from an area of low solute concentration to an area of high solute concentration
  - A solution's osmolality, which is determined by the number of dissolved particles in the fluid, also influences fluid movement
    - In an *isotonic solution*, the dissolved particle concentration equals that of ICF, causing no net water movement
    - In a *hypertonic solution*, the dissolved particle concentration exceeds that of ICF, causing water to move out of the cell to the area of greater concentration; this movement causes cell shriveling
    - In a *hypotonic solution*, the dissolved particle concentration is less than that of ICF, causing water to move into the cell; this movement causes cell swelling
- Organs that regulate fluid movement
  - The kidneys filter 180 L of plasma daily and excrete 1.5 L of urine daily (1 mL/kg/hour)
    - They regulate ECF volume, osmolality, and electrolyte levels by selective retention and excretion of fluids and electrolytes
    - They regulate the pH of ECF by influencing hydrogen ion excretion or retention and the excretion of metabolic wastes and toxic substances
  - The heart and blood vessels affect fluid movement because adequate cardiac output is needed to maintain the renal perfusion pressure required for kidney function; decreased cardiac output decreases renal perfusion pressure
    - Decreased renal perfusion pressure stimulates the stretch receptors in the atria and blood vessels to increase perfusion
    - It also stimulates the release of aldosterone, which increases fluid retention
  - The lungs expel water vapor at the rate of 300 to 400 mL/day
    - Increased respiratory rate or depth increases vapor loss
    - Vapor loss is considered insensible water loss because the actual loss can't be observed or measured
  - Skin affects fluid movement by means of sweat (visible fluid loss) and evaporation
    - The rate of fluid loss by means of sweat, which ranges from 0 to 1,000 mL/hour, is affected by body temperature; temperatures exceeding 101°F (38.3°C) increase the rate of loss, whereas temperatures below 101°F decrease the rate of loss
    - Sweat is considered a sensible water loss because the actual loss can be observed and measured
    - Evaporation of fluid from the skin also accounts for a water loss of 600 mL/day; it occurs as insensible perspiration
  - The GI tract normally loses 100 to 200 mL of fluid daily; diarrhea and fistulas greatly increase this fluid loss
- Hormonal influence
  - ADH, or vasopressin, is a hormone synthesized in the hypothalamus and released by the posterior pituitary; it affects fluid balance by increasing water reabsorption in the renal tubules
    - Increased osmolality and water deficiency stimulate ADH release
    - Decreased osmolality and excess water intake inhibit ADH release
  - Aldosterone is a mineralocorticoid secreted by the adrenal cortex
    - Increased aldosterone levels increase sodium retention, thereby increasing water retention
    - Decreased sodium levels stimulate aldosterone secretion
    - Increased sodium levels inhibit aldosterone secretion
- Thirst
  - The thirst center is located in the anterior hypothalamus; intracellular dehydration stimulates hypothalamus cells, causing a sensation of thirst
  - Thirst leads to increased water intake, which restores ECF volume

- Fluid volume deficit
  - Description
    - Fluid volume deficit (FVD) results from loss of body fluids; isosmolar FVD occurs when equal proportions of water and sodium are lost; hyperosmolar FVD occurs when more water than sodium is lost, resulting in hypovolemia and hypernatremia
    - Isosmolar FVD can result from traumatic injury, rapid blood loss, and decreased fluid intake from nausea, anorexia, fatigue, depression, confusion, neurologic deficits that alter the ability to swallow or detect thirst, and oral or pharyngeal pain
    - Hyperosmolar FVD can result from loss of GI fluids through vomiting, diarrhea, GI suctioning, fistulas, drains, third-space fluid loss, and excessive use of tap water enemas; it also can result from polyuria or excessive urine formation, which is associated with diabetic ketoacidosis, hyperosmolar hyperglycemic nonketotic syndrome, nephritis, and diuretic use
    - Fever can increase fluid loss through diaphoresis and increased respiratory rate; a temperature more than 101°F (38.3°C) requires an extra 500 mL of fluid daily, and more than 103°F (39.4°C) requires an extra 1,000 mL of fluid daily
    - Sweating can contribute to FVD
  - Signs and symptoms
    - Weight loss may be rapid (1 L of fluid equals 2 lb)
    - Skin turgor and elasticity may be decreased
    - The oral cavity may be dry and have a smaller than normal tongue lined with visible longitudinal furrows
    - Urine output may be decreased (less than 30 mL/hour for an adult), but specific gravity may be increased
    - Altered vital signs may include a subnormal body temperature, orthostatic hypotension, and increased heart rate
    - Signs of decreased volume may include decreased central venous pressure (CVP), flattened jugular veins, and slow-filling hand veins
    - Altered sensorium and cold extremities also may occur
    - Laboratory data may include elevated hematocrit, elevated blood urea nitrogen (BUN) level in relation to creatinine level, and serum sodium level greater than 150 mEq/L
  - Medical management
    - Replace fluid loss orally, if possible, or by I.V. infusion (see *Understanding parenteral solutions*, page 69)
    - Correct the deficit's cause
  - Nursing interventions
    - Encourage fluid intake, as appropriate, by providing adequate pain control, relieving nausea, offering fluids, performing frequent skin and mouth care, and consulting the practitioner if the patient can't ingest fluids orally
    - Maintain accurate input and output records to evaluate the effectiveness of interventions
    - Administer parenteral therapy as prescribed, and assess for complications
    - Teach the patient and family about preventing, recognizing, and treating FVD
- Fluid volume excess
  - Description
    - Fluid volume excess (FVE) is the abnormal retention of water
      - When accompanied by altered sodium levels, the condition is referred to as hyperosmolar FVE
      - When water and sodium are retained in equal proportions, the condition is referred to as isosmolar FVE
    - FVE results from compromised regulatory mechanisms, such as those seen in heart failure, renal failure, cirrhosis, and steroid excess
    - It also can result from excessive administration of parenteral fluids (especially those with a high sodium content) and excessive ingestion of sodium chloride or sodium salts
  - Signs and symptoms
    - Rapid weight gain that may be accompanied by peripheral edema
    - Distended neck or peripheral veins and increased CVP
    - Changes in breath sounds, pulmonary edema, ascites, and pleural effusion
    - Bounding pulses
    - Increased urine output
    - Vital signs changes that may include increased pulse rate and blood pressure

○ Shortness of breath and orthopnea
○ Laboratory data that may include a decreased BUN level, decreased hematocrit, and a serum sodium level less than 135 mEq/L

- Medical management
  ○ Reduce sodium intake through diet changes
  ○ Re-evaluate the need for I.V. therapy and the type of I.V. fluids administered
- Nursing interventions
  ○ Monitor daily intake and output
  ○ Encourage strict adherence to diet and fluid orders
  ○ Administer a diuretic as prescribed, and prepare the patient for possible dialysis
  ○ Assess the patient's need for an indwelling urinary catheter during diuresis
  ○ Monitor the patient for complications of diuretic therapy such as alterations in potassium levels
  ○ Check weight daily; weight gain may reflect volume gain
  ○ Check for signs of pitting edema in the extremities, and assess the patient for neck vein distention
  ○ Monitor arterial blood gas (ABG) studies for respiratory alkalosis
  ○ Monitor breath sounds for changes such as crackles, and administer a diuretic as ordered
  ○ Encourage rest periods to relieve shortness of breath and fatigue
  ○ Protect the patient's skin from breakdown caused by the pressure of pitting edema
  ○ Encourage use of the semi-Fowler position to increase lung capacity
  ○ Educate the patient and family about preventing, recognizing, and treating FVE

- Third-space fluid shift
  - Description
    ○ Third-space fluid shift occurs when body fluids move into the interstitial space from which these fluids aren't exchanged readily with ECF
    ○ It can result from acute intestinal obstruction, ascites, acute peritonitis, pancreatitis, acute gastric dilation, postoperative complications, fistulas, trauma, burns, fractures, hypoalbuminemia, lymphatic system blockage, and declamping phenomenon (which occurs when a clamp on the aorta is released during surgery)
  - Phases of third-space fluid shift
    ○ In the *fluid accumulation phase*, fluid shifts from the intravascular space to the interstitial space
      ○ The clinical presentation is similar to that of FVD; fluid is lost from the intravascular space, thus decreasing perfusion
      ○ Fluid losses can't be observed or measured
    ○ In the *fluid shifting phase*, interstitial fluid shifts back to the intravascular space; the clinical presentation is similar to that of FVE when fluid enters the intravascular space and enters the circulation
  - Medical management
    ○ Correct the fluid shift's cause
    ○ Treat the patient for symptoms of FVD or FVE as appropriate
  - Nursing interventions
    ○ For a patient with signs of FVD, see "Fluid volume deficit: Nursing interventions," page 67
    ○ For a patient with signs of FVE, see "Fluid volume excess: Nursing interventions," pages 67–68

Electrolyte Imbalances

- General information
- Electrolytes are substances that dissociate in solution and conduct a weak electrical current
- Intracellular electrolytes include potassium, magnesium, and phosphate
  ○ *Potassium* is the principal intracellular cation; it controls cellular osmotic pressure, influences skeletal and cardiac muscle activity, and is dramatically affected by acid-base imbalance
  ○ *Magnesium*, which also is an intracellular cation, is contained mostly in bone; it activates intracellular enzymes, contributes to carbohydrate and protein metabolism, and acts to dilate vessels and decrease blood pressure; imbalances can trigger ventricular arrhythmias and cardiac arrest
  ○ *Phosphate* is the principal intracellular anion; it's essential for muscle, red blood cell (RBC), and nervous system functioning, and it plays a role in carbohydrate, protein, and fat metabolism
- Extracellular electrolytes include sodium, calcium, bicarbonate, and chloride
  ○ *Sodium* is the principal extracellular cation; it's responsible for the osmotic pressure of ECF, and it doesn't readily cross the cell membrane

Box 6-2: Understanding Parenteral Solutions

Type of Parenteral Solution	Examples	Indications
Hypertonic solution	• Dextrose 5% in normal saline solution • 3% NaCl • Dextrose 10% in water	• To treat severe hyponatremia • To correct severe hyponatremia • To treat hypoglycemia
Hypotonic solution	• Half-normal saline solution	• To expand the intracellular compartment; to replace free water; to replace sodium and chloride
Isotonic solution	• Normal saline solution • Lactated Ringer's solution • Dextrose 5% in water (D5W). (Although D5W is an isotonic solution, it's quickly metabolized to a hypotonic solution.)	• To increase extracellular fluid volume; to maintain fluid volume and treat hypovolemia; to replace sodium and chloride • To treat hypovolemia and fluid lost from burns and GI tract; to provide electrolyte replacement • To maintain fluid volume; to replace mild loss; to provide free water; to treat hypernatremia and hyperkalemia

- ○ *Calcium*, an extracellular cation, is concentrated in the skeletal system; it acts as cell cement, has a sedative effect on nerve cells, regulates muscle contraction and relaxation (including heartbeat), activates enzymes that stimulate chemical reactions, and plays a role in blood coagulation
- ○ *Bicarbonate*, an extracellular anion, plays a role in acid-base balance; it serves as a buffer to keep serum pH within normal limits and is regulated primarily by the kidneys
- ○ *Chloride* is the principal extracellular anion; it helps maintain acid-base balance and works with sodium to help maintain osmotic pressure
- When the body can't maintain the normal level of an electrolyte, an imbalance can result (see *Understanding electrolyte imbalances*, pages 70–73)
- Electrolyte movement
  - Electrolytes move in and out of cells through diffusion, osmosis, active transport, filtration, and plasma colloid osmotic pressure
  - *Diffusion* is the movement of particles from an area of higher concentration to an area of lower concentration across a semipermeable membrane
    - ○ The number of particles diffused depends on permeability, or the relative size of cell membrane pores in relation to the particle's size
    - ○ The greater the difference in particle concentration, the greater the diffusion rate
    - ○ Cell membrane pores are lined with positively charged ions that repel other positive ions and attract negative ions
    - ○ The difference in electric potential helps diffusion occur even without a concentration difference
    - ○ The pressure increase intensifies the molecular forces striking the membrane, which increases the amount of diffusion
  - *Osmosis* is the passive movement of fluid across a membrane from a region of low solute concentration to a region of high solute concentration in an effort to maintain homeostasis
    - ○ Osmolality refers to the specific gravity of body fluids; the higher the specific gravity, the greater the osmotic pressure, which attracts more water to the area
    - ○ Osmolality measures the number of dissolved particles per unit of water; normal osmolality of plasma is 280 to 294 mOsm/kg
  - *Active transport* occurs when the cell membrane must move molecules against their concentration gradient; it requires energy (from cellular chemical reactions) and a carrier substance such as sodium
  - *Filtration* is the movement of fluid through a permeable membrane from a region of high pressure to a region of low pressure
  - *Plasma colloid osmotic pressure* is the osmotic pressure caused by plasma proteins; it results from the selective retention of colloids in plasma, which lowers the concentration of water and electrolytes

Box 6-3: Understanding Electrolyte Imbalances

The following chart summarizes the etiology, signs and symptoms, and nursing care related to various electrolyte imbalances. For all imbalances, treatment goals include diagnosis and correction of the underlying cause, restoration of the normal electrolyte level, prevention of complications associated with the imbalance, and prevention of recurrence.

Cause	Signs and Symptoms	Nursing Care
Hypocalcemia • Hypoparathyroidism, infusion of citrated blood, acute pancreatitis, hyperphosphatemia, inadequate dietary intake of vitamin D, or continuous or long-term use of laxatives • Magnesium deficiency, medullary thyroid carcinoma, low serum albumin levels, or alkalosis • Use of aminoglycosides, caffeine, calcitonin (Miacalcin), corticosteroids, loop diuretics, nicotine, phosphates, radiographic contrast media, or aluminum-containing antacids	• Ionized calcium level below 4.5 mEq/L; serum calcium levels below 8.5 mg/dL • Tingling around the mouth and in the fingertips and feet, numbness, painful muscle spasms, and tetany • Positive Trousseau's and Chvostek's signs • Bronchospasm, laryngospasm, and airway obstruction • Seizures • Changes in cardiac conduction • Hypotension • Depression, impaired memory, confusion, and hallucinations • Dry or scaling skin, brittle nails, dry hair, and cataracts • Skeletal fractures resulting from osteoporosis	• Identify patients at risk for hypocalcemia. • Assess the patient for signs and symptoms of hypocalcemia, especially changes in cardiovascular and neurologic status and in vital signs. • Administer I.V. calcium as prescribed. • Administer vitamin D supplementation as prescribed. • Administer a phosphate-binding antacid. • Review the procedure for eliciting Trousseau's and Chvostek's signs. • Take seizure or emergency precautions as needed. • Encourage a patient with osteoporosis to exercise regularly. • Encourage the patient to increase his intake of foods that are rich in calcium and vitamin D. • Teach the patient and family how to prevent, recognize, and treat hypocalcemia.
Hypercalcemia • Malignant neoplasms, metastatic bone cancer, hyperparathyroidism, immobilization and loss of bone mineral, or thiazide diuretic use • High calcium intake • Hyperthyroidism or hypothyroidism • Drugs, such as calcium-containing antacids, calcium preparations, lithium (Lithane, Lithobid), vitamin A, and vitamin D	• Ionized calcium level above 5.5 mEq/L; serum calcium levels above 10.5 mg/dL • Muscle weakness and lack of coordination • Anorexia, constipation, abdominal pain, nausea, vomiting, peptic ulcers, and abdominal distention • Confusion, impaired memory, slurred speech, and coma • Polyuria and renal colic • Cardiac arrest	• Identify patients at risk for hypercalcemia. • If the patient is receiving digoxin (Lanoxin), assess for signs of digoxin (Lanoxin) toxicity. • Assess the patient for signs and symptoms of hypercalcemia. • Encourage ambulation. • Move the patient carefully to prevent fractures. • Take safety or seizure precautions as needed. • Have emergency equipment available. • Administer phosphate to inhibit GI absorption of calcium. • Administer a loop diuretic to promote calcium excretion. • Force fluids with a high acid-ash concentration, such as cranberry juice, to dilute and absorb calcium. • Reduce dietary calcium. • Teach the patient and family how to prevent, recognize, and treat hypercalcemia, especially if the patient has metastatic cancer.

(continued)

Box 6-3: **Understanding Electrolyte Imbalances (continued)**

Cause	Signs and Symptoms	Nursing Care
Hypokalemia		
• GI losses from diarrhea, laxative abuse, prolonged gastric suctioning, prolonged vomiting, ileostomy, or colostomy • Renal losses related to diuretic use, renal tubular acidosis, renal stenosis, or hyperaldosteronism • Use of certain antibiotics, including penicillin G sodium, carbenicillin (Geocillin), or amphotericin B (Amphotec). • Steroid therapy • Severe perspiration • Hyperalimentation, alkalosis, or excessive blood insulin levels • Poor nutrition • Cushing's syndrome	• Potassium level under 3.5 mEq/L • Fatigue, muscle weakness, and paresthesia • Prolonged cardiac repolarization, decreased strength of myocardial contraction, orthostatic hypotension, reduced sensitivity to digoxin, increased resistance to antiarrhythmics, and cardiac arrest • Flat ST segment and Q wave on electrocardiogram (ECG) • Decreased bowel motility • Suppressed insulin release and aldosterone secretion • Inability to concentrate urine and increased renal phosphate excretion • Respiratory muscle weakness • Metabolic alkalosis, low urine osmolality, slightly elevated glucose level, and myoglobinuria	• Identify patients at risk for hypokalemia. • Assess the patient's diet for a lack of potassium. • Assess the patient for signs and symptoms of hypokalemia. • Administer a potassium replacement as prescribed. • Encourage intake of high-potassium foods, such as bananas, dried fruit, and orange juice. • Monitor the patient for complications. • Have emergency equipment available for cardiopulmonary resuscitation and cardiac defibrillation. • Teach the patient and family how to prevent, recognize, and treat hypokalemia.
Hyperkalemia		
• Decreased renal excretion related to oliguric renal failure, potassium-sparing diuretic use, or adrenal steroid deficiency • High-potassium intake related to the improper use of oral supplements, excessive use of salt substitutes, or rapid infusion of potassium solutions • Acidosis, tissue damage, or malignant cell lysis after chemotherapy	• Potassium level above 5 mEq/L • Cardiac conduction disturbances, ventricular arrhythmias, prolonged depolarization, decreased strength of contraction, and cardiac arrest • Tall, tented T wave, widened QRS complex, and prolonged PR interval on ECG • Muscle weakness and paralysis • Nausea, vomiting, diarrhea, intestinal colic, uremic enteritis, decreased bowel sounds, abdominal distention, and paralytic ileus	• Identify patients at risk for hyperkalemia. • Assess the patient's diet for excess use of salt substitutes. • Assess patient for signs and symptoms of hyperkalemia. • Assess ABG studies for metabolic alkalosis. • Take precautions when drawing blood samples. A falsely elevated potassium level can result from hemolysis or prolonged tourniquet application. • Have emergency equipment available. • Administer calcium gluconate to decrease myocardial irritability. • Administer insulin and I.V. glucose to move potassium back into cells. • Administer sodium polystyrene sulfonate (Kayexalate) with 70% sorbitol to exchange sodium ions for potassium ions in the intestine. • Perform hemodialysis or peritoneal dialysis to remove excess potassium. • Teach the patient and family how to prevent, recognize, and treat hyperkalemia.

(continued)

Box 6-3: Understanding Electrolyte Imbalances (continued)

Cause	Signs and Symptoms	Nursing Care
Hypomagnesemia • Alcoholism, protein-calorie malnutrition, I.V. therapy without magnesium replacement, gastric suctioning, malabsorption syndromes, laxative abuse, bulimia, anorexia, intestinal bypass for obesity, diarrhea, or colonic neoplasms • Hyperaldosteronism or renal disease that impairs magnesium reabsorption • Use of osmotic diuretics or antibiotics (such as ticarcillin-clavulanate [Timentin], gentamicin, carbenicillin [Geocillin], cyclosporine [Sandimmune], and cisplatin [Platinol]) • Overdose of vitamin D or calcium, burns, pancreatitis, sepsis, hypothermia, exchange transfusion, hyperalimentation, or diabetic ketoacidosis	• Magnesium level under 1.5 mEq/L • Muscle weakness, tremors, tetany, and clonic or focal seizures • Laryngeal stridor • Decreased blood pressure, ventricular fibrillation, tachyarrhythmias, and increased susceptibility to digoxin toxicity • Apathy, depression, agitation, confusion, delirium, and hallucinations • Nausea, vomiting, and anorexia • Decreased calcium level • Positive Chvostek's and Trousseau's signs	• Identify patients at risk for hypomagnesemia. • Assess the patient for signs and symptoms of hypomagnesemia. • Administer I.V. magnesium as prescribed. • Encourage the patient to consume magnesium-rich foods. • If the patient is confused or agitated, take safety precautions. • Take seizure precautions as needed. • Have emergency equipment available. Calcium gluconate is used to treat tetany. • Teach the patient and family how to prevent, recognize, and treat hypomagnesemia.
Hypermagnesemia • Renal failure, excessive antacid use (especially in a patient with renal failure), adrenal insufficiency, or diuretic abuse • Excessive magnesium replacement or excessive use of magnesium salts (milk of magnesia) or other magnesium-containing laxative	• Magnesium level above 2.5 mEq/L • Peripheral vasodilation with decreased blood pressure, facial flushing, and sensations of warmth and thirst • Lethargy or drowsiness, apnea, and coma • Loss of deep tendon reflexes, paresis, and paralysis • Cardiac arrest	• Identify patients at risk for hypermagnesemia. • Review all medications for a patient with renal failure. • Assess the patient for signs and symptoms of hypermagnesemia. • Assess reflexes; if absent, notify the practitioner. • Administer calcium gluconate. • Have emergency equipment available. • Prepare the patient for hemodialysis if prescribed. • If the patient is taking an antacid, a laxative, or another drug that contains magnesium, instruct the patient to stop. • Teach the patient and family how to prevent, recognize, and treat hypermagnesemia.
Hyponatremia **Dilutional** • Excessive water gain caused by inappropriate administration of I.V. solutions, syndrome of inappropriate antidiuretic hormone secretion, oxytocin use for labor induction, water intoxication, heart failure, renal failure, or cirrhosis	• Sodium level under 136 mEq/L • Confusion • Nausea, vomiting • Weight gain • Edema • Muscle spasms, convulsions	• Identify patients at risk for hyponatremia. • Assess fluid intake and output. • Assess the patient for signs and symptoms of hyponatremia. • If patient has dilutional hyponatremia, restrict his fluid intake.

(continued)

Box 6-3: Understanding Electrolyte Imbalances (continued)

Cause	Signs and Symptoms	Nursing Care
True • Excessive sodium loss due to GI losses, excessive sweating, diuretic use, adrenal insufficiency, burns, lithium (Lithane, Lithobid) use, or starvation	• Postural hypotension • Tachycardia • Dry mucous membranes • Weight loss • Nausea, vomiting • Oliguria • Muscle twitching and weakness	• If the patient has true hyponatremia, administer isotonic I.V. fluids and observe for hypervolemia. • Teach the patient and family dietary measures that ensure appropriate fluid and sodium intake.
Hypernatremia • Sodium gain that exceeds water gain related to salt intoxication (resulting from sodium bicarbonate use in cardiac arrest), hyperaldosteronism, or use of diuretics, vasopressin, corticosteroids, or some antihypertensives • Water loss that exceeds sodium loss related to profuse sweating, diarrhea, polyuria resulting from diabetes insipidus or diabetes mellitus, high-protein tube feedings, inadequate water intake, or insensible water loss	• Sodium level above 145 mEq/L • Thirst; rough, dry tongue; dry, sticky mucous membranes; flushed skin; oliguria; and low-grade fever that returns to normal when sodium levels return to normal • Restlessness, disorientation, hallucinations, lethargy, seizures, and coma • Muscle weakness and irritability • Serum osmolality above 295 mOsm/kg and urine specific gravity above 1.015	• If the patient is receiving lithium, teach how to prevent alterations in his sodium levels. • If the patient has adrenal insufficiency, teach how to prevent hyponatremia. • Teach the patient and family how to prevent, recognize, and treat hypernatremia.
Hypophosphatemia • Glucose administration or insulin release, nutritional recovery syndrome, overzealous feeding with simple carbohydrates, respiratory alkalosis, alcohol withdrawal, diabetic ketoacidosis, or starvation • Malabsorption syndromes, diarrhea, vomiting, aldosteronism, diuretic therapy, or use of drugs that bind with phosphate, such as aluminum hydroxide (Amphojel) or magnesium salts (milk of magnesia)	• Phosphorus level below 2.5 mg/dL or 0.97 mmol/L • Irritability, apprehension, confusion, decreased LOC, seizures, and coma • Weakness, numbness, and paresthesia • Congestive cardiomyopathy • Respiratory muscle weakness • Hemolytic anemia • Impaired granulocyte function, elevated creatine phosphokinase level, hyperglycemia, and metabolic acidosis	• Identify patients at risk for hypophosphatemia. • Assess the patient for signs and symptoms of hypophosphatemia, especially neurologic and hematologic ones. • Administer phosphate supplements as prescribed. • Note calcium and phosphorus levels because calcium and phosphorus have an inverse relationship. • Gradually introduce hyperalimentation as prescribed. • Teach the patient and family how to prevent, recognize, and treat hypophosphatemia.
Hyperphosphatemia • Renal disease • Hypoparathyroidism or hyperthyroidism • Excessive vitamin D intake • Muscle necrosis, excessive phosphate intake, or chemotherapy	• Phosphorus level above 4.5 mg/dL or 1.45 mmol/L • Soft tissue calcification (chronic hyperphosphatemia) • Hypocalcemia, possibly with tetany • Increased RBC count	• Identify patients at risk for hyperphosphatemia. • Assess the patient for signs and symptoms of hyperphosphatemia and hypocalcemia, including tetany and muscle twitching. • Advise the patient to avoid foods and medications that contain phosphorus. • Administer phosphorus-binding antacids. • Prepare the patient for possible dialysis. • Teach the patient and family how to prevent, recognize, and treat hyperphosphatemia.

Acid-Base Imbalances

- General information
  - An acid is any substance that can donate a hydrogen ion; a base is any substance that can accept or combine with a hydrogen ion
  - Acid-base balance optimizes enzymatic function, nerve conduction, synaptic transmission, and muscle contraction
  - Acids are generated by cellular metabolism of fats and carbohydrates; to maintain acid-base balance, acids must be excreted by the lungs and kidneys at the same rate they're generated
  - Acidemia is a condition in which the blood is too acidic (has a pH below 7.35); acidosis causes acidemia
  - Alkalemia is a condition in which the blood is too alkaline (has a pH above 7.45); alkalosis causes alkalemia (see *Understanding acid-base imbalances*, pages 75–76)
- Regulation of acid-base balance
  - Most of the 12,000 to 20,000 mEq of carbon dioxide produced daily is excreted by the lungs
    - Carbon dioxide is carried from peripheral tissues to the lungs by RBCs, plasma proteins, and plasma (as carbonic acid and bicarbonate)
    - The acid-base balance is regulated by adjustments in ventilation
      - In acidosis, an increased arterial carbon dioxide content or a decreased pH (below 7.35) stimulates hyperventilation; less carbon dioxide results in less carbonic acid and hydrogen ion in the blood, increasing the blood pH
      - In alkalosis, a decreased arterial carbon dioxide content or an increased pH leads to hypoventilation; carbon dioxide retention increases the acid load, thus decreasing the blood pH
  - The kidneys usually excrete 70 mEq of acid daily
    - Renal tubular excretion occurs in several ways
      - Hydrogen ions are directly excreted in exchange for sodium ions
      - Hydrogen ions are indirectly excreted with urine buffers
      - Hydrogen ions are indirectly excreted with the ammonia produced in the distal tubular cells
    - Sodium and bicarbonate are absorbed, and hydrogen is secreted in the proximal tubule
    - Carbonic acid is dissociated into hydrogen ions and bicarbonate in the distal tubule; hydrogen ions are excreted, and bicarbonate moves into the bloodstream
    - Renal compensation for imbalances can take hours to days; in acidosis, the kidneys excrete hydrogen ions and conserve bicarbonate ions; but in alkalosis, the kidneys retain hydrogen ions and excrete bicarbonate ions
- Buffering
  - Buffering is a mechanism that corrects acid-base imbalances by removing or releasing hydrogen
  - Buffers prevent significant pH changes when an acid or a base is added to a solution; they rapidly react with a strong acid or base by replacing it with a relatively weak acid or base
    - Bicarbonate is a buffer for blood and interstitial fluid
      - The normal ratio of bicarbonate to carbonic acid is 20 to 1
      - Carbon dioxide mixed with water becomes carbonic acid
    - Hemoglobin is a buffer for carbon dioxide
    - Phosphates and plasma proteins are intracellular buffers
- Evaluation of ABG studies
  - *pH* is a measure of the acid-base balance in terms of the concentration of free hydrogen ions; the greater the concentration of hydrogen, the more acidic the solution, and the lower the pH
    - A pH of 6.8 to 7.0 indicates severe, life-threatening acidosis
    - A pH of 7.0 to 7.35 indicates acidosis
    - A pH of 7.35 to 7.45 is normal
    - A pH of 7.45 to 7.7 indicates alkalosis
    - A pH of 7.7 to 7.8 indicates severe, life-threatening alkalosis
  - *$PaCO_2$*, or the partial pressure of carbon dioxide in arterial blood, is the best measure of adequate alveolar ventilation
    - A $PaCO_2$ of 34 to 44 mm Hg is normal
    - A $PaCO_2$ above 44 mm Hg indicates hypercapnia resulting from hypoventilation; a $PaCO_2$ below 34 mm Hg indicates hypocapnia resulting from hyperventilation

Box 6-4: Understanding Acid-Base Imbalances

The following chart summarizes the etiology, signs and symptoms, and nursing care related to various acid-base imbalances. Remember that in a mixed acid-base imbalance, the etiology, signs and symptoms, and care will vary with the specific imbalances involved.

Description	Cause	Signs and Symptoms	Nursing Care
Metabolic acidosis Acid-base disturbance characterized by low pH, bicarbonate (HCO_3^-) ion deficit, and excess hydrogen ions in which the lungs compensate with hyperventilation to decrease the partial pressure of arterial carbon dioxide ($PaCO_2$) concentration	Conditions that increase acid production or absorption, such as impaired tissue perfusion, diabetes mellitus, salicylate poisoning, renal insufficiency, methanol or ethylene glycol toxicity, and starvation • Conditions that increase bicarbonate loss, such as diarrhea, intestinal or pancreatic fistula, adrenal insufficiency, ureterosigmoidostomy, renal tubular acidosis, and acetazolamide therapy	Headache, confusion, drowsiness, stupor, and coma • Fruity breath • Nausea and vomiting • Increased respiratory rate and depth (classic Kussmaul's respirations) • Hyperkalemia • Warm, flushed skin • Cardiac arrhythmias • pH below 7.35, HCO_3^- under 22 mEq/L, and normal $PaCO_2$ (34 to 44 mm Hg)	Identify patients at risk for metabolic acidosis. • Assess the patient for signs and symptoms of metabolic acidosis, especially respiratory, neurologic, electrolyte, and ABG changes. • Administer sodium bicarbonate ($NaHCO_3^-$) if necessary. • Evaluate and correct fluid and electrolyte imbalances. • Administer medications for nausea, vomiting, or diarrhea, as prescribed. • If the patient is confused, take safety precautions. • If the patient is diabetic, teach the patient and family about blood glucose monitoring, diet, and drug administration. • Treat the underlying cause—for example, if diabetic ketoacidosis is the cause, administer insulin and fluids.
Metabolic alkalosis Acid-base disturbance characterized by high pH and excess HCO_3^- and base in which the lungs compensate through hypoventilation to increase $PaCO_2$	• Excessive removal or vomiting of gastric acid, nasogastric suctioning, or pyloric stenosis • Hypokalemia • Steroid or diuretic therapy • Abrupt relief of chronic respiratory acidosis • Cushing's syndrome or aldosteronism • Excessive administration of $NaHCO_3$ (during code resuscitation) or bicarbonate-containing antacids	• Tingling in fingers and toes, dizziness, and hypertonicity • Compensatory hypoventilation with decreased respirations • Decreased chloride and potassium levels • Atrial tachycardia • Confusion, irritability • Diarrhea • Nausea, vomiting • Picking at bed clothes (carphology) • pH above 7.45 and HCO_3^- above 26 mEq/L	• Identify patients at risk for metabolic alkalosis. • Assess the patient for signs and symptoms of metabolic alkalosis, especially respiratory, electrolyte, and ABG changes. • Replace electrolytes, such as potassium and chloride, as prescribed, and monitor levels regularly. • Administer an acidifying agent, such as I.V. ammonium chloride. • Replace fluid volume, as prescribed. • Administer an antiemetic, as prescribed. • Prevent complications, such as hypoxemia caused by hypoventilation. • Teach the patient and family how to correctly administer an antacid.

(continued)

Box 6-4: Understanding Acid-Base Imbalances (continued)

Description	Cause	Signs and Symptoms	Nursing Care
Respiratory acidosis Acid-base disturbance characterized by excessive carbonic acid (H_2CO_3), elevated $PaCO_2$, and decreased serum pH that commonly is associated with decreased oxygenation resulting from hypoventilation	*Acute respiratory acidosis* • Pulmonary edema • Aspiration • Atelectasis • Pneumothorax • Sedative overdose • Pneumonia • Cardiac arrest • Laryngospasm • Improperly regulated mechanical ventilation *Chronic respiratory acidosis* • Bronchial asthma • Emphysema • Cystic fibrosis • Advanced multiple sclerosis • Bronchiectasis	*Acute respiratory acidosis* • Dulled sensorium, dizziness, feeling of fullness in head, and unconsciousness • Palpitations, tachycardia, and ventricular fibrillation • Muscle twitching and seizures • Warm, flushed skin, perspiration, and cyanosis • pH below 7.35, $PaCO_2$ above 50 mm Hg, and normal or slightly elevated HCO_3^- *Chronic respiratory acidosis* • Weakness • Dull headache • pH below 7.35, $PaCO_2$ above 42 mm Hg, and HCO_3^- above 26 mEq/L • Symptoms of underlying disease, such as barrel chest and productive cough caused by chronic obstructive pulmonary disease	• Identify patients at risk for respiratory acidosis. • Identify factors that increase the risk of hypoventilation, such as obesity, postoperative pain, tight dressings, and abdominal distention. • Assess the patient for signs and symptoms of respiratory acidosis, especially respiratory, pulse, and neurologic changes. • If the patient has a chronic condition, make sure the patient doesn't receive more than 2 L of oxygen without an order. • Relieve postoperative pain by administering the prescribed analgesic or teaching the patient relaxation techniques. • Maintain an open airway; use suction if the patient can't cough up secretions. • Encourage coughing, deep breathing, and ambulation in a postoperative patient. • Perform chest physiotherapy. • Maintain hydration to keep secretions loose. • Provide food appropriate for the patient's ability to chew and swallow. • If the patient has chronic respiratory acidosis, assist with routine pulmonary care. • If the patient requires ventilator assistance, intervene as needed.
Respiratory alkalosis Acid-base disturbance characterized by low H_2CO_3 and $PaCO_2$ and caused by excessive "blowing off" of carbon dioxide during hyperventilation	• Extreme anxiety (most common cause) • Pulmonary emboli, pulmonary fibrosis, asthma, pneumonia, or injury to the respiratory center • Gram-negative bacteremia and sepsis • High fever • Hypoxemia • Early salicylate intoxication • High altitude • Hyperventilation caused by mechanical ventilation • Pregnancy • Hepatic failure • Heart failure	• Hyperventilation exceeding 40 breaths/minute • Cardiac arrhythmias that fail to respond to conventional treatment • Circumoral or peripheral paresthesia • Carpopedal spasms • Twitching (possibly progressing to tetany) • Seizures • Muscle weakness • Light-headedness, inability to concentrate, dizziness, agitation • pH above 7.45 and normal HCO_3^- level (during an acute episode); normal pH and HCO_3^- below 22 mEq/L (during compensation in an acute episode); and normal pH, HCO_3^- below 22 mEq/L, and $PaCO_2$ below 32 mm Hg (during a chronic episode)	• Identify patients at risk for respiratory alkalosis. • Assess the patient's anxiety level. • Assess the patient for signs of respiratory alkalosis, especially neurologic, electrolyte, and ABG changes. • If the patient is anxious, encourage the patient to breathe slowly. Encourage breathing into a paper bag to increase $PaCO_2$. • Administer a sedative, as prescribed, and take safety measures. • Intervene to decrease hyperthermia. • Teach the patient and family how to perform relaxation techniques and prevent, recognize, and treat hyperventilation. • Teach the patient and family about safety precautions for household medications, especially those containing aspirin.

Interpreting Arterial Blood Gas Levels

- Determine whether the pH value is normal or shows acidosis or alkalosis.
- Determine whether the partial pressure of arterial carbon dioxide ($PaCO_2$) is normal or shows acidosis or alkalosis.
- Determine whether the bicarbonate (HCO_3^-) level is normal or shows acidosis or alkalosis.
- Determine whether the pH value matches the $PaCO_2$ (respiratory) or the HCO_3^- (metabolic) value.
- If the pH value is abnormal and the $PaCO_2$ value, the HCO_3^- value, or both are abnormal, the condition is uncompensated.

If the pH value is normal and the $PaCO_2$ value and the HCO_3^- value are abnormal, the condition is compensated.

- PaO_2, or the partial pressure of oxygen in arterial blood, is a measure of the blood's oxygen content
  - A PaO_2 of 80 to 100 mm Hg is normal
  - A PaO_2 of 70 to 80 mm Hg is borderline hypoxemia; a PaO_2 of 50 to 70 mm Hg indicates hypoxemia; a PaO_2 below 50 mm Hg indicates severe hypoxemia
- HCO_3^- is the level of the buffer bicarbonate
  - An HCO_3^- of 24 mEq/L is normal
  - An HCO_3^- above 26 mEq/L indicates excess bicarbonate; an HCO_3^- below 22 mEq/L indicates inadequate bicarbonate
- Compensation
  - Compensation is the return of an abnormal pH to a normal pH
  - The unaffected system (metabolic or respiratory) is responsible for returning the pH to normal
    - In respiratory acidosis with a high $PaCO_2$, the kidneys compensate by retaining bicarbonate, which changes the $HCO_3^-/PaCO_2$ ratio and returns the pH to normal
    - In respiratory alkalosis with a low $PaCO_2$, the kidneys compensate by excreting bicarbonate, which changes the $HCO_3^-/PaCO_2$ ratio and returns the pH to normal
    - In metabolic acidosis with a low HCO_3^- or base excess, the lungs compensate through hyperventilation, which lowers $PaCO_2$ and returns the pH to normal
    - In metabolic alkalosis with high HCO_3^-, the lungs compensate through hypoventilation, which increases $PaCO_2$ and returns the pH to normal
  - Compensation can be assessed by examining the ABG values
    - Look at the primary system affected ($PaCO_2$ or HCO_3^-)
    - Look at the system not affected ($PaCO_2$ or HCO_3^-)
    - If the ABGs in the unaffected system are moving in the same direction as those in the primary system, compensation is occurring (see *Interpreting arterial blood gas levels*)

Nutrition

- General information
  - Optimal nutrition is important for maintaining health, preventing illness, and promoting recovery from injury
  - Disorders related to nutritional deficiencies (including obesity) are among the leading causes of morbidity and mortality in the United States today
  - As many as 50% of medical-surgical patients have moderate malnutrition; the risk of malnutrition increases with the length of hospitalization
  - Early identification and nutritional support interventions can help prevent malnutrition
- Nutritional assessment
  - Make sure the patient's dietary history includes typical consumption, eating patterns and preferences, use of supplements, and recent changes in appetite or conditions interfering with food ingestion or digestion
  - Compare information obtained from the dietary history with the dietary guidelines outlined in the U.S. Department of Agriculture's Food Guide Pyramid
  - Measure the patient's height and weight and calculate his body mass index (see *Calculating BMI* and *What BMI values mean*, page 78)

Box 6-6: Calculating BMI

You can use one of the formulas below to calculate your patient's body mass index (BMI).

$$BMI = \frac{\text{weight in pounds}}{\text{height in inches} \times \text{height in inches}} \times 703$$

OR

$$BMI = \frac{\text{weight in kilograms}}{\text{height in centimeters} \times \text{height in centimeters}} \times 10{,}000$$

OR

$$BMI = \frac{\text{weight in kilograms}}{\text{height in meters} \times \text{height in meters}}$$

- Malnutrition
  - Clinical signs of malnutrition appear in areas of rapid turnover of epithelial and mucosal cells; signs include dry, flaky, or discolored skin, brittle hair and nails, bleeding gums and swollen tongue, muscle wasting, decreased skin turgor, ascites, and peripheral edema
  - Laboratory studies can indicate nutritional deficits before clinical signs occur
    - Levels of visceral proteins (albumin, transferrin, prealbumin, and retinol-binding protein) are diminished in malnutrition
    - Proteins with shorter half-lives can better indicate acute nutritional changes (see *Visceral proteins and their normal values*, page 79)
  - Other potential indicators of malnutrition include a decreased total lymphocyte count (less than 1,800 cells/mm^3) and a diminished response to skin testing for cell-mediated immunity
  - Nitrogen balance indicates the adequacy of protein intake
    - To determine nitrogen balance, protein intake is measured in conjunction with 24-hour urinary urea nitrogen levels
    - A negative nitrogen balance occurs when losses exceed intake
- Effects of malnutrition
  - Immune function decreases and susceptibility to infection increases
  - Wounds heal poorly and the risk of developing pressure ulcers increases
  - Nutrient losses through the GI tract increase
  - Muscle breakdown results in weakness and fatigue and increases the risk of multiple organ failure
- Malnutrition risks for the medical-surgical patient
  - Underlying disease processes, such as malabsorption syndromes, gastric or bowel resections, pancreatic insufficiency, and vomiting and diarrhea, can interfere with the intake and use of nutrients (see *Normal and hypermetabolic nutritional requirements*, page 79)

Box 6-7: What BMI Values Mean

BMI Value	Correlation
<18.5	Underweight
18.5 to 24.9	Normal weight
25.0 to 29.9	Overweight
30.0 to 39.9	Obese
>40.0	Extremely obese

Box 6-8: Visceral Proteins and Their Normal Values

The chart below shows half-life and normal values for visceral proteins.

Visceral Protein	Half-Life	Normal Value
Albumin	20 days	3.5 to 5 g/dL
Transferrin	10 days	200 to 400 mg/dL
Prealbumin (thyroxine-binding protein)	2 to 3 days	15.7 to 29.6 mg/dL
Retinol-binding protein	12 hours	2.6 to 7.6 mg/dL

- Anorexia, dysphagia, prolonged or frequent nothing-by-mouth status, depression, and advanced age can contribute to inadequate intake of nutrients
- Nutrient losses occur with blood loss, wound drainage, and dialysis
- Increased nutrient needs can occur with the stress response, cancer, surgery, infection, trauma, and burns
- Therapeutic diets
  - Clear liquid diets that minimize residue in the GI tract may be used before or after procedures
    - The diet may include clear juices, broth, tea, popsicles, and soda
    - Because this diet provides inadequate nutrients, it shouldn't be used for more than a few days
  - Full liquid diets serve as an intermediate step between a clear liquid and a soft diet
    - Foods include milk, milk shakes, yogurt, creamed soups, and liquid nutritional supplements
    - Although this diet provides more nutrition than a clear liquid diet, it's considered nutritionally inadequate and shouldn't be used for more than a few days
  - Soft diets are the next step between a liquid and general diet; they're also used when a patient requires food that's easy to chew or swallow
    - Foods are soft and lightly seasoned and moderately low in fiber
    - This diet is nutritionally adequate, and patients may remain on such a diet for a prolonged period
  - Low-residue diets are nutritionally adequate and are used to avoid GI tract irritation and decrease fecal volume
    - Patients with inflammatory bowel disease or regional enteritis and patients who have undergone bowel surgery may be placed on this diet
    - Foods are soft, but the diet limits milk, fruits and vegetables, and whole grains and seeds
  - High-fiber diets are nutritionally adequate; they're used to promote bowel elimination and relieve constipation, diarrhea, and symptoms of diverticular disease
    - Foods include those high in indigestible carbohydrates, such as whole grain cereals and bread as well as fruits and vegetables
  - Renal diets are controlled for fluids, protein, sodium, and potassium and are used for patients with acute or chronic renal failure; the degree of restriction depends on the degree of renal impairment

Box 6-9: Normal and Hypermetabolic Nutritional Requirements

The chart below shows the normal nutritional requirements for calories, protein calories, and nonprotein calories compared with the amount needed during hypermetabolic states.

	Normal Nutritional Requirements	Hypermetabolic Nutritional Requirements
Total calories	25 kcal/kg/day	25 to 30 kcal/kg/day
Protein calories	0.8 g/kg/day	1.2 to 1.5 g/kg/day
Nonprotein calories	2 to 4 g carbohydrate/kg/day; 0.5 to 0.75 g fat/kg/day	2 to 5 g carbohydrate/kg/day; 0.5 to 1.0 g fat/kg/day

- Hepatic diets are controlled for fluid, protein, and sodium to a degree determined by the patient's hepatic impairment; they're used to prevent the catabolism of body proteins and minimize the clinical signs and symptoms of hepatic encephalopathy and ascites
- Sodium- and fluid-restricted diets are used for patients with cardiovascular disease; the extent of the restriction depends on the patient's degree of impairment
- Oral dietary supplements can be used to increase calorie and nutrient intake as needed
- Enteral nutrition
  - Tube feeding may be used for a patient with a functional GI tract who has had inadequate intake for 3 to 5 days
  - Several enteral nutritional products are available and can be tailored to a patient's specific nutritional needs
  - A small-bore nasoenteric tube allows for short-term enteral access (less than 4 weeks); longer-term access (more than 6 weeks) requires placement of a gastroscopy or jejunostomy tube
  - Placement of a nasoenteric tubes must be checked by X-ray or, if inserted endoscopically, by direct visualization before tube feedings can begin
  - The patient can receive gastric feedings as a bolus intermittently over 30 to 60 minutes, or continuously over 12 to 24 hours; postpyloric feedings into the duodenum or jejunum require continuous administration to avoid dumping syndrome
  - To reduce the risk of bacterial contamination of nutritional products, perform hand hygiene before initiating feedings or manipulating the bag or tubing, ensure that formulas are reconstituted in a controlled location such as the pharmacy, and adhere to your facility's guidelines for formula, bag, and apparatus discard times
  - Enteral feedings can result in a variety of complications
    - To prevent the tube from becoming obstructed, gently flush the tube with 30 mL of warm tap water before and after feedings
    - To reduce the risk of aspiration pneumonia, elevate the head of bed 30 degrees during feedings
    - If you suspect that the nasoenteric tube has become dislocated, resulting in inadvertent respiratory tract infusion of formula, stop the feeding and check tube placement by X-ray or the pH of gastric secretions
    - Secure the tube to minimize trauma to the insertion site and decrease the risk of insertion site infection or leakage leading to peritonitis
    - Watch for GI complications, such as diarrhea, delayed gastric emptying, and constipation, as well as such complications as hyperglycemia and fluid and electrolyte imbalance
- Parenteral nutrition
  - Parenteral nutrition is appropriate for patients who require nutritional support for more than 10 days and for whom enteral feedings are contraindicated
  - Peripheral venous nutrition (PVN) provides partial or total nutrition for up to 2 weeks; central venous nutrition (CVN) provides total nutrition for longer periods
  - Both PVN and CVN contain a combination of glucose, amino acids, electrolytes, vitamins, and trace elements, with PVN having formulations of up to 10% glucose and less than 25% amino acids; greater concentrations of glucose and amino acids must be infused centrally
  - Fat emulsions provide essential fatty acids and can be given either peripherally or centrally. Total nutrient admixtures containing proteins, carbohydrates, and lipids in a single I.V. bag are available
  - Four types of central access devices are available
    - Nontunneled or percutaneous catheters such as subclavian lines are indicated for shorter-term nutritional support and can be inserted at the bedside
    - Peripherally inserted central catheters (also called PICC lines) are intended for short-term use; these long catheters are inserted through a peripheral vein and advanced into the superior vena cava
    - Tunneled catheters, such as the Hickman, Broviac, and Groshong, are intended for longer-term use; they're inserted surgically, with the distal end placed in the superior vena cava and the proximal end tunneled through the subcutaneous tissue of the chest wall to exit below the nipple line
    - Implanted vascular access devices such as an implanted infusion port are implanted surgically and contain no external parts; instead, a catheter is placed in the subclavian or internal jugular vein and the access device is implanted in a subcutaneous pocket of the chest wall, with a special access needle used to cannulate the device intermittently
  - Catheter placement should be confirmed by X-ray before initiating any infusions
  - PVN and CVN are usually continuously infused with an infusion pump and a filter; a 0.22-micron filter should be used for CVN alone, and a 1.2-micron filter for CVN with lipids

- Parental nutrition can result in several complications
  - Hypoglycemia and hyperglycemia, fluid overload, and electrolyte imbalances can all occur
  - Infection at the insertion site and sepsis can occur because the high glucose and fat concentrations of the solutions provide an ideal culture medium for bacterial and fungal growth
  - The catheter can become occluded or dislodged
  - Phlebitis can also occur
  - An air embolism can cause such signs as tachypnea, altered mental status, and hypotension; if you suspect an air embolism, position the patient on his left side with his head down to allow bubbles to rise to the right atrium, where they're less likely to obstruct blood flow to the pulmonary artery
- Nursing interventions to improve nutritional outcomes
  - Assess all medical-surgical patients for nutritional status upon admission and at least weekly after that; intervene as quickly as possible if you detect deficits
  - Before discharge, teach patients about maintaining a healthy diet at home; take food preferences and socioeconomic conditions into account
  - Provide individualized nutritional strategies for special populations, such as vegetarians, bariatric surgery patients, and elderly patients
  - For patients who will administer CVN at home, provide appropriate support and teaching to ensure that they and their caregivers understand the equipment required, how to care for the catheter, and how to monitor for complications on an ongoing basis

Obesity

- The prevalence of obesity in the United States has increased markedly over the past two decades
  - In 2017, only Colorado, Hawaii, and the District of Columbia had obesity rates of less than 22%
  - A total of 43 states had obesity rates of 25% or higher; 20 of these states had obesity rates of 30% or higher
- Excess weight substantially increases the risk of diabetes, cardiovascular disease, certain types of cancer, and other diseases, such as gynecologic abnormalities, osteoarthritis, and stress incontinence
- The risk of death from all causes in obese people is 50% to 100% greater than in people of normal weight
- Obesity can increase the risk of morbidity from other pre-existing disorders
  - Obese patients with existing coronary artery disease, type 2 diabetes, stroke, or sleep apnea are at high risk for developing disease-related complications that can lead to death
- Obesity is linked to complications during surgery, pregnancy, and labor and delivery
- A major contributor to preventable deaths, obesity also leads to low self-esteem, negative self-image, hopelessness, and negative social consequences, such as stereotyping, prejudice, social isolation, and discrimination
- Obese patients are more susceptibles to certain complications than nonobese patients
  - The most common complications involve the pulmonary, cardiovascular, GI, and musculoskeletal systems (see *Complications of obesity*, page 82)
- Treatment of obesity can be long and difficult; no single treatment method or combination of methods is guaranteed to produce or maintain weight loss in all patients
- Treatment needs to combine diet therapy and increased physical activity
  - A key element of the current recommendations is a moderate reduction in calories to achieve a slow, progressive weight loss of 1 to 2 lb (0.5 to 1 kg) per week; calories should be reduced only to the level required to achieve the goal weight
  - Exercise plays a critical role in losing and maintaining body weight by increasing energy expenditure, maintaining or increasing lean body mass, and promoting fat loss
- Behavioral therapy serves as adjunct to planned decreases in food intake and increases in physical activity, with the goal of overcoming barriers to compliance with eating and activity habits
  - Various behavior modification strategies must be used because no single method is superior
  - Strategies for behavioral modification include self-monitoring, stress management, stimulus control, problem solving, contingency management, cognitive restructuring, and social support
- If the patient hasn't lost the recommended 1 lb (0.5 kg) per week after 6 months of diet and increased physical activity, drug therapy may be considered
  - Not every patient responds to drug therapy; tests show that initial responders tend to continue to respond, whereas nonresponders are less likely to respond, even with increases in dosage
  - If adverse effects are unmanageable or if therapy is ineffective, drug therapy should be stopped

Box 6-10: Complications of Obesity

Obese patients typically have more complications that affect various body systems. Here are some of the more common complications along with their pathophysiology and related nursing interventions.

System	Pathophysiologic Consequences	Pathophysiologic Problems	Nursing Interventions
Pulmonary	• Decreased diaphragmatic excursion • Decreased vital capacity • Decreased alveolar ventilation • Decreased compliance • Decreased respiratory drive • Chronic carbon dioxide retention	• Increased respiratory rate • Ventilation-perfusion mismatch • Hypoxemia • Respiratory acidosis • Difficulty weaning from the ventilator • Obstructive sleep apnea • Increased risk of aspiration	• Try noninvasive positive-pressure ventilation, such as bilevel positive airway pressure or continuous positive airway pressure. • Be prepared for intubation. • Calculate tidal volume based on ideal weight, not actual weight. • Minimize time the patient spends in a supine position. • Control secretions to maintain airway patency. • Reposition at least every 2 hours.
Cardiovascular	• Left ventricular hypertrophy • Increased total blood volume • Increased stroke volume • Increased cardiac output • Increased cardiac deconditioning	• Right-sided and left-sided heart failure • Hypertension • Myocardial infarction • Stroke • Chronic venous insufficiency • Deep vein thrombosis • Pulmonary embolism	• Encourage mobility as tolerated. • Watch for signs of fluid overload. • Monitor blood pressure. • Administer medications as ordered.
Endocrine	• Increased metabolic requirements • Increased insulin resistance	• Type 2 diabetes • Hyperlipidemia	• Carefully monitor blood glucose levels, especially if the patient is receiving a steroid. • Work with a dietitian to ensure that metabolic needs are met.
GI	• Increased intra-abdominal pressure • Increased gastric volume	• Increased incidence of gastroesophageal reflux disease • Increased risk of aspiration, especially with enteral feedings • Increased constipation • Increased risk of pancreatitis	• Administer medications as ordered. • Keep head of bed at 30 degrees when possible. • Increase fluid and fiber intake. • Monitor amylase and lipase levels. • Be alert for altered pharmacokinetics for some drugs.
Immune	• Impaired immune response • Impaired cell-mediated immunity	• Impaired healing • Increased risk of wound infections • Increased skin breakdown and pressure ulcers • Decreased resistance to infection	• Monitor wounds for early signs of infection. • Reposition the patient at least every 2 hours. • Monitor skin folds for pressure ulcers or skin breakdown. • Work with a dietitian to ensure that metabolic needs are met for proper healing.
Musculoskeletal	• Increased joint trauma • Decreased mobility • Increased atrophy from lack of use • Increased pain with movement	• Osteoarthritis • Rheumatoid arthritis	• Encourage mobilization. • Perform range-of-motion exercises with the patient. • Provide nonpharmacologic pain-relief measures.

- Patients experiencing complications from severe, resistant obesity may benefit from weight-loss surgery if the risk for remaining obese is greater than the risk for surgery
  - Restrictive and malabsorptive-restrictive are the two types of surgeries primarily used to promote weight loss
  - In gastric restriction—also known as vertical banded gastroplasty and adjustable gastric banding—the size of the stomach is surgically decreased so that a patient feels full after eating a small amount of food
  - Malabsorptive-restrictive procedures, which reduce stomach size as well as the number of calories and nutrients the body can absorb, produce better weight-loss results than gastric resection; two types of malabsorptive-restrictive weight-loss surgeries currently performed are the gastric bypass (also known as a Roux-en-Y bypass) and biliopancreatic diversion

Substance Abuse, Dependence, and Addiction

- General information
  - *Substance abuse* is the repeated use of a drug that doesn't result in addiction or lead to withdrawal when discontinued
  - *Substance dependence* is the compulsive use of a drug that results in tolerance to the drug's effects and withdrawal symptoms when the drug is terminated or decreased
  - *Addiction* is characterized by loss of control of substance consumption, substance use despite associated problems, and the tendency to relapse
  - Psychodynamic factors associated with addiction include lack of tolerance for frustration and pain, lack of success in life, lack of affectionate and meaningful relationships, low self-esteem and lack of self-regard, and a risk-taking propensity
  - When taking care of patients with substance abuse disorders, the nurse should be kind, warm, and supportive to help dispel the patient's anxiety and provide a sense of security
  - The nursing process for patients with substance abuse disorders includes a thorough physical and psychosocial assessment, with emphasis on the history of drug use
  - The nurse should document patient's drug of choice, the length of use, and the last use, both to anticipate the patient's risk of developing withdrawal symptoms and to avoid drug interactions
- Alcohol abuse
  - Alcohol is the most commonly abused substance; alcoholism is more common in men, young people, whites, and those who are unmarried
  - Alcohol can affect all organ systems, particularly the central nervous system (CNS) and the GI system
  - GI problems associated with alcoholism include esophagitis, gastritis, pancreatitis, alcoholic hepatitis, and liver cirrhosis
  - Long-term use is commonly associated with tuberculosis, all types of accidents, suicide, and homicide
  - The early signs of alcohol withdrawal occur within a few hours after the last intake and peak in 24 to 48 hours; withdrawal can progress to alcohol withdrawal delirium
  - Signs and symptoms of alcohol withdrawal include hyperalertness, jerky movements, and irritability
  - Alcohol withdrawal delirium usually peaks within 2 to 3 days and is always considered a medical emergency
    - ○ Signs and symptoms of alcohol withdrawal delirium include autonomic hyperactivity, severe disturbance in sensorium, perceptual disturbance, fluctuating LOC, delusions, agitated behaviors, and fever
- Substance abuse
  - Commonly abused CNS stimulants include cocaine and amphetamines
    - ○ Intoxication with CNS stimulants typically causes tachycardia, dilated pupils, increased blood pressure, nausea and vomiting, and insomnia
    - ○ Overdose with CNS stimulants can cause respiratory distress, ataxia, hyperpyrexia, convulsions, coma, stroke, MI, and death
    - ○ Signs and symptoms of withdrawal include fatigues, depression, agitation, apathy, anxiety, sleepiness, disorientation, lethargy, and craving
  - Treatment for individuals with substance abuse includes an assessment phase, treatment of the intoxication and withdrawal when necessary, and the development and implementation of an overall treatment strategy
  - Treatment should include both an interdisciplinary care team and family members; the patient and family should also as receive referrals to support groups

Pain

- General information
  - Pain is a complex phenomenon that involves biological, psychological, cultural, and social factors; it's a primarily subjective experience
  - Margo McCaffery, a pain researcher, defines *pain* as "whatever the experiencing person says it is, existing whenever the experiencing person says it does"
  - The International Association on Pain defines *pain* as unpleasant sensory and emotional experiences related to actual or potential tissue damage
- Pain theories
  - All current pain-control theories are hypothetical; none completely explain the pain experience and all its components
  - The *specificity theory* holds that highly specific structures and pathways exist for pain transmission; this biologically oriented theory doesn't explain pain tolerance and ignores social, cultural, and empirical factors that influence pain
  - The *pattern theory* holds that rapid and slow conduction pathways exist, which relay pain information through the spinal cord to the brain; although this theory addresses the brain's ability to determine the amount, intensity, and type of sensory input, it doesn't address nonbiological influences on pain perception and transmission
  - The *gate control theory* describes a hypothetical gate mechanism in the spinal cord that allows nerve fibers to receive pain sensations; the gate can be closed to pain sensation by occupying the receptor sites with other stimuli
    - This theory has encouraged a holistic approach to pain control and research by considering nonbiological components of pain
    - Pain management techniques, such as cutaneous stimulation, distraction, and acupuncture, are partly based on this theory
- Anatomic and physiologic basis of pain
  - Stimulation of pain receptors in skin and soft tissues typically causes defined, localized pain
  - Stimulation of pain receptors in deep tissues causes dull, poorly localized pain
  - Stimulation of pain receptors in the viscera or organs causes diffuse, sometimes referred pain
  - Pain can be stimulated by mechanical sources such as sharp objects, thermal sources such as fire, or chemical sources such as stomach acids and battery acid
  - Pain travels from the periphery to the spinal cord to the brain by way of a pathway composed of A (delta) fibers (intense pain) and C fibers (dull, aching pain)
  - Pain is processed in the thalamus, midbrain, and cortex
  - Certain neurotransmitters, such as histamine, serotonin, and prostaglandins, enhance pain impulse transmission
  - Other neurotransmitters, such as endogenous opiates, endorphins, and enkephalins, inhibit pain impulse transmission; chronic pain syndrome may be related to a deficiency of these inhibitory neurotransmitters
- Factors that affect pain response
  - Pain is primarily a physical problem that has psychological effects
  - The physical and psychological sources of pain are often complex and intertwined, with causative factors difficult to isolate
  - *Psychogenic pain* is pain without a physiologic basis; this term isn't helpful because all physical causes of pain can't be diagnosed, and all pain is real to the patient
  - *Pain threshold* is the point at which a patient experiences pain
  - *Pain tolerance* is affected by individual, psychosocial, cultural, religious, and environmental factors; it influences pain duration and intensity

Pain Assessment

- General information
  - Pain can be assessed with a subjective pain assessment tool
    - *0 to 10 rating scale:* The patient is asked to rate pain on a scale of 0 to 10, with 0 being no pain and 10 being the worst pain imaginable

○ *Face rating scale:* The patient is shown illustrations of five or more faces demonstrating varying levels of emotion, from happy to sad; by selecting the face that most closely approximates the pain sensation, the patient helps the nurse gauge the effectiveness of interventions

○ *Visual analog scale:* The patient places a mark on the scale, ranging from no pain to pain as bad as it can be, to indicate his current level of pain

○ *Body diagram:* The patient draws the location and radiation of pain on a paper illustration of the body

○ *Questionnaire:* The patient answers questions about the pain's location, intensity, quality, onset, and relieving and aggravating factors

○ *Pain flow chart:* The nurse documents variations in pain, vital signs, and LOC in response to treatments; these forms are particularly useful for monitoring patient response to epidural opioid infusions and for titrating dosages

- Pain also can be assessed by observing for objective signs, such as facial grimacing; elevated blood pressure and increased pulse and respiratory rates; muscle tension; restlessness or an inability to concentrate; decreased interest in surroundings and increased focus on pain; perspiration and pallor; crying, moaning, or verbalizations of pain; and guarding the painful body part

- Pain classification
  - *Acute pain* is mild to severe pain that's rapid in onset and lasts less than 6 months; it can be intermittent or recurrent as in migraine and sinus headaches and gallbladder colic
  - *Chronic pain* lasts beyond the expected healing time and may be difficult to relate to the original injury or tissue damage; it can be further classified as chronic benign pain (as in lower back pain), chronic cancer pain, or pain with ongoing peripheral pathology

- Pharmacologic management of pain
  - Nonopioid drugs, such as nonsteroidal anti-inflammatory drugs (NSAIDs) and acetaminophen (Tylenol), are used to treat acute pain caused by inflammation or tissue destruction and mild to moderate pain; they're useful adjuncts to opioid analgesics for controlling severe, acute pain
  - Opioid analgesics such as narcotic agonist-antagonists relieve pain by occupying opioid receptor sites in the brain and spinal cord; they're used to treat moderate to severe acute pain (postoperative pain and fractures), recurrent acute pain (sickle cell crisis, angina, and renal colic), prolonged time-limited pain (cancer and burns), and pain that requires rapid, short-term relief (procedures such as bone marrow biopsy and thoracentesis)
  - Sometimes, small doses of antidepressants are used as adjuncts to pain control; they affect pain perception and reduce the accompanying anxiety
  - The oral route of administration is the least expensive, easiest for patients to manage, and most widely accepted by patients; most NSAIDs and some opioids can be administered orally
  - Parenteral routes (subcutaneous, intramuscular [I.M.], and intravenous [I.V.]) are widely used to administer opioids
  - Intraspinal (epidural) routes are used for short-term acute pain, such as that caused by abdominal surgery; the opioid's systemic effect is reduced with the intraspinal route compared with other parenteral routes
  - Topical patches, such as those containing fentanyl (Duragesic), are useful during the transition from epidural to oral opioids
  - Rectal administration of opioids may be indicated when a patient can't tolerate oral medications temporarily because of nausea and vomiting
  - Patient-controlled analgesia is the I.V., subcut, or intraspinal administration of opioids by means of an electronic controller that's programmed to respond with small doses when the patient requests medication
  - Scheduled dosing is preferred to "as needed"; around-the-clock dosing controls pain by avoiding the major peaks and valleys of the pain experience

- Nonpharmacologic management of pain
  - *Cutaneous stimulation* is a low-risk, inexpensive, noninvasive, readily available pain management technique that requires little skill to implement; examples include heat application, cold application, massage, pressure, vibration, and transcutaneous electrical nerve stimulation (the application of electric current through skin patches connected to a portable electrical source)
  - *Therapeutic touch* unblocks congested areas of energy in the body; in this technique, the practitioner redirects energy by using touch to promote comfort, relaxation, healing, and a sense of well-being
  - *Acupuncture* is the use of needles of various sizes to stimulate parts of the body to produce analgesia; this centuries-old technique originated in China and is gaining acceptance in Western medicine

- *Cognitive and behavioral pain management* uses imagery, distraction, relaxation techniques, and humor to help patients manage pain
- *Biofeedback* teaches patients to control involuntary body mechanisms, such as heart rate, muscle spasms, and circulation
- Surgical management of pain
  - Surgery seldom is used as a primary treatment for pain but can be considered to manage pain when pharmacologic therapies fail
  - *Nerve blocks* involve the injection of phenol or alcohol to destroy nerve endings in a specific area
  - *Rhizotomy* is the surgical destruction of sensory nerve roots where they enter the spinal cord; *chordotomy* is the transection of spinal cord nerves at the spinal cord's midline portion
  - *Neurectomy* is the resection or partial or total excision of a spinal or cranial nerve
  - *Cryoanalgesia* deactivates a nerve using a cooled probe that causes temporary nerve injury
  - *Radiofrequency lesioning* may affect the nerve from the heat generated, the magnetic field created by the radio waves, or both
  - *Percutaneous electrical nerve stimulation* uses implanted leads and a surface stimulator or implanted generator to block pain impulses by delivering electric charges to a nerve root
  - Spinal nerve blocks, rhizotomy, and chordotomy can impair bladder, bowel, and sexual functioning
- Nursing care of the patient in pain
  - Assess the pain's location, and ask the patient to rate the pain using a pain scale
  - Ask the patient to describe the pain's quality and pattern, including any precipitating or relieving factors
  - Monitor vital signs and note subjective responses to pain, such as facial grimacing and guarding of a body part
  - Administer pain medication around the clock as ordered
  - Provide comfort measures, such as back massage, positioning, linen changes, and oral or skin care
  - Teach the patient noninvasive techniques to control pain, such as relaxation, guided imagery, distraction, and cutaneous stimulation
  - Teach the importance of taking prescribed analgesics before the pain becomes severe
  - Instruct the patient on the need for adequate rest periods and sleep
- Referral to a pain clinic or hospice
  - Patients with chronic benign pain that can't be controlled by nonpharmacologic interventions may benefit from treatment at a pain clinic
  - The clinic's interdisciplinary staff works with the patient to assess the pain and develops a pain-control regimen that helps the patient regain or maintain an acceptable level of functioning
  - Hospice programs give care and support to dying patients and their families; pain control—one of the primary goals—provides the patient with adequate pain relief at home

Review Questions

Question 1. Blood gas values for the patient with advanced respiratory disease with respiratory acidosis is consistent with:

A. retention of CO_2.
B. loss of CO_2.
C. loss of bicarbonate.
D. retention of bicarbonate.

Correct answer: A Advanced respiratory disease causes the retention of CO_2 to the alveolar. Option B loss of CO_2 is seen in respiratory alkalosis. Option C loss of bicarbonate is seen in metabolic acidosis. Option D retention of bicarbonate is seen in metabolic alkalosis.

Question 2. The nurse is caring for a patient who was given pain medication before leaving the recovery room. Upon returning to his room, the patient states they are pain-free. Of the following actions, which would the nurse take?

A. Tell the patient that they must wait 4 hours for more pain medication.
B. Give half of the ordered as-needed dose.
C. Document the patient's pain.
D. Notify the practitioner that the patient is still experiencing pain.

Correct answer: C Document the patient's pain and reassess within 30 minutes.

Option d is incorrect. The practitioner would not be notified unless the patient is still experiencing pain so that new medication orders can be established. Option A is incorrect because patients who have recently undergone surgery shouldn't have to wait 4 hours for pain relief. Option B is incorrect because a nurse can't alter a dose without first consulting the practitioner; doing so could result in a nurse being charged with practicing medicine without a license.

Question 3. A patient is admitted to the health care facility with a possible electrolyte imbalance. The patient is disoriented and weak, has an irregular pulse, and takes hydrochlorothiazide. The patient most likely suffers from:

A. hypernatremia.
B. hyponatremia.
C. hyperkalemia.
D. hypokalemia.

Correct answer: D Signs and symptoms of hypokalemia include GI, cardiac, renal, respiratory, and neurologic symptoms. Options A, B, and C are incorrect because the use of a potassium-wasting diuretic, such as hydrochlorothiazide, without potassium supplement therapy causes hypokalemia.

Question 4. The nurse is assessing a patient who may be in the late stages of dehydration. Late signs and symptoms of dehydration include the following. SELECT ALL THAT APPLY.

A. Coma and seizures
B. Sunken eyeballs and poor skin turgor
C. Increased heart rate with hypotension
D. Thirst and confusion

Correct answer: D is incorrect because early signs and symptoms of dehydration include thirst, irritability, confusion, and dizziness. Options A, B, and C are correct because coma, seizures, sunken eyeballs, poor skin turgor, and increased heart rate with hypotension are all later signs and symptoms of dehydration.

Question 5. The nurse is evaluating a postoperative patient for infection. Which sign or symptom would be most indicative of infection?

A. Presence of an indwelling urinary catheter
B. Rectal temperature of 100°F (37.8°C)
C. Redness, warmth, and tenderness at the incision site
D. WBC count of 8,000/μL

Correct answer: C Redness, warmth, and tenderness at the incision site would lead the nurse to suspect a postoperative infection. Option A is incorrect because the presence of an invasive device predisposes a patient to infection but alone doesn't indicate infection. Option B is incorrect because a rectal temperature of 100°F is a normal finding in a postoperative patient because of the inflammatory response. Option D is incorrect because a normal WBC count ranges from 4,000 to 10,000/μL.

Question 6. When planning the postoperative care of a patient who underwent surgery for repair of a lacerated kidney after a motor vehicle accident, what intervention should take priority in the immediate postoperative period?

A. Monitoring the patient for signs and symptoms of altered mental status
B. Encouraging early ambulation
C. Splinting the abdomen for coughing and deep-breathing exercise
D. Monitoring the patient's renal function

Correct answer: A The nurse's priority should be monitoring the patient for signs and symptoms of mental changes, which usually manifests several hours after trauma. Although encouraging early ambulation (Option B), splinting the abdomen (Option C), and monitoring the patient's renal function (Option D) are important nursing interventions, they don't take priority in the immediate postoperative period.

Question 7. Which diet would be most appropriate for a patient with diverticulosis?

A. A low-fat diet
B. A low-residue diet
C. A high-calorie diet
D. A high-fiber diet

Correct answer: D Option diverticulosis diet should contain such foods as whole grain cereals and fruit. Option B is **incorrect.** A low-residue diet is used to avoid GI tract irritation and decrease fecal volume, appropriate measures for a patient with ulcerative colitis. Such a patient doesn't need to follow a low-fat diet (Option A) or to consume additional calories (Option C).

Question 8. The nurse performs a nutritional assessment on a patient with lung cancer who is in the postoperative period after a lobectomy. Which of the following could be a late sign of malnutrition?

A. A retinal-binding protein level of 2.0 mg/dL
B. Dry, flaky, discolored skin and brittle nails
C. A body mass index (BMI) of 20
D. An albumin level of 4.0 g/dL

Correct answer: B Dry, flaky, discolored skin and brittle nails are later signs of malnutrition. (Option A) Retinal-binding protein has a half-life of 12 hours, so a decrease from the normal values of 2.6 to 7.6 mg/dL could be an early sign of malnutrition. A BMI of 20 (Option C) falls in the normal range. Albumin (Option D) has a half-life of 20 days, and the value falls within the normal acceptable range.

Question 9. The two types of surgery primarily used to promote weight loss are restrictive and malabsorptive-restrictive. Which of the following is an example of restrictive weight-loss surgery?

A. Gastric bypass
B. Adjustable gastric banding
C. Roux-en-Y
D. Biliopancreatic diversion

Correct answer: B Adjustable gastric banding is a type of gastric restriction weight-loss surgery. Malabsorptive-restrictive procedures include gastric bypass (Option A) (also known as a Roux-en-Y bypass [Option C]) and biliopancreatic diversion (Option D).

Question 10. In what type of electrolyte imbalance would the nurse observe tall, tented T waves, a widened QRS complex, and a prolonged PR interval on the patient's ECG?

A. Hypokalemia
B. Hypocalcemia
C. Hypercalcemia
D. Hyperkalemia

Correct answer: D In hyperkalemia, the patient's ECG will show tall, tented T waves, a widened QRS complex, and a prolonged PR interval. In hypokalemia (Option A), the ECG will show a flat ST segment and Q wave. Hypocalcemia (Option B) and hypercalcemia (Option C) won't show T wave, QRS, or PR interval changes on the ECG.

Selected References

Karch, A. M. (2017). *Focus on nursing pharmacology* (7th ed.). Philadelphia, PA: Lippincott Williams & Wilkins.

National Institute of Diabetes and Digestive and Kidney Diseases (2017). *Overweight & obesity statistics*. Retrieved from https://www.niddk.nih.gov/health-information/health-statistics/overweight-obesity.

Porth, C. (2009). *Pathophysiology: Concepts of altered health states (w/CD)* (9th ed.). Philadelphia, PA: Lippincott Williams & Wilkins.

Smeltzer, S. C., & Bare, B. G. (2014). *Brunner & Suddarth's textbook of medical-surgical nursing* (13th ed.). Philadelphia, PA: Lippincott Williams & Wilkins.

Cardiovascular Disorders

Chapter 7

Introduction

- Proper functioning of the cardiovascular system ensures the adequate delivery of nutrients to and the removal of wastes from body cells
- Disruptions in the cardiovascular system can lead to alterations in organ function, disability, and death
- Nursing history
  - The nurse asks the patient about his *chief complaint*
    - The patient with a cardiovascular problem will likely cite a specific complaint, including chest, jaw, arm, or neck pain; irregular heartbeat or palpitations; shortness of breath on exertion, lying down, or at night; cough; cyanosis or pallor; weakness; fatigue; unexplained weight change; swelling of the extremities; dizziness; or high or low blood pressure
    - The patient with a cardiovascular problem may also report peripheral skin changes, such as decreased hair distribution, skin color changes, or a thin, shiny appearance to the skin, and pain in the extremities, such as leg pain or cramps
  - The nurse then questions the patient about his *present illness*
    - Ask the patient about symptoms, including when they started, associated signs and symptoms, location, radiation, intensity, duration, frequency, and precipitating and alleviating factors; if pain is the symptom, ask him to rate it on a scale of 0 to 10 (with 0 being no pain and 10 worst pain experienced)
    - Ask about the use of prescription and over-the-counter drugs, herbal remedies, vitamin and nutritional supplements, and alternative or complementary therapies used
  - The nurse asks about *medical history*
    - Question the patient about other cardiac and related disorders, such as hypertension, diabetes mellitus, hyperlipidemia, stroke, scarlet fever, rheumatic fever, strep throat, anemia, syncope, and congenital heart defects
    - Ask the female patient about the use of oral contraceptives and hormones and whether she is premenopausal or postmenopausal
  - The nurse then assesses the *family history*
    - Ask about a family history of hypertension, coronary artery disease (CAD), vascular disease, congenital heart disease, or hyperlipidemia
    - Also ask about a family history of diabetes mellitus
  - The nurse obtains a *social history*
    - Ask about work, exercise, diet, caffeine intake, use of recreational drugs, alcohol use, and hobbies
    - Also, ask about stress, support systems, coping mechanisms, and his cultural and religious background
- Physical assessment
  - The nurse begins with *inspection*
    - Observe the patient's general appearance: Is the patient thin, cachectic, or obese? Is the patient alert or anxious? What's the patient's respiratory rate and breathing pattern? Check hair distribution
    - Note the skin color: Is it pink, pale, or cyanotic?

- ○ Note any clubbing, edema, and skin lesions
- ○ Observe the chest and thorax: The lateral diameter should be twice the anteroposterior diameter; note any deviations from the typical chest shape
- ○ Inspect the neck for visible pulsations and jugular vein distention
- ○ Look for pulsations, symmetry of movement, retractions, or heaves; note the location of the apical impulse
- Next, the nurse uses *palpation*
  - ○ Palpate the precordium for heaves, thrills, and the point of maximum impulse; also palpate the sternoclavicular, aortic, pulmonic, tricuspid, and epigastric areas
  - ○ Palpate pulses in the extremities and neck for strength, rhythm, and equality, one at a time
  - ○ Palpate the extremities for skin temperature, edema, capillary refill time, and turgor
- Then the nurse *percusses* the heart
  - ○ Percuss the left border of the heart, noting the sound change from resonance to dullness
  - ○ Try to percuss the right border of the heart; in most people, it's under the sternum and can't be percussed
- The nurse continues by *auscultating* the heart and vessels
  - ○ Use the diaphragm of the stethoscope to listen over the mitral or apical area for 1 minute; note heart rate and rhythm
  - ○ Proceed sequentially through the auscultatory landmarks and listen for first and second heart sounds (S_1 and S_2) (see *Auscultatory sequence*)
  - ○ Listen for extra sounds, such as a third and fourth heart sounds (S_3 and S_4), murmurs, clicks, snaps, and rubs
  - ○ Repeat the sequence, using the bell of the stethoscope

Box 7-1: **Auscultatory Sequence**

When auscultating for heart sounds, place the stethoscope over the four different valve sites and at Erb's point. Follow the same auscultation sequence during every cardiovascular assessment:

- First, place the stethoscope in the second intercostal space along the right sternal border, as shown. In the aortic area, blood moves from the left ventricle during systole, crossing the aortic valve and flowing through the aortic arch
- Then move to the pulmonic area, located in the second intercostal space at the left sternal border. In the pulmonic area, blood ejected from the right ventricle during systole crosses the pulmonic valve and flows through the main pulmonary artery
- Next, listen at Erb's point, located in the third intercostal space at the left sternal border. At Erb's point, you'll hear aortic and pulmonic sounds

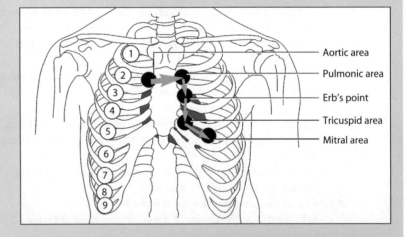

- At the fourth auscultation site, listen over the tricuspid area, which lies in the fifth intercostal space along the left sternal border. In the tricuspid area, sounds reflect blood movement from the right atrium across the tricuspid valve, filling the right ventricle during diastole

- Finally, listen in the mitral area, located in the fifth intercostal space near the midclavicular line. (If the patient's heart is enlarged, the mitral area may be closer to the anterior axillary line.) In the mitral (apical) area, sounds represent blood flow across the mitral valve and left ventricular filling during diastole

○ An S_3 (ventricular gallop) is low pitched and best heard over the apex of the heart; the rhythm is similar to a horse gallop, and the cadence sounds like "Kentucky"

○ An S_4 occurs during atrial contraction, just before S_1; its cadence sounds like "Tennessee"

○ The S_3 and S_4 sounds are best heard with the bell of the stethoscope placed at the apical area while the patient is supine or lying on his left side

○ Auscultate for bruits over the abdominal aorta and the carotid and femoral arteries

Acute Coronary Syndrome

- Description
  - Acute coronary syndrome (ACS) includes three major thrombotic effects of CAD and the resulting myocardial ischemia (see *Acute coronary syndromes*)
    - ○ Unstable angina
    - ○ Non–ST-segment elevation myocardial infarction (non-STEMI)
    - ○ STEMI
  - ACS results when a rupture or erosion of plaque occurs in one or more coronary arteries, resulting in platelet adhesions, activation of thrombin, and clot formation, reducing myocardial blood flow
  - ACS requires prompt evaluation to differentiate noncardiac pain from cardiac pain, so proper treatment can be quickly initiated
  - Complications of myocardial infarction (MI) may include heart failure, mitral valve insufficiency, cardiogenic shock, dysrhythmia, and death

Box 7-2: Acute Coronary Syndromes

Thrombotic Effect	Description	Signs and Symptoms	Diagnosis	Treatment	Nursing Considerations
Unstable angina	• Angina increasing in frequency and severity from patient's baseline • Easily induced • Lasts 5 to 15 minutes	• Burning, squeezing, substernal or retrosternal pain spreading across chest; may radiate to inside of arm, neck, jaw, or shoulder blade • Possible associated symptoms: shortness of breath, dizziness, nausea, palpitations, weakness, and cold sweats • Possible associated signs: hypertension or hypotension, tachycardia or bradycardia • Most often occurs with physical activity • Often relieved by rest or nitrates	• Electrocardiogram (ECG) may be normal or may show ischemia with transient T-wave or ST-segment changes. • Cardiac biomarkers usually remain within normal limits.	• Rest • Nitrates to reduce myocardial oxygen consumption • Beta adrenergic blockers to reduce the workload and oxygen demand • Calcium channel blockers if caused by coronary artery spasm • Oxygen to increase oxygenation of the blood • Antiplatelet drugs to minimize platelet aggregation • Coronary angiography to determine stenosis or obstruction with possible angioplasty or stent placement	• During acute anginal episode, monitor blood pressure and heart rate. • Obtain an ECG before administering nitrates. • Record duration of pain, amount of medication required to relieve pain, and accompanying symptoms. • Obtain cardiac enzyme levels. • Administer oxygen. • Administer medications as ordered.

(continued)

Box 7-2: Acute Coronary Syndromes (continued)

Thrombotic Effect	Description	Signs and Symptoms	Diagnosis	Treatment	Nursing Considerations
Non–ST-segment elevation myocardial infarction (STEMI)	• Myocardial infarction (MI) that usually occurs due to occlusion of coronary vessel • Occlusion may be complete or partial	• Burning, squeezing, substernal or retrosternal pain spreading across chest; may radiate to inside of arm, neck, jaw, or shoulder blade; pain more intense than that of angina • Associated symptoms: shortness of breath, dizziness, nausea, palpitations, weakness, and cold sweats • Associated signs: hypertension or hypotension, tachycardia or bradycardia • Pain not relieved with rest • Difficult to distinguish from angina • S$_3$ and S$_4$ may be present	• Positive cardiac markers • ECG shows ST-segment depression or may be normal. • ECG may have ST-segment elevation for <20 minutes.	• Oxygen to increase oxygenation of the blood • Nonenteric-coated aspirin for antiplatelet effect • Beta adrenergic blockers to reduce the workload and oxygen demand • Angiotensin-converting enzyme (ACE) inhibitor to reduce afterload and preload	• Administer oxygen. • Administer medications as ordered. • Monitor ECG, vital signs, and level of consciousness (LOC). • Obtain cardiac markers. • Monitor cardiopulmonary status frequently and notify practitioner of changes.
ST-segment elevation myocardial infarction (STEMI)	• MI that usually occurs due to complete occlusion of coronary vessel	• Burning, squeezing, substernal or retrosternal pain spreading across chest; may radiate to inside of arm, neck, jaw, or shoulder blade; pain more intense than that of angina • Associated symptoms: shortness of breath, dizziness, nausea, palpitations, weakness, and cold sweats • Associated signs: hypertension or hypotension, tachycardia or bradycardia • Pain not relieved with rest • S$_3$ and S$_4$ may be present	• Positive cardiac markers • ECG shows ST-segment elevation or new left bundle branch block in leads associated with occluded artery. • Nuclear imaging studies show areas of ischemia.	• Oxygen to increase oxygenation of the blood • Non–enteric-coated aspirin for antiplatelet effect • Fibrinolytic therapy for eligible patients • Coronary angioplasty with percutaneous coronary intervention • Beta adrenergic blockers to reduce the workload and oxygen demand • ACE inhibitor to reduce afterload and preload	• Administer oxygen. • Administer medications as ordered. • Monitor ECG, vital signs, and LOC. • Obtain cardiac markers as ordered. • If patient received fibrinolytic, monitor for bleeding. • Monitor cardiopulmonary status frequently and notify practitioner of changes.

Aneurysm, Aortic

- Description
  - An aortic aneurysm is a localized or diffuse dilation of the wall of the aorta, particularly the abdominal aorta below the renal arteries
  - Causes of aortic aneurysm include atherosclerosis, severe hypertension, pregnancy (when hormonal changes affect the smooth muscle and media of the aorta), trauma, congenital abnormalities, infectious arteritis, syphilis, and Marfan syndrome (which increases aortic wall elasticity)
- Signs and symptoms
  - An abdominal aortic aneurysm may cause abdominal pulsations, abdominal aortic bruit, abdominal aching, dull lower back pain with radiation to flank and groin, nausea, and vomiting; if it ruptures, it may produce severe abdominal or lower back pain with nausea and vomiting
  - A thoracic aortic aneurysm (most common site of dissecting aneurysm) may cause cough, hoarseness, dysphagia (from pressure on the esophagus), abrupt loss of radial and femoral pulses and right and left carotid pulses, and dyspnea (from pressure on the trachea); if it ruptures, it may produce sudden, tearing pain in the chest and back
- Diagnosis and treatment
  - Diagnostic tests may include chest or abdominal X-rays, aortography, duplex ultrasonic imaging, computed tomography (CT) scan, and magnetic resonance imaging (MRI); these tests help determine the aneurysm's size, location, and shape
  - Laboratory tests may include complete blood count (CBC) and blood urea nitrogen (BUN) and creatinine levels
  - If the aneurysm is chronic and small, an antihypertensive and a negative inotropic agent may be prescribed to decrease the force of muscle contractions
  - If the aneurysm is at risk to rupture or cause damage to other organs, surgical repair may be required
- Nursing interventions
  - Monitor vital signs
  - Monitor hemodynamic variables; look for hypotension, tachycardia, bradycardia, cool and clammy skin, and tachypnea
  - Reduce anxiety by encouraging the patient to verbalize concerns and by providing emotional support
  - Relieve pain by pharmacologic and nonpharmacologic methods
  - Prepare the patient and family for surgery, if needed; discuss the procedure and their concerns about it

Aneurysm, Femoral and Popliteal

- Description
  - In femoral and popliteal aneurysms, progressive atherosclerotic changes occur in the walls (medial layer) of the femoral and popliteal arteries, resulting in a dilation or outpouching
  - The aneurysms may be fusiform (spindle-shaped) or saccular (pouchlike)
  - These aneurysms are usually progressive, eventually ending in thrombosis, embolization, and gangrene
  - Causes include atherosclerosis, bacterial infection, congenital weakness in the arterial wall (rare), and trauma (blunt or penetrating)
- Signs and symptoms
  - Characteristic signs and symptoms include a pulsating mass that disturbs peripheral circulation distal to it; pain and swelling in the affected extremity, groin, or thigh develop because of pressure on adjacent nerves and veins
  - Other signs and symptoms in the affected extremity include skin changes, a loss of pulse and color, and coldness
  - Distal petechial hemorrhages (from aneurysmal emboli) can form
- Diagnosis and treatment
  - Diagnostic tests include duplex ultrasonography to diagnose the aneurysm and CT angiography to determine its size, length, and extent; arteriography may be performed to evaluate the level of proximal and distal involvement

- Treatment consists of surgical bypass, reconstruction of the artery, or both, usually with an autogenous saphenous vein graft replacement, or replacement grafts or endovascular repair using a stent graft or wall graft (a Dacron or polytetrafluoroethylene graft with external structures made from a variety of materials, such as Nitinol, titanium, and stainless steel, for additional support)
- Nursing interventions
  - Before corrective surgery, evaluate the patient's circulatory status, noting the location and quality of peripheral pulses in the affected arm or leg
  - Administer a prophylactic antibiotic or anticoagulant as ordered
  - Discuss expected postoperative procedures with the patient, and review the surgical procedure
  - After surgery, correlate the condition of the extremity with preoperative circulatory assessment, marking the sites on the patient's skin where pulses are palpable to make repeated checks easier
  - Administer analgesics as ordered for pain
  - Help the patient walk soon after surgery to prevent venostasis and thrombus formation
  - Check the vein donor site for warmth, color, sensation, and pulses

Dysrhythmia

- Description
  - During a cardiac dysrhythmia, abnormal electrical conduction or automaticity changes heart rate and rhythm
  - Dysrhythmias vary in severity, from mild and asymptomatic ones that require no treatment (such as sinus dysrhythmia, in which heart rate increases and decreases with respirations) to catastrophic ventricular fibrillation, requiring immediate resuscitation
  - Dysrhythmias are generally classified according to their origin (atrial or ventricular); their effect on cardiac output and blood pressure, partially influenced by the site of origin, determines their clinical significance (see *The 8-step method of rhythm strip analysis*, pages 95–96)
  - Causes of dysrhythmias include congenital heart disease, degeneration of the conduction system, drug effects or toxicity, heart disease, myocardial ischemia, stress, alcohol, electrolyte imbalance, acid-base imbalances, cellular hypoxia, and conditions such as anemia, anorexia, thyroid dysfunction, adrenal insufficiency, and pulmonary disease (see *Cardiac dysrhythmias*, pages 96–98)
- Signs and symptoms
  - The patient with a dysrhythmia may be asymptomatic or may report palpitations, chest pain, dizziness, weakness, fatigue, and feelings of impending doom
  - Other signs and symptoms include an irregular heart rhythm, bradycardia or tachycardia, hypotension, syncope, reduced level of consciousness (LOC), diaphoresis, pallor, nausea, vomiting, and cold, clammy skin
  - Life-threatening dysrhythmias may result in pulselessness, absence of respirations, and no measurable blood pressure
- Nursing interventions
  - Monitor the pulse for an irregular pattern or an abnormally rapid or slow rate; if the patient is receiving continuous cardiac monitoring, observe him for dysrhythmias
  - Assess the patient for signs and symptoms of hemodynamic compromise
  - If the patient has an dysrhythmia, promptly assess his airway, breathing, and circulation
  - Initiate basic life support measures if indicated, until other advanced cardiac life support measures are available and successful
  - Perform defibrillation early for ventricular tachycardia and ventricular fibrillation
  - Administer medications as needed, and prepare for medical procedures (e.g., cardioversion or pacemaker insertion) if indicated
  - Monitor the patient for fluid and electrolyte imbalance and signs of drug toxicity, especially digoxin; correct the underlying cause and adjust medications as needed
  - Provide adequate oxygen and reduce the heart's workload while carefully maintaining metabolic, neurologic, respiratory, and hemodynamic status
  - Provide support to the patient and family
  - Tell the patient signs and symptoms of dysrhythmia to report, and teach him how to take his pulse
  - Explain all procedures such as pacemaker insertion to the patient

Box 7-3: The 8-Step Method of Rhythm Strip Analysis

Rhythm strip analysis requires a sequential and systematic approach. The following eight steps provide a good outline for you to follow.

Step 1: Determine rhythm

To determine the heart's atrial and ventricular rhythms, use either the pen-and-pencil method or the caliper method.

To determine the atrial rhythm, measure the P-P intervals, the intervals between consecutive P waves. These intervals should occur regularly, with only small variations associated with respirations. Then compare the P-P intervals in several cycles. Consistently similar P-P intervals indicate regular atrial rhythm; dissimilar P-P intervals indicate irregular atrial rhythm.

To determine the ventricular rhythm, measure the intervals between two consecutive R waves in the QRS complexes. If an R wave isn't present, use either Q waves or S waves of consecutive QRS complexes. The R-R intervals should occur regularly. Then compare the R-R intervals in several cycles. As with atrial rhythms, consistently similar intervals mean a regular rhythm; dissimilar intervals point to an irregular rhythm.

After completing your measurements, ask yourself:

- Is the rhythm regular or irregular? Consider a rhythm with only slight variations (up to 0.04 second) to be regular
- If the rhythm is irregular, is it slightly irregular or markedly irregular? Does the irregularity occur in a pattern (a regularly irregular pattern)?

Step 2: Calculate rate

You can use one of three methods to determine the atrial and ventricular heart rates from an electrocardiogram (ECG) waveform. Although these methods can provide accurate information, you shouldn't rely solely on them when assessing your patient. Keep in mind that the ECG waveform represents electrical, not mechanical, activity. Therefore, although an ECG can show that ventricular depolarization has occurred, it doesn't mean that ventricular contraction has occurred. To determine this, you must assess the patient's pulse.

- *Times-ten method.* The simplest, quickest, and most common way to calculate rate is the times-ten method, especially if the rhythm is irregular. ECG paper is marked in increments of 3 seconds, or 15 large boxes. To calculate the atrial rate, obtain a 6-second strip, count the number of P waves that appear on it, and multiply this number by 10. Ten 6-second strips equal 1 minute. Calculate the ventricular rate the same way, using the R waves
- *1,500 method.* If the heart rhythm is regular, use the 1,500 method, so named because 1,500 small squares equal 1 minute. Count the number of small squares between identical points on two consecutive P waves, and then divide 1,500 by that number to determine the atrial rate. To obtain the ventricular rate, use the same method with two consecutive R waves
- *Sequence method.* The third method of estimating heart rate is the sequence method, which requires memorizing a sequence of numbers. For the atrial rate, find a P wave that peaks on a heavy black line, and assign the following numbers to the next six heavy black lines: 300, 150, 100, 75, 60, and 50. Then find the next P-wave peak, and estimate the atrial rate, based on the number assigned to the nearest heavy black line. Estimate the ventricular rate the same way, using the R wave

Step 3: Evaluate P waves

When examining a rhythm strip for P waves, ask yourself:

- Are P waves present?
- Do the P waves have a normal configuration?
- Do all of the P waves have a similar size and shape?
- Is there one P wave for every QRS complex?

Step 4: Determine PR interval duration

To measure the PR interval, count the small squares between the start of the P wave and the start of the QRS complex; then multiply the number of squares by 0.04 second. After you perform this calculation, ask yourself:

- Does the duration of the PR interval fall within normal limits, 0.12 to 0.20 second (or 3 to 5 small squares)?
- Is the PR interval constant?

Step 5: Determine QRS complex duration

When determining QRS complex duration, make sure to measure straight across from the end of the PR interval to the end of the S wave, not just to the peak. Remember, the QRS complex has no horizontal components. To calculate duration, count the number of small squares between the beginning and the end of the QRS complex, and multiply this number by 0.04 second. Then ask yourself the following questions:

- Does the duration of the QRS complex fall within normal limits, 0.06 to 0.10 second?
- Are all QRS complexes the same size and shape? (If not, measure each one and describe them individually.)
- Does a QRS complex appear after every P wave?

(continued)

Box 7-3: The 8-Step Method of Rhythm Strip Analysis (continued)

Step 6: Evaluate T wave

Examine the T waves on the ECG strip. Then ask yourself:

- Are T waves present?
- Do all of the T waves have a normal shape?
- Could a P wave be hidden in a T wave?
- Do all of the T waves have a normal amplitude?
- Do the T waves have the same deflection as the QRS complexes?

Step 7: Determine QT interval duration

Count the number of small squares between the beginning of the QRS complex and the end of the T wave, where the T wave returns to the baseline. Multiply this number by 0.04 second. Ask yourself:

- Does the duration of the QT interval fall within normal limits, 0.36 to 0.44 second?

Step 8: Evaluate other components

Note the presence of ectopic or aberrantly conducted beats or other abnormalities. Also, check the ST segment for abnormalities, and look for the presence of a U wave.

   Next, interpret your findings by classifying the rhythm strip according to one or all of the following features:

- *Site of origin of the rhythm.* For example, sinus node, atria, atrioventricular node, or ventricles
- *Rate.* Normal (60 to 100 beats/minute), bradycardia (less than 60 beats/minute), or tachycardia (greater than 100 beats/minute)
- *Rhythm.* Normal or abnormal; for example, flutter, fibrillation, heart block, escape rhythm, or other dysrhythmias

Box 7-4: Cardiac Dysrhythmias

Normal sinus rhythm

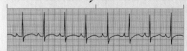

- Ventricular and atrial rates of 60 to 100 beats per minute (BPM)
- QRS complexes and P waves regular and uniform
- PR interval 0.12 to 0.2 second
- Duration of QRS complex less than 0.12 second
- Identical atrial and ventricular rates, with constant PR interval

Sinus tachycardia

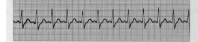

Description

- Rate greater than 100 BPM; rarely greater than 160 BPM
- Every QRS complex follows a P wave

Treatment

- Correction of underlying cause; a beta adrenergic blocker or calcium channel blocker, if symptomatic or cardiac related

Sinus bradycardia

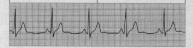

Description

- Rate less than 60 BPM
- QRS complex follows each P wave

Treatment

- For low cardiac output, dizziness, weakness, altered level of consciousness, or low blood pressure, advanced cardiac life support (ACLS) protocol for administration of atropine I.V.
- Dopamine, epinephrine, if atropine fails
- Transcutaneous pacemaker (TCP)

Paroxysmal atrial tachycardia or paroxysmal supraventricular tachycardia

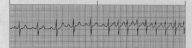

Description

- Heart rate greater than 140 BPM; rarely exceeds 250 BPM

- P waves regular but aberrant; difficult to differentiate from preceding T wave
- Sudden onset and termination of dysrhythmia
- May cause palpitations and light-headedness

Treatment

- Vagal maneuvers
- Adenosine by rapid I.V. push
- Other treatments: beta adrenergic blockers, verapamil, diltiazem, and digoxin (if it isn't the cause of dysrhythmia) to alter atrioventricular (AV) node conduction
- Elective cardioversion, if patient symptomatic and unresponsive to drugs
- Radiofrequency catheter ablation

Atrial flutter

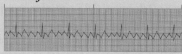

Description

- Ventricular rate depends on degree of AV block (may be 60 to 100 BPM; however, 150 BPM; isn't uncommon)
- Atrial rate 250 to 400 BPM and regular

(continued)

Box 7-4: Cardiac Dysrhythmias (continued)

- QRS complexes uniform in shape, but typically irregular in rate
- P waves may have sawtooth configuration (F waves)

Treatment

- If patient is stable, ACLS protocol for cardioversion and drug therapy including calcium channel blockers, beta adrenergic blockers, or antiarrhythmics
- If patient is unstable with a ventricular rate greater than 150 BPM, immediate cardioversion
- Radiofrequency ablation to control rhythm
- Possible anticoagulation therapy

Atrial fibrillation

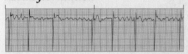

Description

- Atrial rate greater than 400 BPM; ventricular rate varies
- QRS complexes uniform in shape but at irregular intervals
- PR interval indiscernible
- No P waves, or P waves appear as erratic, irregular baseline F waves

Treatment

- If patient is unstable with a ventricular rate greater than 150 BPM, immediate cardioversion
- If patient is stable, ACLS protocol and drug therapy including calcium channel blockers, beta adrenergic blockers, or antiarrhythmics
- In some patients uncontrolled by drugs, radiofrequency ablation
- Anticoagulation therapy to reduce risk of thromboemboli

AV junctional rhythm (nodal rhythm)

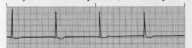

Description

- Ventricular rate usually 40 to 60 BPM (60 to 100 BPM is accelerated junctional rhythm)
- P waves may precede, be hidden within, or follow a QRS complex; if visible, they're altered

- Duration of QRS complex normal, except in aberrant conduction
- Patient may be asymptomatic unless ventricular rate very slow

Treatment

- Correction of underlying cause
- Atropine or pacemaker for slow rate
- If patient taking digoxin, it is discontinued

First-degree AV block

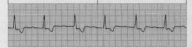

Description

- PR interval prolonged greater than 0.20 second
- QRS complex normal

Treatment

- Digoxin (cautiously)
- Correction of underlying cause; otherwise, monitoring for increasing block
- Possibly atropine, if severe symptomatic bradycardia develops

Second-degree AV block Mobitz type I (Wenckebach)

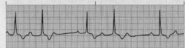

Description

- PR interval becomes progressively longer with each cycle until QRS complex disappears (dropped beat); after a dropped beat, PR interval shorter
- Ventricular rate irregular; atrial rhythm regular

Treatment

- Atropine, if patient symptomatic
- May discontinue digoxin
- Temporary pacing, if ventricular rate slow

Second-degree AV block Mobitz type II

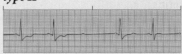

Description

- PR interval constant, with QRS complexes dropped
- Ventricular rhythm may be irregular, with varying degree of block
- Atrial rate regular

Treatment

- Temporary pacemaker, sometimes followed by permanent pacemaker
- If patient taking digoxin, it is discontinued
- Atropine, dopamine, or epinephrine for symptomatic bradycardia

Third-degree AV block (complete heart block)

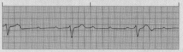

Description

- Atrial rate regular; ventricular rate slow and regular
- No relationship between P waves and QRS complexes
- No constant PR interval
- QRS interval normal (nodal pacemaker); wide and bizarre (ventricular pacemaker)

Treatment

- Usually requires TCP, followed by permanent pacemaker
- Dopamine and epinephrine to maintain blood pressure
- Atropine for symptomatic bradycardia
- Cardiopulmonary resuscitation (CPR) until pacing initiated

Premature ventricular contraction

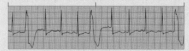

Description

- Beat occurs prematurely, usually followed by complete compensatory pause after a premature ventricular contraction (PVC); irregular pulse
- QRS complex wide and distorted
- Can occur singly, in pairs, or in threes; can alternate with normal beats; focus can be from one or more sites
- PVCs most ominous when clustered, multifocal, and with R wave on T pattern

(continued)

Box 7-4: Cardiac Dysrhythmias (continued)

Treatment
- May not be treated if patient's condition is stable
- If warranted, lidocaine, amiodarone, or procainamide I.V.
- If induced by digoxin, cessation of drug; if induced by hypokalemia, potassium chloride I.V.; if induced by hypomagnesemia, magnesium sulfate I.V.
- An oral type III agent (such as amiodarone or sotalol), if maintenance therapy necessary

Ventricular tachycardia

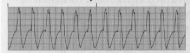

Description
- Ventricular rate 100 to 220 BPM; may be regular
- Three or more PVCs in a row
- QRS complexes wide, bizarre, and independent of P wave
- QRS complexes may be monomorphic (look alike) or polymorphic (look different)
- Usually no visible P waves
- Can produce chest pain, anxiety, palpitations, dyspnea, shock, coma, and death

Treatment
- If pulses are absent, CPR, following ACLS protocol for defibrillation and administration of epinephrine I.V. or vasopressin, followed by amiodarone, lidocaine, magnesium, or procainamide
- If pulse present with polymorphic QRS complexes and normal QT interval, beta adrenergic blockers, lidocaine, amiodarone, procainamide, or sotalol (following ACLS protocol); if drug unsuccessful, cardioversion
- If pulse present with polymorphic QRS and prolonged QT interval, magnesium I.V., then overdrive pacing if rhythm persists
- If pulse present and patient's condition stable with monomorphic QRS complexes, procainamide, sotalol, amiodarone, or lidocaine (follow ACLS protocol); if drugs ineffective, cardioversion
- Correction of underlying cause
- Maintenance therapy with drugs, such as amiodarone and sotalol
- Implanted cardiovert tachycardia defibrillator if recurrent ventricular tachycardia

Ventricular fibrillation

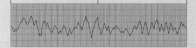

Description
- Ventricular rhythm rapid and chaotic
- No QRS complexes; no visible P waves
- Loss of consciousness, with no peripheral pulses, blood pressure, or respirations; possible seizures; sudden death

Treatment
- CPR, following ACLS protocol for defibrillation and administration of epinephrine, vasopressin, amiodarone, or lidocaine and, if ineffective, magnesium sulfate or procainamide

- Implanted cardioverter defibrillator if risk for recurrent ventricular fibrillation

Pulseless electrical activity (electromechanical dissociation)

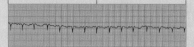

Description
- Organized electrical activity without pulse or other evidence of effective myocardial contraction
- Any rhythm possible

Treatment
- CPR
- Epinephrine
- Atropine for bradycardia
- Correction of underlying cause

Ventricular standstill (asystole)

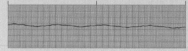

Description
- *Primary ventricular standstill:* regular P waves, no QRS complexes
- *Secondary ventricular standstill:* QRS complexes wide and slurred, occurring at irregular intervals; agonal heart rhythm
- Loss of consciousness, no peripheral pulses, blood pressure, or respirations

Treatment
- CPR
- ACLS protocol for endotracheal intubation, TCP, and epinephrine and atropine administration

Arterial Occlusive Disease

- Description
  - Arterial occlusive disease is an obstructive, usually degenerative arterial disorder representing a late stage of arteriosclerosis; it is the most common form of obstructive disease after age 30
  - Occlusion that occurs rapidly, completely and unexpectedly may be caused by atheromas such as thrombosis, embolism, and arteritis
  - Risk factors include smoking, advanced age, hypertension, hyperlipidemia, diabetes mellitus, and genetic predisposition
  - In arterial occlusive disease, atheromas partially or completely occlude arteries; the aorta and its major branches, along with the carotid, vertebral, femoral, iliac, and other arteries, may be involved; arteries in the legs are the most commonly affected

- This disorder produces symptoms when the arteries can no longer provide enough blood to supply oxygen and nutrients to the limbs and remove the waste products of metabolism
- Signs and symptoms
  - Acute arterial occlusion may produce the following five classic signs: paralysis, pain, paresthesia, pallor, and pulselessness
  - Other characteristic symptoms of arterial occlusive disease include intermittent claudication and pain in the affected limb that occurs with exercise and is relieved with 1 to 5 minutes of rest
  - Signs and symptoms can also include cool feet and hands with poor hair growth, differences in the color and size of the lower legs, altered arterial pulsations and bruits over the affected area, ischemic ulcers, a burning sensation in the feet and toes, changes to nails, and decreased or absent pulses
- Diagnosis and treatment
  - Diagnostic tests may include arteriography, Doppler ultrasonography, CT scan, and MRI
  - Treatment aims to prevent circulatory compromise
    - ○ Encourage patients to stop smoking
    - ○ Encouraged to exercise, eat a proper diet, and lose weight, if necessary
    - ○ Advise on proper posture and the need to wear nonconstrictive clothing
    - ○ Medications such as pentoxifylline (Trental, Pentoxil) may be prescribed to improve blood flow through the capillaries
    - ○ Control hypertension through drug therapy and lifestyle modifications
    - ○ An antilipemic may be necessary to lower elevated cholesterol levels; antiplatelets may also be prescribed along with antihypertensives
    - ○ Thrombolytic therapy may be given to treat arterial thrombosis
  - Surgery is used to correct the obstruction if the disease progresses rapidly and the patient otherwise is in good health
    - ○ Angioplasty and laser therapy may be performed to reestablish blood flow
    - ○ Bypass grafting may use an artificial or autologous graft
    - ○ Patch grafting replaces a damaged segment of the artery with a vein patch
    - ○ Endarterectomy strips plaques from the intimal lining
- Nursing interventions
  - Check arterial pulses frequently
  - Have the patient sleep with the head of the bed slightly elevated to aid perfusion to the lower extremities
  - Don't massage the affected extremities because massage could further damage tissue
  - Instruct to dress warmly and to avoid exposing the affected extremity to extreme temperatures
  - Discuss gradual exercise programs, proper diet, and skin care
  - Perform appropriate postoperative care
    - ○ Assess the affected extremity and check distal and proximal pulses
    - ○ Maintain the patient on bed rest for 12 to 24 hours after surgery
    - ○ Avoid sharp flexion of the affected extremity
    - ○ Assess for signs and symptoms of infection

Buerger's Disease

- Description
  - Buerger's disease, also called thromboangiitis obliterans, is an inflammatory, nonatheromatous occlusive condition that causes segmental lesions and subsequent thrombus formation in the small and medium arteries (and sometimes the veins), resulting in decreased blood flow to the feet and legs
  - It usually occurs in men between ages 20 and 40 and in heavy smokers; and recently, women and people over 50 have been added as at risk
- Signs and symptoms
  - Buerger's disease typically causes intermittent claudication of the instep, legs, arms, or hands, which is aggravated by exercise and relieved by rest
  - Pulses are diminished or absent, and the patient may experience coldness, numbness, tingling, or burning in the affected extremity

- As the disease progresses, redness, heat, tingling, or cyanosis may appear when the extremity is in a dependent position, and ulcers and gangrene may appear
- Diagnosis and treatment
  - Angiography is the most common imaging used to diagnose Buerger's disease
  - For patients with severe disease, lumbar sympathectomy may improve blood flow through vasodilation
  - Amputation may be necessary for nonhealing ulcers, intractable pain, or gangrene
  - Vasodilator therapy hasn't proved to be effective, but pentoxifylline (Pentoxil), calcium channel blockers, and thromboxane inhibitors may be helpful, especially if vasospasm is present
  - Smoking cessation is the single most effective treatment for Buerger's disease
- Nursing interventions
  - Educate about smoking cessation to minimize impact on symptoms
  - Teach to avoid excessive cold temperatures to reduce vasoconstriction
  - Avoid the use of vasoconstricting medications
  - Teach the patient to take measures to protect the extremities from trauma and infection
  - Encourage the patient to participate in progressive exercise

Cardiomyopathy

- Description
  - Cardiomyopathy is a disease of the heart muscle, reducing cardiac output and eventually resulting in heart failure
  - Cardiomyopathy is classified by the structural and functional abnormalities of the heart muscle; types include dilated, or congestive (most common form; dilated cardiac chambers contract poorly, causing blood to pool and thrombi to form); hypertrophic obstructive (hypertrophied left ventricle is small, unable to relax and fill properly); restrictive (rare form; stiff ventricles are resistant to filling); arrhythmogenic right ventricular; and unclassified
  - Causes of dilated cardiomyopathy include chronic alcoholism, viral or bacterial infection, metabolic and immunologic disorders, and pregnancy and postpartum disorders; causes of hypertrophic cardiomyopathy include congenital disorders and hypertension; restrictive cardiomyopathy may be idiopathic, or it may stem from amyloidosis, cancer, or heart transplant; arrhythmogenic right ventricular cardiomyopathy most likely has a genetic cause and results from the infiltration of fibrous and adipose tissue into the myocardium; unclassified cardiomyopathy doesn't fit into other categories and can have various causes
  - Cardiomyopathy may also be genetic
- Signs and symptoms
  - Signs and symptoms of heart failure are present, including tachycardia, S_3 and S_4 heart sounds, exertional dyspnea, paroxysmal nocturnal dyspnea, cough, fatigue, jugular venous distention, dependent pitting edema, peripheral cyanosis, and hepatomegaly
  - Heart murmurs and dysrhythmias may also occur
- Diagnosis and treatment
  - Diagnostic tests include electrocardiogram (ECG), echocardiogram, cardiac catheterization, radionuclide studies, and chest X-ray
  - Medications for dilated cardiomyopathy include an angiotensin-converting enzyme (ACE) inhibitor or hydralazine plus a nitrate (the mainstay of therapy), a beta adrenergic blocker, digoxin, a diuretic, and an anticoagulant
  - Medications for hypertrophic cardiomyopathy include a beta adrenergic blocker and a calcium channel blocker
  - No specific medications are used to treat restrictive cardiomyopathy; however, diuretics, digoxin, nitrates, and other vasodilators can worsen the condition and should be avoided
  - An antiarrhythmic, a pacemaker, or an implantable cardiac defibrillator may be necessary to control dysrhythmias
  - Surgery, such as heart transplantation or cardiomyoplasty (for dilated cardiomyopathy) or ventricular myotomy or myectomy (for hypertrophic obstructive cardiomyopathy), may be indicated if medications fail

- Nursing interventions
  - Monitor ECG results, cardiovascular status, vital signs, and hemodynamic variables to detect heart failure and dysrhythmias and assess the patient's response to medications
  - If the patient is receiving a diuretic, monitor his serum electrolyte levels to detect abnormalities such as hypokalemia
  - Administer oxygen and keep the patient in semi-Fowler's position to promote oxygenation
  - Make sure the patient restricts activity if necessary to reduce oxygen demands on the heart
  - Teach the patient the signs and symptoms of heart failure to report to the practitioner
  - Explain the importance of checking weight daily and reporting an increase of 3 lb (1.4 kg) or more (1 L of fluid equals 1 kg or 2.2 lb)
  - Encourage the patient to express feelings, such as a fear of dying

Coronary Heart Disease

- Description
  - In coronary heart disease (CHD), plaque, a thick, oily substance in the blood, builds up and partially or totally occludes the coronary artery vasculature; it is the leading cause of death and disease in the United States
  - Some risk factors for CHD can't be modified: old age, male gender, and family history of heart disease
  - Other risk factors can be modified: increased levels of triglycerides, low-density lipoprotein, and very-low-density lipoprotein; high-fat diet; hypertension; obesity; diabetes; cigarette smoking; sedentary lifestyle; and high stress level
  - CHD begins when endothelial cells in the arterial lining are injured, making them permeable to lipoproteins
    - ○ Clot-forming platelets adhere to the injury site, and lipoproteins build up around smooth muscle cells, causing fatty streaks
    - ○ Fibrofatty plaques form from repeated injury to the endothelial cells; as the process is repeated, the vessel progressively narrows
    - ○ Plaques can rupture, causing emboli, or can worsen and compromise myocardial oxygenation and blood flow, thus precipitating angina or MI
- Signs and symptoms
  - Anginal pain is a classic symptom of CHD (see *Angina*, page 102)
  - Others include the secondary effects of CHD, such as MI, heart failure, sudden cardiac death, cardiomegaly, valvular insufficiencies, cardiogenic shock, and stroke
- Diagnosis and treatment
  - Diagnostic tests may include ECG, exercise ECG (stress test), cardiac catheterization, coronary angiography, intravascular ultrasound, myocardial perfusion imaging, and echocardiography
  - Laboratory tests for cardiac isoenzymes (CK-MB and LD_1), troponin, myoglobin, cholesterol, lipoproteins, and triglycerides also may be performed
  - Treatment aims to modify risk factors for CHD to prevent acute myocardial events (e.g., smoking cessation, decreased intake of dietary fat, and increased activity level); treatment may also include medication for anginal pain as well as beta adrenergic blockers, calcium channel blockers, antiplatelet, antilipemic, antihypertensive drugs, and oxygen therapy
  - Surgical treatment, such as angioplasty, rotational atherectomy or stent placement, percutaneous transluminal coronary angioplasty, or coronary artery bypass grafting (CABG), may be required to prevent progression to MI (see *Nursing care of the cardiac surgical patient requiring CABG*, page 103)
- Nursing interventions
  - Increase the patient's knowledge of the relationship between risk factors and the development of CHD
  - Teach the patient and family how to modify risk factors
  - Encourage the patient to establish healthful habits, such as regular exercise and a low-fat diet
  - Encourage participation in a smoking cessation program
  - Emphasize the importance of prevention in treating heart disease
  - Administer medication for anginal pain as ordered

Box 7-5: Angina

Description

- Four types of angina exist: stable (angina that hasn't increased in severity or frequency over several months), unstable (angina that has increased in frequency, severity, or duration or has changed in quality and occurs with minimal exertion and rest), Prinzmetal's or variant (angina that occurs at rest, long after exercise, or during sleep), and microvascular (angina-like chest pain due to impairment of vasodilator reserve in patients with normal coronary arteries)
- Angina may result from atherosclerosis of coronary arteries, vasospasm, or hypotension that decreases blood flow through these arteries

Signs and symptoms

- The major symptom is substernal or anterior chest pain that may radiate to the arms, neck, jaw, and shoulders; it may be described as mild-to-moderate pressure, tightness, squeezing, burning, smothering, indigestion, choking, or mild soreness; the patient may exhibit Levine's sign (clenched fist over sternum)
- Atypical chest pain, such as arm or shoulder pain; jaw, neck, or throat pain; toothache; back pain; or pain under the breastbone or in the stomach is likely to be seen in women
- Related signs and symptoms include shortness of breath, diaphoresis, nausea, increased heart rate, pallor, weak or numb feelings in the arms and hands, and unexplained anxiety

Diagnosis and treatment

- Diagnostic tests may include electrocardiogram (ECG) (a patient with stable or unstable angina may have ST-segment depression; a patient with Prinzmetal's angina, ST-segment elevation), exercise ECG (stress test), cardiac catheterization, radioisotope imaging, and echocardiogram
- Laboratory tests may include levels of cardiac isoenzymes (creatine kinase [CK], CK-MB, and lactate dehydrogenase), troponin, myoglobin, cholesterol, lipoproteins, triglycerides, high-sensitivity C-reactive protein, and homocysteine
- Treatment aims to decrease myocardial oxygen demand and increase myocardial oxygen supply
- Precipitating factors—such as exercise, overexertion, emotional upset, cold weather, and large meals—are identified and avoided if possible
- Exercise programs are prescribed to build collateral circulation and increase myocardial efficiency
- A nitrate (e.g., nitroglycerin in oral, sublingual, spray, ointment, or patch forms; isosorbide dinitrate; or isosorbide mononitrate), a beta adrenergic blocker, a calcium channel blocker, or an antiplatelet drug (e.g., aspirin, clopidogrel [Plavix], or ticlopidine [Ticlid]) also may be prescribed to relieve symptoms
- A calcium channel blocker may be useful for a patient with Prinzmetal's or variant angina (see *Nursing implications in clinical pharmacology*, pages 348–362)
- Angioplasty, stent placement, laser therapy, or atherectomy may be necessary to treat stable but debilitating anginal pain

Nursing interventions

- Tell the patient to call an ambulance and seek medical attention immediately if the angina persists or changes in quality or severity or if other symptoms develop
- Inform the patient and family that angina is more easily evoked in cold weather and in times of emotional upset or extreme stress; these conditions should be avoided if possible
- Discuss structured exercise regimens, and encourage family support
- Instruct the patient to plan rest periods between activities to prevent fatigue
- Tell the patient to take medications exactly as prescribed and not to change the medications without first consulting the practitioner
- Educate the patient about nitroglycerin
- Teach the patient how to take nitroglycerin before certain activities to prevent angina and how to take it for acute anginal episodes (e.g., to sit down when taking the tablet, to take one tablet at 5-minute intervals but not to exceed three tablets, and to be aware that a burning sensation will be felt under the tongue)
- Tell the patient to dispose of nitroglycerin that has been open for more than 6 months and to keep the tablets in a container protected from heat, light, and moisture
- Tell the patient and family to carry antianginal medications and nitroglycerin when traveling, even on short trips
- Emphasize to the family the importance of learning cardiopulmonary resuscitation and basic life support
- Prepare the patient and family for surgery (if indicated), and offer psychological and emotional support
- Reinforce the importance of lifestyle modifications, such as diet, exercise, stress reduction, and smoking cessation

Box 7-6: Nursing Care of the Cardiac Surgical Patient Requiring CABG

The medical-surgical nurse is an integral part of the multidisciplinary team caring for the patient undergoing coronary artery bypass grafting (CABG). The nurse's astute assessments and prompt interventions can affect the patient's experience of and recovery from CABG.

Preoperative Care

- Obtain an accurate and complete medical history. The degree of cardiac impairment is demonstrated by the patient's lifestyle limitations
- Assess the patient's physiologic status before surgery. Baseline vital signs, integrity of pulses and extremities, neurologic status, respiratory status, height, weight, nutritional status, elimination patterns, and psychological status should be assessed and recorded
- Teach the patient and family about the surgery and the immediate postoperative period in the intensive care unit. Prepare them for postoperative equipment that will be used, such as pulmonary artery lines, chest tubes, I.V. lines, indwelling urinary catheters, and equipment for mechanical ventilation and cardiac monitoring
- Discuss specific issues with the patient and family. For example, the patient should always report pain. (Reassure a patient who will be intubated and unable to speak that pain will be detected by facial grimaces and other physiologic measures.) Bloody drainage in the chest tube is normal, as is feeling the need to void while the urinary catheter is in place. The tubes and lines may restrict patient movement, but the nurse should help the patient to prevent injury
- Ask if the patient has an advanced directive in place

Intraoperative Procedure

- The patient is placed on a cardiopulmonary bypass machine, which drains blood from the left ventricle and atrium and passes it through a pulsatile or roller pump to the femoral artery or descending aorta. Pulmonary circulation isn't interrupted
- Myocardial tissue is preserved during surgery by arresting the heart with a cardioplegic solution, which usually is cold (39.4°F [4.1°C]). External cooling also may be achieved with a slush saline solution administered into the pericardium
- After the patient is cooled sufficiently, bypass grafts, which are usually harvested from saphenous veins in the legs, are placed surgically from the aorta to sites distal to the occlusions on coronary arteries. The internal mammary artery may also be rerouted to bypass an occlusion
- After the procedure is completed, the blood in the bypass machine is slowly warmed, and the patient's body temperature is returned to normal. While the incisions are closed, epicardial pacing wires are placed and grounded, and chest tubes are inserted

Postoperative Care

- Achieve and maintain body temperature. Monitor cardiovascular function with serial blood pressure, hemodynamic monitoring (cardiac output, central venous pressure, pulmonary artery wedge pressure, systemic vascular resistance), and electrocardiogram evaluations, and maintain it with various medications. Monitor drainage from chest tubes in the mediastinal area, and assess peripheral pulses
- Turn the patient every 2 hours to promote drainage. A sudden change in drainage color to bright red, hemorrhaging that lasts more than 1 minute, or cessation of drainage are abnormal; report them to the practitioner immediately
- Monitor respiratory status. Maintain an open airway at all times. Promote aggressive pulmonary hygiene
- Inform the practitioner if the patient doesn't awaken 1 to 3 hours after surgery. Report any neurologic change from the baseline value
- Maintain adequate renal circulation. Postoperative renal insufficiency is caused by complications of extracorporeal circulation during surgery and can lead to the need for hemodialysis if permanent damage occurs
- Document daily weight and fluid intake and output. Monitor serum electrolytes frequently
- Make the patient as comfortable as possible; for example, by administering an opioid analgesic or positioning for comfort
- Organize activities so that the patient can rest frequently. A structured program of early, progressive ambulation and activity can be helpful, but must allow for individual differences
- Provide a program of cardiac risk modification. Encourage participation in a cardiac rehabilitation program

Endocarditis

- Description
  - Endocarditis is an infection of the lining of the endocardium, heart valves, or a cardiac prosthesis resulting from bacterial (particularly streptococci, staphylococci, or enterococci) or fungal invasion
  - Conditions that increase the risk of endocarditis are having a prosthetic heart valve or having a damaged heart valve—for example, from rheumatic fever, syphilis, a congenital heart or heart valve defect, mitral valve prolapse with a murmur, hypertrophic cardiomyopathy, Marfan syndrome, or I.V. drug abuse
- Signs and symptoms
  - Nonspecific signs and symptoms include chills, diaphoresis, fatigue, weakness, anorexia, weight loss, pleuritic pain, and arthralgia (intermittent fever and night sweats may recur for weeks)
  - The classic physical sign of endocarditis is a loud, regurgitant heart murmur, or sudden change in an existing murmur, or the discovery of a new murmur along with fever
  - Other signs include petechiae of the skin and mucous membranes and splinter hemorrhages under the nails
  - Rarely, endocarditis produces Osler's nodes (tender, raised subcutaneous lesions on the fingers or toes), Roth's spots (hemorrhagic areas with white centers on the retina), and Janeway lesions (purplish macules on the palms or soles)
  - Embolization from vegetating lesions or diseased valve tissues may produce specific signs and symptoms of infarction of splenic, renal, cerebral, pulmonary, or peripheral vascular infarction
- Diagnosis and treatment
  - Diagnostic tests may include echocardiogram and ECG
  - Laboratory tests may include white blood cell (WBC) count, erythrocyte sedimentation rate, and serum rheumatoid factor
  - Three or more blood cultures in a 24- to 48-hour period identify the causative organism
  - An antibiotic is prescribed, based on the infecting organism; an I.V. antibiotic lasting 4 to 6 weeks is usually prescribed, followed by a course of oral antibiotics
  - Surgery may be necessary to repair or replace a defective heart valve
- Nursing interventions
  - Make sure the patient maintains bed rest to reduce myocardial oxygen demands
  - Encourage adequate fluid intake
  - Watch for signs and symptoms of embolization (such as hematuria, flank pain, pleuritic chest pain, dyspnea, left upper quadrant pain, neurologic deficits, and numbness and tingling of the extremities)
  - Assess the patient for signs and symptoms of heart failure, such as dyspnea, tachycardia, tachypnea, crackles, neck vein distention, edema, and weight gain
  - Suggest quiet diversionary activities to prevent excessive physical exertion
  - Teach the patient about the need for prophylactic antibiotics when undergoing invasive procedures, such as dental work; genitourinary, GI, or gynecologic procedures; or childbirth
  - Tell the patient about signs and symptoms of endocarditis that should immediately be reported to the practitioner

Heart Failure

- Description
  - Heart failure is a condition in which the heart can no longer pump enough blood to meet the body's demands
  - Left-sided heart failure may be caused by anterior MI, ventricular septal defect, cardiomyopathy, cardiac tamponade, constrictive pericarditis, increased circulating blood volume, aortic stenosis and insufficiency, or mitral stenosis and insufficiency
  - Right-sided heart failure may be caused by left-sided heart failure, a right ventricular MI, atrial septal defect, fluid overload and sodium retention, mitral stenosis, pulmonary embolism, pulmonary outflow stenosis, chronic obstructive pulmonary disease, pulmonary hypertension (cor pulmonale), or thyrotoxicosis
  - With left-sided heart failure, the diseased left ventricle can't pump effectively because of decreased cardiac output, decreased contractility, increased volume, and increased left ventricular pressure
    - The left atrium can't empty into the left ventricle, causing increased pressure in the left atrium; this pressure increase affects the lungs, causing pulmonary congestion that leads to decreased oxygenation
    - Increased pressure in the lungs causes increased right-sided heart pressure; the right ventricle can't relieve the pressure by emptying into the lungs, which impairs venous return to the right side of the heart
    - As systemic pressure builds, body organs become congested with venous blood

- Heart failure may also be classified as systolic or diastolic dysfunction
  - With systolic dysfunction, poor ventricular contraction results in inadequate emptying of the ventricle
  - With diastolic dysfunction, reduced ventricular compliance results in increased resistance to ventricular filling
- High-output failure may occur in high-output states, such as anemia, pregnancy, thyrotoxicosis, beriberi, and arteriovenous fistula
  - High-output failure results in high cardiac output and leads to ventricular dysfunction
  - Despite increased cardiac output, the heart is unable to meet the body's increased metabolic needs
- Signs and symptoms
  - Both right- and left-sided heart failure may cause chest discomfort, shortness of breath, paroxysmal nocturnal dyspnea, bloating, edema in the extremities, jugular venous distention, and decreased urine output
  - Left-sided heart failure also may produce anxiety, orthopnea, dyspnea on exertion and at night, Cheyne-Stokes respirations, cough with frothy sputum, diaphoresis, crackles, rhonchi, cyanosis of extremities, respiratory acidosis, hypoxia, increased pulmonary artery pressures (determined with a pulmonary artery catheter), mental confusion, abnormal heart sounds (S_3 and S_4), fatigue, lethargy, mitral insufficiency murmur, oliguria, edema, anoxia, and nausea
  - Right-sided heart failure also may produce hepatomegaly, anorexia, nausea, splenomegaly, dependent edema, hepatojugular reflex, bounding peripheral pulses, oliguria, dysrhythmias, increased right- and left-sided heart pressures (determined with a pulmonary artery catheter), Kussmaul's respirations, abnormal heart sounds (S_3 and S_4), fatigue, lethargy, abdominal pain, and weight gain
- Diagnosis and treatment
  - Diagnostic tests may include ECG, chest X-ray, echocardiography, pulmonary artery catheter insertion, and arterial blood gas studies
  - Laboratory tests may include a CBC; liver function tests; serum creatinine, BUN, electrolyte, and glucose; albumin levels (patients with atrial fibrillation should have thyroid function tests performed); and B-type natriuretic peptide
  - The goals of treatment are to decrease cardiac workload, increase cardiac output and contractility, decrease fluid and sodium retention, and decrease venous congestion
  - Activity is restricted to decrease cardiac workload
  - Oxygen may be administered to counteract desaturation
    Chronically symptomatic patients with reduced cardiac output should be treated with an ACE inhibitor or and angiotensin receptor blocker and angiotensin receptor-neprilysin inhibitor (ARNI; valsartan), with a beta adrenergic blocker and an aldosterone antagonist
    - Diuretics and vasodilators should be avoided in patients with diastolic dysfunction because they may not be able to tolerate reduced blood pressure or reduced volume
    - Other drugs that may be useful in treating heart failure include vasodilators (such as hydralazine) combined with a nitrate (such as isosorbide), angiotensin II receptor blockers in patients who can't tolerate ACE inhibitors, or nesiritide (a human B-type natriuretic peptide) to augment diuresis and decrease afterload
    - ACE inhibitors should never be given to patients who have experienced angioedema
    - Patients with acute pulmonary edema may also be treated with nitroglycerin I.V., morphine sulfate, oxygen, and mechanical ventilation
  - If the patient has high-output failure, correct the underlying cause
- Nursing interventions
  - Monitor the patient for common signs and symptoms of heart failure, such as chest discomfort, shortness of breath, and paroxysmal nocturnal dyspnea
  - Also watch for signs and symptoms of left-sided heart failure, such as anxiety, orthopnea, and abnormal breath sounds
  - Monitor for signs and symptoms of right-sided heart failure, such as jugular venous distension, hepatomegaly, splenomegaly, peripheral edema, and bounding peripheral pulses
  - Encourage bed rest in semi-Fowler's position for ease of breathing
  - Provide rest intervals between periods of activity
  - Restrict fluids as prescribed
  - Administer medications as prescribed, and monitor for their therapeutic and adverse effects (see *Nursing implications in clinical pharmacology*, pages 348–362)
  - Monitor fluid intake and output
  - Administer oxygen as prescribed

- Monitor vital signs carefully, especially when administering vasoactive drugs
- Check the patient's weight daily
- Frequently assess for cardiac and respiratory signs of heart failure
- Note changes that suggest worsening of heart failure or fluid imbalance
- Explain procedures and provide reassurance to decrease patient and family anxiety
- Teach the patient and family about medications and the importance of careful management of fluids, sodium intake, and weight

Hypertension

- Description
  - Hypertension is persistent high blood pressure, usually defined as a systolic pressure of 140 mm Hg or higher, or a diastolic pressure above 90 mm Hg based on two or more consecutive readings over a 2-week period (see *Classifying blood pressure readings*, page 107)
  - Three types of hypertension exist: essential or idiopathic (elevated blood pressure of unknown cause), secondary (elevated blood pressure of known cause, such as renovascular disease, pregnancy, and coarctation of the aorta), and malignant (severe, fulminant form with a diastolic pressure above 140 mm Hg)
  - Hypertension may result from renovascular disease, toxemia of pregnancy, pheochromocytoma, pituitary tumor, coarctation of the aorta, adrenocortical hyperfunction, Cushing's syndrome, polycythemia, atherosclerosis, and some medications; a genetic predisposition, smoking, diabetes, stress, sedentary lifestyle, and obesity increase the risk of developing hypertension
- Signs and symptoms
  - The cardinal sign is consistently elevated blood pressure although there may be no other symptoms or physical findings
  - Related signs and symptoms may include headache (usually in the morning), dizziness, bruits, flushed face, epistaxis, blurred vision, retinopathy, retinal hemorrhages, restlessness, crackles, and dyspnea (if the lungs are involved)
- Diagnosis and treatment
  - Diagnostic tests depend on the suspected cause or effects of hypertension
    - For example, kidney function tests, such as urinalysis and creatinine and BUN levels, may be performed because renal damage can cause hypertension
    - ECG, chest X-ray, and echocardiography may be done to determine if hypertension has affected cardiac function
    - Ophthalmic examination may reflect retinal damage
  - Diet, exercise, and lifestyle modifications (such as smoking cessation, reducing alcohol intake, stress management, and weight reduction) are recommended first
  - If nonpharmacologic measures fail to maintain blood pressure within normal limits, antihypertensives, such as diuretics, ACE inhibitors, beta adrenergic blockers, calcium channel blockers, angiotensin II receptor blockers, alpha adrenergic blockers, and combined alpha and beta adrenergic blockers, are prescribed
- Nursing interventions
  - Monitor the patient's blood pressure regularly, and assess for other signs and symptoms of hypertension, such as headache and retinal hemorrhages
  - Provide a calm, quiet environment
  - Teach the patient and family about weight control, stress reduction, and smoking cessation
  - Discuss the importance of a low-sodium diet; include the dietitian in teaching low-sodium recipes and recipe modification for the patient and the person who does the cooking
  - Instruct the patient on how to take blood pressure
  - Administer antihypertensive medications as prescribed; teach the patient to take medications at the same time every day
  - Advise the patient to stand up slowly when on antihypertensive therapy because antihypertensive medications can cause dizziness
  - Emphasize the importance of adhering to the medication regimen
  - Advise to avoid alcohol during antihypertensive therapy

Box 7-7: Classifying Blood Pressure Readings

In 2015, the National Institutes of Health updated recommendations first reported in the Seventh Report of the Joint National Committee on Prevention, Detection, Evaluation, and Treatment of High Blood Pressure. Categories now are normal, prehypertension, and stages 1 and 2 hypertension.

The revised categories are based on the average of two or more readings taken on separate visits after an initial screening. They apply to adults age 18 and older. (If the systolic and diastolic pressures fall into different categories, use the higher of the two readings to classify the readings.)

Patients with prehypertension are at increased risk of developing hypertension and should follow health-promoting lifestyle modifications to prevent cardiovascular disease. Patients with diabetes mellitus or chronic renal disease should be treated to keep their blood pressure below 130/80 to help prevent complications of these diseases.

Stages	Systolic (Top Number)		Diastolic (Bottom Number)
Prehypertension	120 to 139	OR	80 to 89
High blood pressure stage 1	140 to 159	OR	90 to 99
High blood pressure stage 2	160 or higher	OR	100 or higher

Myocarditis

- Description
  - Myocarditis is a focal or diffuse inflammatory process involving the myocardium; it may be acute or chronic
  - The underlying cause is most often an infectious organism that triggers an autoimmune, cellular, and humoral reaction; the heart muscle weakens and contractility decreases; the conduction system can also be affected
  - The disorder can result in heart dilation, heart failure, thrombi on the heart wall (mural thrombi), infiltration of circulating blood cells around coronary vessels and between muscle fibers, and degeneration of the muscle fibers themselves
  - Most patients with mild signs and symptoms recover completely, but some develop cardiomyopathy, heart failure, and dysrhythmias
- Signs and symptoms
  - The signs and symptoms of acute myocarditis depend on the type of infection, the degree of myocardial damage, and the capacity of the myocardium to recover
  - Patients may be asymptomatic, with an infection that resolves on its own
  - Initially, flulike signs and symptoms typically occur
  - Mild-to-moderate symptoms include fatigue, dyspnea, palpitations, and occasional discomfort in the chest and upper abdomen
  - Severe congestive heart failure can quickly develop, and sudden cardiac death can occur
- Diagnosis and treatment
  - Laboratory tests include cardiac enzyme levels, including creatine kinase (CK), CK-MB, aspartate aminotransferase, and lactate dehydrogenase, which are elevated; troponin T and I levels are also elevated
  - WBC count, C-reactive protein, and erythrocyte sedimentation rate are all elevated
  - Antibody titers such as antistreptolysin-O titer in rheumatic fever are elevated
  - Stool cultures, throat or pharyngeal washings, and other body fluid cultures show the causative bacteria or virus
  - Diagnostic tests include two-dimensional echocardiography, which may reveal impaired systolic or diastolic ventricular function or both
  - A chest X-ray may show cardiomegaly, pulmonary edema, and possible pleural effusions
  - Cardiac angiography helps rule out cardiac ischemia as a cause
  - MRI reveals the extent of inflammation and cellular edema
  - Biopsy of the endomyocardium can confirm the diagnosis

- Although electrocardiography can produce highly variable results, it may show sinus tachycardia; diffuse ST segments; T-wave abnormalities, such as T-wave inversion, ST-segment elevation, and bundle branch block; conduction defects (prolonged PR interval); and ventricular and supraventricular ectopic dysrhythmias
- Nursing interventions
  - Assess the patient for resolution of tachycardia, fever, and any other clinical manifestations
  - Focus your cardiovascular assessment on signs and symptoms of heart failure and dysrhythmias
  - For a patient with dysrhythmias, provide continuous cardiac monitoring, with personnel and equipment readily available to treat life-threatening dysrhythmias
  - Provide ventricular assistance if needed
  - Closely monitor patients prescribed digoxin for indications of digitalis toxicity, such as dysrhythmias, anorexia, nausea, vomiting, headache, and malaise, since patients with myocarditis are sensitive to digitalis
  - Use antiembolism stockings and provide passive and active range-of-motion exercises for patients on bed rest to help prevent embolization from venous thrombosis and mural thrombi

Pericarditis

- Description
  - Pericarditis refers to an inflammation and irritation of the pericardium, the fibroserous sac that envelops, supports, and protects the heart
  - It may develop as a primary illness or secondary to medical disorders or surgical procedures and may be classified as acute or chronic
  - The acute form is characterized by serous, purulent, or hemorrhagic exudates; the chronic form is characterized by dense, fibrous pericardial thickening that constricts the heart
  - Pericarditis may be idiopathic, or it may result from infection that causes inflammation, connective tissue disorders, immune reactions, MI, pneumonia, pleural disease, cancer, trauma, or renal failure
  - Complications include pericardial effusion, cardiac tamponade, and heart failure
- Signs and symptoms
  - Pericarditis may be asymptomatic; when symptoms do occur, the most common is a sharp, piercing, sudden chest pain that typically starts over the sternum and radiates to the neck, shoulders, back, and arms
  - Other symptoms include pleuritic pain that increases with laying down or deep inspiration and decreases when the patient sits up and leans forward, dyspnea, dry cough, low-grade fever, pericardial friction rub, hypotension, and tachycardia
- Diagnosis and treatment
  - Diagnostic tests may include echocardiography, which shows the extent of pericardial effusion; cardiac MRI to show changes in the endocardium; chest X-ray to determine heart size and amount of fluid in the pericardium; and ECG, which may show ST-segment elevation in multiple leads
  - Laboratory tests may include WBC count, sedimentation rate, and C-reactive protein, which are all elevated
  - Identifying and treating the underlying cause guide therapy
  - Drug therapy may include analgesics and nonsteroidal anti-inflammatory drugs, such as aspirin or ibuprofen (Motrin), for pain relief during the acute phase
  - Pericardiocentesis removes some of the pericardial fluid, reduces pressure, and can be cultured to reveal the causative infectious agent
  - Surgical removal of the tough encasing pericardium (pericardiectomy) may be necessary to release both ventricles from the constrictive and restrictive inflammation and scarring
- Nursing interventions
  - Administer pain medications as needed as well as steroids and other anti-inflammatory agents; give with food to minimize the risk of GI complications
  - Administer an antibiotic or antifungal agent based on the underlying causative organism
  - Prepare the patient for pericardiocentesis if signs and symptoms of cardiac tamponade develop, which may begin with shortness of breath, chest tightness, or dizziness; developing signs include progressive restlessness and a drop of 10 mm Hg or more in the systolic blood pressure during inspiration (pulsus paradoxus)
  - Prepare the patient for pericardiectomy or pericardiotomy (pericardial window)

- Provide appropriate postoperative care
- Supply oxygen therapy as needed
- Monitor the patient's hemodynamics
- Place the patient upright to relieve dyspnea and chest pain; allow for frequent rest periods, and cluster activities to reduce energy expenditure and oxygen demand
- Encourage the patient to express concerns about the effects of activity restrictions on his normal routines and responsibilities

Raynaud's Disease

- Description
  - Raynaud's disease is characterized by episodic vasospasm in the small peripheral arteries and arterioles, precipitated by exposure to cold or stress
  - This disease is most prevalent in women and usually develops between puberty and age 40
  - Raynaud's disease may be primary or secondary; primary disease is idiopathic, and symptoms occur without an underlying disease or associated condition
  - Secondary Raynaud's disease is a condition commonly associated with connective tissue disorders—such as scleroderma, systemic lupus erythematosus, and polymyositis—and has a progressive course, leading to ischemia, gangrene, and amputation
- Signs and symptoms
  - After exposure to cold or stress, the skin of the fingers typically blanches and then becomes cyanotic before changing to red; numbness and tingling may also occur
  - In long-standing disease, trophic changes, such as sclerodactyly, ulcerations, or chronic paronychia, may result (ulceration and gangrene are rare)
- Diagnosis and treatment
  - Diagnostic tests may include Doppler studies, arteriography, plethysmography, and antinuclear antibody titer
  - Drug treatment includes vasodilators, such as phenoxybenzamine, calcium channel blockers, and adrenergic blockers; pentoxifylline may also be effective
  - Sympathectomy may be performed if conservative measures fail to prevent ischemic ulcers
- Nursing interventions
  - Teach the patient to avoid exposure to the cold
  - Advise the patient to avoid stressful situations and to stop smoking; teach the patient biofeedback and relaxation exercises
  - Teach the patient to inspect the skin and to seek immediate treatment for signs of skin breakdown or infection

Thrombophlebitis

- Description
  - Thrombophlebitis is marked by inflammation of the venous wall and thrombus formation of the deep or superficial veins
  - Deep vein thrombophlebitis may lead to occlusion of the vessels or systemic embolization such as pulmonary embolism
  - Several conditions may lead to thrombophlebitis, including hypercoagulability (such as from cancer, blood dyscrasias, or oral contraceptives), injury to the venous wall (such as from I.V. injections, fractures, antibiotics, or infection), and venous stasis (such as from varicose veins, pregnancy, heart failure, or prolonged bed rest)
- Signs and symptoms
  - Deep vein thrombophlebitis will sometimes cause no clinical symptoms or physical findings; when they do occur, they may include cramping pain, edema, positive Homans' sign, tenderness to touch, fever, chills, and malaise
  - Superficial thrombophlebitis produces visible and palpable signs, such as heat, pain, swelling, rubor, tenderness, and induration along the affected vein's length

- Diagnosis and treatment
  - Diagnostic tests may include photoplethysmography, Doppler ultrasonography, and venography; laboratory tests include a CBC
  - Superficial thrombophlebitis may require no specific therapy other than treatment for symptoms
  - An anticoagulant (initially I.V. heparin or low-molecular-weight heparin followed by oral warfarin [Coumadin]) or newer anticoagulants such as Pradaxa (dabigatran) is administered to prolong clotting time
  - Thrombolytic therapy (such as streptokinase [Streptase]) is indicated for acute, extensive deep vein thrombophlebitis
  - Embolectomy, venous ligation, or insertion of a vena caval umbrella or filter may also be indicated
- Nursing interventions
  - If the patient is receiving a thrombolytic, heparin, or warfarin (Coumadin), monitor for signs and symptoms of bleeding
  - If the patient is receiving heparin, measure partial thromboplastin time (PTT) regularly; if the patient is receiving warfarin, measure prothrombin time (PT) and international normalized ratio (INR) (therapeutic values for PTT and PT are 1½ to 2 times control values; for INR, between 2 and 3); no monitoring is needed for Pradaxa
  - Assess the patient for signs and symptoms of pulmonary embolism, such as crackles, dyspnea, tachypnea, hemoptysis, tachycardia, and chest pain
  - Make sure the patient maintains bed rest and elevates the affected extremity
  - Apply moist, warm compresses to improve circulation to the affected area and relieve pain
  - Tell the patient to avoid prolonged sitting and standing to help prevent recurrence
  - Teach the patient how to properly apply and use antiembolism stockings
  - To prevent thrombophlebitis in high-risk patients, perform range-of-motion exercises while the patient is on bed rest, use intermittent pneumatic calf massage during lengthy surgical or diagnostic procedures, apply antiembolism stockings or pneumatic compression devices postoperatively, and encourage early ambulation

Valvular Heart Disease

- Description
  - Three types of mechanical disruption can occur in patients with valvular heart disease: narrowing (stenosis) of the valve opening, incomplete closure of the valve (insufficiency), or prolapse of the valve
  - Valvular heart disease may result from conditions such as endocarditis (most common), rheumatic fever, congenital defects, or inflammation and can lead to heart failure
  - The most common forms of valvular heart disease include mitral stenosis, mitral insufficiency, mitral valve prolapse, aortic stenosis, aortic insufficiency, and tricuspid insufficiency (see *Types of valvular heart disease*, pages 111–113)
- Treatment
  - Medications are administered to treat heart failure and dysrhythmias
  - An anticoagulant may be prescribed to prevent thrombus formation around diseased or replaced valves
  - Surgery to repair or replace valves is indicated when medical management can no longer control symptoms
- Nursing interventions
  - Offer a low-sodium diet, and maintain fluid restrictions
  - Place the patient in an upright position to relieve dyspnea
  - Instruct the patient on the use of anticoagulants, including signs and symptoms of bleeding to report, the need for frequent monitoring, and precautions to take while taking the drug
  - If the patient has an artificial valve, or a history of having infective endocarditis, explain that prophylactic antibiotics are needed before undergoing dental work, surgery, or other invasive procedures

Box 7-8: Types of Valvular Heart Disease

Causes and Incidence	Clinical Features	Diagnostic Measures
Aortic insufficiency		
• Results from rheumatic fever, syphilis, hypertension, or endocarditis, or may be idiopathic • Associated with Marfan syndrome • Most common in males • Associated with ventricular septal defect, even after surgical closure	• Dyspnea, cough, fatigue, palpitations, angina, syncope • Pulmonary vein congestion, heart failure, pulmonary edema (left-sided heart failure), "pulsating" nail beds (Quincke's sign) • Rapidly rising and collapsing pulses (pulsus bisferiens), cardiac dysrhythmias, wide pulse pressure in severe insufficiency • Auscultation reveals a third heart sound (S_3) and a diastolic blowing murmur at left sternal border • Palpation and visualization of apical impulse in chronic disease	• Cardiac catheterization: reduction in arterial diastolic pressures, aortic insufficiency, other valvular abnormalities, and increased left ventricular end-diastolic pressure • X-ray: left ventricular enlargement, pulmonary vein congestion • Echocardiography: left ventricular enlargement, alterations in mitral valve movement (indirect indication of aortic valve disease), and mitral thickening • Electrocardiography (ECG): sinus tachycardia, left ventricular hypertrophy, and left atrial hypertrophy in severe disease
Aortic stenosis		
• Results from congenital aortic bicuspid valve (associated with coarctation of the aorta), congenital stenosis of valve cusps, degenerative calcifications caused by mechanical stress, diabetes mellitus, hypercholesterolemia, or hypertension • Most common in males	• Exertional dyspnea, paroxysmal nocturnal dyspnea, fatigue, syncope, angina, palpitations • Pulmonary vein congestion, heart failure, pulmonary edema • Diminished carotid pulses, decreased cardiac output, cardiac dysrhythmias; may have pulsus alternans • Auscultation reveals systolic murmur at base or in carotids and, possibly, a fourth heart sound (S_4)	• Cardiac catheterization: pressure gradient across valve (indicating obstruction), increased left ventricular end-diastolic pressures • X-ray: valvular calcification, left ventricular enlargement, and pulmonary venous congestion • Echocardiography: thickened aortic valve and left ventricular wall • ECG: left ventricular hypertrophy
Mitral insufficiency		
• Results from rheumatic fever, hypertrophic cardiomyopathy, mitral valve prolapse, myocardial infarction, severe left-sided heart failure, or ruptured chordae tendineae • Associated with other congenital anomalies such as transposition of the great arteries • Rare in children without other congenital anomalies	• Orthopnea, dyspnea, fatigue, angina, palpitations • Peripheral edema, jugular vein distention, hepatomegaly (right-sided heart failure) • Tachycardia, crackles, pulmonary edema • Auscultation reveals a holosystolic murmur at the apex, possible split second heart sound (S_2), and an S_3	• Cardiac catheterization: mitral insufficiency with increased left ventricular end-diastolic volume and pressure, increased atrial pressure and pulmonary artery wedge pressure (PAWP), and decreased cardiac output • X-ray: left atrial and ventricular enlargement, pulmonary venous congestion • Echocardiography: abnormal valve leaflet motion, left atrial enlargement • ECG: may show left atrial and ventricular hypertrophy, sinus tachycardia, and atrial fibrillation

(continued)

Box 7-8: Types of Valvular Heart Disease (continued)

Causes and Incidence	Clinical Features	Diagnostic Measures
Mitral stenosis • Results from rheumatic fever (most common cause), atrial myxoma, or endocarditis • Most common in females • May be associated with other congenital anomalies	• Exertional dyspnea, paroxysmal nocturnal dyspnea, orthopnea, weakness, fatigue, palpitations • Peripheral edema, jugular vein distention, ascites, hepatomegaly (right-sided heart failure in severe pulmonary hypertension) • Crackles, cardiac dysrhythmias (atrial fibrillation), signs of systemic emboli • Auscultation reveals a loud first heart sound (S_1) or opening snap and a diastolic murmur at the apex	• Cardiac catheterization: diastolic pressure gradient across valve, elevated left atrial pressure and PAWP with severe pulmonary hypertension and pulmonary artery pressures, elevated right-sided heart pressure, decreased cardiac output, and abnormal contraction of the left ventricle • X-ray: left atrial and ventricular enlargement, enlarged pulmonary arteries, and mitral valve calcification • Echocardiography: thickened mitral valve leaflets, left atrial enlargement • ECG: left atrial hypertrophy, atrial fibrillation, right ventricular hypertrophy, and right axis deviation
Mitral valve prolapse syndrome • Cause unknown; researchers speculate that metabolic or neuroendocrine factors cause constellation of signs and symptoms • Most commonly affects young women but may occur in both sexes and in all age groups	• May produce no signs or may produce signs and symptoms of mitral insufficiency • Chest pain, palpitations, headache, fatigue, exercise intolerance, dyspnea, syncope, light-headedness, mood swings, anxiety, panic attacks • Auscultation typically reveals a mobile, midsystolic click, with or without a mid-to-late systolic murmur	• Two-dimensional echocardiography: prolapse of mitral valve leaflets into left atrium • Color-flow Doppler studies: mitral insufficiency • Resting ECG: ST-segment changes, biphasic or inverted T waves in leads II, III, or A_V • Exercise ECG: evaluates chest pain and dysrhythmias
Pulmonic insufficiency • May be congenital or may result from pulmonary hypertension • May rarely result from prolonged use of pressure monitoring catheter in the pulmonary artery	• Dyspnea, weakness, fatigue, chest pain • Peripheral edema, jugular vein distention, hepatomegaly (right-sided heart failure) • Auscultation reveals diastolic murmur in pulmonic area	• Cardiac catheterization: pulmonic insufficiency, increased right ventricular pressure, and associated cardiac defects • X-ray: right ventricular and pulmonary arterial enlargement • ECG: right ventricular or right atrial enlargement
Pulmonic stenosis • Results from congenital stenosis of valve cusp or rheumatic heart disease (infrequent) • Associated with other congenital heart defects such as tetralogy of Fallot	• Asymptomatic or symptomatic with exertional dyspnea, fatigue, chest pain, syncope • May lead to peripheral edema, jugular vein distention, hepatomegaly (right-sided heart failure) • Auscultation reveals a systolic murmur at the left sternal border, a split S_2 with a delayed or absent pulmonic component	• Cardiac catheterization: increased right ventricular pressure, decreased pulmonary artery pressure, and abnormal valve orifice • ECG: may show right ventricular hypertrophy, right axis deviation, right atrial hypertrophy, and atrial fibrillation

(continued)

Box 7-8: Types of Valvular Heart Disease (continued)

Causes and Incidence	Clinical Features	Diagnostic Measures
Tricuspid insufficiency		
• Results from right-sided heart failure, rheumatic fever, and, rarely, trauma and endocarditis • Associated with congenital disorders	• Dyspnea and fatigue • May lead to peripheral edema, jugular vein distention, hepatomegaly, ascites (right-sided heart failure) • Auscultation reveals possible S_3 and systolic murmur at lower left sternal border that increases with inspiration	• Right-sided heart catheterization: high atrial pressure, tricuspid insufficiency, and decreased or normal cardiac output • X-ray: right atrial dilation, right ventricular enlargement • Echocardiography: shows systolic prolapse of tricuspid valve, right atrial enlargement • ECG: right atrial or right ventricular hypertrophy, atrial fibrillation
Tricuspid stenosis		
• Results from rheumatic fever • May be congenital • Associated with mitral or aortic valve disease • Most common in females	• May be symptomatic with dyspnea, fatigue, syncope • Possibly peripheral edema, jugular vein distention, hepatomegaly, ascites (right-sided heart failure) • Auscultation reveals diastolic murmur at lower left sternal border that increases with inspiration	• Cardiac catheterization: increased pressure gradient across valve, increased right atrial pressure, and decreased cardiac output • X-ray: right atrial enlargement • Echocardiography: leaflet abnormality, right atrial enlargement • ECG: right atrial hypertrophy, right or left ventricular hypertrophy, and atrial fibrillation

Review Questions

Question 1. Which of the following describes cardiac dysrhythmias?

A. Always severe; the patient can feel them when they happen.
B. Classified according to origin and effect on cardiac output.
C. Caused by dietary deficiencies.
D. No dysrhythmia is life threatening.

Correct answer: B Dysrhythmias are classified according to where they originate and how they affect cardiac output. They can be mild to severe (Option A), and some can be life threatening (Option D). Causes for dysrhythmias are cardiac in nature and not directly related to deficiency of certain nutrients.

Question 2. Which of the following nursing interventions is most appropriate for a patient on anticoagulants for thrombophlebitis?

A. Encourage ambulation; avoid prolonged sitting.
B. Assess for pulmonary embolism; use ice for pain control in limbs.
C. Monitor for signs of bleeding; apply warm compresses to affected area.
D. Elevate affected extremity; avoid use of antiembolism stockings.

Correct answer: C Monitoring a patient for bleeding and using warm compresses for pain relief in extremities is a nursing intervention for a patient on anticoagulation for thromboembolism. Options A, B, and D have some appropriate interventions in their responses, but patients with thromboembolism should not be encouraged to walk. Ice slows down blood flow and can cause formation of additional thrombi. Antiembolism stockings are used to help with prevention of thromboembolism formation and support of veins in legs.

Question 3. Which statement does the nurse know is true about valvular heart disease?

A. Surgery is the first step to control symptoms in valvular heart disease.
B. Anticoagulants may be prescribed to prevent thrombus formation.
C. Valvular heart disease means a cardiac valve is sealed shut by plaque.
D. Common forms of valvular heart disease include atrial fibrillation and ventricular tachycardia.

Correct answer: B Anticoagulants help prevent formation of clots around diseased natural and artificial valves. Medication is the first step to controlling valvular heart disease, and surgery is an option when medications failed (Option A). Valvular heart disease is a term that means the valves may be narrowed or have incomplete closure or prolapse (Option C). Atrial fibrillation and ventricular tachycardia are dysrhythmias.

Question 4. A patient with pericarditis questions the order for ibuprofen (Motrin) to control pain. Which statement best addresses this patient's concern?

A. This is just a starting point. I can ask the provider for a stronger pain killer.
B. Pericarditis is an inflammatory process; ibuprofen fights inflammation while it relieves pain.
C. Ibuprofen will not make you fall asleep or become constipated.
D. It is inexpensive and will make you feel better. You will be able to continue this at home.

Correct answer: B The anti-inflammatory effect of ibuprofen addresses the reason for the pain while relieving pain. Option A avoids answering why the medication was prescribed. While Options C and D has correct information, it does not address why ibuprofen was ordered specifically for pericarditis.

Question 5. A person is learning about hypertension. Which statement shows good understanding of this disease process?

A. Hypertension medications need to be taken daily for the rest of the patient's life.
B. The heart will be damaged by uncontrolled high blood pressure, but nothing else will.
C. Weight loss, smoking cessation, and exercise may help a person get off hypertension medications.
D. A person will get a bad headache and that will alert them that their blood pressure is up.

Correct answer: C Lifestyle changes of aerobic exercise, smoking cessation, and weight loss can replace medications in some patients (Option A). Many organ

systems are damaged by hypertension, including eyes and kidneys (Option C). Hypertension is a silent killer, meaning there are no warning signs that blood pressure is elevated (Option D).

Question 6. When evaluating an ECG strip of a patient on a telemetry unit, the nurse notices the patient is having atrial flutter. What criterion on the ECG strip does the nurse use to evaluate the presence of atrial flutter?

A. An indiscernible PR interval
B. P waves that appear erratic
C. P waves that have a sawtooth configuration
D. A QRS complex followed by a compensatory pause

Correct answer: C P waves that make a sawtooth formation on the strip are hallmark for atrial flutter. In PVCs, the ECG shows a QRS complex followed by a compensatory pause that ends when the underlying rhythm resumes (Option D). Options A and B are ECG criteria used to evaluate atrial fibrillation.

Question 7. When locating the correct spot to hear mitral sounds, the nurse should place the stethoscope at the:

A. fifth intercostal space near the midclavicular line.
B. fifth intercostal space along the left sternal border.
C. second intercostal space at the left sternal border.
D. third intercostal space at the left sternal border.

Correct answer: A The fifth intercostal space near the midclavicular line is used to listen to the mitral area. Erb's point is located at the third intercostal space at the left sternal border (Option D). The fifth intercostal space along the left sternal border (Option B) is the location for the tricuspid area. The second intercostal space at the left sternal border (Option C) is the location for the pulmonic area.

Question 8. Which patient is most at risk for coronary heart disease?

A. A 55-year-old male, sedentary, with no family history.
B. A 78-year-old female, active, whose sister recently had a myocardial infarction.
C. A 70-year-old female, mildly active, diabetes type 2 for 25 years and history of angina.
D. A 65-year-old male, moderately active, with a high stress job and no past medical history. "It's best to wear tight socks instead of no socks."

Correct answer: C This patient has the most risk factors with a personal history of cardiac disease, diabetes mellitus, and older age. Options A, B, and D have risk factors, like being sedentary, first-degree relative with cardiac disease, and high stress jobs.

Question 9. After an acute myocardial infarction, the nurse knows it is important to reduce preload and afterload of the heart. Which class of medication will the nurse give?

A. Antiplatelet medication
B. ACE inhibitors
C. Nitrates
D. Beta adrenergic blockers

Correct answer: B ACE inhibitors reduce preload and afterload. Antiplatelet drugs minimize platelet aggregation (Option A). Nitrates reduce myocardial oxygen consumption (Option C). Beta adrenergic blockers reduce the workload of the heart and myocardial oxygen demand (Option D).

Question 10. Which of the following conditions can be caused by an atrial septal defect?

A. A ventricular septal defect
B. Left heart failure
C. Right heart failure
D. Constrictive pericarditis

Correct answer: C An atrial septal defect can lead to right-sided heart failure. Left-sided heart failure can result from a ventricular septal defect, an anterior MI, or constrictive pericarditis (Option B). Ventricular septal defects (Option A) are usually congenital. Constrictive pericarditis (Option D) is caused by inflammation.

Selected References

American Heart Association. (2016, March). Symptoms and diagnosis of pericarditis. Retrieved from http://www.heart.org/HEARTORG/Conditions/More/Symptoms-and-Diagnosis-of-Pericarditis_UCM_444932_Article.jsp#.WQ-19YWcFPY

American Heart Association. (2016, April). Coronary heart disease. Retrieved from http://www.heart.org/HEARTORG/Conditions/More/MyHeartandStrokeNews/Coronary-Artery-Disease---Coronary-Heart-Disease_UCM_436416_Article.jsp#.WQ-bM4WcFPY

Buerger's disease. (2017). Retrieved from https://www.hopkinsvasculitis.org/types-vasculitis/buergers-disease/

Buerger's disease. (1998–2017). Retrieved from http://www.mayoclinic.org/diseases-conditions/buergers-disease/symptoms-causes/dxc-20179162

Description of high blood pressure. (2015, September 10). Retrieved from https://www.nhlbi.nih.gov/health/health-topics/topics/hbp

Fleisher, L. A., Fleischmann, K. E., Auerbach, A. D., Barnason, S. A., Beckman, J. A., Bozkurt, B., … Wijeysundera, D. N. (2014). 2014 ACC/AHA guideline on perioperative cardiovascular evaluation and management of patients undergoing noncardiac surgery. *Journal of the American College of Cardiology, 64*, 2. doi: 10.1016/j.jacc.2014.07.944.

Hallet, J. W. (2017). Occlusive peripheral arterial disease. Retrieved from http://www.merckmanuals.com/home/heart-and-blood-vessel-disorders/peripheral-arterial-disease/occlusive-peripheral-arterial-disease

Heart Failure Society of America. (2016, May). ACC/AHA/HFSA guideline for management of heart failure update. Retrieved from http://www.hfsa.org/accahahfsa-guideline-management-heart-failure-update/

Huckell, V. F. (2016). Infective endocarditis. Retrieved from http://www.merckmanuals.com/professional/cardiovascular-disorders/endocarditis/infective-endocarditis

Nishimura, R. A., Otto, C. M., Bonow, R. O., Carabello, B. A., Erwin, J. P., Fleisher, L. A., … Thompson, A. (2017). 2017 AHA/ACC focused update of the 2014 AHA/ACC guideline for the management of patients with valvular heart disease: A report of the American College of Cardiology/American Heart Association task force on clinical practice guidelines. *Circulation,135*(25),e1159–e1195. Retrieved from http://circ.ahajournals.org/content/early/2017/03/14/CIR.0000000000000503

Rivera-Bou, W. L. (2016). Thrombolytic therapy. Retrieved from http://emedicine.medscape.com/article/811234-overview#a2

Sexton, D. J. (2017, March 16). Patient education: Antibiotics before procedures (beyond the basics). Retrieved from https://www.uptodate.com/contents/antibiotics-before-procedures-beyond-the-basics

Thrombophlebitis. (1998–2017). Retrieved on May 5, 2017 from http://www.mayoclinic.org/diseases-conditions/thrombophlebitis/home/ovc-20251852

What is cardiomyopathy? (2016, June 22). Retrieved from https://www.nhlbi.nih.gov/health/health-topics/topics/cm

What is coronary heart disease? (2016, June 22). Retrieved from https://www.nhlbi.nih.gov/health/health-topics/topics/cad

What is Raynaud's phenomenon? Fast facts: An easy-to-read series of publications for the public. (2014, November). Retrieved from https://www.niams.nih.gov/Health_Info/Raynauds_Phenomenon/raynauds_ff.asp

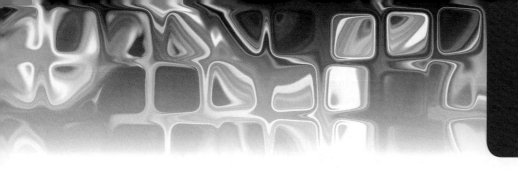

Chapter 8

Hematologic Disorders

Introduction

- The average human adult has more than 5 L (6 qt) of blood in their body
- Blood circulates in the cardiovascular system, carrying oxygen and removing waste from cells
- The continuous movement of blood also provides a defense against infection and injury, which are more likely to occur with stasis
- The cellular components of red blood cells (RBCs), white blood cells (WBCs), and platelets are subject to pathologic alterations that can cause severe disruptions in homeostasis
- Nursing history
  - The nurse asks the patient about their *chief complaint*
  - A patient with a hematologic disorder may report any of the following signs or symptoms: aching bones, anorexia, bleeding gums, bruising, dyspnea, fatigue, infection, lethargy, malaise, nausea, nosebleeds, numbness, paresthesia, swollen and tender lymph nodes, tarry stools, tingling, vomiting, and, in women, heavy menses
  - The nurse then questions the patient about his *present illness*
    - Ask the patient about his symptoms, including when they started, associated symptoms, location, radiation, intensity, duration, and frequency
    - Question the patient about what factors make the symptoms feel better or worse
  - The nurse asks about *medical history*
    - Ask about the present and past use of prescription and over-the-counter drugs, herbal remedies, and vitamin and nutritional supplements because many of these products can interfere with hematologic function
    - Ask the patient about previous problems, such as anemia, leukemia, enlarged lymph nodes, malabsorption, and spleen or liver disorders
    - Ask about previous treatments, such as blood transfusions and radiation treatments
    - Question the patient about their diet, and look for deficiencies—for example, in folic acid, iron, or vitamin B_{12}
  - The nurse then assesses the *family history*
    - Ask about a family history of blood and lymph disorders, acquired and genetic
    - Ask about a family history of cancers involving the blood or lymph systems
  - The nurse obtains a *social history*
    - Ask about ethnic background and race
    - Question the patient about use of cigarettes, alcohol, and recreational drugs
    - Ask him about occupational or household exposure to radiation or chemicals
- Physical assessment
  - The nurse begins with *inspection*
    - Observe the patient's general appearance. Does he appear alert, confused, tired, or irritable?
    - Note the patient's skin color; look for ecchymosis, diaphoresis, dyspnea, lesions, petechiae, and swelling of the lymph nodes
    - Note the size and color of his tongue
    - Ask the patient whether his abdominal girth is enlarged

- The nurse uses *auscultation*
  - Listen to heart sounds, noting abnormal sounds, rhythms, or tachycardia
  - Auscultate the abdomen, noting bowel sounds, bruits, friction rubs, or venous hums
  - Listen to lung sounds, noting any abnormal sounds
- Next, the nurse uses *palpation*
  - Palpate peripheral pulses, noting strength, rhythm, and rate
  - Palpate the lymph nodes, noting consistency, mobility, shape, size, and tenderness; compare nodes on one side of the body with those on the other side
  - Palpate the abdomen, noting ascites, enlarged organs, or tenderness
- The nurse then uses *percussion*
  - Percuss the liver and spleen to estimate size
  - Note the size and location of other abdominal organs

Anemias

- Anemia exists when the number of RBC is less than normal or when RBCs do not have enough hemoglobin
- Types of anemia include blood loss or hemolysis and aplastic, iron deficiency, and megaloblastic anemias (see *Types of anemia*, pages 118–119)

Disseminated Intravascular Coagulation

- Description
  - Disseminated intravascular coagulation (DIC) is a serious blood coagulation disorder that occurs as a complication of conditions that accelerate blood clotting.
  - It is characterized by suppression of the fibrinolytic system and the development of small clots in the microcirculation, which consumes clotting factors, resulting in excessive bleeding
  - The disorder can result from septicemia, obstetric complications (abruptio placentae and amniotic fluid embolism), cancer, blood transfusion reactions, and liver disease
  - Altered tissue profusion and multiple organ failure can occur; the mortality rate can exceed 80%
- Signs and symptoms
  - The main sign is abnormal bleeding, evidenced by cutaneous oozing, petechiae, ecchymosis, hematomas, GI bleeding, and bleeding from wounds and I.V. sites
  - Signs of organ compromise include dyspnea, oliguria, and muscle or abdominal pain; shock can also occur
- Diagnosis and treatment
  - Laboratory tests show a steadily decreasing platelet count, elevated prothrombin time (PT) and partial thromboplastin time (PTT), elevated fibrin degradation products, and decreased hemoglobin and hematocrit
  - Medical management aims to identify and treat the underlying disorder, promote oxygenation, replace fluids and electrolytes, and provide hemodynamic support
  - Treatments include clotting factor and blood replacement and I.V. heparin
- Nursing interventions
  - Early recognition of DIC improves patient outcomes, so closely monitor patients at risk, watching for signs and symptoms
  - For a patient with DIC, avoid trauma to skin or wounds to minimize bleeding, protect the patient from injury, and avoid dislodging clots
  - Apply pressure to puncture sites until bleeding stops
  - Monitor the patient's vital signs, and administer I.V. fluids and blood products as ordered
  - Monitor the patient's intake and output carefully and record blood loss
  - Watch for signs of tissue ischemia and failure
  - Provide emotional support to the patient and family

Hemophilia

- Description
  - Hemophilia is a hereditary bleeding disorder that results from the lack of specific clotting factors

Box 8-1: Types of Anemia

This chart summarizes the etiology, signs and symptoms, medical management, and nursing interventions for each type of anemia, which is defined as a decreased number of red blood cells (RBCs).

Description and Etiology	Signs and Symptoms	Medical Management	Nursing Interventions
Anemia from blood loss			
Anemia resulting from the loss of more than 500 mL of blood • Acute blood loss, as in trauma or surgery • Chronic blood loss, as in menstrual or GI bleeding	• RBC count below normal on serum blood tests • _With acute blood loss:_ sudden onset of symptoms, such as hypovolemia, hypotension, hypoxemia, irritability, stupor, weakness, tachycardia, and cool, moist skin • _With chronic blood loss:_ gradual and vague symptoms, such as exertional dyspnea, increased fatigue, and pallor	• The source of the bleeding is identified and controlled through medical or surgical means. • Transfusion and iron supplementation may be needed. Packed RBCs are typically used if a blood transfusion is required. • Shock must be treated if it occurs.	• Help determine the cause of bleeding by testing stool, urine, vomitus, or sputum for blood. • Help control blood loss by applying pressure to obvious bleeding sites, assessing the patient for internal bleeding, and performing dressing changes as needed to assess blood loss.
Aplastic anemia			
Anemia characterized by a decreased hemoglobin level and pancytopenia • Unknown etiology or an autoimmune disturbance (50% of cases) • Drug therapy with a chemotherapeutic drug, chloramphenicol, mephenytoin, phenylbutazone, or a sulfonamide • Exposure to environmental or occupational hazards, such as benzene, insecticides, or radiation • Infection, such as cytomegalovirus, Epstein-Barr virus, hepatitis, parvovirus B19, HIV, or miliary tuberculosis • Congenital causes	• Exertional dyspnea, fatigue, infections, pallor, and palpitations • Hemorrhage—for example, bleeding (nasal, oral, rectal, or vaginal), ecchymosis, petechiae, or purpura • Low platelet, RBC, and WBC counts • Dry bone marrow—low number of stem cells found upon aspiration	• Initial treatment involves removing the causative agent, if possible, and administering blood component transfusions. • Medications such as antithymocyte globulin (ATG), cyclosporine (CSA), granulocyte colony–stimulating factors, and granulocyte-monocyte colony–stimulating factor may be administered. • The idiopathic form of the disease is treated with steroids. • If the anemia can't be reversed or if it results from an autoimmune disturbance, bone marrow/stem cell transplantation is recommended; this treatment is more effective if the patient doesn't receive blood products first and is younger than age 30.	• Help identify the causative agent. • Assist a weak patient with daily activities. • If the patient has pancytopenia, take safety precautions and steps to control infection and bleeding because his ability to fight infection and sustain clotting is decreased. • Help the patient and family cope with the severity of the illness and its prognosis. (Death may result from infection or hemorrhage.) • If the patient is receiving ATG, perform skin testing, and monitor him for allergic reaction.
Congenital hemolytic anemia: Sickle cell anemia			
Anemia characterized by RBC destruction beyond the bone marrow's ability to produce these cells and misshapen hemoglobin and RBCs • Inherited (found primarily in persons of African descent due to heredity)	• Abnormally shaped blood cells found on blood smear • Painful vasoocclusive events in the extremities or affected organs (sickle cell crisis) • Other symptoms similar to other chronic anemias	• No cure or prevention is available. • Hydroxyurea (Droxia or Hydrea) is a chemotherapeutic drug that is used to reduce frequency of sickle cell crisis. • Supportive interventions are used to prevent infection, relieve pain, and provide fluid and oxygen during a sickle cell crisis, which can cause massive organ damage.	• If the patient has sickle cell anemia, provide genetic counseling and possible gene replacement therapy. • Teach the patient to avoid factors that may precipitate sickle cell crisis, such as cold exposure, dehydration, excessive exercise, high altitudes, and smoking. • Monitor patient closely during sickle cell crisis, especially related to pain management and oxygenation.

Box 8-1: Types of Anemia (continued)

Description and Etiology	Signs and Symptoms	Medical Management	Nursing Interventions
Congenital hemolytic anemia: Thalassemia **Anemia characterized by RBC destruction beyond the bone marrow's ability to produce these cells and mutated hemoglobin** • Inherited (primarily affects people of African, Asian, and Mediterranean descent)	• Cardiac problems, such as cardiomegaly, heart failure, and murmurs • Excessive hematopoiesis and iron overload • Other symptoms similar to other chronic anemias	• Blood product transfusions are the primary treatment. • Chelating agents are used to remove excess iron from the blood after multiple transfusions have been administered. • Splenectomy may be required for severe thalassemia. • Bone marrow/stem cell transplant also is an option.	• If the patient has thalassemia, provide genetic counseling. • Monitor for activity intolerance due to impaired oxygenation.
Iron deficiency anemia **Anemia caused by inadequate iron supplies** • Chronic blood loss without iron replacement • Poor nutrition • Decreased iron absorption from the intestines • Increased need for iron, such as during childhood or pregnancy	• Fatigue due to RBC lack of ability to carry oxygen • Shortness of breath, pallor, dizziness, and headache • Cold sensitivity related to iron's role in regulating body temperature • Brittle, spoon-shaped nails with longitudinal ridges; cheilosis (painful mouth cracks or sores) and red, shiny tongue • Hypochromic, microcytic anemia (on blood smears); low serum iron level; and elevated serum iron-binding capacities	• The cause of blood loss or nutritional deficits is identified and corrected. • An oral iron supplement may be prescribed. If the patient is unable to tolerate it, a parenteral iron formulation may be administered I.M. via the Z-track method or I.V. • In extreme cases, blood transfusions may be administered.	• Help determine the cause of bleeding by testing stool, urine, vomitus, and sputum for blood. • Teach the patient how to take oral iron. Advise the patient to take iron pills with meals to reduce GI irritation and to continue therapy until the underlying problem is corrected. • Teach the patient about adverse reactions to oral iron therapy, such as black stools, constipation or diarrhea, and GI disturbances. • Educate the patient about nutrition, including the need for iron-rich foods and adequate vitamin C to enhance iron absorption.
Megaloblastic anemia **Anemia characterized by a predominance of megaloblasts and a relative lack of normoblasts; includes pernicious, vitamin B_{12} deficiency, and folic acid deficiency anemias** • Gastric surgery, particularly of the terminal ileum where vitamin B_{12} is absorbed; strict vegetarian diets; and prolonged exposure to nitrous oxide • Aging and long-term gastritis (pernicious anemia) • Alcoholic malnutrition and malabsorption (folic acid deficiency anemia)	• Fatigue, loss of coordination, neuropathy, and paresthesia of the extremities • Gastritis, glossitis (red, beefy tongue), and malabsorption with anorexia and weight loss • Decreased RBC and platelet counts	• Monthly administration of parenteral vitamin B_{12} typically is required for pernicious and vitamin B_{12} deficiency anemias. • An oral folic acid supplement and dietary improvement typically are required for a patient with folic acid deficiency, which commonly results from nutritional deficits.	• Provide care for oral mucous membranes to help relieve glossitis. • Teach the patient how to increase dietary intake of folic acid and vitamin B_{12}. • Refer the patient with anemia related to alcohol abuse to an alcohol rehabilitation clinic. • If the patient has a vitamin B_{12} deficiency, teach him about long-term treatment with an oral or parenteral vitamin B_{12} supplement. Treatment typically calls for monthly I.M. administration of cyanocobalamin (B_{12}).

- Two main forms exist: hemophilia A, called "classic hemophilia," results from deficiency of factor VIII and is seen in 80% of cases, and hemophilia B, called "Christmas disease," results from deficiency of factor IX and is seen in 15% of cases; the two types are clinically indistinguishable
- Hemophilia A and B are X-linked recessive traits; female carriers have a 50% chance of transmitting the gene to each child; sons who receive the gene have the disease, whereas daughters who receive the gene are carriers; patients with the disease are usually identified in childhood
- Hemophilia produces bleeding, with the degree of bleeding varying depending on the degree of clotting factor deficiency
  - Mild hemophilia usually causes bleeding only during major surgery or trauma
  - Moderate hemophilia occasionally causes spontaneous bleeding in addition to bleeding during surgery and from trauma
  - Severe hemophilia causes spontaneous bleeding; bleeding from minor trauma may be severe
- Signs and symptoms
  - Signs of hemophilia include excessive bleeding from wound and puncture sites, hematomas, ecchymosis, spontaneous bleeding (such as nosebleeds), and GI bleeding
  - Bleeding into joints is a common occurrence; this can lead to joint pain and stiffness
  - A change in level of consciousness can signal intracranial bleeding
- Diagnosis and treatment
  - Laboratory tests include abnormal clotting factor assays, which confirm diagnosis; prolonged PTT with normal PT and normal platelet count may also occur
  - Treatment typically consists of replacement of deficient clotting factors (VIII or IX); however, patients can develop antibodies to factor concentrates, which reduces their effectiveness
  - Aminocaproic acid inhibits fibrinolysis and can be used to stabilize clots
  - Desmopressin (DDAVP) can be used to induce a transient rise in factor VIII
- Nursing interventions
  - During bleeding episodes, administer the deficient clotting factors or plasma as ordered
  - Prevent trauma, and limit activity when bleeding occurs
  - Minimize injections and apply pressure for at least 10 minutes to puncture sites
  - Monitor vital signs and be alert for hemodynamic changes
  - Administer analgesics and cold packs for joint pain; promote joint mobility when bleeding is controlled
  - Teach the patient and family about the disease process, monitoring, treatment, and genetic testing

Hodgkin's Lymphoma

- Description
  - Hodgkin's lymphoma is a malignant B lymphocyte cell line disease of the lymph system that primarily affects those between ages 15 and 30 and those older than age 55
  - The malignant cell associated with Hodgkin's lymphoma is the Reed-Sternberg cell, a giant, morphologically unique cell that's most likely of immature lymphoid origin
  - Although the cause is unknown, this cancer is associated with viral infections (Epstein-Barr) and prolonged immunosuppression; a genetic and environmental association may also exist
  - It is among the most treatable of adult cancers and has a better prognosis than malignant or non-Hodgkin's lymphoma
- Signs and symptoms
  - This cancer is characterized by greatly enlarged, painless, movable lymph nodes in the cervical or supraclavicular area
  - The patient may also experience fever, night sweats, and weight loss (referred to as "B" or systemic symptoms)
  - Symptoms resulting from compression by the enlarged lymph nodes depend on the area involved
- Diagnosis and treatment
  - Lymph node biopsy showing Reed-Sternberg cells supports the diagnosis
  - Staging is done after the initial diagnosis of Hodgkin's lymphoma is confirmed
    - The stage of disease is determined by biopsies of distant lymph nodes, bilateral bone marrow biopsies, lymphangiography, computed tomography scan (CT) or magnetic resonance imaging (MRI) of the thorax and abdomen, gallium scan, positron emission tomography (PET), chest X-ray, a complete blood count (CBC), and serum alkaline phosphatase
    - A splenectomy is usually done during staging

- Hodgkin's lymphoma has four stages (see *Staging lymphomas*)
- Generally, all stages of Hodgkin's lymphoma are treated with a combination of chemotherapy and radiation
- Autologous bone marrow/stem cell transplantation and immunotherapy are used for disease resistant to standard treatment
  - Nursing interventions
    - Provide supportive care related to the adverse effects of radiation therapy and chemotherapy (see *Nursing implications in oncology care*, pages 341–347)
    - Provide psychological support to help the patient cope with the diagnosis, treatment, and effects of treatment
    - Provide education to the patient and his family regarding the diagnosis of Hodgkin's lymphoma and its treatment

Leukemia

- Description
  - Leukemia is a group of malignant disorders of the hematopoietic system that involves the bone marrow and lymph nodes and is characterized by the uncontrolled proliferation of immature WBCs
  - Leukemias are classified by onset and severity of symptoms (acute or chronic) and by the precursor cell (myeloid or lymphoid) involved in the formation of the abnormal cells (see *Types of leukemia*, page 123)

Box 8-2: **Staging Lymphomas**

Hodgkin's lymphoma and non-Hodgkin's lymphoma are classified into stages so that treatment protocols can be established and outcomes predicted. The Ann Arbor classification system is used.

Stages

Stage I
- Involvement of a single lymph node region

or

- Localized involvement of a single extranodal organ or site

Stage II
- Involvement of two or more lymph node regions on the same side of the diaphragm

or

- Localized involvement to a single associated extranodal organ or site and its regional lymph nodes with or without other lymph node regions on the same side of the diaphragm

Stage III
- Involvement of lymph node regions on both sides of the diaphragm that may also be accompanied by localized involvement of an extranodal organ or site, by involvement of the spleen, or by both

Stage IV
- Disseminated involvement of one or more extralymphatic sites with or without associated lymph node involvement

or

- Isolated extralymphatic organ involvement with distant (nonregional) nodal involvement

Extralymphatic sites include the liver, lungs, bone marrow, pleurae, bone, and skin as well as tissues separate from but near to major lymphatic clusters. The spleen is considered a lymphatic site.

Letter Designation

The stages are also accompanied by a letter designation that refers to patient symptoms as follows:
- **A** means absence of the specific symptoms listed in **B** but may include other common symptoms such as pruritus
- **B** includes the presence of at least one of the following three symptoms:
  - Temperature greater than 100.4°F (38°C)
  - Unexplained loss of more than 10% of body weight in the preceding 6 months
  - Drenching night sweats

- Although the cause of leukemia is unknown, it has been linked to genetic damage to cells, which transforms normal cells into malignant cells—chronic exposure to chemicals such as benzene, use of drugs that cause aplastic anemia, radiation exposure, and chemotherapy; it is also linked to Down's syndrome and other chromosomal abnormalities
- In leukemia, WBC (leukocyte) proliferation interferes with the production of other cells, leading to thrombocytopenia and anemia; the immature leukocytes decrease immunocompetence and increase susceptibility to infection
- Signs and symptoms
  - A patient with either acute or chronic leukemia may report vague signs and symptoms, such as fatigue, malaise, petechiae, night sweats, bone or joint pain, and weight loss
  - Acute leukemia produces anemia, bleeding, and symptoms of infection such as sudden onset of high fever
  - Hepatosplenomegaly and lymphadenopathy may also be present; chronic leukemia causes milder anemia and splenomegaly; however, many patients are asymptomatic at the time of diagnosis
  - Additional signs and symptoms depend on the organ or tissue involved—for example, central nervous system involvement may cause headache and vomiting
- Diagnosis and treatment
  - Diagnosis is usually based on bone marrow examination that reveals leukemic blast cells and on a CBC
  - Chemotherapy, with or without stem cell transplantation, is standard treatment for leukemia (see *Nursing implications in oncology care*, pages 341–347)
  - Radiation, immunotherapy, and targeted therapy are also used to augment leukemia treatment
  - Patients with low-risk chronic lymphocytic leukemia may not receive treatment if they're asymptomatic
  - Stem cell transplantation is used to treat leukemia
    - In *allogenic transplantation*, donor stem cells are transplanted into the patient
      - Before transplantation, the patient undergoes chemotherapy and total body radiation to eliminate the leukemic cells; these procedures destroy all the patient's bone marrow in preparation for grafting from the donor
      - The principal complication of this type of transplantation is graft-versus-host disease (GVHD), a type of organ rejection in which the transplanted cells reject the patient
    - An alternative method is to harvest the patient's own stem cells during remission, treat the cells to remove residual tumor cells, and reinfuse them after the patient undergoes immunosuppressant chemotherapy and radiation therapy; this method, called *autologous stem cell transplantation*, avoids GVHD because the patient receives his own cells
  - Blood component transfusions may be necessary to treat severe thrombocytopenia, leukopenia, and anemia resulting from the disease process or from treatment (see *Blood and plasma transfusion compatibility*, page 124)
    - Most RBC transfusions involve 250 to 300 mL/unit of packed RBCs; whole blood is seldom transfused to treat leukemia
      - The blood must be refrigerated until it's used
      - The nurse must take baseline vital signs before transfusion, monitor cardiac status before and during transfusion, confirm blood product compatibility with the patient's blood type, administer blood through a filter (only with normal saline solution), check the blood according to facility policy with another professional nurse, infuse it slowly (2 to 4 hours/unit), observe for reactions, and record vital signs at least hourly and at the end of the transfusion (see *Guide to immediate transfusion reactions*, pages 124–125)
    - Platelet transfusions may be prescribed; a 6-unit I.V. bolus of platelets should be infused over 20 to 30 minutes
      - Platelets shouldn't be refrigerated
      - The nurse must take baseline vital signs before transfusion; premedicate with steroids or antihistamines, as prescribed, to prevent reactions; and administer platelets through a filter (only with normal saline solution)
    - WBC transfusions, though rarely used, must be infused within 24 hours of collection; the process for WBC transfusions is similar to that for RBC transfusions
- Nursing interventions
  - Follow infection control procedures if the WBC count is low, also known as neutropenia—for example, place a severely neutropenic patient in a private room, with no flowers, plants, or fresh fruits; avoid unnecessary invasive procedures; limit patient contact with infected personnel or visitors; and teach hand hygiene techniques to the patient, family, and visitors

- If the patient has a low platelet count, monitor blood counts and take precautions to prevent bleeding—for example, avoid parenteral injections, limit frequent venipuncture, and advise the patient to use an electric razor for shaving and a soft toothbrush for brushing teeth
- Prevent or manage stomatitis (oral/GI mucosa breakdown) by inspecting the oral cavity daily and encouraging oral care with peroxide or saline solution on a regular basis
- Teach the patient how to care for an indwelling vascular access device and how to detect signs of infection
- Educate patients undergoing chemotherapy about the effects, adverse effects, and length of treatment
- Provide supplemental feedings as prescribed
- Conserve the patient's energy, but promote his independence
- Provide emotional support to the patient and family, and encourage them to verbalize feelings

Multiple Myeloma

- Description
  - Multiple myeloma is a malignancy of plasma cells that can invade the bone marrow, lymph nodes, liver, spleen, and kidneys and leads to bone destruction throughout the body
  - The malignant plasma cells produce an increased amount of a specific nonfunctional immunoglobulin
  - This type of cancer is two times more likely in black males between ages 50 and 70; men are 50% more likely to develop the disease than women
  - Other risks include radiation exposure, family history, obesity, and occupational exposure in petroleum-related industries

Box 8-3: Types of Leukemia

The following chart compares the incidence and signs and symptoms for various types of leukemia.

Leukemia	Incidence	Signs and Symptoms
Acute leukemias		
Acute lymphoblastic leukemia (ALL)	• Primarily affects children under the age of 5. Incidence declines dramatically after age 10. Survival rates are higher in children than adults, and the prognosis for ALL is better than that of acute myeloblastic leukemia (AML).	• Anemia with fatigue and pallor • Bleeding, such as ecchymosis, gingival or rectal bleeding, and petechiae • Fever • Hepatosplenomegaly • Decreased hematocrit, hemoglobin level, and platelet count; lymphoblasts present on peripheral blood smear
Acute myelogenous leukemia (AML)	• Primarily affects those over 40; the incidence increases with age. • Survival rates for AML have improved with the use of autologous and allogenic bone marrow transplants.	• Infections, particularly those of the mucous membranes, respiratory tract, and skin • Normal, decreased, or increased WBC count • Bone or joint pain, fever without infection, hepatosplenomegaly, lymphadenopathy, and weight loss
Chronic leukemias		
Chronic lymphocytic leukemia (CLL)	• Primarily affects men, with 72 being the average age at diagnosis. • CLL runs a long course (4 to 10 years) and rarely progresses to acute leukemia.	• Enlarged spleen • Lymphadenopathy • Lymphocytosis (on peripheral blood smear)
Chronic myelogenous leukemia (CML)	• The median age at diagnosis is ~50.	• Hepatosplenomegaly • Anemia and increased WBC and platelet counts • Presence of Philadelphia chromosome on genetic screening

Box 8-4: Blood and Plasma Transfusion Compatibility

For a blood or plasma transfusion to be safe, the patient and donor must have compatible blood types. The chart below allows you to determine compatibility. Keep in mind that, before transfusing begins, the blood product *must* be crossmatched to fully establish donor-recipient compatibility.

Blood Product Compatibility Chart

Recipient Blood Type	Compatible Whole Blood Type	Compatible Red Blood Cell Type	Compatible Plasma Type (Rh Match Not Needed)
O Rh+	**O** Rh+, **O** Rh–	**O** Rh+, **O** Rh–	**O, A, B, AB**
O Rh–	**O** Rh–	**O** Rh–	**O, A, B, AB**
A Rh+	**A** Rh+, **A** Rh–	**A** Rh+, **A** Rh–, **O** Rh+, **O** Rh–	**A, AB**
A Rh–	**A** Rh–	**A** Rh–, **O** Rh–	**A, AB**
B Rh+	**B** Rh+, **B** Rh–	**B** Rh+, **B** Rh–, **O** Rh+, **O** Rh–	**B, AB**
B Rh–	**B** Rh–	**B** Rh–, **O** Rh–	**B, AB**
AB Rh+	**AB** Rh+, **AB** Rh–	**AB** Rh+, **AB** Rh–, **A** Rh+, **A** Rh–, **B** Rh+, **B** Rh–, **O** Rh+, **O** Rh–	**AB**
AB Rh–	**AB** Rh–	**AB** Rh–, **A** Rh–, **B** Rh–, **O** Rh–	**AB**

Box 8-5: Guide to Immediate Transfusion Reactions

Any patient receiving a transfusion of blood or blood products is at risk for a transfusion reaction. An immediate reaction may occur during the transfusion itself or several hours after the transfusion. The chart below describes immediate reactions.

Reaction	Cause	Signs and Symptoms	Nursing Interventions
Acute hemolytic	• Administration of incompatible blood	• Chest pain • Dyspnea • Facial flushing • Fever • Chills • Hypotension • Flank pain • Bloody oozing at the infusion or surgical incision site • Nausea • Tachycardia	• Monitor the patient carefully, especially during the first 15 minutes of any transfusion. If you see signs of a reaction, stop the transfusion immediately. • Administer I.V. fluids, oxygen, epinephrine, and a vasopressor, as ordered. • Observe the patient for signs of coagulopathy.
Bacterial contamination	• Contamination of blood product	• Chills • Fever • Vomiting • Abdominal cramping • Diarrhea • Shock	• Provide broad-spectrum antibiotics, as prescribed. • Monitor the patient for fever for several hours after completion of the transfusion. • Obtain blood cultures from a site other than I.V. infusion site. • Keep all blood bags and tubing and send them to the blood bank.

Reaction	Cause	Signs and Symptoms	Nursing Interventions
Febrile nonhemolytic	• Cytokines from leukocytes in transfused red cell or other blood components cause a reaction in the recipient.	• Fever within 2 hours of transfusion • Chills • Rigor • Headache • Palpitation • Cough • Tachycardia	• Relieve signs and symptoms with an antipyretic. • If the patient requires further transfusions, consider using a leukocyte removal filter.
Transfusion-related acute lung injury (TRALI)	• Granulocyte antibodies in the donor or recipient react with one another and subsequently cause pulmonary edema in the recipient	• Severe respiratory distress within 6 hours of transfusion • Fever • Chills • Cyanosis • Hypotension	• Stop the transfusion immediately. • Provide oxygen as needed. • Monitor pulse oximetry. • Prepare for intubation and ventilatory support and hemodynamic monitoring.
Allergic reaction	• Allergic reaction to the allogenic proteins in the donor's plasma	• Urticaria • Fever • Nausea and vomiting • Anaphylaxis (facial swelling, laryngeal edema, respiratory distress) in extreme cases	• Stop the transfusion and administer antihistamine, corticosteroid, or epinephrine, as ordered. • Prepare for intubation and respiratory support if the patient develops anaphylaxis.
Transfusion-associated circulatory overload	• Rapid infusion of blood or excessive volume of transfusion	• Chest tightness • Chills • Dyspnea • Tachypnea • Hypoxemia • Hypertension and jugular vein distention that occurs 2 to 6 hours after transfusion	• Monitor intake and output, breath sounds, and blood pressure. • Administer diuretics as needed. • Watch elderly patients and those with a history of cardiac disease carefully because they are at higher risk.

Box 8-5: Guide to Immediate Transfusion Reactions (continued)

- Signs and symptoms
  - Severe bone pain, confusion, weakness, dizziness, weight loss, fractures, renal failure, frequent infections, and skeletal deformities
  - Anemia, leukopenia, and thrombocytopenia—with resulting bleeding, infection, shortness of breath, weakness, and protein in blood and urine—may also occur
- Diagnosis and treatment
  - Serum and urine protein electrophoresis showing immunoglobulin or beta$_2$-microglobulin are indicative of multiple myeloma; urine studies may show Bence Jones proteins and hypercalciuria
  - Bone X-rays or MRI may show bone destruction
  - Bone marrow aspiration and biopsy may show an increased number of immature plasma cells
  - Chemotherapy suppresses plasma cell growth, and radiation therapy may be used to treat bone lesions and relieve pain
  - Radiation therapy may be used to damage myeloma cells and stop growth
  - Patients with multiple myeloma may also receive interferon to slow the growth of the myeloma cells and thalidomide (Thalomid) to inhibit angiogenesis
  - Biologic agents including lenalidomide (Revlimid) and pomalidomide (Pomalyst) utilize the body's immune system to attack the myeloma cells
  - Autologous bone marrow transplantation isn't a cure but may put the patient into remission for a period; allogenic transplantation carries a higher risk of serious complications but produces longer-lasting remissions
  - Plasmapheresis is sometimes used to temporarily remove the high-myeloma protein and thereby improve symptoms

- Hypercalcemia may be managed with a diuretic, hydration, or a phosphate
- Other treatments include targeted therapies including bortezomib (Velcade) and carfilzomib (Kyprolis) for resistant forms
- Nursing interventions
  - Educate the patient and family about diagnostic and treatment procedures and adverse effects
  - Assess the patient for pain, and administer an analgesic regularly
  - Instruct the patient on safety measures to prevent fractures of affected bones; direct the patient not to walk without assistance; have the patient use devices, such as splints or braces, to prevent injury and reduce pain
  - Encourage the patient to drink plenty of fluids, or administer I.V. fluids, to dilute calcium, prevent dehydration, and prevent renal precipitates
  - Assess the patient for signs and symptoms of infection and bleeding, and take measures to prevent their occurrence

Non-Hodgkin's Lymphoma

- Description
  - Non-Hodgkin's lymphoma describes a group of malignant neoplasms arising from abnormal lymphocytes that affect the immune system; this disease is usually disseminated when diagnosed and produces systemic symptoms
  - It may be associated with viral infection, congenital immunodeficiency, or immunosuppression after organ transplantation
  - The prognosis is poor but depends on the histologic type and progression of the disease
- Signs and symptoms
  - Non-Hodgkin's lymphoma can affect any organ or tissue and produces a wide range of symptoms
  - Signs and symptoms resemble those of Hodgkin's lymphoma
  - Fever, painless lymphadenopathy, profuse sweating (especially at night), severe pruritus, abdominal pain or swelling, and weight loss are common signs and symptoms
- Diagnosis and treatment
  - Diagnostic procedures are similar to those for Hodgkin's lymphoma; however, Reed-Sternberg cells are not present
  - Staging is similar to Hodgkin's lymphoma (see *Staging lymphomas*, page 121)
  - Radiation therapy, chemotherapy, and stem cell transplantation are the principal treatments
  - Biological response modifiers, such as interferon and monoclonal antibodies, also may be used to change the tumor-host relationship
  - Targeted radioimmunotherapy may also be used
- Nursing interventions
  - Educate the patient and family about transfusions, chemotherapy, and stem cell transplantation
  - Initiate interventions similar to those for leukemia and Hodgkin's lymphoma
  - Prevent infection
  - Support nutritional status

Polycythemia Vera

- Description
  - Polycythemia vera is a proliferative disorder of myeloid stem cells that primarily results in elevated levels of RBCs but also can impact WBCs and platelets
  - In the early phase and for 10 or more years, hematocrit is elevated; in later stages, the bone marrow becomes fibrotic, with the resulting inability to produce as many cells, while the spleen resumes its embryonic function of hematopoiesis and enlarges
  - The disease may eventually progress to myeloid metaplasia with myelofibrosis or acute myelogenous leukemia (AML)
  - The median age at onset is 65, and the median survival is between 10 and 15 years after diagnosis
  - Death results from thrombosis, hemorrhage, or complications of AML
- Signs and symptoms
  - Patients typically have a ruddy complexion

- Splenomegaly
- Symptoms of increased blood volume or increased blood viscosity include headache, dizziness, tinnitus, fatigue, paresthesia, blurred vision, angina, claudication, dyspnea, thrombophlebitis, and hypertension
- Pruritus, gout, and burning in the fingers and toes may also occur
- Complications include stroke, myocardial infarction (MI), thrombotic events, and bleeding related to dysfunctional platelets
- Diagnosis and treatment
  - Laboratory tests include hematocrit, which can initially exceed 60%; leukocyte and platelet counts are elevated, and uric acid levels are often increased
  - Treatment aims to reduce the high blood cell mass; regular phlebotomy is performed to keep hematocrit below 45%
  - Drug therapy may include chemotherapeutics agents including hydroxyurea (Hydrea or Droxia) to suppress bone marrow function, as well as platelet inhibitors like aspirin
- Nursing interventions
  - Be alert for thrombotic complications such as deep vein thrombosis, and observe for excessive bleeding
  - Monitor for signs and symptoms of infection
  - Provide supportive care, keep pain under control and treat pruritus with warm or cool baths and antihistamines as ordered
  - Teach the patient and family about the disease process and how to prevent complications
  - Provide emotional support

Thrombocytopenia

- Description
  - Thrombocytopenia is an abnormally low level of circulating platelets (less than 100,000/mm^3) due to decreased production, decreased survival, increased destruction, or increased sequestration of platelets in the spleen
  - It may result from antibody production (idiopathic thrombocytopenic purpura [ITP]), bone marrow radiation, excessive alcohol use, folate deficiency, or a disease, such as aplastic anemia or leukemia, DIC, hypothermia, or an autoimmune disorder
  - It also may result from drug therapy with an analgesic, an antibiotic (resulting in ITP), a chemotherapeutic drug, an anti-inflammatory, or a thiazide diuretic; although the platelet count may return to normal 1 to 2 weeks after the drug is withdrawn, more than 90% of adults don't go into spontaneous remission
- Signs and symptoms
  - Ecchymosis, petechiae, and purpura may affect the skin
  - Epistaxis, gingival bleeding, severe hemorrhage, and menorrhagia also may occur
- Diagnosis and treatment
  - The diagnosis is made by examining the CBC, especially the platelet count, blood smear, PT/PTT (clotting times), and bone marrow to determine whether the platelet loss is caused by lack of production or increased destruction
  - Treatment focuses on correcting the underlying cause
  - For ITP, the principal treatment is corticosteroid therapy; for severe or resistant cases, immunosuppressant therapy or splenectomy may be used; platelet transfusions aren't helpful because of continued platelet destruction
  - For other types of thrombocytopenia, platelet transfusions are indicated for supportive care until the underlying cause can be treated
- Nursing interventions
  - Monitor platelet counts; the patient is more susceptible to injury and bleeding when the platelet count falls below 60,000/mm^3 and may develop spontaneous hemorrhage, particularly cerebral hemorrhage when the platelet count drops below 20,000/mm^3
  - Test all stools and urine for blood
  - Avoid taking the patient's temperature rectally and giving injections I.M.
  - Apply pressure to venipuncture and arterial puncture sites
  - Provide meticulous oral care to prevent stomatitis
  - Tell the patient to use only an electric razor and a soft toothbrush and to avoid contact sports, elective surgery, tooth extraction, and the use of aspirin and ibuprofen

Review Questions

Question 1. When assessing a patient who has been diagnosed with megaloblastic anemia, which of the following signs/symptoms would the nurse expect to find?

A. Sudden onset of symptoms, hypotension, and tachycardia
B. Brittle "spoon-shaped" nails
C. Bloody stool
D. Glossitis, neuropathy, and loss of coordination

Correct answer: D All of these are symptoms specific to megaloblastic anemia. Option A presents compensatory symptoms associated with anemia attributed to acute blood loss or an anemia that occurs suddenly. Option B is a sign of iron deficiency anemia. Option C would be a sign of active bleeding related to anemia of blood loss.

Question 2. When teaching neutropenic precautions to a patient who is leukopenic/neutropenic, the nurse should include which of the following directives?

A. Eat foods high in iron.
B. Avoid products that contain aspirin.
C. Avoid people with respiratory tract infections.
D. Eat lots of raw vegetables.

Correct answer: C People with low WBC and neutrophil counts have decreased ability to fight infection and should avoid people who are sick and could transmit the infection to them. Option A would be important to teach the patient with anemia. Option B would be significant for a patient with a low platelet count/thrombocytopenia. Option D is incorrect because those on neutropenic precautions should avoid raw or unwashed vegetables due to exposure to bacteria.

Question 3. When assessing the patient with multiple myeloma, the nurse knows that the body system least affected by multiple myeloma is the

_____:

A. skeletal system.
B. renal system.
C. nervous system.
D. cardiovascular system.

Correct answer: D Multiple myeloma usually doesn't have a direct effect on the heart. Options A, B, and C are incorrect because multiple myeloma usually affects the skeletal, renal, and nervous systems.

Question 4. A nurse is caring for a patient diagnosed with stage IIB Hodgkin's lymphoma. The "B" after the stage indicates the patient has the following:

A. Involvement of a single lymph node region
B. Involvement of extralymphatic sites
C. Unexplained loss of more than 10% of body weight in the past 6 months
D. Uncontrolled itching and skin irritation

Correct answer: C Unexplained weight loss is one of the three "B" or systemic symptoms that helps providers to determine the stage and prognosis. The other "B" symptoms include a temperature above 100.4°F (38°C) and drenching night sweats. Options A and B describe findings that are used to determine the stage of the illness. Option D can be a symptom of Hodgkin's lymphoma but is not considered a "B" or systemic symptom.

Question 5. A 50-year-old male patient recently diagnosed with AML voices that he "isn't sure he wants to go through the hassle of treatment." His nurse should first:

A. give the patient facts about treatment and how it works.
B. offer to call pastoral care.
C. listen to the patient's concerns about treatment and his questions.
D. tell the patient he has to get treatment or he will die.

Correct answer: C The most pertinent need for this patient is to have someone to listen to his concerns. When patients are under stress, big decisions can be hard to process, and therapeutic communication is key. Option A is incorrect because it is not the first thing the nurse should do. Facts can be very useful in this situation, but not as a first action. Option B is incorrect because offering to call pastoral care may be helpful for some patients but should be done after the nurse has spent time with the patient. Option D is incorrect because using scare tactics to get the patient to change his mind does not benefit the therapeutic relationship.

Question 6. A patient with blood type A can receive a transfusion of what type of RBCs?

A. Type A or type O
B. Type B or type O
C. Type AB or type O
D. Type A or type B

Correct answer: A Type A blood contains A antigens and anti-B antibodies, but no anti-A antibodies. Therefore, a patient with type A blood can receive type A or type O RBCs, which contain neither anti-A nor anti-B antibodies. Options B, C, and D are incorrect because blood type A contains anti-B antibodies.

Question 7. Which type of anemia results from deficiency of all the blood's formed elements, caused by failure of the bone marrow to generate enough new cells?

A. Sickle cell anemia
B. Folic acid deficiency anemia
C. Aplastic anemia
D. Iron deficiency anemia

Correct answer: C Aplastic anemia usually develops when damaged or destroyed stem cells inhibit RBC production. Option A, sickle cell anemia, is a genetic disorder that causes malformation of RBCs. Option B, folic acid deficiency anemia, and option D, iron deficiency anemia, are not related to bone marrow failure.

Question 8. Which disorder results from a lack of particular clotting factors?

A. Hemophilia
B. Sickle cell anemia
C. Thalassemia
D. Thrombocytopenia

Correct answer: A Hemophilia is a hereditary bleeding disorder that results from the lack of specific clotting factors. Option B, sickle cell anemia, is a genetic disorder that causes malformation of RBCs. Option C, thalassemia, is an anemia characterized by RBC destruction beyond the bone marrow's ability to produce these cells. Option D, thrombocytopenia, is a disorder defined by a low level of circulating platelets.

Question 9. A patient with Hodgkin's disease has lymph node involvement in the neck and armpit area with spots found on the lungs. According to the Ann Harbor classification system, what stage of lymphoma does this patient have?

A. Stage I
B. Stage II
C. Stage III
D. Stage IV

Correct answer: B Stage II involves two or more lymph node regions on one side of the diaphragm and also regional involvement of one extranodal cite of disease. Option A, stage I, involves a single lymph node regions. Option C, stage III, involves lymph nodes on both sides of the diaphragm with splenic disease. Option D, stage IV, may involve isolated extralymphatic organs as well as nonregional nodes.

Question 10. A patient comes to your unit after losing at least a liter of blood after a car accident. What assessment findings would the nurse expect to find?

A. Night sweats, weight loss, and diarrhea
B. Dyspnea, tachycardia, and pallor
C. Nausea, vomiting, and anorexia
D. Itching, rash, and jaundice

Correct answer: B Signs of anemia from acute blood loss include dyspnea, tachycardia, and pallor, as well as fatigue and irritability. Option A, night sweats, weight loss, and diarrhea, may signal acquired immunodeficiency syndrome. Option C, nausea, vomiting, and anorexia, may be signs of hepatitis B. Option D, itching, rash, and jaundice, may result from an allergic or hemolytic reaction.

Selected References

Lash, B. W., & Argiris, A. (2017). Hodgkin's lymphoma treatment and management. Retrieved on April 28, 2017 from http://emedicine.medscape.com/article/201886.

Mayo Clinic. (2015). Multiple myeloma. Retrieved on May 11, 2017 from http://www.mayoclinic.org/diseases-conditions/multiple-myeloma/basics/definition/con-20026607.

Mayo Clinic. (2016). Leukemia. Retrieved on May 10, 2017 from http://www.mayoclinic.org/diseases-conditions/leukemia/basics/definition/con-20024914.

National Heart, Lung and Blood Institute. (2014). What is iron-deficiency anemia? Retrieved on May 20, 2017 from https://www.nhlbi.nih.gov/health/health-topics/topics/ida.

PDQ® Adult Treatment Editorial Board. (2017). PDQ adult Hodgkin's lymphoma treatment. Bethesda, MD: National Cancer Institute. Retrieved on April 30, 2017 from https://www.cancer.gov/types/lymphoma/patient/adult-hodgkin-treatment-pdq.

Rai, K. R., & Stilgenbauer, S. (2017). Clinical presentation, pathologic features, diagnosis, and differential diagnosis of chronic lymphocytic leukemia. In R. A. Larson & R. A. Connor (Eds.), UptoDate. Retrieved on May 20, 2017 from https://www.uptodate.com/contents/clinical-presentation-pathologic-features-diagnosis-and-differential-diagnosis-of-chronic-lymphocytic-leukemia.

Tefferi, A. (2017). Prognosis and treatment of polycythemia vera. In A. G. Rosemarin & S. L. Schrier (Eds.), UptoDate. Retrieved on May 12, 2017 from https://www.uptodate.com/contents/prognosis-and-treatment-of-polycythemia-vera.

U.S. National Library of Medicine. (2016). Adult Hodgkin's lymphoma. In Medline.com. Retrieved on April 24, 2017 from https://www.ncbi.nlm.nih.gov/pubmedhealth/PMHT0024534/.

U.S. National Library of Medicine. (2016). Thalassemia. Retrieved on May 20, 2017 from https://medlineplus.gov/ency/article/000587.htm.

Van Etten, R. A. (2017). Clinical manifestations and diagnosis of chronic myeloid leukemia. In A. G. Rosemarin & R. A. Larson (Eds.), Uptodate. Retrieved on May 20, 2017 from https://www.uptodate.com/contents/clinical-manifestations-and-diagnosis-of-chronic-myeloid-leukemia.

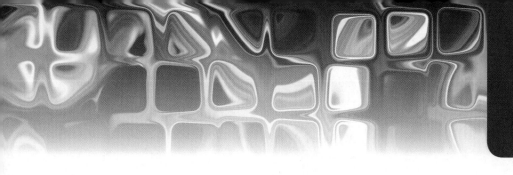

Chapter 9

Respiratory Disorders

Introduction

- The function of the respiratory system is to exchange gases (oxygen and carbon dioxide) with the external environment; the respiratory system maintains the level of these gases within a narrow range, regardless of the demand for oxygen
- Respiration, which the central nervous system controls, is regulated by metabolic demands and cardiac output
- Nursing history
  - The nurse asks the patient about their *chief complaint*
    - A patient with a respiratory disorder may report the following signs or symptoms: chest pain, cough, dyspnea, orthopnea, shortness of breath, or wheezing
    - The patient may also report hemoptysis, increased sputum production, or a change in the characteristics of his sputum
  - The nurse then questions the patient about his *present illness*
    - Ask the patient about symptoms, including when it started, associated symptoms, location, duration, frequency, and precipitating and alleviating factors
    - If the patient has dyspnea, ask the patient to rate it on a scale of 0 to 10, in which 0 means no dyspnea and 10 means the worst dyspnea experienced
    - If the patient has orthopnea, ask how many pillows are being used to sleep
    - Ask if the patient's cough is productive or nonproductive. Is the cough recent? If not recent, how long the patient has been experiencing it? Has it changed recently?
    - When a patient produces sputum, ask for an estimated amount produced in teaspoons or another common measurement; ask at what time of day coughing occurs the most; question about the color and consistency of sputum; ask whether its character has changed recently. If so, how? Do they cough up blood?
    - If a patient wheezes, ask when the wheezing occurs. What makes the patient wheeze? Is the patient wheezing loudly enough for others to hear it? What helps stop the wheezing?
    - If the patient has chest pain, ask where the pain is located, what it feels like, what characteristics it has, whether it moves or radiates, how long it lasts, what causes it to occur, and what makes it better; have patient rate the pain on a scale of 0 to 10 (with 0 being no pain and 10 worst pain experienced)
    - Ask about the use of prescription and over-the-counter drugs, herbal remedies, vitamin and nutritional supplements, and alternative or complementary therapies used
  - The nurse asks about *medical history*
    - Question the patient about other respiratory disorders—such as allergies, asthma, cystic fibrosis, pneumonia, tuberculosis, and upper respiratory tract infections
    - Ask the patient if he has undergone chest or lung surgery
  - The nurse then assesses the *family history*
    - Ask about a family history of chronic obstructive pulmonary disease (COPD), pneumonia, or tuberculosis
    - Determine if there's a family history of lung cancer
  - The nurse obtains a *social history*
    - Ask about smoking habits and environmental exposure to irritants such as asbestos
    - Question the patient about his tolerance for exercise

130

- Physical assessment
  - The nurse begins with *inspection*
    - Observe the patient's general appearance; note the patient's position. Is he sitting upright? Leaning forward? In a tripod position?
    - Take note of level of awareness and general appearance. Does the patient appear relaxed? Anxious? Uncomfortable? Having trouble breathing?
    - Note deformities, masses, or scars of the chest; look for chest wall symmetry at rest and with inspiration; note the anteroposterior chest diameter; observe chest wall movement. Is it paradoxical, or uneven?
    - Note tracheal deviation; look for spinal abnormalities such as kyphosis; note whether the costal angle is enlarged
    - Observe the patient's respirations, noting rate, depth, rhythm, and inspiratory-expiratory ratio; look for the use of accessory muscles with breathing, pursed-lip breathing, nostril flaring, and retracting
    - Observe the color of the patient's skin, lips, mucous membranes, and nail beds; check nails for clubbing
  - Next, the nurse uses *palpation*
    - Palpate the chest for temperature, dryness, crepitus, pain, and tactile fremitus
    - Check for respiratory excursion
  - Then the nurse *percusses* the heart
    - Percuss the anterior and posterior chest, noting lung boundaries and movement of the diaphragm
    - Also note percussion sounds; describe any abnormal ones, including the location and size of the area
  - The nurse continues with *auscultation*
    - Auscultate the anterior, posterior, and lateral chest, comparing breath sounds
    - Classify each sound according to its intensity, location, pitch, duration, and characteristic; note whether the sound occurs during inhalation, exhalation, or both
    - Auscultate for vocal fremitus, noting bronchophony, egophony, and whispered pectoriloquy

Acute Respiratory Distress Syndrome

- Description
  - Acute respiratory distress syndrome (ARDS), a severe form of lung injury, occurs when the lungs can't maintain the oxygen–carbon dioxide balance
  - Although its exact cause is unknown, ARDS occurs as a result of diffuse alveolar damage; its mortality rate is 50% or higher; death is usually due to a multisystem failure or an infection
  - Risk factors for ARDS include aspiration pneumonia, drug overdose, fat or amniotic emboli, head injury, hemorrhagic shock, massive blood transfusions or transfusion reactions, near drowning, pulmonary contusion, sepsis, smoke inhalation, and trauma
  - With ARDS, capillaries leak, causing interstitial edema; this decreases blood flow to the lungs and causes platelet aggregation
    - The respiratory membrane becomes inflamed; alveolar edema develops, leading to pulmonary edema
    - Lung compliance decreases, and patches of atelectasis develop; the patient hyperventilates, thereby causing hypocapnia and hypoxemia and leading to multisystem organ dysfunction syndrome
    - A ventilation-perfusion mismatch occurs
- Signs and symptoms
  - Vital sign measurements reveal increased blood pressure, tachycardia, and tachypnea (along with increased respiratory effort and accessory muscle use)
  - Other signs and symptoms may include barotrauma symptoms, bibasilar crackles, crepitus, cyanosis, decreased breath sounds, diaphoresis, dyspnea, progressive hypoxemia despite oxygen therapy, restlessness, and thick, frothy sputum
- Diagnosis and treatment
  - Early diagnosis and prompt treatment allow for successful management of ARDS
  - Arterial blood gas (ABG) studies reveal decreased partial pressure of arterial oxygen (PaO_2) unresponsive to supplemental oxygen
  - A pulmonary artery (PA) catheter inserted to measure pressures reveals pulmonary artery wedge pressure (PAWP) of less than 18 mm Hg
  - Chest X-ray shows bilateral infiltrates (in early stages) and lung fields with ground-glass appearance, irreversible hypoxemia, and massive consolidation seen as "white lung" (in later stages)

- Mechanical ventilation may be necessary
  - Raising the fraction of inspired oxygen (FIO_2) with a ventilator helps to reverse hypoxemia but may increase the risk of oxygen toxicity and pulmonary fibrosis
  - Supplementing mechanical ventilation with positive end–expiratory pressure (PEEP) provides a constant pressure that prevents the alveoli from collapsing
  - PEEP allows the use of a lower FIO_2 to obtain an adequate PaO_2
  - Pressure control ventilation that prevents overdistention of the alveoli and inverse ratio ventilation in which inspiration is longer than expiration may also be used
- A diuretic may be administered to reduce pulmonary edema
- An antibiotic is used to treat any respiratory tract infection or underlying systemic infection
- Pharmacologic paralysis is used to decrease oxygen consumption; the patient must be sedated for this treatment
- Vasopressors are given to maintain blood pressure
- Electrolyte and acid-base imbalances are corrected to maintain cellular integrity
- Nursing interventions
  - Make sure the patient maintains bed rest in semi-Fowler's or the prone position, if possible, to improve oxygenation
  - Provide oxygen therapy (and mechanical ventilation, if indicated) to maintain PaO_2 above 60 mm Hg; this will maintain oxygenation and help to reverse hypoxemia
  - Implement chest physiotherapy to loosen secretions
  - If the patient isn't on mechanical ventilation, teach him effective coughing and deep breathing exercises to maximize lung expansion and reexpand collapsed alveoli
  - Suction the patient's airway as needed to maintain patency and to clear secretions; sterile technique prevents bacterial contamination of lower airways
  - Administer drugs to relieve pain and discomfort as needed
  - If the patient is on mechanical ventilation, administer a paralyzant and a sedative as necessary
  - Monitor fluid intake and output to determine the effectiveness of diuretic therapy
  - Frequently reposition the patient to prevent complications of immobility, help loosen secretions, and promote lung perfusion
  - Provide 2,500 calories daily to prevent weakness and increase immune response; use enteral or parenteral feeding if needed
  - Teach relaxation techniques, and encourage the patient not to fight the ventilator
  - Because a mechanically ventilated patient can't speak, provide communication alternatives, such as letter and picture boards

Acute Respiratory Failure

- Description
  - In acute respiratory failure, the lungs' inability to adequately maintain arterial oxygenation or eliminate carbon dioxide results in inadequate ventilation
  - The disorder is classified as hypoxemic (type I) or hypercapnic (type II)
  - Primarily hypercapnic respiratory failure results from inadequate alveolar ventilation caused by a ventilation-perfusion ($\dot{V}/\dot{Q}$) mismatch and shunting
  - Primarily hypoxemic respiratory failure results from inadequate oxygen exchange between the alveoli and capillaries
  - The disorder also commonly occurs as a combination of hypercapnic and hypoxemic respiratory failure
  - Causes include accumulated secretions secondary to cough suppression; airway irritants; any condition that increases the work of breathing and decreases the respiratory drive of patients with COPD; bronchospasm; central nervous system depression; disorders of the peripheral nervous system, respiratory muscles, and chest wall; endocrine or metabolic disorders; gas exchange failure; heart failure; myocardial infarction (MI); and pulmonary embolism
- Signs and symptoms
  - Signs include changes in mental status, such as confusion, somnolence, and cyanosis of the oral mucosa, lips, and nail beds
  - Assessment may reveal absent breath sounds, wheezes, rhonchi, and crackles in the lung fields
  - Other signs and symptoms include yawning and use of accessory muscles, pursed-lip breathing, nasal flaring, ashen skin, and tachypnea

- Diagnosis and treatment
  - ABG analysis reveals hypercapnia (partial pressure of arterial carbon dioxide [$Paco_2$] greater than 50 mm Hg) and hypoxemia (Pao_2 less than 60 mm Hg) on room air
  - If a bacterial infection is involved, laboratory tests show an increased serum white blood cell (WBC) count; blood cultures, Gram stain, and sputum cultures reveal the pathogen
  - Serum hemoglobin and hematocrit show decreased oxygen-carrying capacity
  - Chest X-rays may reveal underlying pulmonary diseases or conditions, such as emphysema, atelectasis, lesions, pneumothorax, infiltrates, and effusions
  - Electrocardiography (ECG) may show arrhythmias, cor pulmonale, or myocardial ischemia
  - Pulse oximetry may show decreased arterial oxygen saturation
  - Treatment may include mechanical ventilation with an endotracheal or a tracheostomy tube
  - If the underlying cause is heart failure, the patient will need fluid restriction
  - Initially, the patient is maintained on bed rest, progressing to activity as tolerated
  - Oxygen therapy increases the pressure of arterial oxygen
  - Antibiotics treat any underlying infection
  - Bronchodilators, such as terbutaline (Brethine), albuterol sulfate (Ventolin, Proventil), theophylline (Theo-24), aclidinium (Tudorza), arformoterol (Brovana), and ipratropium bromide (Atrovent), alleviate obstruction and bronchospasm
  - Corticosteroids reduce inflammation
  - Positive inotropic agents, such as dopamine or dobutamine, maintain perfusion
  - Nitrates, such as nitroglycerin or nitroprusside (Nitropress), reduce myocardial oxygen demand
  - Morphine serves as an adjunct treatment for acute pulmonary edema
  - Diuretics alleviate heart failure
- Nursing interventions
  - Monitor the patient's vital signs, pulse oximetry readings, and ECG
  - Administer prescribed drugs as indicated (via inhalation, the oral route, nebulization, or I.V., as appropriate)
  - Orient the patient frequently
  - Administer humidified, supplemental oxygen as ordered
  - Maintain a patent airway
  - Help clear the patient's secretions with postural drainage and chest physiotherapy; also suction as necessary
  - Encourage pursed-lip breathing
  - Encourage the use of an incentive spirometer to promote lung expansion
  - Reposition the patient every 1 to 2 hours to help mobilize secretions
  - Perform or assist with oral hygiene
  - Position the patient for comfort, with the head of the bed elevated, if appropriate, to promote optimal gas exchange
  - Maintain a normal body temperature with antipyretics
  - Cluster nursing activities and schedule care to provide frequent rest periods
  - Prepare for intubation and mechanical ventilation if needed
  - Provide sedation as necessary
  - Provide education and emotional support to the patient and family

Asthma

- Description
  - Asthma is a chronic reactive airway disorder that involves episodic, reversible airway obstruction resulting from bronchospasms, increased mucus secretions, and mucosal edema
  - It's characterized by airway inflammation, intermittent airflow obstruction, and bronchial hyperresponsiveness
  - Asthma can result from several types of triggers
    - Exposure to tobacco or wood smoke
    - Breathing polluted air
    - Inhaling other respiratory irritants, such as perfumes or cleaning products
    - Exposure to airway irritants at the workplace
    - Breathing in allergy-causing substances (allergens), such as molds, dust, or animal dander
    - Upper respiratory tract infection, such as a cold, influenza, sinusitis, or bronchitis
    - Exposure to cold

○ Dry weather

○ Emotional excitement or stress

○ Physical exertion or exercise (exercise-induced asthma)

○ Reflux of stomach acid (gastroesophageal reflux disease, or GERD)

○ Ingestion of sulfites, an additive found in some foods and wine

- Comorbidities include GERD, drug-induced asthma, and other allergic reactions, such as eczema, rashes, and temporary edema

● Signs and symptoms

- Overall signs and symptoms of asthma range from mild wheezing and dyspnea to life-threatening respiratory failure; signs and symptoms of bronchial airway obstruction may persist between acute episodes

- An asthma attack may begin dramatically, with simultaneous onset of severe, multiple signs and symptoms, or insidiously, with gradually increasing respiratory distress (see *Determining Asthma's Severity*, pages 135–136)

- Exposure to a particular allergen is followed by a sudden onset of dyspnea and wheezing and by tightness in the chest accompanied by a cough that produces thick, clear, or yellow sputum (cough, dyspnea, and wheezing are the three most common signs and symptoms of asthma)

- An attack often starts during the night or in the early morning

- Physical findings may include visible dyspnea, use of accessory respiratory muscles, complaints of chest tightness, diaphoresis, increased anteroposterior thoracic diameter, and hyperresonance

- Tachycardia, tachypnea, mild systolic hypertension, and pulsus paradoxus may occur as the exacerbation progresses

- Inspiratory and expiratory wheezes may occur, along with wheezing and coughing (which may be exercise-induced), a prolonged expiratory phase of respiration, and diminished breath sounds

- The occurrence of cyanosis, confusion, and lethargy indicate the onset of life-threatening status asthmaticus and respiratory failure

● Diagnosis and treatment

- ABG analysis provides the best indication of an attack's severity and may reveal hypoxemia during an acute attack; in acutely severe asthma, PaO_2 is less than 60 mm Hg, $PaCO_2$ is 40 mm Hg or more, and pH is usually decreased; normal $PaCO_2$ during an acute attack may signal impending respiratory failure

- Radioallergosorbent testing shows increased serum immunoglobulin E levels as a result of an allergic reaction

- A complete blood count (CBC) including WBC count and differential shows increased eosinophil count in acute phases

- Chest X-rays may show hyperinflation, flattened diaphragms, areas of focal atelectasis, pneumothorax, or pneumomediastinum

- Pulmonary function tests commonly show decreased peak flow rates and forced expiratory volume in 1 second, low-normal or decreased vital capacity, and increased total lung and residual capacities, although results may be normal between attacks

- Skin testing may identify specific allergens

- Bronchial challenge testing shows the clinical significance of allergens identified by skin testing

- Pulse oximetry measurements may show decreased oxygen saturation

- Peak flow monitoring reveals a result of less than 80% of personal best; a reading below 50% of personal best indicates a severe exacerbation

- Treatment involves identifying and avoiding precipitating factors and desensitizing the patient to specific antigens

- Generally, asthma medications are divided into two categories: quick relief for relief of immediate symptoms and long-acting medications to control the underlying inflammation

○ Quick-relief bronchodilators include an albuterol sulfate (Ventolin, Proventil) and arformoterol (Brovana) inhaler used as needed

○ Quick-relief anticholinergics for bronchospasms include ipratropium bromide (Atrovent)

○ Corticosteroids, such as systemic methylprednisolone, prednisolone, and prednisone, prevent exacerbation and progression during moderate or severe exacerbations

○ Corticosteroids for persistent asthma include inhaled corticosteroid of fluticasone (Flovent), beclomethasone (QVAR), budesonide inhaled (Pulmicort Turbuhaler), and mometasone inhaled (Asmanex)

○ Long-acting beta-agonist or combination drugs include salmeterol inhaled (Serevent), formoterol inhaled (Foradil), fluticasone and salmeterol inhaled (Advair), and budesonide and formoterol inhaled (Symbicort)

○ Leukotriene antagonists (antileukotrienes) include montelukast (Singulair)

○ Anticholinergic bronchodilators include tiotropium inhaled (Spiriva)

○ Monoclonal antibodies such as omalizumab (Xolair) and anti-inflammatory agents such as nedocromil sodium (Tilade) inhaled before exercise reduce bronchospasm

- Nursing interventions
  - Give prescribed inhalers and asthma medications
  - Place the patient in high Fowler's position
  - Encourage pursed-lip and diaphragmatic breathing
  - Administer prescribed humidified oxygen
  - Adjust oxygen according to the patient's vital signs and ABG values
  - Assist with intubation and mechanical ventilation, if appropriate
  - Perform postural drainage and chest percussion, if tolerated
  - If the patient is intubated, suction as needed
  - Treat the patient's dehydration with I.V. or oral fluids as tolerated
  - Keep the room temperature comfortable
  - Use an air conditioner or a fan in hot, humid weather
  - Monitor the patient's vital signs, intake and output, response to treatment, signs and symptoms of theophylline toxicity, breath sounds, ABG results, pulmonary function test results, pulse oximetry, complications of corticosteroid treatment, and anxiety level

Box 9-1: Determining Asthma's Severity

The severity of asthma is classified by the:
- Frequency, severity, and duration of symptoms
- Degree of airflow obstruction (spirometry measure) or peak expiratory flow (PEF)
- Frequency of nighttime symptoms and the degree that the asthma interferes with daily activities

Severity can change over time, and even milder cases can become severe in an uncontrolled attack. Long-term therapy depends on whether the patient's asthma is classified as mild intermittent, mild persistent, moderate persistent, or severe persistent. For all patients, quick relief can be obtained by using a short-acting bronchodilator (two to four puffs of a short-acting inhaled beta 2 adrenergic agonist as needed for symptoms). However, the use of a short-acting bronchodilator more than twice a week in patients with intermittent asthma or daily or increasing use in patients with persistent asthma may indicate the need to initiate or increase long-term control therapy.

Mild intermittent asthma

The signs and symptoms of mild intermittent asthma include:
- Daytime symptoms that occur no more than twice a week
- Nighttime symptoms that occur no more than twice a month
- Lung function testing (either PEF or forced expiratory volume in 1 second) of 80% of predicted value or higher
- PEF that varies no more than 20%

Severe exacerbations, separated by long, symptomless periods of normal lung function, indicate mild intermittent asthma. A course of systemic corticosteroids is recommended for these exacerbations; otherwise, daily medication isn't required.

Mild persistent asthma

The signs and symptoms of mild persistent asthma include:
- Daytime symptoms that occur 3 to 6 days a week
- Nighttime symptoms that occur three to four times a month
- Lung function testing of 80% of predicted value or higher
- PEF that varies between 20% and 30%

The preferred treatment for mild persistent asthma is low-dose inhaled corticosteroids, but alternative treatments include cromolyn, leukotriene modifier, nedocromil, and sustained-release theophylline.

Moderate persistent asthma

The signs and symptoms of moderate persistent asthma include:
- Daily daytime symptoms
- Nighttime symptoms that occur at least weekly
- Lung function testing of 60% to 80% of predicted value
- PEF that varies more than 30%

The preferred treatment for moderate persistent asthma is low- or medium-dose inhaled corticosteroids combined with a long-acting inhaled beta 2 adrenergic agonist. Alternative treatments include increasing inhaled corticosteroids within the medium-dose range or low- or medium-dose inhaled corticosteroids with either leukotriene modifier or theophylline.

Box 9-1: Determining Asthma's Severity (continued)

For recurring exacerbations, the preferred treatment is to increase inhaled corticosteroids within the medium-dose range and add a long-acting inhaled beta 2 adrenergic agonist. The alternative treatment is to increase inhaled corticosteroids within the medium-dose range and add either leukotriene modifier or theophylline.

Severe persistent asthma

The signs and symptoms of severe persistent asthma include:
- Continual daytime symptoms
- Frequent nighttime symptoms
- Lung function testing of 60% of predicted value or lower
- PEF that varies more than 30%

The preferred treatment for severe persistent asthma includes high-dose inhaled corticosteroids combined with long-acting inhaled beta 2 adrenergic agonists. Long-term administration of corticosteroid tablets or syrup (2 mg/kg/day, not to exceed 60 mg/day) may be used to reduce the need for systemic corticosteroid therapy.

Atelectasis

- Description
  - Atelectasis is the partial or total collapse of the functioning alveoli
  - Airway obstruction, COPD, ascites, and lung compression resulting from hemothorax, pneumothorax, or tumor can cause atelectasis; atelectasis also is a common complication of thoracic and upper abdominal surgery that can occur 24 to 48 hours postoperatively
  - General anesthesia, immobility, lung disease, obesity, opioid use, pain, and smoking increase the risk of atelectasis
  - A patient with atelectasis has decreased ventilation because the collapsed alveoli can't exchange gases; this decreased ventilation leads to hypoxemia
  - Stasis of mucus leads to bacterial growth and pneumonia
- Signs and symptoms
  - Vital sign assessment typically reveals fever (which may occur 24 to 48 hours postoperatively), tachycardia, and tachypnea
  - Auscultation may reveal crackles and decreased breath sounds over the affected area
  - Other effects may include cyanosis, dyspnea, and increased sputum production
- Diagnosis and treatment
  - The patient should undergo ABG studies, chest X-ray, and sputum culture
  - A bronchodilator is administered to dilate bronchioles and promote secretion removal
  - An antibiotic is administered to treat infection
  - If present, tumors are removed surgically or treated with radiation therapy
  - A chest tube is inserted for a patient with hemothorax (to drain blood) or pneumothorax (to reinflate the lung)
- Nursing interventions
  - Encourage the patient to cough and breathe deeply to maximize lung expansion and reexpand collapsed alveoli; use an incentive spirometer hourly after surgery
  - Provide adequate hydration to liquefy secretions; thin secretions are easier to expectorate
  - Implement chest physiotherapy to help clear secretions; postural drainage uses gravity to clear secretions, whereas percussion and vibration loosen secretions, making them easier to cough up
  - Suction the patient's airway to maintain patency and to clear secretions
  - Provide oxygen therapy to improve PaO_2 and maintain adequate oxygenation
  - Medicate for pain or discomfort as needed, which will allow the patient to cough and deep-breathe effectively
  - Teach the patient to use a pillow to splint abdominal and chest incisions during coughing exercises
  - Encourage early ambulation and frequent position changes to prevent complications of immobility and promote lung expansion

Cancer, Laryngeal

- Description
  - Laryngeal cancer affects the epithelial lining of the mucous membrane of the larynx, most commonly as squamous cell carcinoma; it usually affects men in their 60s and 70s
  - Although laryngeal cancer has no proven cause, two major risk factors are cigarette smoking and alcohol consumption; other risk factors include frequent laryngitis, poor nutrition, and compromised immunity
- Signs and symptoms
  - Hoarseness for more than 2 weeks, an early warning sign, may become progressively worse
  - Dysphagia, dyspnea, and hemoptysis may be present
  - Pain may be referred to the ear or throat if ulceration occurs
  - Cervical lymph nodes may be enlarged
- Diagnosis and treatment
  - Laryngoscopy shows nodules on the vocal cords, and nodule biopsy reveals cancer cells
  - Radiation therapy and surgery may be used alone or together
    - Partial laryngectomy changes the voice and preserves the respiratory tract
    - Total laryngectomy produces a complete loss of voice and creates a permanent tracheostomy opening
- Nursing interventions
  - Encourage deep breathing to maintain respiratory function
  - Suction the patient's airway as needed to maintain patency and to clear secretions
  - Administer oxygen to improve PaO_2 and maintain adequate oxygenation
  - Provide tracheostomy care to prevent infection and maintain the airway
  - Ensure adequate hydration and nutrition while preventing aspiration and aspiration-induced infection
    - Have the patient eat slowly and in the sitting position only
    - Provide frequent small meals, and advance the diet as tolerated
    - Have suction equipment readily available
  - Provide pain relief as needed to reduce anxiety, and encourage deep breathing and activity
  - If needed, teach the patient and family alternative methods of communication, such as an alphabet board or gesturing
  - Discuss and initiate speech therapy, if appropriate, to maximize remaining vocal function

Cancer, Lung

- Description
  - Lung cancers are classified into two major categories: small-cell carcinomas and non–small-cell carcinomas
  - Small-cell carcinoma accounts for 15% to 20% of lung cancers; non–small-cell carcinomas account for 80% of lung cancers
  - Non–small-cell carcinomas include squamous cell carcinoma (20% to 30%), large-cell carcinoma (15%), and adenocarcinoma (40%)
  - Up to 40% of lung cancers are metastatic; breast, GI, prostate, and renal cancers commonly metastasize to the lungs
  - Risk factors for lung cancer include cigarette smoking, environmental factors such as air pollution, genetic factors, and occupational exposure to carcinogens
  - Adenocarcinoma tends to grow slowly and is peripherally located; this well-circumscribed tumor seldom cavitates but spreads early to regional lymph nodes
  - Large-cell carcinoma produces large necrotic masses that tend to grow rapidly and are peripherally located; it tends to cavitate, metastasizes early, and spreads extensively
  - Small-cell carcinoma, the most aggressive lung cancer, tends to grow rapidly and is centrally located; it rapidly metastasizes through lymph and blood systems but responds to chemotherapy
  - Squamous cell carcinoma, the most common lung cancer, tends to grow slowly and is centrally located; it produces early local symptoms, tends to cavitate, and metastasizes to intrathoracic sites first
- Signs and symptoms
  - Some lung cancers are asymptomatic; symptoms arise from metastasis to other body areas
  - Dyspnea may range from mild dyspnea during extreme exertion to severe dyspnea at rest
  - Auscultation may reveal decreased breath sounds, localized wheezing, and pleural rub (with pleural effusion)
  - A chronic cough may be nonproductive; however, hemoptysis is common
  - Enlarged lymph nodes and fatigue may occur

- Finger clubbing may be a late sign of lung cancer
- Weight loss may occur
- The patient may report bone pain, chest pain or tightness, joint aching, and shoulder and arm pain
- Superior vena cava syndrome may cause edema of the face, neck, and upper torso as well as dilated veins in the abdomen and chest
- Diagnosis and treatment
  - Chest X-ray, computed tomography (CT) scan, MRI, bronchoscopy, sputum cytology, pulmonary function tests, ABG studies, brain and bone scans, and lymph node biopsy may be prescribed
  - Specimens may be obtained for culture by way of bronchoscopy, transthoracic needle biopsy, mediastinoscopy, open lung biopsy (thoracotomy), or thoracentesis
  - Surgical procedures—such as lobectomy, pneumonectomy, and wedge resection—are used to treat lung cancer
  - Chemotherapy, immunosuppressant therapy, and radiation therapy also may be used (see *Nursing Implications in Oncology Care*, pages 341–347)
  - Serial thoracentesis or chest tube placement is used for recurrent pleural effusions
  - Laser therapy through a bronchoscope is a palliative measure that relieves endobronchial obstructions caused by nonresectable tumors
- Nursing interventions
  - Monitor a patient who has undergone surgery
    - Assess the incision for signs of infection
    - Check the dressing for drainage and the chest tube for proper functioning, air leakage, and amount of drainage
    - Assess lungs for signs of atelectasis
    - Assess the intensity, quality, and location of pain
    - Assess the patient for heart failure caused by fluid overload, hyponatremia, and renal failure
    - Monitor electrolyte levels to detect hyponatremia or hyperkalemia
    - Monitor the patient's CBC for anemia and leukopenia
    - Assess fluid intake and output
    - Assess nutritional status
  - Administer oxygen to improve PaO_2, and maintain adequate oxygenation
  - Suction the patient's airway as needed to maintain patency and to clear secretions
  - Provide pain relief as needed to reduce anxiety, and encourage coughing, deep breathing, and early ambulation
  - Position the patient for comfort and adequate respiration
  - Teach relaxation techniques to alleviate anxiety
  - Intervene appropriately for a postoperative patient
    - Ensure adequate hydration to liquefy secretions; thin secretions are easier to expectorate
    - Provide chest physiotherapy; postural drainage uses gravity to clear secretions, and percussion and vibration loosen secretions, making them easier to expectorate
    - Teach effective coughing and deep breathing to promote lung expansion and prevent atelectasis
    - Encourage early ambulation and frequent position changes to prevent complications and promote lung expansion
    - Increase the patient's caloric intake to 2,500 calories daily
      - Although patients may have a poor appetite, their metabolic needs are increased
      - Administer medications to control diarrhea, nausea, and vomiting
      - Encourage the patient to eat frequent, small meals
      - Encourage family members and friends to provide nutritious food that the patient likes
    - Have a patient who has undergone thoracotomy practice arm exercises to promote lung expansion and maintain arm mobility
    - Encourage the patient to express concerns to reduce anxiety, decrease pain, and promote healing
    - If the patient is a smoker, discuss the effects of smoking, and help get him into a smoking cessation program
    - Teach the patient how to improve his quality of life by conserving energy and reorganizing the home so that frequently used items are within reach, and consider employing a homemaking service

Chest Trauma

- Description
  - *Rib fracture* can result from a blunt or penetrating injury; fractures commonly involve multiple ribs
  - *Flail chest* is usually caused by blunt trauma; it results when two or more ribs are fractured at two different places on each rib, leaving a rib section that isn't connected at either end

- *Pneumothorax*, which can be caused by blunt or penetrating trauma, means that air has entered the pleural cavity; the air causes complete or partial collapse of the lung
  - *Tension pneumothorax* can be caused by blunt trauma and is life-threatening if untreated because of its effects on respiratory and cardiac function
  - *Cardiac tamponade* is the accumulation of blood in the pericardial sac, resulting from blunt or penetrating injury to the pericardium or heart; it's life-threatening if untreated (see *Comparing Types of Chest Trauma*)
- Pathophysiology
  - With a rib fracture, pain may cause hypoventilation that leads to atelectasis
  - With a flail chest, the flail segment moves in a manner opposite that of normal rib movement during respirations; as a result, the lungs can't fully expand
  - Pneumothorax can result when a fractured rib or penetrating trauma perforates a lung
    - ○ Air escapes from the lung into the pleural cavity
    - ○ The lung can't fully expand, gas exchange is compromised, normal intrathoracic pressure is disturbed, and the lung may collapse
  - With tension pneumothorax, trauma causes air to escape from the lung into the pleural cavity, where the air becomes trapped
    - ○ Pressure builds in the thoracic cavity, causing lung collapse
    - ○ The mediastinum shifts to the opposite side, compromising the other lung, and the vena cava becomes depressed, causing impaired venous return
  - With cardiac tamponade, intrapericardial pressure increases, compressing the heart; cardiac output decreases, and cardiogenic shock occurs

Box 9-2: Comparing Types of Chest Trauma

Signs and Symptoms	Diagnosis and Treatment	Nursing Care
Cardiac tamponade		
• Varied symptoms, depending on speed of blood accumulation • Chest pain, hypotension, muffled heart sounds, and tachycardia • Cyanosis, diaphoresis, dyspnea, and restlessness • Distended neck veins • Narrowed pulse pressure and paradoxical pulse • When tamponade develops more slowly: ascites, edema in arms and legs, liver enlargement	• Echocardiography can be used to diagnose cardiac tamponade. • Central venous pressure, which is elevated in patients with cardiac tamponade, is monitored. • Pericardiocentesis is used to remove fluid from the pericardial sac. • The injured area is repaired surgically. • I.V. fluids are rapidly infused. • Inotropic drugs are given to improve myocardial contractility.	• Administer oxygen to maintain adequate oxygenation, improve partial pressure of arterial oxygen (PaO_2), and reverse the hypoxemia. • Watch for complications, such as ventricular fibrillation, vasovagal response, or cardiac compression.
Flail chest		
• Cyanosis and dyspnea • Hypercapnia and hypoxemia • Increased respiratory effort • Pain on inspiration and on palpation of the injured area • Paradoxical movement of the flail segment	• Chest X-ray and arterial blood gas (ABG) studies typically are ordered. • Several types of analgesia may be used to relieve pain: patient-controlled analgesia, transcutaneous electrical nerve stimulation, or intercostal nerve block. • A chest tube may be inserted to treat hemothorax or pneumothorax. • Endotracheal intubation and mechanical ventilation may be used to stabilize the chest wall. • The flail segment may need to be repaired surgically.	• Teach the patient techniques for effective coughing and deep breathing to improve airway clearance. • Medicate for pain to promote effective coughing and deep breathing. • Provide hydration to liquefy secretions; thin secretions are easier to cough up. • Administer oxygen to improve PaO_2 and reverse hypoxemia. • Suction the patient's airway as needed to maintain patency and to clear secretions. • Provide pillows and teach the patient to support and splint the flail segment to minimize pain and to allow maximum lung expansion.

(continued)

Box 9-2: Comparing Types of Chest Trauma (continued)

Signs and Symptoms	Diagnosis and Treatment	Nursing Care
Pneumothorax		
• Asymmetrical lung expansion • Chest pain, crepitus, and dyspnea • Decreased or absent breath sounds on the affected side • Restlessness • Signs of mediastinal shift and tension pneumothorax	• Chest X-ray and ABG studies typically are ordered. • Analgesia is provided to relieve pain. • A chest tube may be inserted and attached to a suction device. In a three-chamber device, the first chamber allows for fluid drainage, the second one is a water seal that acts as a one-way valve to prevent air from entering the pleural cavity, and the third one controls the amount of suction, which is needed to remove air from the pleural cavity. • In an emergency, a Cook catheter with a Heimlich valve may be used to prevent air from entering the pleural cavity.	• Administer oxygen to improve PaO_2 and reverse hypoxemia. • Teach the patient techniques for effective coughing and deep breathing to prevent atelectasis and promote lung expansion. • Maintain the integrity of the chest tube system to facilitate air drainage from around the lung and promote lung expansion. Crepitus near the tube insertion site reflects air leakage into tissue and a possible leak in the chest tube system. When an air leak is no longer evident, the lung has healed itself and sealed off the injured area. If the chest drainage system is impaired and loses its seal, place the end of the chest tube in a container of sterile water. • Encourage frequent position changes to prevent complications of immobility and promote lung expansion and perfusion. • Provide an analgesic as needed to reduce anxiety and encourage coughing and deep breathing.
Rib fractures		
• Pain on inspiration • Pain and tenderness of injured area upon palpation • Ineffective ventilation and retention of secretions • Signs of other injury such as soft tissue injury	• Chest X-ray and ABG studies typically are ordered. • Analgesia is given to relieve pain. • An epidural catheter may be inserted for administration of narcotic analgesia. • A nerve block into the intercostal nerves above and below the fractured ribs may be used to relieve severe pain.	• Tell the patient not to wear tight or constrictive clothing, which can inhibit lung expansion and decrease effective ventilation. • Encourage the patient to breathe deeply and use an incentive spirometer hourly to maximize lung expansion and re-expand collapsed alveoli. • Medicate for pain or discomfort as needed, which will allow the patient to deep-breathe effectively. • Implement chest physiotherapy, unless contraindicated, to loosen secretions, which makes them easier to expectorate. • Provide adequate hydration to liquefy secretions; thin secretions are easier to cough up.
Tension pneumothorax		
• Asymmetrical lung expansion and tracheal deviation to affected side • Cyanosis, hypotension, and tachycardia • Decreased or absent breath sounds on the affected side • Distended neck veins • Severe chest pain and respiratory distress • Subcutaneous emphysema	• Chest X-ray and ABG studies typically are ordered. • Needle decompression is used for emergency air removal. • A chest tube may be inserted and attached to a suction device, such as a three-chamber device.	• Administer oxygen to improve PaO_2, reverse hypoxemia, and promote lung expansion. • Teach the patient techniques for effective coughing and deep breathing to prevent atelectasis and promote lung expansion. • Maintain the integrity of the chest tube system to facilitate air drainage from around the lung and promote lung expansion, as in pneumothorax. • Encourage frequent position changes to prevent complications of immobility and promote lung expansion and perfusion. • Provide an analgesic as needed to reduce anxiety and encourage coughing and deep breathing.

Chronic Obstructive Pulmonary Disease

- Description
  - COPD is the term used for preventable and treatable disorders that block the normal flow of air through the lungs, thereby trapping air in the alveoli
  - Chronic bronchitis, and emphysema are types of COPD; asthma, once classified as a type of COPD, is now considered a distinct restrictive rather than obstructive disorder (see *Comparing Chronic Obstructive Pulmonary Diseases*)
- Chronic bronchitis
  - Chronic bronchitis affects the lung parenchyma; it's characterized by a productive cough for at least 3 months a year for 2 or more consecutive years
  - It results from lung irritants, such as air pollution and smoking, as well as from genetic factors
  - With chronic bronchitis, increased bronchial mucus gland production and goblet cell hyperplasia result in increased sputum production; ciliary damage and epithelial metaplasia may occur
  - Bronchial irritants or infection may cause bronchial edema, bronchospasm, impaired mucociliary clearance, impaired ventilation (especially during expiration), increased secretions, and small airway blockage
  - Impaired diffusion is caused by decreased airflow, mucus plugs, and secondary infection; cyanosis and polycythemia develop as a result of hypoxemia
  - Signs of emphysema may be present, and as the disease progresses, cor pulmonale and pulmonary hypertension may develop
- Emphysema
  - Emphysema is a disease of the lung parenchyma characterized by changes in the alveolar wall and enlarged alveoli distal to the nonrespiratory bronchioles

Box 9-3: Comparing Chronic Obstructive Pulmonary Diseases

Chronic bronchitis and emphysema have distinctive signs and symptoms and require specific treatments and nursing care.

Signs and Symptoms	Diagnosis and Treatments	Nursing Care
Chronic bronchitis • Accessory muscle use, slight increase in anteroposterior chest diameter • Anxiety and depression • Bronchospasm • Chronic productive cough for thick, tenacious sputum that isn't clear and may have mucus plugs • Cyanosis and dyspnea • Decreased activity tolerance • Heart failure, hyponatremia, and renal failure caused by fluid overload late in disease • Lung hyperresonance, decreased breath sounds, diffuse wheezes, crackles and rhonchi, and prolonged expiration • Signs of right-sided heart failure (cor pulmonale)	• Chest X-ray, pulmonary function tests, arterial blood gas (ABG) studies, complete blood count, electrolyte levels, electrocardiogram, and sputum analysis typically are ordered. • An inhaled anticholinergic and an inhaled beta 2 adrenergic agonist are the mainstay of therapy; they're delivered by metered-dose inhaler (MDI) or nebulizer to enlarge the airways. • Aminophylline or another methylxanthine is given orally or I.V. to relax bronchial spasms. • An antibiotic is used to prevent or treat infection. • An inhaled or oral steroid is used to decrease the inflammatory response, thus decreasing bronchial edema during acute exacerbations.	• Administer oxygen to maintain a partial pressure of arterial oxygen (PaO_2) of 60 mm Hg or an arterial oxygen saturation of 90%. • Provide adequate hydration to liquefy secretions. Thin secretions are easier to expectorate. • Implement chest physical therapy. Postural drainage uses gravity to clear secretions; percussion and vibration loosen secretions, making them easier to cough up. • Teach the patient how to cough effectively to help clear secretions and to use diaphragmatic and pursed-lip breathing. • Teach the patient how to use an MDI with spacer correctly to ensure delivery of accurate doses to the small airways and to prevent overuse. • Educate the patient about the signs of respiratory tract infections, such as fever, change in sputum color or amount, and increased shortness of breath. Untreated infections may lead to acute respiratory failure. • Teach about proper and safe use of home oxygen equipment. • Teach the patient about the effects of smoking, and help the patient quit. • Recommend yearly influenza vaccines and pneumococcal vaccines every 5 years to reduce the risk of these infections.

(continued)

Box 9-3: Comparing Chronic Obstructive Pulmonary Diseases (continued)

Signs and Symptoms	Diagnosis and Treatments	Nursing Care
Emphysema		
• Accessory muscle use, increased anteroposterior diameter (barrel chest), lowered diaphragm, and reduced chest excursion • Anxiety and depression • Characteristic patient positioning—that is, leaning slightly forward with arms resting on the sides of the chair • Decreased activity tolerance • Dyspnea • Fatigue from increased work of breathing • Pursed-lip breathing and hyperventilation • Lung hyperresonance, decreased breath sounds, expiratory wheezes, and prolonged expiration	• Chest X-ray, pulmonary function tests, ABG studies, and sputum analysis typically are ordered. • The patient is immunized against the flu to prevent infection. If infection occurs, an antibiotic is the treatment of choice. • Smoking cessation is encouraged to prevent continued alveolar damage. • See *"Chronic Bronchitis: Diagnosis and Treatments,"* page 141, for specific therapies.	• Administer oxygen to a hypoxemic patient to maintain a PaO_2 of 60 mm Hg. Be aware that excessive oxygenation may cause loss of the incentive to breathe. • Teach about pursed-lip and abdominal breathing, which prevent small airway collapse during exhalation by slowing respiration and increasing bronchiole pressure. • Encourage activity to help prevent muscle wasting, but schedule frequent rest periods to avoid tiring the patient. • Teach the patient to conserve energy by sitting for activities when possible and alternating hard and easy tasks. • Teach relaxation and stress reduction techniques to prevent anxiety, which can exacerbate the disease. • Provide information about prescribed drugs. • Explain the importance of adequate fluid intake, which liquefies secretions, and a balanced diet, which prevents muscle wasting. • Instruct the patient to eat frequent small meals to prevent constipation and to avoid gas-forming foods to prevent pressure on the diaphragm and increased shortness of breath. • Help prevent infections by telling the patient to avoid crowds, small children, and exposure to persons with respiratory tract infections. • Teach the patient about the symptoms of respiratory tract infections. Untreated infections can lead to acute respiratory failure. • Teach the patient about the effects of smoking, and help the patient quit. • Recommend yearly influenza vaccines and a pneumococcal vaccine every 5 years. • Arrange for home oxygen therapy if needed.

- It results from alpha$_1$-antitrypsin deficiency and is associated with smoking and air pollution
- Emphysema impairs ventilation by decreasing lung elasticity, collapsing small airways during exhalation, trapping air, and causing poor gas exchange in the alveoli
- It impairs diffusion by enlarging distal air spaces (which increases the distance for diffusion) and causing loss of capillary membranes and pulmonary vasoconstriction
- It impairs perfusion by causing loss of pulmonary vasculature, pulmonary hypertension, and cor pulmonale

Cor Pulmonale

- Description
  - In cor pulmonale, hypertrophy and dilation of the right ventricle secondary to disease affect the structure or function of the lungs or their vasculature, resulting in right-sided heart failure
  - The disorder can occur at the end stage of various chronic disorders of the lungs, pulmonary vessels, chest wall, and respiratory control center

- Pulmonary hypertension increases the heart's workload
- To compensate, the right ventricle hypertrophies to force blood through the lungs
- In response to hypoxia, the bone marrow produces more red blood cells, causing polycythemia; the resulting increased viscosity further aggravates pulmonary hypertension and increases right ventricular workload
- Causes include primary pulmonary hypertension, pulmonary embolism, asthma, connective tissue disorders, COPD (the cause in more than half of all cases), chronic severe tricuspid regurgitation, disorders affecting the pulmonary parenchyma, and neuromuscular disease
- Cor pulmonale accounts for approximately 6% to 8% of all types of heart disease in adults in the United States
- Patients with cor pulmonale are typically older than age 45; males are more likely to be affected than females
- Signs and symptoms
  - Signs and symptoms include a history of dyspnea, chronic productive cough, fatigue, and weakness
  - Other signs and symptoms include tachypnea, wheezing, chest wall retractions, hemoptysis, pitting edema in the extremities, distended jugular veins, an enlarged liver, and tachycardia with pansystolic murmur at the lower left sternal border
- Diagnosis and treatment
  - ABG analysis reveals decreased PaO_2 (usually less than 70 mm Hg and rarely more than 90 mm Hg), hypercapnia, and hypoxia
  - Hematocrit is typically over 50%
  - Serum liver enzyme levels may show an elevated level of aspartate aminotransferase
  - Brain natriuretic peptide level may be elevated
  - Chest X-ray, echocardiography, angiography, and magnetic resonance imaging (MRI) demonstrate right ventricular enlargement
  - An ECG shows arrhythmias and may show atrial fibrillation and right bundle-branch block
  - Pulmonary function studies reflect underlying pulmonary disease
  - A hemodynamic profile shows increased pulmonary vascular resistance
  - The key to treatment is correcting the underlying problem
  - Oxygen therapy improves oxygenation
  - Phlebotomy is indicated for patients with COPD with a hematocrit of 55% or more
  - Continuous positive airway pressure or biphasic positive air pressure is indicated for sleep apnea
  - The patient should be on moderate sodium restriction and diuretics
  - Patients should limit activity as tolerated; during the acute phase, patients should be on bed rest
  - Beta selective agonists, such as epoprostenol (Flolan), treprostinil (Remodulin), and iloprost (Ventavis), are used to treat primary pulmonary hypertension
  - Bronchodilators administered by nebulizer include ipratropium (Atrovent), metaproterenol, and albuterol (Ventolin, Proventil)
  - For patients with persistent disease, vasodilators include hydralazine (apresoline), nifedipine (Procardia), diltiazem (Cardizem), and prazosin (Minipress)
  - The endothelin-1 receptor antagonists bosentan can help patients with pulmonary hypertension and severe symptoms to improve exertional tolerance and increase walking distance
  - Antibiotics treat acute respiratory infections
  - Anticoagulants help prevent thromboembolism
- Nursing interventions
  - Monitor the patient's vital signs, and pay attention to his cardiac and respiratory status
  - Reposition the patient often; elevate the head of the bed to increase thoracic expansion and ease the work of breathing
  - Administer oxygen as ordered based on oxygen saturation levels obtained with pulse oximetry and ABG results
  - Give prescribed drugs; if the patient will receive I.V. diuretics, ensure patent I.V. access
  - Encourage the patient to take slow, deep breaths when using nebulized medications, as appropriate
  - Provide frequent rest periods; cluster nursing activities to minimize oxygen and metabolic demands
  - Teach the patient and family about the disorder, the patient's diagnosis, the underlying cause and its relationship to the patient's current condition, treatment, and follow-up care

Hemothorax

- Description
  - Hemothorax is the presence of blood in the pleural cavity; it typically accompanies pneumothorax
  - It may result from chest trauma, lacerated liver, penetrating trauma, perforated blood vessels, perforated diaphragm, pleural damage that causes bleeding, or rib fracture
  - In hemothorax, blood collects in the pleural layer, compressing the lung on the affected side; this lung compression compromises gas exchange
- Signs and symptoms
  - Chest pain, cyanosis, dyspnea, and tachypnea commonly occur
  - With marked blood loss, hypertension and shock may occur
  - Asymmetrical lung expansion is accompanied by decreased breath sounds on the affected side
- Diagnosis and treatment
  - Chest X-ray, CBC, and ABG studies are commonly prescribed
  - A chest tube is inserted, and a water seal or suction is used to facilitate drainage
  - Thoracotomy may be indicated if blood loss is severe
  - If total blood loss is severe, the patient is treated with I.V. fluids and transfusion
- Nursing interventions
  - Administer oxygen to maintain adequate oxygenation, improve Pao_2, and reverse hypoxemia
  - Teach techniques for effective coughing and deep breathing to prevent atelectasis and promote lung expansion
  - Maintain the integrity of the chest tube system to facilitate blood drainage from around the lung and promote lung expansion
  - Check the chest tube insertion site for crepitus, which indicates air leakage into tissue and may indicate a leak in the chest tube system
    - An air leak in the system may indicate that the lung is damaged, causing air to leak from the lung into the pleural space
    - If the air leak is outside the chest cavity (such as from the chest tube), air entering the system may increase air accumulation in the pleural space
  - Encourage frequent position changes to prevent complications of immobility and promote lung expansion
  - Provide an analgesic as needed to reduce anxiety, relieve pain, and ease coughing and deep breathing

Influenza

- Description
  - Influenza is an infectious disease caused by ribonucleic acid (RNA) viruses that can affect humans, birds, and other mammals
  - Influenza A, influenza B, and influenza C can all infect humans
  - H1N1 is a subtypes of influenza A; strains are endemic in pigs (swine) and in birds (avian)
- Avian influenza
  - Infected migratory and domestic birds shed the virus in their saliva, nasal secretions, and feces
  - The strain is known as H5N1
  - Transmission has been limited to people, and some animals such as cats, in contact with infected birds
  - Should this virus become more easily transmissible person-to-person, it may lead to a pandemic
- Signs and symptoms
  - Symptoms range from typical human influenza-like symptoms, such as fever, cough, sore throat, and muscle aches, to eye infections, pneumonia, and acute respiratory distress
  - Diarrhea, vomiting, and abdominal pain may occur
- Diagnosis and treatment
  - Chest X-ray may show pneumonia, infiltrates, or consolidations
  - Sputum Gram stains and culture isolate the virus
  - Neuraminidase inhibitor class drugs, such as oseltamivir (Tamiflu), peramivir (Rapivab), and zanamivir (Relenza), can reduce the severity and duration of illness caused by seasonal influenza; efficacy depends on early administration

- M2 inhibitors amantadine and rimantadine (Flumadine) could possibly be used for pandemic influenza, but resistance to these drugs may develop
- The patient may require treatment to maintain fluid and electrolyte balance
- The patient may need mechanical ventilation for acute respiratory distress
- Nursing interventions
  - Follow standard and contact precautions, wear a fit-tested ventilator, and perform frequent hand hygiene
  - Wear eye protection within 3 feet of the patient
  - Maintain a patent airway, suctioning the patient when necessary
  - Notify the National Respiratory and Enteric Virus Surveillance System

Pleural Effusion

- Description
  - Pleural effusion is an accumulation of fluid in the pleural space (the thin space between the visceral and parietal pleura); although it isn't a disease itself, it occurs secondary to other disease states
  - Empyema is the accumulation of pus and necrotic tissue in the pleural space; blood (hemothorax) and chyle (chylothorax) may also collect in this space
  - A pleural effusion can be classified either as exudative (caused by inflammation of the pleura) or transudative (caused by excessive hydrostatic pressure or decreased osmotic pressure)
    - Common causes of exudative effusions are bacterial or fungal empyema or pneumonitis, chest trauma, collagen disease, malignancy, myxedema, pancreatitis, pulmonary embolism, subphrenic abscess, and tuberculosis
    - Common causes of transudative effusions are heart failure, hepatic disease with ascites, hypoalbuminemia, and peritoneal dialysis
- Signs and symptoms
  - The most common symptoms are pleuritic pain and dyspnea
  - Physical examination may reveal decreased chest wall movement, decreased breath sounds over the affected area, and dullness on percussion
  - Infection from empyema may produce cough, fever, and night sweats
- Diagnosis and treatment
  - Chest X-ray can diagnose pleural effusion; other tests that may be prescribed include CT scan of the chest, bronchoscopy, pleurocentesis, and ultrasonography
  - The underlying cause should be treated if it can be identified
  - Thoracentesis is performed to remove fluid; chest tubes may be placed for continued drainage
  - Thoracotomy may be needed if thoracentesis isn't effective
  - An antibiotic is prescribed to treat empyema; the specific antibiotic used depends on the causative organism
- Nursing interventions
  - Explain thoracentesis to the patient, and support him during the procedure
  - Watch for respiratory distress or pneumothorax after thoracentesis
  - Administer oxygen to improve oxygenation
  - Encourage deep breathing exercises and incentive spirometry to promote lung expansion
  - Maintain the integrity of the chest tube drainage system; monitor the amount, color, and consistency of drainage; and check for air leaks

Pneumonia

- Description
  - Pneumonia is an acute lung infection with inflammation accompanied by accumulation of exudate in the alveoli (see *Pneumocystis jiroveci Pneumonia*, page 146)
  - The risk of pneumonia increases with aspiration, central nervous system depression, chronic illness, COPD, dehydration, existence of a tracheostomy opening, immobility, immunosuppression, intubation, pain in the thoracic cavity, and use of general anesthesia
  - It may result from a bacterial, fungal, or viral infection or from exposure to a chemical irritant, through aspiration or gas inhalation
  - Pneumonia remains a major cause of morbidity and mortality among elderly and chronically ill people

Box 9-4: *Pneumocystis jiroveci* Pneumonia

Pneumocystis jiroveci pneumonia (PCP) commonly results from a fungal infection of *P. jiroveci* in an immunocompromised patient. PCP is one of the most frequent and severe opportunistic infection in patients with weakened immune system, particularly patients with HIV or AIDS. Its onset is abrupt and may be a flareup of a latent disease. Its signs and symptoms may include crackles over the affected areas, cyanosis, dyspnea or tachypnea, fever, hypoxemia, irritability or restlessness, and dry nonproductive cough.

Diagnostic tests may include chest X-ray, arterial blood gas analysis to check for hypoxemia, induced sputum sample and/or bronchoalveolar lavage, and needle or open biopsy to obtain lung tissue specimens for culture. The drugs of choice for treating this type of pneumonia are pentamidine isethionate (Nebupent, Pentam), an inhaled antibiotic, and co-trimoxazole (also known as sulfamethoxazole-trimethoprim) (Bactrim, Septra; TMP-SMX).

Care for a patient with *P. jiroveci* pneumonia resembles that of a patient with other types of pneumonia. Key nursing interventions include administering oxygen and an analgesic as needed, practicing good hand hygiene throughout care, limiting activity and encouraging rest periods, and teaching techniques to reduce the spread of infection and reduce stress.

- Signs and symptoms
  - Dyspnea or tachypnea, fatigue, and fever commonly occur
  - Signs of cyanosis or hypoxia may occur in those with advanced disease
  - Irritability or restlessness may signal cerebral hypoxia
  - Sputum may vary in amount, color, and consistency, depending on the causative agent
  - Lung auscultation may reveal crackles, rhonchi, bronchial breath sounds over areas of consolidation, or wheezes over the affected areas; breath sounds may be decreased in those with advanced disease
- Diagnosis and treatment
  - Chest X-ray, ABG studies, sputum culture (for bacterial infection), and serologic testing (for viral infection) may be prescribed
  - Needle or open biopsy may obtain lung tissue specimens (for fungal infection), and cold agglutinins may reveal antibodies associated with *Mycoplasma pneumoniae* infection
  - Pneumonia is treated with antibiotics to eradicate the infecting organism
  - A bronchodilator is used to open narrowed airways
- Nursing interventions
  - Teach effective coughing and deep breathing to improve airway clearance
  - Provide adequate hydration to liquefy secretions; thin secretions are easier to expectorate
  - Implement chest physiotherapy; postural drainage uses gravity to clear secretions, and percussion and vibration loosen secretions, making them easier to cough up
  - Administer oxygen to aid ventilation, improve PaO_2, and preserve oxygenation
  - Suction the patient's airway as needed to maintain patency and to clear secretions
  - Advise the patient to limit activity and to rest for long periods to decrease oxygen consumption
  - Provide pain medication as needed to allow effective coughing and deep breathing
  - Maintain adequate nutrition to offset the increased use of calories secondary to infection
  - Teach the patient how to contain secretions to reduce the risk of spreading infection
  - Practice good hand hygiene techniques to reduce the risk of spreading infection
  - Teach relaxation and stress reduction techniques; anxiety can compromise the immune system and increase the risk of infection

Pulmonary Edema

- Description
  - Pulmonary edema is the collection of fluid in the interstitium and alveoli of the lungs as pressure rises in the pulmonary vessels
  - It can result from ARDS, fluid overload, left-sided heart failure, mitral stenosis, MI, or pulmonary emboli
  - With pulmonary edema, the left ventricle can't effectively pump blood from the heart
    - With increased resistance to left ventricular filling, fluid backs up into the lungs
    - Surface tension increases, the alveoli shrink, and the lungs become stiff, making breathing more difficult
    - Hypoxemia and an altered $\dot{V}/\dot{Q}$ ratio develop
    - Fluid moves into the larger airways, where it's coughed up as pink, frothy sputum

- Signs and symptoms
  - Tachycardia and tachypnea may be accompanied by narrowed pulse pressures and hypotension; third and fourth heart sounds may be present; skin may be cold and clammy
  - Dyspnea, increased respiratory rate, orthopnea, and pulmonary hypertension may occur
  - Jugular veins may be distended, and PAWP may be elevated
  - Coughing may produce blood-tinged or pink, frothy sputum
  - Lung auscultation may reveal dependent crackles
  - Other signs and symptoms may include confusion, decreased urine output, diaphoresis, drowsiness, lethargy, and restlessness
- Diagnosis and treatment
  - Chest X-ray, pulse oximetry, and ABG studies typically are prescribed
  - A PA catheter is inserted to measure pressures
  - A diuretic is administered to decrease edema
  - Other drugs that may be administered include an inotropic drug to increase myocardial contractility, nitroglycerin to reduce preload and afterload, I.V. nitroprusside to reduce preload and afterload, and a vasopressor to maintain blood pressure
  - Intubation and mechanical ventilation may be necessary to treat respiratory distress
  - Morphine is administered to decrease preload, respiratory rate, and anxiety
  - Patients who don't respond to drug therapy may be treated with an intra-aortic balloon pump, which temporarily assists the failed left ventricle, or with surgery (such as angioplasty, coronary artery bypass grafting, or valve repair), depending on the underlying heart condition
- Nursing interventions
  - Administer oxygen to aid ventilation, improve PaO_2, and reverse hypoxemia
  - Place the patient in semi-Fowler's position to maximize oxygenation and increase comfort
  - Carefully monitor fluid intake and output to assess the effectiveness of diuretic therapy and prevent sudden increases in venous return caused by oral and I.V. intake
  - Medicate for pain as needed to reduce anxiety and increase comfort
  - Frequently change the patient's position to prevent pressure ulcers and encourage lung expansion

Pulmonary Embolism

- Description
  - Pulmonary embolism is a blockage in the pulmonary vasculature
  - Risk factors include atrial fibrillation; COPD; a family history of pulmonary embolism; oral contraceptive use; prior thromboembolic disease; venous injury caused by abdominal, pelvic, or thoracic surgery or leg or pelvic trauma; and venous stasis caused by age (older than age 55), burns, obesity, pregnancy, or prolonged immobility
  - Pulmonary embolism is commonly caused by dislodged thrombi from deep veins in the pelvis or legs or from any systemic veins
  - In this disorder, an embolism lodges in a branch of the pulmonary vasculature; the embolism may consist of bone, air, fat, amniotic fluid, a thrombus, or a foreign object
    - The area of the lung below the embolism isn't perfused, causing altered $\dot{V}/\dot{Q}$ ratio, which can cause alveolar collapse and lead to atelectasis and hypoxemia
    - Pulmonary infarction may occur, destroying lung tissue
    - A massive pulmonary embolism can cause pulmonary hypertension as a result of increased vascular resistance, right-sided heart failure as a result of increased right ventricular workload, or ventricular hypertrophy as a result of increased right ventricular workload
- Signs and symptoms
  - Dyspnea may occur suddenly, accompanied by chest pain
  - Pleuritic chest pain may indicate pulmonary infarction
  - Cough may produce hemoptysis
  - Anxiety, increased restlessness, hypotension, and tachycardia may occur
  - Lung auscultation may reveal crackles, pleural friction rub, and wheezes
  - Low-grade fever and tachypnea may occur
  - Signs of cor pulmonale and right-sided heart failure may develop
  - If the patient has a massive pulmonary embolism, he may experience arrhythmias, cyanosis, or diaphoresis

- If the patient has a fat embolism, he may experience confusion, dyspnea, or petechiae on his chest and axillae
- The patient's legs may have signs and symptoms of deep vein thrombosis, such as edema, redness, tenderness, and warmth
- Diagnosis and treatment
  - Several tests are used to diagnose pulmonary embolism: ABG studies, chest X-ray, ECG, lung scintigraphy, MRI, pulmonary angiography, and $\dot{V}/\dot{Q}$ lung scanning
  - Several tests are used to diagnose deep vein thrombosis, which can lead to pulmonary embolism: contrast venography, Doppler ultrasonography, impedance plethysmography, and leg scan after injection of fibrinogen
  - After an initial I.V. bolus of heparin, a therapeutic heparin infusion is given to inhibit clot formation, prevent emboli development, and maintain the partial thromboplastin time (PTT) between 1.5 and 2 times the control (60 to 70 seconds)
  - If the patient needs long-term therapy, warfarin (Coumadin) is administered to maintain the prothrombin time (PT) between 1.5 and 2 times the control (11 to 12 seconds) or the international normalized ratio (INR) between 2 and 3; once the therapeutic dose of warfarin is achieved, the heparin infusion may be discontinued
  - If the patient has a life-threatening embolism, a thrombolytic is administered, or a surgical embolectomy is performed
  - If the patient can't tolerate anticoagulant therapy or continues to develop clots despite taking these drugs, surgical insertion of a vena caval filter may be needed
  - A diuretic may be prescribed for a patient with a fat embolism; an antibiotic, for a patient with a septic embolism
  - An antiarrhythmic may be used to correct heart rhythm disturbances caused by ischemia
- Nursing interventions
  - Administer oxygen to improve PaO_2, reverse hypoxemia, and promote lung expansion
  - If the patient requires mechanical ventilation, assist as needed
  - Teach effective coughing and deep breathing to help clear secretions and prevent atelectasis
  - Provide adequate hydration to liquefy secretions; thin secretions are easier to expectorate
  - Encourage early ambulation to prevent clot formation in deep veins; encourage range-of-motion (ROM) exercises or perform passive ROM exercises if the patient can't walk
  - Use antiembolism stockings or a compression device to divert blood flow to the large veins, prevent emboli formation, and promote venous return
  - Don't raise the patient's knees; this obstructs venous flow and increases the risk of deep vein thrombosis
  - Elevate the patient's legs to prevent venous stasis
  - Maintain the heparin infusion, and monitor the PTT
  - Administer warfarin daily, as prescribed, and monitor the PT or INR
  - Test all stool for blood caused by anticoagulant-induced GI bleeding
  - Provide analgesia and comfort measures to reduce anxiety
  - Teach the patient about anticoagulant therapy to reduce the risk of bleeding, and help the patient maintain therapeutic PT or INR
  - Have the family or home health nurse check the home for hazards, especially those that may cause falls; a safe environment is necessary because a patient receiving an anticoagulant has an increased tendency to bleed
  - Instruct the patient not to cross his legs, sit for long periods, or wear restrictive clothing; these activities inhibit venous return and promote clot formation

Severe Acute Respiratory Syndrome

- Description
  - Severe acute respiratory syndrome (SARS) is a life-threatening viral infection believed to be coronavirus
  - A theory suggests that coronavirus may have mutated from pigs, birds, and other animals, allowing transmission to and infection of humans
  - The incubation period is estimated to range from 2 to 7 days (average is 3 to 5 days)
  - Risk factors include close contact with an infected person, contact with exhaled droplets and bodily secretions from an infected person, or travel to endemic areas
- Signs and symptoms
  - In early stages, signs and symptoms include nonproductive cough, rash, high fever, headache, body aches, and pneumonia
  - Shortness of breath and respiratory distress occur in later stages
- Diagnosis and treatment
  - Serum electrophoresis detects antibodies to the coronavirus

- Sputum Gram stain and culture isolates the coronavirus
- SARS-specific polymerase chain reaction tests detect SARS-CoV RNA
- Isolation (strict respiratory and mucosal barrier) prevents the spread of disease
- Antivirals treat viral infection, and a combination of corticosteroids and antimicrobials treat inflammation and infection
- Mechanical ventilation treats respiratory failure
- Nursing interventions
  - Maintain isolation for the patient
  - Practice good hygiene to prevent further transmission
  - Maintain a patent airway through suctioning if the patient requires mechanical ventilation
  - Monitor the patient's vital signs and nutritional, fluid, and respiratory status

Tuberculosis

- Description
  - Tuberculosis (TB) is an infectious disease that commonly affects the lungs; it typically occurs only after repeated, close contact with a person infected with *Mycobacterium tuberculosis*
  - Risk factors for TB include alcoholism, immunosuppression, low economic status, and malnutrition; elderly people, populations in crowded areas (e.g., shelters and prisons), and immigrants from areas with high incidences of TB (such as Africa, Southeast Asia, and the Caribbean islands) are also more susceptible
  - The incidence of TB has increased in proportion to the increase in patients who are infected with the human immunodeficiency virus
  - *M. tuberculosis* is spread by way of infected airborne droplets; after infected droplets are inhaled into the terminal bronchioles, localized pneumonia develops, initiating an inflammatory response
    - Bacilli are phagocytized by macrophages but remain viable within the phagocyte
    - Tubercles form and grow in the lungs
    - The lesion center forms a yellow, cheesy mass called caseous necrosis
    - Healing begins, walling off the initial infection, and adenopathy occurs
    - Systemic infection may develop in the absence of appropriate treatment
  - Within 6 weeks of exposure to the infected droplets, cellular immunity occurs, and skin test results become positive
  - Latent TB infection can become active TB disease years after exposure, when resistance is lowered
- Signs and symptoms
  - Anorexia, weight loss, chills, fever, chest pain, coughing up blood or sputum, and night sweats may occur in patients with active TB disease
  - Lung auscultation may reveal crackles, pleural effusions, and rhonchi.
- Diagnosis and treatment
  - The Mantoux TB skin test or the QuantiFERON-TB Gold test, a gamma interferon blood test for TB, can be used to test for *M. tuberculosis* infection
  - Abnormalities seen during a chest X-ray may suggest TB, but can't be used to diagnose TB
  - The presence of acid-fast bacilli on a sputum smear or other specimen after indicates disease
  - A positive culture for *M. tuberculosis* confirms the diagnosis of active TB disease
  - Preventive treatment with isoniazid for 9 to 12 months is recommended for other members of the patient's household, those with recently converted positive skin tests, and those with positive skin tests (depending on medical history)
  - If the patient has active TB disease, an antituberculotic is used for 6 to 9 months; isoniazid (INH) with rifampin (Rifadin) usually is the first choice; other antituberculotics include ethambutol (Myambutol) and pyrazinamide
- Nursing interventions
  - Teach the patient how to contain airborne droplets and secretions to reduce the risk of spreading the infection
  - Practice good hand hygiene techniques to reduce the risk of spreading the infection
  - Explain disease transmission to the patient and the need for prolonged therapy to help increase his compliance with the treatment plan
  - Teach the patient about the prescribed drugs, including how to recognize adverse reactions (especially the symptoms of hepatotoxicity)
  - Encourage the patient to maintain adequate dietary intake to maintain nutritional status, build strength, and improve the body's defense mechanisms
  - Weigh the patient daily to assess nutritional status

Review Questions

Question 1. A patient with pneumonia in the right lower lobe is prescribed percussion and postural drainage. When performing percussion and postural drainage, the nurse should position him:

A. in semi-Fowler's position with his knees bent.
B. in a right sidelying position with the foot of his bed elevated.
C. in a prone or supine position with the foot of his bed elevated higher than his head.
D. bent at the waist leaning slightly forward.

Correct answer: C The aim of percussion and postural drainage is to mobilize pulmonary secretions, so they can be effectively expectorated. When a patient has pneumonia in the right lower lobe, the nurse should position him with his right side up or lower lobes elevated above the upper lobes so that gravity can help mobilize pulmonary secretions. Options A and D are incorrect because semi-Fowler's position and being bent forward at the waist would hamper mobilization of secretions from the right lower lobe. Option B is incorrect because the patient should be positioned with his right side up.

Question 2. A patient with acquired immunodeficiency syndrome (AIDS) develops *P. jiroveci* pneumonia. Which nursing diagnosis has the highest priority for this patient?

A. Impaired gas exchange
B. Impaired oral mucous membranes
C. Imbalanced nutrition: Less than body requirements
D. Activity intolerance

Correct answer: A Although all these nursing diagnoses are appropriate for a patient with AIDS, *Impaired gas exchange* is the priority nursing diagnosis for the patient with *P. jiroveci* pneumonia. Airway, breathing, and circulation take top priority for any patient.

Question 3. A patient has emphysema. The nurse is teaching him breathing exercises. Which point should the nurse include in her teaching?

A. Make inhalation longer than exhalation.
B. Exhale through an open mouth.
C. Use pursed-lip breathing.
D. Use chest breathing.

Correct answer: C In patients with emphysema, air trapped at alveoli, pursed-lip breathing improves exchange of oxygen and carbon dioxide and maximizes ventilation. Option A is incorrect because exhalation should be no longer than inhalation to prevent collapse of the bronchioles. Because a patient with chronic bronchitis should exhale through pursed lips to prolong expiration, keep the bronchioles from collapsing, and prevent air trapping, Option B is incorrect. Option D is incorrect because diaphragmatic breathing, not chest breathing, increases lung expansion.

Question 4. A patient with ARDS is intubated and placed on mechanical ventilation. His PaO_2 is 60 mm Hg on 1.0 FIO_2. To improve his PaO_2 without raising the FIO_2, the patient will most likely be placed on:

A. time-cycled ventilation.
B. volume-cycled ventilation.
C. pressure support.
D. PEEP.

Correct answer: D PEEP is widely used during mechanical ventilation of the patient with ARDS to improve gas exchange over the alveolar capillary membrane. Time- or volume-cycled ventilation, Options A and B, are less likely to be used for a patient with ARDS than pressure-cycled ventilation. Pressure support, Option C, depends on the patient's inspiratory effort and isn't as effective as PEEP in treating ARDS.

Question 5. When auscultating the chest of a patient with pneumonia, the nurse should expect to hear which type of sounds over areas of consolidation?

A. Bronchial
B. Bronchovesicular
C. Tubular
D. Vesicular

Correct answer: A Chest auscultation reveals bronchial breath sounds over areas of consolidation. Bronchovesicular breath sounds (Option B) are normal over midlobe lung regions, tubular sounds (Option C) are commonly heard over large airways, and vesicular breath sounds (Option D) are commonly heard in the bases of the lung fields.

Question 6. A patient's history reveals that he suffers from continual daytime symptoms of asthma. How would his asthma severity be described?

A. Mild intermittent
B. Mild persistent
C. Moderate persistent
D. Severe persistent

Correct answer: D In severe persistent asthma the patient has continual daytime symptoms. In mild persistent asthma, the patient's daytime symptoms of asthma occur 3 to 6 days a week (Option B). In mild intermittent asthma (Option A), the patient's daytime symptoms occur no more than twice a week. In moderate persistent asthma (Option C), the patient has daily daytime symptoms.

Question 7. A 66-year-old patient has marked dyspnea at rest, is thin, and uses accessory muscles to breathe. He is tachypneic, with a prolonged expiratory phase. He has no cough. He leans forward with his arms braced on his knees to support his chest and shoulders for breathing. This patient has signs and symptoms of which respiratory disorder?

A. ARDS
B. Asthma
C. Chronic obstructive bronchitis
D. Emphysema

Correct answer: D These are classic signs and symptoms of a patient with emphysema. Patients with ARDS (Option A) are acutely short of breath and require emergency care; those with asthma (Option B) are also acutely short of breath during an attack and appear very frightened. Patients with chronic obstructive bronchitis (Option C) appear bloated and cyanotic.

Question 8. A nurse is preparing to reinforce the teaching plan for a patient who has recently been diagnosed with squamous cell carcinoma of the left lung. Which statement by the nurse is correct?

A. "You have a slow-growing cancer that rarely spreads."
B. "In terms of prognosis, you may have only a few months to live."
C. "Squamous cell cancer is a very rapidly growing cancer."
D. "The cancer has generally metastasized by the time diagnosis is made."

Correct answer: A Squamous cell carcinoma is a type of cancer that grows slowly and rarely metastasizes. It has the best prognosis of all lung cancer types. It's not appropriate for the nurse to tell the patient how long he has to live (Option B). Squamous cell carcinoma does not grow rapidly (Option C) and rarely metastasizes (Option D).

Question 9. Which respiratory disorder is most common in the first 24 to 48 hours after surgery?

A. Atelectasis
B. Bronchitis
C. Pneumonia
D. Pneumothorax

Correct answer: A Atelectasis develops when there's interference with the normal negative pressure that promotes lung expansion. Patients in the postoperative phase often splint their breathing because of pain and positioning, which causes hypoxia. It's uncommon for any of the other respiratory disorders (Options B, C, and D) to develop.

Question 10. A patient with acute asthma showing inspiratory and expiratory wheezes and a decreased forced expiratory volume should be treated immediately with which class of medication?

A. Beta 1 adrenergic blockers
B. Inhaled beta 2 adrenergic agonists
C. Inhaled corticosteroids
D. Oral corticosteroids

Correct answer: B Inhaled beta 2 adrenergic agonists are the first line of treatment for asthma because bronchoconstriction is the cause of reduced airflow. Beta 1 adrenergic blockers (Option A), which can cause bronchoconstriction, aren't used to treat asthma. Inhaled or oral corticosteroids (Options C and D) may be given to reduce the inflammation but aren't used for emergency relief.

Selected References

Centers for Disease Control and Prevention. (2017). Tuberculosis. Retrieved from https://www.cdc.gov/TB.

Karch, A. M. (2017). *Focus on nursing pharmacology* (7th ed.). Philadelphia, PA: Lippincott Williams & Wilkins.

Smeltzer, S. C., & Bare, B. G. (2014). *Brunner & Suddarth's textbook of medical-surgical nursing* (13th ed.). Philadelphia, PA: Lippincott Williams & Wilkins.

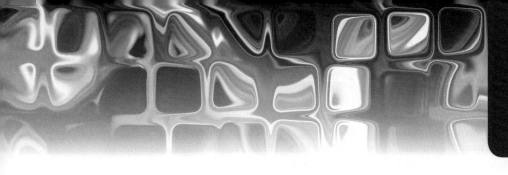

Chapter 10

Neurologic Disorders

Introduction

- The nervous system is the communications center of the body
- It coordinates all sensory and motor activities essential to proper physiologic functioning; it also plays a significant role in maintaining homeostasis
- Nursing history
  - The nurse asks the patient about the *chief complaint*
    - The most common complaints concerning the neurologic system include changes in level of consciousness (LOC), confusion, memory loss, dizziness, faintness, headache, numbness and tingling in extremities, seizures, weakness, and difficulty walking or moving
    - The patient may also report a change in balance or gait
  - The nurse then questions the patient about the *present illness*
    - Ask the patient about symptom, including when it started, associated signs and symptoms, location, radiation, intensity, duration, frequency, and precipitating and alleviating factors
    - Ask the patient about any dizziness, numbness, paralysis, seizures, tingling, tremors, or weakness
    - Question about sensory problems or with maintaining balance, swallowing, urinating, or walking
    - Ask about headaches and photophobia
    - Ask the patient to rate memory and ability to concentrate
    - Question about trouble speaking or understanding people
    - Ask about difficulties reading or writing
  - The nurse asks about *medical history*
    - Question the patient about other neurologic disorders
    - Ask about chronic diseases, major illnesses, accidents, injuries, surgeries, and allergies
  - The nurse then assesses the *family history*
    - Ask about a family history of neurologic diseases, such as amyotrophic lateral sclerosis (ALS), cerebrovascular accident (stroke), migraines, and seizures
    - Question the patient about a family history of diabetes mellitus, coronary artery disease, and hypertension
  - The nurse obtains a *social history*
    - Ask about work, exercise, diet, use of recreational drugs, alcohol, and hobbies
    - Also ask about stress, support systems, and coping mechanisms
- Physical assessment
  - The nurse assesses neurologic function in these five areas: mental status and speech, cranial nerve function, sensory function, motor function, and reflexes
  - The nurse assesses *mental status* and *speech*
    - Note the patient's appearance, mannerisms, posture, facial expression, grooming, emotions, speech, and tone of voice
    - Check for orientation to person, place, and time and for memory of recent and past events
    - To test intellect, ask the patient to count backward from 100 by 7s, to read aloud, or to interpret a common proverb, and see how well the patient understands and follows commands
    - Describe the patient's response to verbal, motor, and sensory stimuli; use the Glasgow Coma Scale for a standardized assessment

- The nurse assesses cranial nerve function
  - ○ Assess each of the 12 pairs of cranial nerves
  - ○ Note whether the patient has motor or sensory deficits or both
- The nurse assesses *sensory function*
  - ○ Assess the patient for sensation to superficial pain, light touch, vibration, position, and discrimination
  - ○ Compare the patient's responses bilaterally
  - ○ For patients with diabetes, test for neurosensory loss using a thin, single filament on noncalloused skin of the feet. Assess for ability to feel the monofilament and compare the responses bilaterally.
- The nurse assesses *motor function*
  - ○ To test cerebellar function, inspect muscle size, contour, and symmetry, observing the patient for abnormal movements, such as tics, tremors, and fasciculations; note coordination, gait, and balance
  - ○ Assess the patient's muscle tone and strength
  - ○ Compare assessment findings bilaterally
- The nurse assesses *reflexes*
  - ○ Test the patient's deep tendon, superficial, and primitive reflexes
  - ○ Compare the findings bilaterally

Alzheimer's Disease

- Description
  - Alzheimer's disease is a progressive, degenerative disorder of the cerebral cortex; it's irreversible
  - Alzheimer's affects 60% to 80% of all patients with dementia
  - It's associated with brain cell atrophy, decreased levels of acetylcholine, enlarged ventricles, neuritic plaques in brain tissue, and neurofibrillar tangles
  - The exact cause is unknown; it may be caused by abnormal protein in the brain, environmental toxins, genetic factors (e.g., a variant of apolipoprotein E), and inadequate cerebral blood flow
- Signs and symptoms
  - Altered behavior and memory may include recent memory loss and impaired judgment (see *Stages of Alzheimer's disease*, page 154)
  - Muscle rigidity, myoclonic jerks, and restlessness may occur
  - Obsessive behaviors may develop
  - The patient may develop anomia (inability to remember one's name) and aphasia (impaired ability to communicate verbally or in writing due to brain center dysfunctions)
  - During the final stages, the patient loses almost all mental abilities, including self-care skills, speech, and voluntary movement
- Diagnosis and treatment
  - Alzheimer's disease typically is diagnosed when other dementia-producing conditions have been ruled out
  - A definitive diagnosis can be made only if neuritic plaques and neurofibrillar tangles are found in the brain during a postmortem examination
  - Treatment calls for supportive measures, such as relieving specific symptoms, providing for patient safety, and providing emotional support to the patient and family

Age-Related Changes Versus Alzheimer's Symptoms

Signs of Alzheimer's/Dementia	Typical Age-Related Changes
Consistent poor judgment and decision-making	Occasional bad decisions
Inability to manage a budget	Occasionally missing a monthly payment
Inability to recognize season or track the date	Occasionally forgetting the date but having later recall
Conversational difficulty	Occasionally forgetting which word to use in conversation
Misplacing items with inability to later find them with retracing steps	Occasional misplacing items but finding upon later retracing steps

- The anticholinergics donepezil (Aricept) and memantine (Namenda) may improve memory in the early stages of the disease
- Nursing interventions
  - Make sure the patient carries identification, such as an ID card or bracelet, which can help if the patient wanders away from home
  - Speak in calm, friendly tones; even if the patient can't understand the content of what's being said, nonverbal communication is nonthreatening
  - Give simple instructions; the patient may become frustrated trying to follow complicated directions
  - Plan a full schedule of daily activities, especially music therapy and stretching to music, to facilitate sleep at night and provide diversion from an otherwise monotonous day
  - Provide a quiet, calm environment. Most Alzheimer's patients can't tolerate overstimulation, including bright colors and noises
  - Maintain the patient's nutritional status; the patient may not eat unless reminded to do so, may not be able to use utensils, and may need help preparing food and eating
  - Assist the patient with dressing and toileting
  - Give the patient and family information about Alzheimer's disease; refer family members to a local support group to enhance their ability to cope
  - Provide a safe environment for the patient and discuss with the family the possible need for a home care aide; the patient may lack the judgment to drive safely, use appliances, or manage personal finances
  - As soon as a diagnosis is made, discuss the possibility of power of attorney with the patient and family
  - Provide emotional support and affection; the family may be so exhausted and frustrated that they can't display affection toward the patient

Amyotrophic Lateral Sclerosis

- Description
  - Amyotrophic lateral sclerosis (ALS)—also known as Lou Gehrig disease—is a chronic, rapidly progressive, and debilitating neurologic disease that's incurable and invariably fatal
  - In ALS, motor neurons located in the anterior horns of the spinal column degenerate and the muscles they serve begin to atrophy
  - The disease is characterized by weakness that begins in the upper extremities; it progressively involves the neck and throat, eventually leading to disability, respiratory failure, and death
  - The exact cause is unknown, but factors associated with ALS include an autoimmune mechanism, viral infection, autosomal-dominant inheritance, and metabolic interference in nucleic acid production by the nerve fibers
  - Factors that precipitate acute deterioration include stress, trauma, infections, and exhaustion
  - The disease affects more men than women
  - Complications include respiratory infections and (ultimately) respiratory failure, complications of immobility, and aspiration

Box 10-1: Stages of Alzheimer's Disease

Early Stage	Intermediate Stage	End Stage
• Recent memory loss • Inability to learn and retain new information • Difficulty finding words • Personality changes and mood swings • Progressive difficulty performing activities of daily living	• Inability to learn and recall new information • Reduced ability to remember past events • Increased need for assistance with activities of daily living • Wandering • Agitation, hostility, or physical aggressiveness • Lack of orientation to time and place • Bladder and bowel incontinence	• Inability to walk • Total incontinence • No recent or remote memory • Inability to swallow and eat • No intelligible speech

- Signs and symptoms
  - Signs and symptoms include twitching and involuntary movements accompanied by atrophy and weakness in the muscles of the forearms, hands, legs, and trunk
  - Focal wasting of muscle groups also occurs
  - The patient may have slurred speech, difficulty chewing and swallowing, and drooling
  - Other symptoms include dyspnea and shortness of breath
- Diagnosis and treatment
  - Levels of glutamate in cerebrospinal fluid (CSF) and serum are increased
  - Electromyography and muscle biopsy may help diagnosis ALS
  - Magnetic resonance imaging (MRI) helps rule out spinal cord or spinal column problems that mimic ALS
  - Treatment is supportive and aims to prevent complications; rehabilitative measures include occupational, physical, and speech therapy
  - High treatment priorities include airway protection and preventing aspiration and respiratory infections; patients may ultimately need mechanical ventilation
  - Assisted coughing helps clear airways and prevent mucus plugs
  - Muscle relaxants, mucolytics, antidepressants, and anxiolytics may be used
  - Riluzole, a glutamate antagonist, may help slow disease progression
- Nursing interventions
  - Implement a rehabilitation program that helps the patient maintain as much independence as possible for as long as possible
  - Help obtain supportive equipment, such as a walker or wheelchair, as needed
  - Prevent complications of immobility; help the patient change position frequently and perform active range-of-motion (ROM) activities
  - Monitor the patient's respiratory status, and provide supplemental oxygen as needed
  - Initiate a diet of easy-to-swallow soft foods, and monitor for potential aspiration
  - Provide supportive care to both the patient and family, and teach them about the disease process and treatment options

Arteriovenous Malformations

- Description
  - Arteriovenous malformations (AVMs) are tangled masses of thin-walled, dilated blood vessels that form abnormal connections between arteries and veins; AVMs range in size from a few millimeters to large malformations that extend from the cerebral cortex to the ventricles; typically, more than one AVM is present
  - AVMs are primarily located in the posterior portion of the cerebral hemispheres
  - Most AVMs result from congenital defects in capillary development; traumatic injury may also be a cause
  - Most AVMs are present at birth; however, symptoms typically don't occur until young adulthood
  - Typically, high-pressured arterial flow moves into the venous system through the connecting channels to increase venous pressure, engorging and dilating the venous structures
  - If the AVM is large enough, the shunting can deprive the surrounding tissue of adequate blood flow
  - Thin-walled vessels may develop aneurysms and ooze small amounts of blood or actually rupture, causing hemorrhage into the brain or subarachnoid space
- Signs and symptoms
  - AVMs can cause persistent headaches unresponsive to treatment
  - Other signs and symptoms include changes in mental status and intellectual acuity, dizziness, and visual disturbances
  - Seizures and neurologic deficits may also occur
- Diagnosis and treatment
  - Cerebral arteriography confirms the presence of AVMs and evaluates blood flow
  - Doppler ultrasonography of the cerebrovascular system indicates abnormal, turbulent blood flow
  - Computed tomography (CT) scanning and MRI can help differentiate an AVM from a clot or tumor
  - EEG can help localize the AVM
  - Treatment depends on the size and location of the AVM, the feeder vessels supplying it, and the patient's condition
  - Treatments include embolization, proton beam radioablation, laser surgery, and surgical excision

- Nursing interventions
  - Provide supportive measures, including aneurysm precautions (placing the patient on bed rest or with limited activity, maintaining a quiet atmosphere, and keeping the patient calm [with sedatives, if needed]) to prevent possible rupture
  - Institute seizure precautions, and monitor for signs of increased intracranial pressure
  - Prepare for surgery, and administer I.V. fluids and medications as ordered
  - Postoperatively, control hypertension, monitor the patient's neurologic status, and provide pain relief
  - Teach the patient and family about the disorder, including the signs and symptoms of complications
  - If the patient develops deficits from the AVM, provide for adaptive measures

Encephalitis

- Description
  - Encephalitis is a severe, acute inflammation of the brain
  - In this disorder, intense lymphocytic infiltration of brain tissues and the leptomeninges results in cerebral edema, degeneration of the brain's ganglion cells, and diffuse nerve cell destruction (gray more than white matter)
  - Causes include adenoviruses, enteroviruses in urban areas (such as coxsackievirus, poliovirus, and echovirus), herpesvirus, human immunodeficiency virus, arboviruses, mumps and measles viruses, and amebic infection. Some seasonal variation occurs, with arboviruses typically occurring in spring and summer, enteroviruses peaking in later summer or early fall, and mumps and varicella occurring in spring
  - Determining the true incidence of encephalitis is difficult because reporting policies vary
  - Males and females appear to be affected equally; the very young and very old are at highest risk
  - Complications may include paralysis, epilepsy, mental deterioration, parkinsonism, and death
- Signs and symptoms
  - Signs and symptoms include fever, malaise, myalgias, headache, muscle stiffness, photophobia
  - Altered LOC, confusion, seizures, and other signs of increased intracranial pressure (ICP) can all occur
  - Other signs and symptoms include nausea and vomiting, exaggerated deep tendon reflexes and absent superficial reflexes, paresis or paralysis of the extremities, a positive Brudzinski's sign, and aggression
  - Certain anthropoid-borne viruses may cause a rash
- Diagnosis and treatment
  - CSF may contain elevated white blood cell and protein levels and decreased glucose levels; the causative organism may also be cultured from CSF
  - Polymerase chain reaction (PCR) testing checks for viral DNA
  - MRI may demonstrate inflammation in affected areas in the brain
  - EEG shows changes in encephalitis
  - Treatment focuses on correcting the underlying cause and preventing injury from increased ICP
- Nursing interventions
  - Monitor for signs of increasing ICP to allow for early control and management
  - Administer nonopioid analgesics, and provide a quiet, nonstimulating environment
  - Administer anti-infective agents as ordered, and watch for therapy-related complications
  - Administer antipyretics and antiseizure medications as ordered
  - Teach the patient and family about the disease process and treatment, and provide supportive care

Guillain-Barré Syndrome

- Description
  - Guillain-Barré syndrome is an acute, rapidly progressing, and potentially fatal form of polyneuritis
  - In this syndrome, the body's autoimmune system attacks peripheral nerve myelin, resulting in rapid segmental demyelination of peripheral nerves and some cranial nerves; this produces ascending weakness with dyskinesias (inability to execute voluntary movements), hyporeflexia, and paresthesias
  - A viral infection often precedes the clinical presentation
  - Guillain-Barré syndrome is the most common cause of acute flaccid paralysis in the United States; it most often affects males between the ages of 16 to 25 and 45 to 60

- The syndrome has a mortality rate of about 5%; up to 75% of patients recover completely over the course of a few months to several years
- Complications include paralysis, permanent muscle weakness, contractures, muscle wasting, and respiratory and cardiac compromise
- Signs and symptoms
  - Minor febrile illness (respiratory or diarrheal) may precede signs and symptoms of Guillain-Barré by 1 to 3 weeks
  - Symptoms of Guillain-Barré include tingling and numbness (paresthesia) in the legs; symptom progress to the arms, trunk, and, finally, the face
  - Other signs and symptoms include stiffness and pain in the legs and back; acute, symmetrical ascending weakness of the limbs; sensory loss, usually in the legs and spreading to the arms; difficulty talking, chewing, and swallowing; paralysis of the ocular, facial, and oropharyngeal muscles; loss of position sense; and diminished or absent deep tendon reflexes
  - Heart rate may be increased and blood pressure can be abnormally high or low
- Diagnosis and treatment
  - CSF shows elevated protein levels
  - Evoked potential studies may show a progressive loss of nerve conduction velocity
  - Because Guillain-Barré is a medical emergency, with rapid progression and neuromuscular respiratory failure, treatment may include aggressive respiratory therapy and mechanical ventilation along with oxygen support
  - Treatment includes supportive hemodynamic measures
  - The patient may also require plasmapheresis
- Nursing interventions
  - Monitor the patient's cardiac and respiratory status
  - Administer oxygen as needed
  - If possible, establish a means of communication before the patient requires intubation
  - Monitor the patient's intake and output
  - Take measures to prevent complications of immobility, such as deep vein thrombosis, pressure ulcer formation, and muscle wasting
  - Provide adequate nutrition
  - Provide supportive care to the patient and family

Traumatic Brain Injury

- Description
  - Traumatic brain injury (TBI), a term that encompasses several types of injuries, is the leading cause of disability
  - TBIs a general term for any impact injury to the head that impacts normal brain function, ranging from a minor concussion to life-threatening hematoma and herniation
  - Primary injuries are directly caused by the trauma; secondary injuries are indirectly caused by the trauma (see *Types of head injury*, page 159)
- Signs and symptoms
  - Depending on the severity and location of the injury, the patient will have varying neurologic deficits, such as motor and sensory changes, pupillary changes, reduced LOC, and seizures
  - If the patient has increased ICP, bradycardia, decerebrate or decorticate posturing, focal neurologic signs, headache, increased blood pressure, pupillary changes (including sluggish or absent response to light and unequal size), reduced LOC (including agitation, coma, confusion, lethargy, and restlessness), seizures, vomiting, and widened pulse pressure may be experienced
  - If CSF leakage occurs, the patient may experience frequent swallowing, otorrhea, and rhinorrhea
- Diagnosis and treatment
  - Diagnosis may be based on skull X-ray, CT scan of the head and cervical spine, MRI, lumbar puncture, cerebral angiography, and EEG
  - A cervical collar may be placed on the patient's neck until a cervical injury is ruled out
  - Treatment depends on the severity of the injury
    - For a concussion, neurologic function is monitored for 24 hours

○ For a contusion, neurologic function is monitored in a controlled environment for possibly increased ICP

○ For laceration, diagnostic procedures are implemented for early identification of secondary injuries

● Continuous ICP monitoring may be indicated

● If present, clots are removed surgically; hematomas may need to be evacuated; in the presence of hydrocephalus, a drain may be placed in the ventricles

● Supportive measures—such as drug therapy for increased ICP (see *Increased intracranial pressure*, pages 161–162), intubation and mechanical ventilation, invasive hemodynamic monitoring, and invasive ICP monitoring—are initiated

● Nursing interventions

● Monitor vital signs every 15 minutes until the patient's condition is stable to detect increased ICP

● Perform neurologic assessments every 15 minutes until the patient's condition is stable to detect increased ICP; assess LOC according to the Glasgow Coma Scale (see *Using the Glasgow Coma Scale*, page 160)

● Initiate I.V. therapy while strictly monitoring intake and output to maintain hydration and prevent cerebral edema

○ Excessive urine output may indicate diabetes insipidus (antidiuretic hormone deficiency) due to pituitary gland damage; it's treated with vasopressin

○ Fluid retention may indicate syndrome of inappropriate antidiuretic hormone (SIADH) due to craniocerebral trauma; it's treated with fluid restriction

● Provide respiratory care to maintain a patent airway and adequate ventilation; turn and encourage frequent deep breathing in a nonintubated patient, suction an intubated patient, and remember that hypoxemia and hypercapnia increase ICP

● Provide a safe, quiet, dimly lit environment

● Take seizure precautions and keep emergency equipment nearby; a patient with head trauma is at risk for seizures and respiratory insufficiency

● Provide bed rest with positioning appropriate to the injury

○ Elevate the head of the bed as prescribed to reduce cerebral edema; immediately after cranial surgery, the patient may need to lie in a supine position for 24 hours; early elevation of the head of the bed after infratentorial craniotomy can increase the risk of postoperative herniation

○ Change the patient's position frequently to prevent complications stemming from immobility, and position accordingly for comfort and to prevent deformity

● Watch for signs of acute respiratory distress syndrome and traumatic delirium; if the patient experienced an open head injury, look for signs of infection, which could point to meningitis or brain abscess

● Initiate ROM exercises (unless contraindicated by increased ICP) to prevent complications of immobility

● Provide appropriate nutritional support, including enteral or parenteral feedings if the patient can't eat; nutritional deficits impede healing and lead to muscle wasting; check cough and gag reflexes to prevent aspiration

● Provide emotional support to the patient and his family; remember that the injury may be fatal or severely alter the patient's lifestyle and that the patient may require extensive rehabilitation

Huntington's Disease

● Description

● Huntington's disease (also called Huntington's chorea, hereditary chorea, chronic progressive chorea, and adult chorea) is a degenerative disease of the brain that causes dementia

● Death usually occurs 15 to 20 years after the onset of the disease

● Degeneration in the cerebral cortex and basal ganglia leads to chronic progressive chorea (dancelike movements); the exact disease mechanism is still under investigation

● It's transmitted as an autosomal-dominant trait (transmitted and inherited by either sex)

● About 1 in every 10,000 people of both sexes and all races may develop Huntington's disease in midlife; the juvenile form of the disease typically occurs before age 20, and life expectancy after diagnosis is 10 to 15 years

● Signs and symptoms

● Huntington's disease is characterized by abnormal, involuntary body movements and, often, emotional disturbances

● As the disease progresses, patients develop a constant writhing, twisting, uncontrollable series of movements that may involve the entire body, including the face, resulting in tics and grimaces; the gait is also affected

Box 10-2: Types of Head Injury

Primary and secondary head injuries result from trauma in different ways.

Injury	Description	Mechanisms
Primary injuries		
Concussion	Brief period of cerebral paralysis; full recovery usually occurs in 12 hours, but postconcussion syndrome (characterized by difficulty concentrating, fatigue, headache, and photophobia) sometimes occurs	Sudden blow to the head that causes anterograde and retrograde brain injury
Contusion	Bruising of the brain; may be a *coup* injury (hemorrhage and edema under the injury site) or a *contrecoup* injury (hemorrhage and edema opposite from the injury site)	Sudden impact, commonly resulting from acceleration-deceleration forces, that displaces cerebrospinal fluid and causes the brain to hit the inside of the skull
Laceration	Tearing of the cortical surface	High-velocity acceleration-deceleration injury or a penetrating trauma, such as a stab wound or gunshot wound
Secondary injuries		
Cerebellar herniation	Pushing of the cerebellar tonsils through the foramen magnum	Force that pushes the brain contents into another compartment, compressing the medulla
Epidural hemorrhage or hematoma	Arterial bleeding between the dura and the skull; initially causes loss of consciousness, followed by a brief lucid period and progressive neurologic deterioration	Tearing of the medial meningeal artery by a temporal bone fracture
Intracerebral hemorrhage or hematoma	Bleeding within the cerebrum; may lead to increased intracranial pressure and permanent neurologic damage	Contusion or laceration
Subarachnoid hemorrhage or hematoma	Arterial bleeding in the subarachnoid space; sudden symptoms can include chills, decreased level of consciousness, diaphoresis, dizziness, nausea, severe headache, and vomiting	Force that causes bleeding immediately or long after an injury
Subdural hemorrhage	Venous bleeding between the dura and the arachnoid membrane	Acute process (causing symptoms within 48 hours of injury), subacute process (causing symptoms within 2 to 14 days), or chronic process (causing symptoms 2 or more weeks after the injury)
Supratentorial (central) herniation	Pushing of the cerebral ventricles through the incisura of tentorium	Force, such as a supratentorial mass, that pushes the brain contents into another compartment, compressing the diencephalon and midbrain
Uncal (lateral transtentorial) herniation	Shifting of the temporal lobe across the tentorium into the posterior fossa	Force that shifts the brain contents into another compartment, compressing the midbrain and brain stem

Box 10-3: Using the Glasgow Coma Scale

The Glasgow Coma Scale provides an easy way to describe a patient's baseline mental status and to help detect and interpret changes from baseline findings. To use the scale, test the patient's ability to respond to verbal, motor, and sensory stimulation and grade your findings according to the scale. If a patient is alert, can follow simple commands, and is oriented to person, place, and time, his score will total 15 points, the highest possible score. A low score in one or more categories may signal an impending neurologic crisis. A total score of 7 or less indicates severe neurologic damage.

Test	Score	Patient's Response
Eye opening response		
Spontaneously	4	Opens eyes spontaneously
To speech	3	Opens eyes when told to
To pain	2	Opens eyes only on painful stimulus
Never	1	Doesn't open eyes in response to stimulus
Motor response		
Obeys commands	6	Shows two fingers when asked
Localizes pain	5	Reaches toward painful stimulus and tries to remove it
Withdraws	4	Moves away from painful stimulus
Abnormal flexion	3	Assumes a decorticate posture (in which the hands are toward the cord, shown below)

Test	Score	Patient's Response
Abnormal extension	2	Assumes a decerebrate posture (shown below)

Test	Score	Patient's Response
None	1	No response; just lies flaccid (an ominous sign)
Verbal response		
Oriented	5	Tells correct date
Confused conversation	4	Tells incorrect year
Inappropriate words	3	Replies randomly with incorrect words
Incomprehensible	2	Moans or screams
None	1	No response
Total score		

- Speech becomes slurred, hesitant, and explosive
- Chewing and swallowing become difficult
- Patients lose bowel and bladder function
- Personality changes occur, with impairment progressing until dementia ensues
- Diagnosis and treatment
  - Diagnosis depends on the patient's clinical presentation, a positive family history or a genetic marker, and the exclusion of other diagnoses
  - CT scans and MRI reveal brain atrophy
  - Positron emission tomography scans may show reduced glucose use and lowered dopamine receptor binding
  - Because no known cure exists, treatment aims to control signs and symptoms
  - Tranquilizers and antidepressants may be used along with psychotherapy
  - Thiothixene hydrochloride (Navane) and haloperidol decanoate (Haldol) block dopamine receptors and may improve chorea in some patients
  - Levodopa and other antiparkinsonian medications may be used for patients with rigidity
- Nursing interventions
  - Provide psychological support to the patient and family; allow them time to verbalize their concerns and feelings, and assist with positive coping strategies
  - Educate families about genetic testing and family planning options to prevent passing on Huntington's disease to the next generation
  - Identify self-care deficits; assist with activities of daily living as necessary, and encourage the patient's participation as much as possible
  - Encourage the patient to be independent
  - Provide communication aids, speak slowly and clearly to the patient, allow time for the patient to respond, and ensure that the patient has understood what was said
  - Provide assistance with ambulation; encourage the use of assistive devices, such as a cane or walker, as indicated
  - If the patient is on bed rest, maintain a turning schedule, repositioning the patient at least every 2 hours; pad bony prominences, perform passive ROM exercises on the extremities to maintain joint function and mobility, and encourage the patient to participate as able
  - Provide adequate nutrition and provide for increased calorie needs
  - Elevate the head of the bed while the patient is eating to help prevent choking and aspiration
  - Give medications as ordered
  - Monitor the patient's mental status, and be alert for neurologic changes

Increased Intracranial Pressure

- Description
  - ICP is a measure of the pressure in the cranial cavity; 0 to 15 mm Hg is normal, 16 to 20 mm Hg is mildly elevated, 21 to 30 mm Hg is moderately elevated, and 31 mm Hg or more is severely elevated
  - The adult skull has a fixed volume of intracranial components, which consist of 80% brain tissue, 10% blood, and 10% CSF
    - According to the Monro-Kellie doctrine, an increase in any of the three components must be offset by a decrease in the others
    - If this balancing out doesn't occur, ICP increases
  - Autoregulation adjusts cerebral blood flow and CSF production and reabsorption to maintain normal ICP; it can no longer maintain normal pressure when ICP exceeds 33 mm Hg or the mean arterial pressure (MAP) exceeds 160 mm Hg
  - Cerebral perfusion pressure (CPP) is the pressure at which the brain cells are perfused; CPP = MAP − ICP; CPP is normally 70 to 100 mm Hg
  - Several factors may increase ICP: cerebral edema resulting from infection, intracranial or subarachnoid bleeding, or brain tumor; cytotoxic cerebral edema resulting from a metabolic disorder; interstitial cerebral edema caused by blocked CSF reabsorption; intracranial or subarachnoid bleeding; or vasogenic cerebral edema caused by trauma

- Signs and symptoms
  - An altered LOC is usually the earliest sign of increased ICP
    - ○ The patient may exhibit partial or total loss of motor and sensory function
    - ○ Pupillary changes may occur, such as unequal size, constriction, dilation, or reduced or absent responses to light
    - ○ Cushing's triad (bradycardia, bradypnea, and hypertension) is a late sign of increased ICP
  - Other signs and symptoms include changes in respiratory patterns, headache, seizures, vomiting, and a widening pulse pressure
- Diagnosis and treatment
  - Diagnosis is based on CT scan, skull X-rays, and ICP monitoring
  - The goal of treatment is to normalize ICP and avoid complications, such as brain herniation, diabetes insipidus, and SIADH
  - Pressures are carefully monitored by means of epidural monitoring, subarachnoid screw and bolt, or intraventricular monitoring
  - CSF blockage is corrected by surgical placement of shunts; a tumor or hematoma also is removed surgically; craniectomy or burr holes may be required for decompression
  - Drug therapy may include an antibiotic to treat or prevent infection, an anticonvulsant to prevent seizures, and a diuretic to prevent cerebral edema
  - Hyperventilation therapy is used to reduce the partial pressure of carbon dioxide in arterial blood level, which decreases cerebral edema and ICP
  - Metabolic disorders are corrected
  - Lumbar puncture is contraindicated in a patient with increased ICP because it can cause life-threatening herniation (shifting of brain contents into another compartment)
- Nursing interventions
  - Provide bed rest, with the head of the bed elevated 30 to 45 degrees to promote venous drainage from the cranium
  - Avoid neck extension, flexion, and rotation to promote optimal venous drainage
  - Avoid hip flexion above 60 degrees, which can lead to increased intra-abdominal pressure that increases ICP
  - Monitor and document fluid intake and output until the patient's condition is stable to ensure proper hydration
    - ○ Excessive urine output may indicate diabetes insipidus due to posterior pituitary gland damage; it's treated with vasopressin
    - ○ Fluid retention may indicate SIADH due to craniocerebral trauma; it's treated with fluid restriction
  - Slowly infuse I.V. bolus medications; rapid infusion can trigger an abrupt increase in brain fluid volume
  - Administer an analgesic, an antibiotic, an anticonvulsant, and a diuretic as prescribed
  - Perform neurologic assessments hourly until the patient's condition is stable to help prevent complications and then every 4 hours or as prescribed; watch for changes in LOC and motor responses using the Glasgow Coma Scale (see *Using the Glasgow Coma Scale*, page 160)
  - Monitor vital signs hourly until the patient's condition is stable
  - Monitor the patient for signs of bleeding and hypovolemia—for example, by checking stools, urine, and vomitus for occult blood; systemic bleeding may signal coagulopathy, which increases the risk of intracranial bleeding
  - Place pads loosely over the ears or under the nose to absorb leaking CSF (a clear liquid that leaves yellow halos on linen and tests positive for glucose); change pads frequently to prevent pathogens from migrating through the CSF to the brain
  - Use aseptic technique to prevent systemic or intracranial infection, which increases the risk of further increases in ICP
  - Closely monitor respiratory status by auscultating breath sounds and checking tissue oxygenation with noninvasive pulse oximeters; encourage deep breathing
    - ○ Hypoxemia and hypercapnia further elevate ICP; coughing and inspired spirometry temporarily increase ICP
    - ○ Bed rest and altered LOC increase the risks of atelectasis and pneumonia
  - Assist with turning in bed, and teach the patient to breathe while moving to avoid straining, which can increase ICP

- Maintain a quiet environment: limit noise, light, visitors, and emotional stress; overstimulation can increase ICP
- Provide nutritional support as appropriate to maintain normal fluid and electrolyte balance; tube feedings may be required
- Teach the patient to avoid performing Valsalva's maneuver; also, instruct to avoid coughing, holding his breath while lifting, sneezing, straining during defecation, and vomiting; since these actions increase ICP
- Provide emotional support to the patient and his family

Meningitis

- Description
  - Meningitis is an inflammation of the subarachnoid space and meninges; it can be classified as septic (caused by bacterial infection) or aseptic (caused by viral infection)
  - Exudate formation causes meningeal irritation and increased ICP
  - Meningococcal meningitis is caused by *Neisseria meningitidis*, a highly contagious organism
  - *Haemophilus influenzae* meningitis is the most common bacterial meningitis in infants and children
  - Pneumococcal meningitis is caused by *Streptococcus pneumoniae*; it can be a severe complication of an upper respiratory tract infection, is the most common type of meningitis after neurosurgery, and has a high mortality rate
  - Tuberculous meningitis is a bacterial infection caused by *Mycobacterium tuberculosis*; it's generally self-limiting and benign
  - Meningitis can be spread in different ways, depending on the infecting organism, by droplets, through the birth process, by the fecal-oral route, or in food.
- Signs and symptoms
  - The cardinal signs and symptoms of meningitis are those of infection (including chills, fever, and malaise) and those of increased ICP (including headache and vomiting)
  - Other signs and symptoms include changes in LOC, irritability, and seizures
  - Signs and symptoms of brain and spinal cord irritation may include Brudzinski's sign (leg adduction and flexion when the neck is flexed), Kernig's sign (resistance to extension when thigh is flexed up to the abdomen), nuchal rigidity, and severe headache
  - Irritation of cranial nerve (CN) II may cause blindness and papilledema; of CN III, IV, and VI, diplopia, impaired ocular movement, ptosis, and unequal pupils; of CN V, photophobia; of CN VII, facial paresis; and of CN VIII, tinnitus or deafness and vertigo
- Diagnosis and treatment
  - Diagnosis may be based on physical examination findings and the results of lumbar puncture, serologic studies, and cultures of blood, urine, nasal or pharyngeal mucosa, sputum, and skin lesions
  - Meningitis is treated with organism-specific antibiotic therapy
  - An anticonvulsant may be administered to decrease the risk of seizures; an analgesic may be given to reduce headache, which is common with meningitis
  - Prophylactic antibiotic therapy may be prescribed for family members and other people who have had close contact with a patient who has bacterial meningitis
  - Supportive measures include reducing fever, ensuring adequate hydration and nutrition, providing mechanical ventilation, if necessary, and preventing and treating increased ICP
  - Vaccinations are available to prevent some bacterial causes of meningitis, such as *N. meningitidis*, *S. pneumoniae*, and Hib.
- Nursing interventions
  - Perform neurologic examinations, and check vital signs hourly; early detection of increased ICP, hyperthermia, hydrocephalus, and shock can help prevent complications
  - Implement isolation techniques if the causative agent is highly contagious; bacterial meningitis is transmitted by direct and sometimes indirect contact with respiratory droplets from infected people and carriers
  - Report meningococcal meningitis to local health authorities; report other bacterial meningitis in endemic areas only
  - Monitor fluid intake and output to prevent overhydration, which can lead to cerebral edema and increased ICP

- Provide nutritional support to maintain immune response and fluid and electrolyte balance; enteral feedings may be required
- Provide proper positioning, skin care, and ROM exercises to prevent complications of immobility, such as contracture deformities, muscle wasting, pneumonia, and pressure ulcers
- Provide a comfortable, quiet, dimly lit environment to help prevent seizures and to reduce the discomfort of photophobia
- Give emotional support to the patient and family
- Provide referrals for rehabilitation if neurologic deficits are permanent

Multiple Sclerosis

- Description
  - Multiple sclerosis is a progressive neurologic immune-mediated process that causes destruction, injury, or malformation of the myelin sheaths that cover nerves
  - Plaques (areas of demyelination) can occur anywhere in the nervous system but are most common on the white matter of the brain and spinal cord and the optic nerves; plaques slow or stop saltatory conduction, the normally rapid conduction of nerve impulses
  - Although the exact cause is unknown, multiple sclerosis may be triggered by a slow, progressive viral disease, an autoimmune disorder, or an allergic reaction to an infection
  - Multiple sclerosis is characterized by unpredictable exacerbations and remissions; symptoms worsen with each episode
- Signs and symptoms
  - Symptoms of multiple sclerosis may be transient, variable, and bizarre
  - The first symptoms are usually sensory and visual problems, such as burning, electrical sensations, and pins and needles
  - Ocular disturbances may include blurred vision, diplopia, nystagmus, ophthalmoplegia, and optic neuritis
  - Muscle dysfunction—including gait ataxia, hyperreflexia, intention tremor, paralysis ranging from monoplegia to quadriplegia, spasticity, and weakness—may also occur
  - Urinary disturbances may include frequency, incontinence, urgency, and frequent infections
  - Bowel problems include constipation and involuntary evacuation
  - Fatigue is usually the most debilitating symptom; speech disturbance may also occur
- Diagnosis and treatment
  - Diagnostic tests may include lumbar puncture, evoked response, and MRI of the brain and spinal cord to detect plaques from multiple sclerosis; optic atrophy typically is present, and evoked potential of the brain stem and rolandic somatosensory responses may be abnormal
  - Because multiple sclerosis has no cure, treatment aims to decrease the length and severity of exacerbations and diminish or reverse the deficits caused by exacerbations
  - Drug therapy consists of a corticosteroid and a muscle relaxant; interferon beta-1b may be used to reduce the frequency of exacerbations in patients with relapsing-remitting multiple sclerosis; glatiramer acetate may also be helpful in reducing the frequency of relapses in such patients
  - Occupational, physical, and speech therapies and nutritional counseling are used to help the patient manage the disorder's effects
  - The patient may also need home care or to stay in an extended-care facility
- Nursing interventions
  - Teach the patient and family about the disease and strategies for avoiding stress, fatigue, and infections, factors that can exacerbate it
  - Administer carbamazepine, phenytoin, or amitriptyline to control pain from dysesthesias or other pain syndromes such as trigeminal neuralgia; transcutaneous electrical nerve stimulation and alternative measures such as relaxation techniques can also help
  - Encourage the patient to participate in physical therapy to maintain muscle strength and decrease spasms
  - Encourage the patient to eat a balanced diet to maintain proper functioning of the immune system and avoid constipation
  - Initiate bowel and bladder training; loss of muscle and sphincter tone may require self-catheterization and daily suppositories

- Encourage good respiratory hygiene; tell the patient and family to contact the health care provider if the patient develops dyspnea, shortness of breath, or pulmonary infection
- Teach the patient and caregivers how to prevent complications of immobility; if bed rest or a wheelchair is required, discuss transfer techniques and proper turning and positioning to prevent deformity
- Develop alternative forms of communication for use during exacerbations, such as eyelid blinking or using letter or picture boards
- Teach the patient to alternate rest and activity, avoid temperature extremes, and reduce stress
- Refer the patient to a support group or a local chapter of the Multiple Sclerosis Society

Myasthenia Gravis

- Description
  - Myasthenia gravis is a chronic autoimmune disorder of neuromuscular transmission characterized by extreme, abnormal voluntary muscle weakness during activity; weakness can be relieved by rest
  - It may be caused by a defect of the postsynaptic receptor sites or acetylcholine deficiency
  - It affects neuromuscular transmission at the myoneural junction, leaving sensation intact and preventing muscle atrophy
- Signs and symptoms
  - The dominant symptoms of myasthenia gravis are skeletal muscle fatigability and weakness; typically, muscles are strongest in the morning but weaken throughout the day, especially after exercise
  - The first indications may include weak eye closure, diplopia, and ptosis
  - The face may be blank and expressionless; the voice, nasal
  - Problems with chewing and swallowing may be present. Weakened respiratory muscles may make breathing difficult, leading to respiratory distress
- Diagnosis and treatment
  - Diagnostic tests may include thymus MRI or CT (to rule out the presence of thymoma and thymic hyperplasia, both of which are associated with myasthenia gravis), chest X-ray, electromyography, and the Tensilon test (to evaluate muscle contractility); if the Tensilon test is inconclusive, a neostigmine test is done
  - Pulmonary function testing to assess ventilation
  - An anticholinesterase alleviates symptoms but is ineffective during a crisis
  - Corticosteroid and immunosuppressive therapy and thymectomy (if thymomas are present) may alter the course of the disease
  - Intravenous immunoglobulin (IVIg) may be ordered to increase antibodies in the bloodstream
  - Plasmapheresis may relieve symptoms; it may be used to prepare the patient for thymectomy and during a respiratory crisis
  - Ventilator support may be needed during a myasthenic crisis
- Nursing interventions
  - Support respiratory function, encourage coughing and deep breathing, and use nasotracheal or oral tracheal suction when necessary to keep the airway open; use mechanical ventilation or a tracheostomy tube, if prescribed
  - Schedule activity 20 to 30 minutes after medication is given, when strength is greatest, and space activities to avoid fatigue
  - If the patient can't chew and swallow solid food, provide a semisoft diet; observe and intervene for choking on liquids due to cranial nerve weakness
  - Assess the patient for signs and symptoms of myasthenic crisis, such as anxiety, fever, increased weakness, problems with chewing and swallowing, and respiratory distress
  - Assess the patient for signs and symptoms of cholinergic crisis, such as abdominal cramps, bradycardia, diarrhea, dyspnea, general weakness, lacrimation, muscle cramps, myasthenic crisis, nausea, respiratory distress, salivation, sweating, vomiting, and wheezing
  - Teach the patient and his family about the disease, and suggest lifestyle changes such as scheduling activities during energy peaks
  - Teach the patient and family the signs of anticholinesterase toxicity—such as diaphoresis, dyspnea, increased muscle weakness, nausea, and ptosis—to ensure prompt intervention
  - Teach the patient and family the signs of respiratory distress and failure
  - Provide emotional support, and refer the patient to the Myasthenia Gravis Foundation of America

Parkinson's Disease

- Description
  - Parkinson's disease is a chronic, degenerative disease of the basal ganglia, substantia nigra, and corpus striatum of the brain; it's associated with a deficiency of the neurotransmitter dopamine after 60% to 80% of the cells that produce dopamine are damaged
  - Although the exact cause of Parkinson's disease is unknown, possible causes include exposure to a toxic agent such as carbon monoxide and manganese, genetic factors, vascular (arteriosclerotic) changes, and viral infection
  - Iatrogenic Parkinson's disease can result from the use of major tranquilizers, methyldopa, and reserpine; it's generally reversible within 2 weeks of discontinuing the drug
- Signs and symptoms
  - Parkinson's disease presents with four main motor symptoms. Bradykinesia, or slowness in movement affects the ability to do daily activities or speak; involuntary tremor at rest of hands, limbs, lips, or jaw may improve when actively using affected muscle groups (includes "pill rolling"); stiffness of limbs and trunk may cause aches and difficulty with ambulation; and postural instability will cause difficulty with walking, balance, and turning (includes festination, or speeding up with each step to compensate for displaced center of gravity)
  - Other symptoms include decreased blinking; dysarthria; dysphagia; excessive drooling; micrographia (handwriting that becomes progressively smaller); oculogyric crisis (involuntary deviation and fixation of the eyeballs); slow, slurred, monotone speech; and a wide-eyed, blank facial expression, and freezing in place when trying to walk
- Diagnosis and treatment
  - Physical examination and health history findings may be confirmed by electromyography
  - Treatment aims at slowing the progression of symptoms and providing supportive care
  - Antiparkinsonians are prescribed: levodopa decreases muscle rigidity and an anticholinergic decreases rigidity and tremors
  - The antiviral amantadine is used early on to reduce tremors and rigidity
  - The dopamine receptor agonists bromocriptine (Parlodel), pergolide, pramipexole dihydrochloride (Mirapex), and ropinirole (Requip) activate dopamine receptors in the basal ganglia
  - The monoamine oxidase type B inhibitor selegiline allows conservation of dopamine and enhances the therapeutic effect of levodopa
  - The catechol-*O*-methyltransferase inhibitors entacapone (Comtan) and tolcapone (Tasmar) inhibit the breakdown of dopamine and may be useful as adjuncts to levodopa
  - Patients may benefit from physical therapy
  - Referrals may be provided for home health assistants, visiting nurses, adult day care, or nursing home placement
- Nursing interventions
  - Administer medications as prescribed
  - Encourage physical therapy to maintain muscle function for as long as possible
  - Teach the patient and family about the disease and the drugs' adverse effects
  - Teach the patient and family about home safety; suggest removal of throw rugs and loose carpeting and install grab bars and elevated toilet seats in the bathrooms; recommend the use of a cane or walker for a patient in the later stages of Parkinson's disease
  - Teach the patient and family about preventing constipation by encouraging adequate nutrition and hydration; stress the importance of establishing a regular pattern of elimination
  - Provide emotional support for the patient and family, and refer them to Parkinson's disease support groups

Seizure Disorders

- Description
  - Seizures are sudden paroxysmal discharges of a group of neurons that interfere with normal mental and behavioral activities
  - Seizures may be triggered by toxic states, electrolyte imbalances, tumors, anoxia, CNS inflammation, increased ICP, or idiopathic causes
  - Epilepsy is a seizure disorder associated with brain disorders like malformations, stroke, and tumors

- Signs and symptoms
  - Seizure symptoms vary with the type of seizure (see *Differentiating seizures*, page 168)
  - Seizures have three phases
    - The prodromal phase occurs before the seizure and produces auras (sensory signals that warn of an approaching seizure), such as a flash of light, mood or behavior changes, or a sudden sensation of smell or taste; this phase lasts from seconds to days
    - The ictal phase is the seizure itself
    - The postictal phase occurs after the seizure and may produce amnesia, confusion, inability to be aroused for minutes or hours, or sleepiness
- Diagnosis and treatment
  - Diagnosis may be based on CT scan or MRI, EEG, cerebral angiography, medical history, drug use history or toxicology results, and neurologic examination
  - Lumbar puncture may be performed to rule out an infectious cause
  - An anticonvulsant is prescribed to prevent seizures
  - If the seizures are not controlled by two or more drugs, surgery may be necessary
  - Brain tumors, if present, are surgically removed
  - The optimal goal is to eliminate the cause of seizure activity
- Nursing interventions
  - Take seizure precautions during hospitalization to prevent injury
  - Protect the patient during a seizure
    - Never insert a tongue blade or other foreign object into the patient's mouth during an active seizure; forcing one in may break his teeth and lead to aspiration
    - Safeguard the patient from nearby objects, but don't restrain; restraining limbs can fracture bones; loosen tight clothing
    - To maintain a patent airway, turn the patient to his side to prevent aspiration of saliva or stomach contents
  - After a seizure occurs, document your observations
    - Note prodromal signs and the time of onset
    - Write down the specific types of movements and the order in which they occurred, including body parts involved
    - Note changes in the patient's respiratory pattern
    - Document eye deviation and pupillary response
    - Record the time the seizure stopped and any postictal response
  - Teach the patient and family about the therapeutic and adverse effects of the prescribed anticonvulsant, the importance of taking medications exactly as prescribed to maintain therapeutic levels, and the need to return for laboratory work to monitor serum drug levels and detect adverse reactions
  - Advise the patient to avoid oral thermometers, which can be swallowed or broken if a seizure occurs
  - Instruct the patient to avoid alcohol and nicotine; these stimulants can precipitate a seizure
  - Tell the patient to always carry identification, which explains that the patient has seizures and listing the name and phone number of the practitioner
  - Refer the patient to the Epilepsy Foundation for additional support and strategies for living with epilepsy

Spinal Cord Injury

- Description
  - Spinal cord injury usually results from traumatic force on the vertebral column, which, in turn, injures the spinal cord
  - Spinal cord injury includes concussion, contusion, hemorrhage, herniated disk syndrome, laceration, transection, and vertebral fractures (see *Types of spinal cord injury*, page 171)
  - *Complete spinal cord injury* or lesion causes loss of voluntary motor function, all sensations, and proprioception below the level of the lesion
    - Paraplegia (paralysis of both legs) results from spinal cord injuries from the level of T1 down
    - Quadriplegia (paralysis of all arms and legs) results from spinal cord injuries of one or more cervical vertebrae

Box 10-4: Differentiating Seizures

Seizures can be classified as partial or generalized. Some patients may be affected by more than one type.

Partial seizures

Partial seizures arise from a localized area in the brain and cause specific symptoms. In some patients, partial seizure activity spreads to the entire brain, causing a generalized seizure. Partial seizures include simple partial (Jacksonian motor-type and sensory-type), complex partial (psychomotor or temporal lobe), and secondarily generalized partial seizures.

Simple Partial (Jacksonian Motor-Type) Seizure

A simple partial seizure begins as a localized motor seizure, which is characterized by a spread of abnormal activity to adjacent areas of the brain. Typically, the patient experiences a stiffening or jerking in one extremity, accompanied by a tingling sensation in the same area. For example, the seizure may start in the thumb and spread to the entire hand and arm. The patient seldom loses consciousness, although the seizure may secondarily progress to a generalized tonic-clonic seizure.

Simple Partial (Sensory-Type) Seizure

Perception is distorted in a simple partial seizure. Symptoms can include hallucinations, flashing lights, tingling sensations, a foul odor, vertigo, or déjà vu (the feeling of having experienced something before).

Complex Partial (Psychomotor or Temporal Lobe) Seizure

Symptoms of a complex partial seizure vary but usually include purposeless behavior. The patient may experience an aura and exhibit overt signs, including a glassy stare, picking at his clothes, aimless wandering, lip-smacking or chewing motions, and unintelligible speech. The seizure may last for a few seconds or as long as 20 minutes. Afterward, mental confusion may last for several minutes; as a result, an observer may mistakenly suspect psychosis or intoxication with alcohol or drugs. The patient has no memory of his actions during the seizure.

Secondarily Generalized Partial Seizure

A secondarily generalized partial seizure can be either simple or complex and can progress to generalized seizures. An aura may precede the progression. Loss of consciousness occurs immediately or within 1 to 2 minutes of the start of the progression.

Generalized seizures

As the term suggests, generalized seizures cause a generalized electrical abnormality in the brain. They include several distinct types, including absence (petit mal), myoclonic, generalized tonic-clonic (grand mal), and akinetic.

Absence (Petit Mal) Seizure

An absence seizure commonly occurs in children but also may affect adults. It usually begins with a brief change in the level of consciousness, indicated by blinking or rolling of the eyes, a blank stare, and slight mouth movements. The patient retains his posture and continues preseizure activity without difficulty. Typically, the seizure lasts from 1 to 10 seconds. The impairment is so brief that the patient is sometimes unaware of it. If not properly treated, these seizures can recur as often as 100 times a day. An absence seizure can progress to a generalized tonic-clonic seizure.

Myoclonic Seizure

A myoclonic seizure—also called bilateral massive epileptic myoclonus—is marked by brief, involuntary muscular jerks of the body or extremities, which may occur in a rhythmic manner, and a brief loss of consciousness.

Generalized Tonic-Clonic (Grand Mal) Seizure

Typically, a generalized tonic-clonic seizure begins with a loud cry, precipitated by air rushing from the lungs through the vocal cords. The patient falls to the ground, losing consciousness. The body stiffens (tonic phase) and then alternates between episodes of muscle spasm and relaxation (clonic phase). Tongue biting, incontinence, labored breathing, apnea, and subsequent cyanosis may also occur. The seizure stops in 2 to 5 minutes, when abnormal electrical conduction of the neurons is completed. The patient then regains consciousness but is somewhat confused and may have difficulty talking. If able to talk, the patient may complain of drowsiness, fatigue, headache, muscle soreness, and arm or leg weakness. Then patient may fall into a deep sleep after the seizure.

Akinetic Seizure

An akinetic seizure is characterized by a general loss of postural tone and a temporary loss of consciousness. This type of seizure occurs in young children. Sometimes, it's called a drop attack because it causes the child to fall.

- *Incomplete spinal cord injury* or lesion leaves some motor or sensory function intact
  - ○ Central cord syndrome is damage to the central fibers of the spinal cord; it commonly results from a forced hyperextension injury, causes arterial disruption to the spinal cord, and leads to motor function deficit in the arms and, possibly, the legs
  - ○ Anterior cord syndrome is damage to the anterior two-thirds of the spinal cord; it usually results from a flexion injury, disrupts the anterior spinal artery, and leads to paralysis and loss of pain and temperature sensation below the lesion (senses of touch, vibration, position, and motion remain intact)
  - ○ Posterior cord syndrome is damage to the posterior gray and white matter of the spinal cord; it usually results from an extension injury and impairs vibratory sensation, light touch, and proprioception (motor function, pain, and temperature sensation remain intact)
  - ○ Brown-Séquard syndrome is damage to one side of the spinal cord; it results from a penetrating injury (such as a gunshot or stab wound)
    - ○ Rotation-flexion injury causes unilateral damage
    - ○ Ipsilateral damage below the lesion affects motor function, pressure and touch sensations, and the senses of vibration and position
    - ○ Contralateral damage causes loss of pain and temperature sensations
  - ○ Horner syndrome can occur as part of Brown-Séquard syndrome or result from damage to the midbrain; it occurs ipsilaterally to a cervical lesion and causes anhidrosis (lack of sweat), ptosis, and pupillary contraction on the affected side of the face
  - Spinal cord injury may result from trauma (see *Mechanisms of spinal cord injury*, page 171); it also can result from organic causes, such as AVM, emboli, hematoma, infection, and tumor
- Motor loss caused by spinal cord injury
  - Paralysis is a temporary or permanent loss of function
    - ○ Spastic paralysis is the loss of voluntary movement caused by damage to upper motor neurons; the lower motor neurons may be intact, in which case, the reflex arc remains intact
    - ○ Flaccid paralysis is the loss of voluntary movement caused by damage to the lower motor neurons; reflexes, including deep tendon reflexes, are lost
  - Deep tendon reflexes include the biceps reflex, triceps reflex, brachioradialis reflex, patellar reflex, and Achilles tendon reflex; they're graded as 0 (absent), 1+ (diminished), 2+ (normal), 3+ (increased), or 4+ (hyperactive)
  - Superficial reflexes comprise the abdominal reflex, cremasteric reflex, plantar reflex, and gluteal reflex; they're graded as 0 (absent), +/− (diminished or inconsistent), or + (normal)
- Level of spinal cord injury and associated motor loss
  - Injury above the cord at the C1 to C3 level causes quadriplegia and loss of respiratory function
  - Injury to the cord at the C4 level causes quadriplegia and may affect respiratory function if edema damages the phrenic nerve
  - Injury to the cord at the C5 to C6 level causes quadriplegia; gross motor movement of the arms remains intact with use of the scapular elevators; diaphragmatic breathing remains intact but may not be able to support ventilation because of the loss of intercostal muscle innervation
  - Injury to the cord at the C6 to C7 level causes quadriplegia; diaphragmatic breathing remains intact but may not be able to support ventilation; arm muscles remain innervated and capable of elbow flexion, wrist extension, and weak thumb grasp
  - Injury to the cord at the C7 to C8 level causes quadriplegia; diaphragmatic breathing remains intact, but ventilation and airway secretion removal may be compromised because of loss of intercostal muscle innervation; biceps and triceps muscles respond to voluntary control, and wrist flexion may be possible
  - Injury to the cord between the T1 and L1 to L2 levels causes paraplegia; voluntary motor function of the arms remains intact; loss of some intercostal muscle innervation may impede ventilation and secretion removal
  - Injury to the cauda equina causes mixed loss of motor, sensory, bowel, bladder, and sexual function and depends on which roots are damaged
  - Injury to the sacral spinal nerves causes loss of bowel, bladder, and sexual function
- Spinal shock
  - Spinal shock is caused by sudden, severe spinal cord damage and initially produces flaccid paralysis; areflexia below the level of the lesion and loss of cutaneous and proprioceptive sensations occur in the first few hours and may last for weeks
  - Recovery occurs over time; reflex activity returns in 3 to 6 weeks; flexion spasms affect paralyzed limbs 6 to 16 weeks after injury; alternating flexion and extension spasms affect paralyzed limbs about 6 months after injury; extension spasms predominate after 6 months

- Autonomic dysreflexia
  - Autonomic dysreflexia is a complication of complete spinal cord injury
  - Injuries at or above T6 present the greatest risk, but autonomic dysreflexia has been observed in injuries occurring at the T8 level
  - Autonomic dysreflexia is a clinical emergency and is caused by stimulation of the autonomic reflexes below the level of the lesion
  - Autonomic dysreflexia causes decreased heart rate, pallor, pilomotor spasm (goose bumps and hair erection), and severe, persistent hypertension
  - Other findings include blotchy skin, diaphoresis, flushing, nasal congestion, pounding headache, and vasodilation above the lesion
  - Autonomic dysreflexia can be precipitated by various sensory stimuli, including a full bladder or rectum, painful stimuli (such as pressure on the skin, pressure ulcers, and surgical incisions), other skin stimulation (such as pressure on the glans penis or perianal or periurethral area), and visceral contractions (such as bladder spasms and uterine contractions of pregnancy)
  - Treatment aims to control blood pressure while locating and removing the sensory stimulus
- Diagnosis and treatment
  - Diagnosis is based on anterior and lateral X-rays of the spine, CT scan, and MRI
  - Emergency life support is required to maintain vital function and avoid further injury; priorities include maintaining a patent airway; ensuring adequate ventilation (spontaneous or mechanical); maintaining adequate circulation; and performing neurologic assessments
  - To prevent further injury, the spine is immobilized with a cervical collar, cervical traction or cervical tongs (such as Gardner-Wells, Crutchfield, Barton, Cone, and Vinke), kinetic bed with cervical tongs for skeletal traction, halo brace with vest (for long-term use), or surgery (by means of Harrington rods, Weiss springs, laminectomy, or spinal fusion)
  - Clots, fragments, and tumors are surgically decompressed
  - A steroid is administered for the first 24 hours after the injury to reduce edema and inflammatory response
  - An analgesic and an opioid may be administered to control pain
  - A muscle relaxant is given to reduce muscle spasm
  - Proton pump inhibitors like omeprazole (Prilosec) or a histamine H2 receptor blocker like ranitidine (Zantac) are given to prevent gastric ulcers (traumatic events, such as spinal cord injury, can precipitate gastric ulcer formation)
  - Anticoagulant therapy is initiated to prevent deep vein thrombosis; therapy may include low doses of heparin, thigh-high antiembolism stockings (which compress superficial veins and prevent peripheral blood pooling), and sequential pneumatic compression devices (which massage the veins, mimic muscle action, and prevent peripheral blood pooling and thrombus formation)
  - Rehabilitative management includes surgical release of tendons for persistent muscle spasm of paralyzed muscles and surgical correction for cervical support (laminectomy and spinal fusions)
  - Rehabilitation referrals include those for occupational and physical therapies, nutritional counseling, social services, and psychiatric evaluation and assistance
- Nursing interventions
  - Provide respiratory support for a patient with a spinal cord injury above L1 to L2; support ranges from deep-breathing exercises to diaphragmatic coughing (exertion of abdominal pressure during coughing) to mechanical ventilation
  - Continuously monitor and assess neurologic function to detect early signs of deterioration
  - Modify the patient's environment to decrease dependence on others and increase his feelings of self-worth; discuss modifications with the patient and his family before discharge; modifications may include manual or electric wheelchairs, ramps, widened doorways, structural changes to bathroom facilities, and home care aides
  - Provide frequent and proper positioning, skin care, and proper hydration and nutrition to prevent complications of immobility
  - Teach the patient and his family about the recovery process, therapeutic and adverse effects of prescribed drugs, possible drug interactions, nutritional needs, exercise, bowel and bladder training, ways to prevent constipation and urinary tract infection, self-catheterization techniques, skin care, proper positioning, ways to avoid infection (especially respiratory infection), symptoms to report to the practitioner, and local support groups
  - Provide emotional support to the patient and family; permanent physical disabilities can be devastating to self-concept, relationships, and lifestyle; emotional support, particularly from others with similar experiences, can facilitate healing

Box 10-5: Types of Spinal Cord Injury

Different spinal cord injuries produce different effects.

Injury	Description	Possible effects
Concussion	Severe shaking	Temporary loss of function for 24 to 48 hours
Contusion	Bruising of the spinal cord	Spinal cord compression by bleeding and edema, causing varying degrees of damage
Dislocated vertebrae	Rupture of spinal ligaments and disruption of vertebral alignment	Spinal cord disruption
Hemorrhage	Bleeding from an aneurysm or other rupture	Spinal cord irritation by blood and edema, causing neurologic deficits
Herniated disk syndrome	Anterior, lateral, or posterior displacement of intervertebral disk, especially in lumbar and lumbosacral areas	Spinal cord injury caused by displaced tissue that compresses nerve roots and narrows the spinal canal
Laceration	Tear in the spinal cord	Spinal cord compression by bleeding and edema, causing permanent damage
Transection	Severing of the spinal cord	Complete or incomplete loss of spinal cord function
Vertebral fracture		
• Comminuted (burst)	Shattering of vertebrae	Fragment penetration of spinal cord
• Compressed	Compression or anterior wedging of vertebrae	Spinal cord compression
• Odontoid (hangman's)	Fracture of odontoid process of second cervical vertebra	Typically fatal injury of spinal cord and all organs below the fracture
• Simple	Single break, usually of a transverse or spinous process	Spinal cord unaffected if vertebrae remain aligned
• Stable	Fracture without bone displacement	No permanent damage if properly immobilized
• Unstable	Fracture with bone displacement	Spinal cord injury, instant quadriplegia, and loss of respiratory function

Box 10-6: Mechanisms of Spinal Cord Injury

Spinal cord injury may result from various types of trauma.

Mechanism	Possible effects
Compression injury Caused by vertical fall, such as diving into shallow water	• Vertebral and spinal cord damage
Flexion Caused by violent impact to back of head	• Anterior dislocation of vertebrae • Rupture of posterior ligaments
Hyperextension (whiplash) Caused by violent impact to the chin	• Rupture of anterior ligaments • Rupture of intervertebral disks and vertebrae
Penetrating injury Caused by a gunshot wound or stab injury	• Spinal cord damage that disrupts tissue function
Rotation injury Caused by violent rotation in opposite directions of top and bottom of body	• Rupture of ligaments, vertebrae, and disks

Stroke

- Description
  - Stroke is a disruption in cerebral circulation, causing permanent neurologic deficits
  - An embolic stroke may result from atherosclerotic plaque, an embolism, or vasospasm
  - A thrombotic ischemic stroke occurs when the occlusion evolves from partial to complete and may be heralded by a transient ischemic attack (TIA)
  - A hemorrhagic stroke may result from a ruptured or leaking aneurysm, an AVM, a bleeding disorder, trauma, or an arterial rupture (as caused by hypertension)
  - A TIA is a temporary disruption in the blood supply to the brain and symptoms last for 5 minutes or less. TIAs still require emergency treatment and are warning signs for future strokes
- Signs and symptoms
  - Symptoms of stroke vary with the affected artery (see *Signs and symptoms of stroke*, page 173)
  - Symptoms also vary according to the severity of the damage and the extent of collateral circulation
  - Generally, consider stroke if the patient experiences sudden numbness in face or limbs, trouble seeing, walking or talking, or a sudden severe headache
- Diagnosis and treatment
  - CT scan, MRI, cerebral arteriography, lumbar puncture, Doppler flow studies, and EEG may be used to diagnose stroke
  - Carotid endarterectomy removes plaque to improve cerebral blood flow
  - Surgical evacuation of the clot or hematoma relieves increased ICP
  - Although anticoagulants are contraindicated in a patient with a hemorrhagic stroke, they may be useful in a patient with a nonhemorrhagic thrombolytic event
  - An anticonvulsant is used to prevent or treat seizures
  - Tissue plasminogen activator can improve neurologic function when given within 3 hours of the onset of symptoms in a patient with a thrombotic stroke
  - An analgesic is used to relieve discomfort such as headache
  - An antihypertensive is used to lower blood pressure and, thus, prevent additional bleeding
  - A diuretic is used to lower blood pressure and reduce cerebral edema
  - Physical therapy and occupational therapy help maintain muscle and joint function, while teaching the patient needed home management techniques
- Nursing interventions
  - Provide emergency care; the patient may require lifesaving measures because of cardiopulmonary arrest triggered by the injury; administer oxygen, if needed, to promote oxygenation within the cerebral tissue
  - Maintain a patent airway; the patient may be unable to protect his airway because of impaired cough and gag reflexes and inability to support his head; suction the patient as necessary
  - Make sure the patient maintains bed rest until the cause of the stroke is known because activity can cause bleeding to recur
  - Position the patient to prevent deformity; loss of muscle tone leads to flexion contractures; turn and position every 2 hours to prevent pressure ulcers
  - Implement physical therapy to maintain strength and prevent contractures; provide passive ROM exercises to prevent venous thrombosis and contractures
  - Speak slowly and simply; the patient may not be able to understand rapid speech and may become confused
  - Monitor vital signs at least hourly until the patient's condition is stable; alterations can indicate further injury
  - Assess neurologic status hourly until the patient's condition is stable; early identification and treatment of increased ICP (signs include abnormal posturing, bradycardia, decreased LOC, decreased motor response, increased systolic blood pressure, and widened pulse pressure) may prevent further injury
  - Monitor fluid input and output hourly to ensure hydration until the patient's condition is stable
  - Ensure nutritional status by helping the patient to eat or by providing enteral or parenteral feedings when necessary
  - Provide for toileting needs; use aseptic technique with indwelling urinary catheters to prevent infections, and begin a bowel retraining program to reestablish continence
  - Modify nursing care for left and right hemisphere stroke

Box 10-7: Signs and Symptoms of Stroke

Signs and symptoms of stroke vary with the artery affected, the severity of the damage, and the extent of collateral circulation. Typical arteries affected and their associated signs and symptoms are described below.

Middle cerebral artery

When a stroke occurs in the middle cerebral artery, the patient may experience the following:
- Altered level of consciousness (LOC)
- Aphasia
- Contralateral hemiparesis (more severe in the face and arm than in the leg)
- Contralateral sensory deficit
- Dysgraphia
- Dysphagia
- Dyslexia
- Visual field cuts

Carotid artery

When a stroke occurs in the carotid artery, the patient may experience the following:

- Altered LOC
- Aphasia
- Bruits over the carotid artery
- Headaches
- Numbness, paralysis, sensory changes, transient vision loss, and weakness on the affected side
- Ptosis

Vertebrobasilar artery

When a stroke occurs in the vertebrobasilar artery, the patient may experience the following:
- Amnesia
- Ataxia
- Diplopia
- Dizziness
- Dysphagia
- Numbness around the lips and mouth
- Poor coordination
- Slurred speech
- Visual field cuts
- Weakness on the affected side

Anterior cerebral artery

When a stroke occurs in the anterior cerebral artery, the patient may experience the following:
- Confusion
- Impaired motor and sensory function
- Incontinence
- Loss of coordination
- Numbness and weakness on the affected side
- Personality changes

Posterior cerebral arteries

When a stroke occurs in the posterior cerebral arteries, paralysis is usually absent; however, the patient may experience the following:
- Coma
- Cortical blindness
- Dyslexia
- Sensory impairment
- Visual field cuts

- ○ Left hemisphere stroke causes expressive, global, or receptive aphasia (in most people, the left side is dominant for speech); right-sided hemiparesis or hemiplegia; right visual field deficit; and slow, cautious behavior
  - ○ Right hemisphere stroke causes apparent unawareness of the deficits of the affected side, leading to accidents; distractibility, impulsive behavior, and poor judgment; left-sided hemiparesis or hemiplegia; left visual field deficit; and spatial-perceptual deficits
- Teach the patient and his family how to use assistive devices, such as walkers and braces
- Refer the patient and his family to the American Stroke Association for support groups

Tumors, Brain

- Description
  - Brain tumors, which grow in the cranial cavity, can be malignant or benign, primary or metastatic
  - Brain tumors may cause serious consequences as they compress or invade adjacent tissue; symptoms are caused by the destruction of neurons, displacement of brain structures, and increased ICP
  - Common primary sites for metastatic cranial tumors are the lungs, breasts, and colon
  - The most common primary brain tumors in adults are gliomas and meningiomas
- Signs and symptoms
  - Symptoms vary not only by cell type but also by tumor location
  - Generalized signs and symptoms include dizziness, headache, mental changes, progressive neurologic deficits, and seizures
  - Signs and symptoms of increased ICP include alteration in LOC, bradycardia, difficulty with temperature regulation, headache, nausea and vomiting, personality changes, pupillary changes, respiratory pattern alterations, visual disturbances, and widened pulse pressure
  - Frontal tumors can lead to expressive aphasia, memory loss, and personality changes; occipital tumors, to visual changes or blindness; temporal tumors, to seizures that are precipitated by olfactory or visual auras, receptive aphasia, or dysarthria; tumors in the dominant hemisphere, to communication problems; tumors near the optic tract, to visual difficulties; acoustic tumors, to hearing difficulties; and pituitary tumors, to symptoms of hormonal disruption
- Diagnosis and treatment
  - Diagnosis of brain tumors involves various tests, including CT scan, EEG, MRI, and skull X-ray
  - Stereotactic surgery is the definitive diagnostic method to acquire tumor tissue and make an exact tissue diagnosis
  - Specific treatments vary with the tumor's histologic type, radiosensitivity, and location and may include surgery, radiation therapy, chemotherapy, and decompression of increased ICP with drugs or shunting of CSF
- Nursing interventions
  - Assess neurologic status, including signs of increased ICP to establish a baseline and facilitate early intervention
  - Maintain a patent airway to ensure adequate oxygenation; monitor and report respiratory changes
  - Maintain seizure precautions, and administer an anticonvulsant as ordered
  - Monitor the patient's temperature; fever commonly follows hypothalamic anoxia, but it can also indicate meningitis; use hypothermia blankets before and after surgery to keep the patient's temperature down and minimize cerebral metabolic demands
  - Turn and position the patient for comfort every 2 hours to prevent pressure ulcer development and encourage lung expansion
  - After surgery, monitor the patient's neurologic status, and be alert for signs of increasing ICP, such as changes in LOC; after supratentorial craniotomy, position the patient with the head of the bed elevated about 30 degrees to promote venous drainage; after infratentorial craniotomy, keep the patient flat for 48 hours
  - Consult with occupational and physical therapists to encourage independence in daily activities; assist with self-care as required; if the patient is aphasic, arrange for consultation with a speech pathologist
  - Provide emotional support to the patient and his family to help them cope with the diagnosis, treatment, potential disabilities, and changes in lifestyle

Review Questions

Question 1. What symptoms would a nurse watch for in a patient with a spinal cord injury at the C7 level?

A. Bradycardia, elevated blood pressure, and sweating
B. Tachycardia, constipation, and diaphoresis
C. Hypotension, change in LOC, and diarrhea
D. Urinary incontinence, hypertension, and polydipsia

Correct answer: A Bradycardia, hypertension, and sweating are signs of autonomic dysreflexia, a complication that may occur with a spinal cord injury at or above T6. Because a distended bladder is one of the most common causes of autonomic dysreflexia, the nurse should palpate the patient's bladder for fullness. If the patient has an indwelling urinary catheter, the nurse should check it for patency and kinks. Sometimes, constipation can also cause autonomic dysreflexia. Options B, C, and D are incorrect because tachycardia, hypotension, and urinary incontinence are not associated with autonomic dysreflexia. Excessive thirst is not related.

Question 2. Which best describes parts of the assessment of neurological function?

A. Test reflexes, heart rate, and bilateral muscle strength
B. Assess gait, balance, and sensation of light touch
C. Evaluate understanding of commands, speech, and blood pressure
D. Observe mood, posture, and mannerisms

Correct answer: B Balance, gait, and sensation of light touch are all parts of the neurological assessment. Also part of the assessment are reflexes, bilateral muscle strength, understanding of commands, assessment of speech, posture, and mannerisms. Heart rate, blood pressure, and mood are not part of the neurological exam (Options A, C, and D).

Question 3. When educating the patient's family, which is the best statement about Alzheimer's disease?

A. The ability to do activities of daily living will be lost suddenly.
B. Alzheimer's is a diagnosis of exclusion.
C. Bowel and bladder incontinence starts early in the disease process.
D. Teach your loved one new things to replace the ones forgotten.

Correct answer: B Alzheimer's is diagnosed after other reasons for dementia have been ruled out. Loss of ability to do self-care is a gradual process (Option A). Incontinence begins in the late stages of the disease (Option C). Patients with Alzheimer's cannot learn new things.

Question 4. When teaching a patient with multiple sclerosis, which is the most appropriate statement by the nurse? What techniques have helped you decrease stress in the past?

A. It's OK to continue babysitting your group of preschoolers in your home every day.
B. Physical therapy helps some people, but your medicine will do the same thing for you.
C. Continue with your normal toileting habits. Nothing there will change.

Correct answer: A Decreasing stress and fatigue will help prevent exacerbations of MS. Preschoolers are often ill, due to exposure to illness at daycares, preschools, and with the general public. Considering options to avoid contracting illnesses is beneficial to the patient with MS (Option B). Physical therapy helps maintain muscle strength and decrease spasm, beyond what medication alone can provide (Option C). As muscle and sphincter tone is lost, toilet training including self-catheterization and daily suppositories may be necessary.

Question 5. The nurse is providing care for a patient with a seizure disorder. What is the best explanation for the patient's statement, "I see flashing lights that are not there before I have a seizure."

A. This prodromal symptom indicates that the seizure will be worse than the last.
B. This is the initial part of the ictal phase of the seizure.
C. This is an abnormal finding and should be reported to the provider.
D. This is an aura and is a normal part of the prodromal phase of a seizure.

Correct answer: D Auras before seizure are normal and include flashing lights or perception of odors (Option C). The aura does not predict the intensity of the seizure (Option A). The aura starts before the seizure; the ictal phase is when the patient is actively seizing.

Question 6. An elderly patient has just suffered a stroke that damaged the vertebrobasilar artery. Which symptom should the nurse prepare the patient's family to expect?

A. Transient visual loss
B. Impaired motor and sensory function
C. Amnesia
D. Contralateral hemiparesis

Correct answer: C Damage to the vertebrobasilar artery can produce amnesia. Damage to the carotid artery can cause transient visual loss (Option C). Damage to the anterior cerebral arteries can cause impaired motor function (Option C), and damage to the middle cerebral artery can cause contralateral hemiparesis.

Question 7. Atrial fibrillation can cause which neurological condition?

A. Embolic stroke
B. Multiple sclerosis
C. Parkinson's disease
D. Traumatic brain injury

Correct answer: A Atrial fibrillation results from the irregular and rapid discharge from multiple ectopic atrial foci that causes quivering of the atria without atrial systole. This asynchronous atrial contraction predisposes the patient to mural thrombi, which may embolize, leading to an embolic stroke. No other neurological conditions correlate with atrial fibrillation.

Question 8. If a patient is experiencing difficulty with heart rate, body temperature, and breathing after a stroke, which area of the brain does the nurse suspect was damaged?

A. Lobar
B. Brain stem
C. Anterior CVA
D. Posterior

Correct answer: B The brain stem contains the medulla and the vital cardiac, vasomotor, and respiratory centers. A brain stem infarction leads to vital sign changes such

as bradypnea. Aphasia (Option A) is associated with lobar strokes in the cerebral hemispheres. Anterior and posterior strokes do not generally affect involuntary body systems.

Question 9. In a patient with meningitis, what symptoms would indicate irritation to CN III, IV, and VI?

A. Photophobia, impaired eye movements, and ptosis
B. Ptosis, photophobia, and presbyopia
C. Diplopia, astigmatism, and impaired eye movements
D. Impaired ocular movement, diplopia, and anisocoria

Correct answer: D Irritation to CN III (Option A), IV (Option B), and VI (Option D) may cause diplopia, impaired ocular movement, ptosis, and unequal pupils. Irritation to CN V may cause photophobia. Presbyopia is an age-related ocular change and astigmatism is a visual deficit due to an irregularity in the eye surface.

Question 10. Which of the following does the nurse know is not true about brain tumors?

A. They can be benign, malignant, or metastasized.
B. Symptoms come from neuronal destruction, increased ICP, and displacement of structures.
C. Gliomas and meningiomas are uncommon in adult patients with brain tumors.
D. Brain tumors may be metastasized from breast, lung, or colon cancer.

Correct answer: C Gliomas and meningiomas are common in adult patients. Options A, B, and D are all true about brain tumors.

Selected References

Adamolekun, B. (2017). Seizure disorders. Retrieved from http://www.merckmanuals.com/professional/neurologic-disorders/seizure-disorders/seizure-disorders

Alzheimer's Association. (2017). Alzheimer's disease. Retrieved from http://www.alz.org/alzheimers_disease_what_is_alzheimers.asp

Amyotrophic lateral sclerosis. (2016, September 22). Retrieved from http://www.mayoclinic.org/diseases-conditions/amyotrophic-lateral-sclerosis/diagnosis-treatment/diagnosis/dxc-20247217

Arteriovenous malformations. (2016, July 27). Retrieved from https://medlineplus.gov/arteriovenousmalformations.html

Bruce, J. (2016, December 13). Brain cancer treatment protocols. Retrieved from http://emedicine.medscape.com/article/2005182-overview

Carney, N., Totten, A. M., O'Reilly, C., Ullman, J. S., Hawryluk, G. W., Bell, M. J., … Ghajar, J. (2016). Guidelines for the management of severe traumatic brain injury. 4th ed. Retrieved from https://braintrauma.org/uploads/03/12/Guidelines_for_Management_of_Severe_TBI_4th_Edition.pdf

Christopher & Dana Reeve Foundation. (2017). Spinal cord injury. Retrieved from https://www.christopherreeve.org/living-with-paralysis/health/causes-of-paralysis/spinal-cord-injury

Encephalitis. (2016, August 31). Retrieved from https://medlineplus.gov/ency/article/001415.htm

Goldberg, C. (2015). A practical guide to clinical medicine: The neurological examination. Retrieved from https://meded.ucsd.edu/clinicalmed/neuro2.htm

Guillain-Barré syndrome. (2016, January 1). Retrieved from http://www.mayoclinic.org/diseases-conditions/guillain-barre-syndrome/basics/definition/CON-20025832

Huntington's disease. (2017, May 16). Retrieved from https://ghr.nlm.nih.gov/condition/huntington-disease#diagnosis

Increased intracranial pressure. (2017, May 9). Retrieved from https://medlineplus.gov/ency/article/000793.htm

Kantor, D., Zieve, D., & Ogilvie, I. (2015). Myasthenia gravis. Retrieved from https://medlineplus.gov/ency/article/000712.htm

Meningitis. (2017, April 10). Retrieved from https://www.cdc.gov/meningitis/index.html

Multiple Sclerosis. (2017, March 3). Retrieved from https://medlineplus.gov/multiplesclerosis.html

Muscular Dystrophy Association. (2017). ALS: Amyotrophic lateral sclerosis. Retrieved from https://www.mda.org/disease/amyotrophic-lateral-sclerosis

Muscular Dystrophy Association. (2017). Myasthenia gravis. Retrieved from https://www.mda.org/disease/myasthenia-gravis

National Parkinson Foundation. (2017). Understanding Parkinson's. Retrieved from http://www.parkinson.org/understanding-parkinsons/

Nordqvist, C. (2016). Encephalitis: Diagnosis, symptoms and treatment. *Medical News Today*. Retrieved from http://www.medicalnewstoday.com/articles/168997.php

Parkinson's Disease Foundation. (2017). What is Parkinson's disease? Retrieved from http://www.pdf.org/about_pd

Roopali, G.; Laroni, A., & Weiner, H. (2011). Role of the innate immune system in the pathogenesis of multiple sclerosis. *Journal of Neuroimmunology, 221*(1–2), 7–14. doi: 10.1016/j.jneuroim.2009.10.015

Stroke. (2017, February 6). Retrieved from https://www.cdc.gov/stroke/index.htm

Traumatic brain injury and concussion. (2017, April 27). Retrieved from https://www.cdc.gov/traumaticbraininjury/get_the_facts.html

Chapter 11

Musculoskeletal Disorders

Introduction

- The musculoskeletal system provides the structure and leverage that permits mobility. The parts that make up the system are bones, joints, and muscles. This system is important for the human body to be able to move, to stand erect, to protect the organs, and to aid in making red blood cells located in the body's bone marrow and as a reservoir for minerals like phosphorus and calcium
  - Alterations in the musculoskeletal system can result from soft tissue injury, bone fractures, infections, and tumors
- Various tests are used to assess musculoskeletal integrity

Nursing History

- The nurse asks the patient about the *chief complaint*
  - The patient with a joint injury may report a joint deformity, pain, stiffness, swelling, or sensory alteration
  - A patient with a fracture may report deformity or pain
  - A patient with a muscular injury may report pain, swelling, weakness, or sensory alteration
- The nurse then questions the patient about the *present illness*
  - Ask the patient about the symptom, including when it started, associated symptoms, location, radiation, intensity, duration, frequency, and precipitating and alleviating factors
  - Ask the patient if activities of daily living (ADLs) are affected; ask questions to determine if assistive devices are used, such as a cane, walker, or crutches
  - Ask about the use of prescription and over-the-counter drugs, herbal remedies, and vitamin and nutritional supplements
- The nurse asks about *medical history*
  - Question the patient about other musculoskeletal disorders, such as arthritis, gout, osteoporosis, and trauma
  - Ask the female patient whether she uses an oral contraceptive or is undergoing hormone therapy and whether she's premenopausal or postmenopausal
- The nurse then assesses the *family history*
  - Ask about a family history of musculoskeletal problems
  - Also ask about a family history of chronic and genetic disorders
- The nurse obtains a *social history*
  - Ask about work, exercise, diet, use of recreational drugs and alcohol, and hobbies
  - Also ask about stress, support systems, and coping mechanisms
  - Assess how the patient functions at home; determine his ability to get around, climb stairs, and drive
- Physical assessment
  - The nurse begins with *inspection*
    - Note the size and shape of joints, limbs, and body regions; note body symmetry
    - Inspect the skin and tissues around the joint, limb, or body region for color, swelling, masses, and deformities
    - Observe how the patient stands and moves; watch them walk, noting gait, posture, arm movements, and coordination
    - Inspect the curvature of the spine
    - To check range of motion (ROM), ask the patient to abduct, adduct, and flex or extend affected joints

○ Inspect major muscle groups for tone, strength, symmetry, and abnormalities; note contractures and abnormal movements, such as spasms, tics, tremors, and fasciculations
- Next, the nurse uses *palpation*
  ○ Palpate the patient's bones, noting any deformities, masses, or tenderness
  ○ Evaluate the patient's muscle tone, mass, and strength
  ○ Palpate joints for tenderness, nodes, crepitus, and temperature at rest and during passive ROM
  ○ Palpate arterial pulses and check capillary refill time
  ○ Check neurovascular status, including movement and sensation

Bursitis and Tendinitis

- Description
  - *Tendinitis* (also called *tendinopathy*) is an inflammatory process that affects the tendons and tendon-muscle attachments; it most commonly affects the shoulder rotator cuff, Achilles' tendon, hip, elbow, and knee
  - Tendinitis is caused by abnormal body development, hypermobility in calcific tendinitis, musculoskeletal disorders (such as rheumatic diseases and congenital defects), postural malalignment, and trauma (such as overuse or straining during sports activities)
  - *Bursitis* is a painful inflammation of one or more bursae; it most commonly affects the subdeltoid, subacromial, olecranon, trochanteric, calcaneal, prepatellar, and radiohumeral bursae
  - Types of bursitis include septic, calcific, acute, and chronic
  - Causes include common stressors (such as repetitive kneeling, prolonged sitting, or jogging in shoes without proper support) and recurrent trauma; septic bursitis can result from wound infection
  - Both bursitis and tendonitis typically occur in patients ages 15 to 50; overuse injuries are more likely to occur in high-risk populations, older adults, and athletes
  - Complications result from scar tissue with subsequent disability
- Signs and symptoms
  - Signs and symptoms of tendinitis include pain on palpation over the affected muscle-tendon unit, warmth (in acute tendinitis), and restricted movement; in the elbow, tenderness may occur over the lateral epicondyle; in the knee, palpable tenderness may occur in the hamstring when the knee is flexed at a 90-degree angle; and in the foot, crepitus may occur when the patient moves their foot
  - Signs and symptoms of bursitis include tenderness over the affected site, erythema, and swelling (with severe bursitis)
- Diagnosis and treatment
  - Various serum and urine tests rule out other disorders
  - X-rays in tendinitis may show bony fragments, osteophyte sclerosis, or calcium deposits
  - X-rays in calcific bursitis may show calcium deposits in the joint
  - Ultrasonography in tendinitis reveals increased tendon diameter, localized tendon swelling and thickening, and tendon sheath swelling
  - MRI in tendinitis shows tendon thickening, edema, and any tears in the tendon
  - Arthrocentesis may identify causative microorganisms and other causes of inflammation to rule out tendinitis
  - Arthrography is usually normal in tendinitis, showing only minor irregularities on the tendon under the surface
  - Treatment of both tendonitis and bursitis involves resting the affected area and providing symptomatic management
  - Medications include nonsteroidal anti-inflammatory drugs (NSAIDs) and corticosteroids for inflammation and analgesics for pain
  - Antibiotics are used to treat septic bursitis
  - Physical therapy may be prescribed
- Nursing interventions
  - Apply cold or heat therapies as ordered; protect the patient's skin when applying therapies
  - Encourage rest of the affected area, including immobilization if indicated
  - Elevate the affected area and apply gentle compression (elastic bandage or compression or neoprene sleeve)
  - Inspect the area for changes in swelling or erythema
  - Encourage the patient to participate in self-care to the extent possible and provide extra time for activities and assistance as necessary

- Administer medications, such as NSAIDs and analgesics, as ordered
- Encourage the use of active ROM exercises; reinforce participation in physical therapy as appropriate and indicated
- Teach the patient about the disease and how to prevent future episodes

Dislocations

- Description
  - A dislocation occurs when the articulating surfaces of a joint come out of position
  - Dislocations may result from trauma, diseases that affect the joint, or congenital weaknesses
  - Dislocations may cause injury to blood vessels and nerves and change in the contour of the joint, length of the extremity, and axis of the dislocated bones
- Signs and symptoms
  - The patient experiences pain at the affected joint
  - Neurovascular compromise may occur, including loss of movement, paresthesia, and pulselessness
- Diagnosis and treatment
  - Diagnosis is based on patient history, physical examination, and X-rays
  - Treatment consists of open or closed reduction, activity limitations as indicated, and pain relief
- Nursing interventions
  - Immobilize and elevate the affected joint; apply cold compresses as indicated
  - Assess neurovascular status before and after reduction, including strength of the pulse, capillary refill time, sensation, movement, pain, and color of the skin

Fractures, Femoral

- Description
  - A femoral fracture is a break in the femur anywhere along its shaft
  - Transverse, oblique, and comminuted fractures are the most common types of femoral fractures and may be open or closed (see *Types and Causes of Fractures*, page 181)
  - A femoral fracture can occur at any age, as a result of a fall, an accident, a gunshot wound, or other injury
- Signs and symptoms
  - Pain occurs at the fracture site
  - Discoloration and deformity may also be present
  - The fractured limb can't bear weight and may be shortened and externally rotated
  - Other findings may include an open wound, edema, and bruising
  - Leg fractures may produce any or all of the five Ps: pain, pallor, paralysis, paresthesia, and pulselessness
- Diagnosis and treatment
  - Diagnosis is based on patient history, physical examination, and X-rays that show the type and severity of the fracture
  - Cold therapy is applied to the fracture site
  - An opioid analgesic and a muscle relaxant are given to relieve pain
  - If the patient has an open fracture or has undergone surgery to correct the fracture, an antibiotic is administered; tetanus prophylaxis may also be required
  - Reduction of the fracture restores the displaced bone segments to their normal position
    - ○ With closed reduction, the bones are aligned by manual manipulation or traction; immobilization is by splint, cast, or traction
    - ○ With open reduction, the fracture is surgically reduced and immobilized with rods, plates, screws, and an immobilization device
- When a splint or cast fails to maintain the reduction, immobilization requires skin or skeletal traction, using a series of weights and pulleys (see *Skeletal and Skin Tractions*, pages 182–183)
  - With skin traction, elastic bandages and moleskin coverings are used to attach the traction devices to the patient's skin
  - With skeletal traction, a pin or wire is inserted through the bone distal to the fracture and attached to a weight, allowing more prolonged traction
- Nursing interventions
  - Perform neurovascular checks, which will provide data needed to formulate a care plan (see *Neurovascular Checks*, page 184)

- Assess vital signs, and monitor the patient for signs of shock because significant blood loss may occur with a femur fracture
- Assess the patient for signs of fat embolism—including confusion, dyspnea, hypotension, petechiae on the trunk, tachycardia, and tachypnea—which can occur following the fracture of a long bone
- Apply cold packs to the fracture site; cold causes vasoconstriction, which decreases bleeding and edema and lessens pain
- Check and maintain the traction setup, if used (see *Nursing Considerations for Patients in Skeletal or Skin Traction*, page 184)
- Provide good cast care to prevent skin breakdown and other complications
- Provide appropriate postoperative care
  - Keep the fractured leg elevated on a pillow to reduce edema by increasing venous return
  - Apply cold therapy to reduce bleeding and edema
  - Help the patient sit in a chair with his leg elevated; upright positions increase peripheral circulation, which decreases edema
  - Help the patient use an ambulatory aid when prescribed; weightbearing is restricted until some bone union occurs
  - Administer an opioid analgesic, or monitor the use of patient-controlled analgesia
  - Encourage the patient to perform leg and foot exercises to maintain muscle and joint strength and decrease venous stasis
  - Change dressings as needed, using strict aseptic technique, and administer an antibiotic, if prescribed; the patient is susceptible to wound infection and, possibly, osteomyelitis
  - Provide good pin care by cleaning the insertion site daily with chlorhexidine solution and assess pin site for signs of inflammation or infection
  - Assess patient for signs of compartment syndrome (e.g., pallor; paresthesia; paralysis; and pain that is throbbing, intensifies with elevation, is unrelenting, and is uncontrolled with analgesics)
  - Monitor fluid intake and output to ensure fluid balance
- Help with discharge planning by anticipating the patient's discharge needs

Box 11-1: Types and Causes of Fractures

Type of Fracture	Description	Force Causing the Fracture
Avulsion	Fracture that pulls bone and other tissues from their usual attachments	Direct force with resisted extension of the bone and joint
Closed (nondisplaced)	Skin is closed, but bone is fractured	Minor force
Compression	Fracture in which the bone is squeezed or wedged together at one side	Compressive, axial force applied directly above the fracture site
Greenstick	Break in only one cortex of the bone	Minor direct or indirect force
Impacted	Fracture with one end wedged into the opposite end or into the fractured fragment	Compressive, axial force applied directly to the distal fragment
Linear	Fracture line runs parallel to bone's axis	Minor or moderate direct force applied to the bone
Oblique	Fracture at an oblique angle across both cortices	Direct or indirect force with angulation and some compression
Open (compound)	Skin is open, bone is fractured, and soft tissue trauma may occur	Moderate to severe force that is continuous and exceeds tissue tolerances
Pathologic	Transverse, oblique, or spiral fracture of a bone weakened by tumor	Minor direct or indirect force
Spiral	Fracture curves around both cortices	Direct or indirect twisting force, with the distal part of the bone held or unable to move
Stress (fatigue)	Crack in one cortex of a bone	Repetitive direct force, as from jogging, running, or osteoporosis
Transverse	Horizontal break through the bone	Direct or indirect force toward the bone

Box 11-2: Skeletal and Skin Tractions

Type and Description	Purpose	Nursing Considerations
Skeletal traction		
Balanced suspension to femur Used in patients age 3 and older on the upper tibia and thigh with 20 to 35 lb (9 to 16 kg) of weight	• Realignment of fractures of the femur • Relief of muscle spasms associated with femoral fractures	• A Steinmann pin or Kirschner wire is inserted through the upper tibia. The thigh and leg are suspended in a splint and leg attachment. • Thigh and leg suspension is counterbalanced by traction to the top of the thigh splint. • The patient should be recumbent, but he can turn about 30 degrees to either side briefly for back care or lift himself up using the trapeze and the uninjured leg and foot. • Neurovascular checks are vital to assess circulatory status and prevent compartmental syndrome. • Tissue pressure monitoring is performed.
Cervical traction via skull tongs Used in patients of any age, but especially in young adults, bilaterally on skull bones with 20 to 30 lb (9 to 14 kg) of weight	• Realignment of fractures of cervical vertebrae • Relief of pressure on cervical nerves	• Patients may be severely injured and may have quadriplegia.
Halo-pelvic traction Used in adolescents and young adults on the skull and pelvis with no weight (bars extending between the skull and pelvic portions hold the body in the desired position)	• Preoperative straightening of scoliosis curvature	• Pins are inserted into the skull in four areas to hold the halo. Pins are inserted through the iliac pelvic bones to hold the pelvis. • Straightening is accomplished by tightening the bars, which overcomes muscle contractions. • Traction is "comfortable" after the patient has recovered from the insertional trauma. • Dressing is complicated because the vertical bars interfere with clothing. • Traction may remain in place postoperatively to be replaced by a brace or cast. • Halo-pelvic traction is a variant of halo-femoral traction, in which the pins are inserted through the distal femurs instead of the pelvic bones, and the skull pins pull away from the femoral pins.
Skin traction		
Buck's extension Most commonly used in adults on one or both legs with 5 to 8 lb (2.5 to 3.5 kg) of weight per leg	• Preoperative traction for hip fractures • "Pulling" contracted muscles • Relief of leg or back muscle spasms	• Patient generally lies recumbent. • Patient may be turned to either side if no fracture is present or turned to the unaffected side if fracture is present. • An older patient's skin is more friable and subject to loosening because of less subcutaneous fat. • Patient may complain of burning under tape, moleskin, or traction boot. • Traction may be removed for skin care even if fracture is present.

(continued)

Box 11-2: Skeletal and Skin Tractions (continued)

Type and Description	Purpose	Nursing Considerations
Cervical head halter Used in adults under the chin and around the face and back of the head with 5 to 15 lb (2.5 to 7 kg) of weight	• Relief of muscle spasms caused by degenerative or arthritic conditions of the cervical vertebrae or by muscle strain	• Halter should be applied so that the pull comes from the occipital area, not through the chin portion. • Patients may be in low- or high-Fowler's position, depending on the purpose of the traction. • If the patient complains of pain in the chin, teeth, or temporomandibular joint, the halter may be incorrectly positioned. Side straps should be adjusted to relieve these complaints. • Patients should be removed from traction for sleeping. • Patients can use this type of traction at home for cervical arthritic conditions.
Cotrel's traction Used in adolescents and young adults with a head halter (5 to 7 lb [2.5 to 3 kg] of weight) and a pelvic belt (10 to 20 lb [4.5 to 9 kg] of weight)	• Preoperative muscle stretching in patients with scoliosis	• Pulling in opposite directions may cause pain or discomfort. • Traction can be removed briefly for massage and skin care.
Dunlop's traction Used in adolescents and young adults on the lower humerus (5 to 7 lb of weight) and forearm (3 to 5 lb [1.5 to 2.5 kg] of weight)	• Realignment of fractures of the humerus	• Body is used for countertraction by slightly elevating side of bed of arm in traction. • Forearm is held at a right angle to the humerus for comfort, by using Buck's extension on the forearm. • Dunlop's traction can be used for skin traction (using Buck's extension to the humerus) or skeletal traction (using a Steinmann pin inserted through the distal humerus); use of skin or skeletal traction depends on the patient's injury. • Traction to the forearm should be removed daily for skin care.
Pelvic belt or girdle Used in older adolescents and adults on the abdomen or pelvis with 20 to 35 lb of weight	• Relief of muscle spasms and pain associated with disk conditions	• Pull comes from iliac crests to relieve spasm. • Patient may be placed in the William's position, which permits 45-degree knee and hip flexion to relax the lumbosacral muscles. • Orders typically are "in traction 2 hours, out 2 hours" and out of traction at night. • Traction straps shouldn't put pressure on sciatic nerves.
Pelvic sling Used in adults under the pelvis and buttocks like a hammock with 20 to 35 lb of weight	• Holding of fractured pelvic bones	• Buttocks must be slightly off the bed. • Patients are comfortable in the sling even with extensive pelvic bruising. • They may become dependent on the sling and may require gradual weaning. • The sling should be kept clean and dry. • Patients can be removed from the sling for care and toileting if facility policy permits.
Russell traction Used in patients age 5 and older on one or both legs with 2 to 5 lb (1 to 2.5 kg) of weight per leg	• Preoperative traction for hip fractures • "Pulling" contracted muscles • Treatment of Legg-Calvé-Perthes disease	• Pulley placement and amount of weight used are based on the principle that "for every force in one direction, there is an equal force in the opposite direction." • Patient is positioned on back for most effective pull. • Knee sling can be loosened for skin care and checking pulses in popliteal area.

Box 11-3: Neurovascular Checks

Fractures may cause nerve or arterial damage, producing any or all of the five Ps: pain, pallor, paralysis, paresthesia, and pulselessness. When performing a neurovascular check, compare findings bilaterally and above and below the fracture.

Pain

Ask the patient if they are having pain. Assess the location, severity, and quality of the pain as well as anything that seems to relieve or worsen it. Pain that is unrelieved by an opioid or that worsens with elevating the limb (elevation reduces circulation and worsens ischemia) may indicate compartment syndrome.

Pallor

Paleness, discoloration, and coolness of the injured site may indicate neurovascular compromise from decreased blood supply to the area. Check capillary refill time. Tissues should return to normal color within 3 seconds. Palpate skin temperature with the back of your hand.

Paralysis

Note any deficits in movement or strength. If the patient can't move the affected area or if movement causes severe pain and muscle spasms, they might have nerve or tendon damage. For a femoral fracture, assess peroneal nerve injury by checking for sensation over the top of the foot between the first and second toes.

Paresthesia

Ask the patient about changes in sensation, such as numbness or tingling. Check for loss of sensation by touching the injured area with the tip of an open safety pin or the point of a paper clip. Abnormal sensation or loss of sensation indicates neurovascular involvement.

Pulselessness

Palpate peripheral pulses distal to the injury, noting rate and quality. If a pulse is decreased or absent, blood supply to the area is reduced.

Box 11-4: Nursing Considerations for Patients in Skeletal or Skin Traction

Nursing Action	Rationale
Check ropes, knots, pulleys, freedom of movement, and intactness.	These actions help ensure that the traction is functioning properly.
Check the entire traction setup, pin site, and all suspension apparatus for tightness or signs of loosening.	These actions help ensure that the traction is functioning properly.
Check weights to ensure that they're hanging freely.	This action helps ensure that there is a proper amount of traction.
Make sure the weights aren't "lifted" during care.	This action helps to avoid pain caused by sudden muscle contraction and disrupted fragments of the injured or fractured bone. (Patients in skeletal traction should be moved for position changes without lifting or releasing the weights.)
Take care not to bump the weights or weight holders.	This action helps to avoid pain caused by rope movements that affect the traction bow and pin.
Check all skin surfaces for signs of tolerance or pressure areas (especially on the occipital area of the head, shoulder blades, elbows, coccyx, and heels).	These actions may uncover signs of pressure, which include redness, tenderness or pain, soreness caused by excoriation, and numbness.
Provide physical and psychological comfort. Answer questions honestly, answer the call light promptly, provide prompt and thorough care, encourage patient participation in care, provide diversionary activities, and prepare the patient and family for discharge.	These actions help ensure that the patient participates in and is prepared for self-care.

Fractures, Hip

- Description
  - Hip fracture is a fracture of the head, neck, trochanteric, or subtrochanteric regions of the femur
    - ○ *Intracapsular* fractures are those of the femoral head and neck, which are inside the hip capsule; the hip capsule is made up of ligaments surrounding the hip joint
    - ○ *Extracapsular* fractures are those of the femoral trochanteric and subtrochanteric regions, which lie outside the ligaments of the hip capsule
  - Hip fractures are most common in older people, particularly elderly women; many are associated with osteoporosis and falls
- Signs and symptoms
  - The fractured limb is shortened and rotated externally; it can't bear weight
  - Other findings include hip discoloration, pain, and tenderness
- Diagnosis and treatment
  - Diagnosis is based on patient history, physical examination, and X-rays
  - Intracapsular fracture requires open reduction with prosthetic replacement because of the high risk of loss of blood supply to the head of the femur, which leads to avascular necrosis
  - Extracapsular fracture requires insertion of a sliding compression hip nail, hip nail with side plate, or multiple pins
- Preoperative nursing interventions
  - Monitor traction setup and functioning; skin traction may be used as a temporary measure to reduce muscle spasms and increase patient comfort and safety
  - Monitor neurovascular status; trauma disrupts arterial and venous vessels, leading to bruising, edema, pain, and color changes
  - Monitor vital signs; fluctuating vital signs may be caused by shock (up to 1,000 mL of blood may be lost into the hip joint), trauma, or a pre-existing vascular condition; temperature typically is below normal unless a urinary or respiratory tract infection exists
  - Perform other preoperative care, such as giving the patient nothing by mouth, having them empty the bladder, and checking vital signs
  - Send an abduction pillow to the operating room if the patient is receiving a prosthesis; the pillow helps keep the prosthesis in the hip joint until muscles and ligaments heal
- Postoperative nursing interventions
  - Monitor vital signs and neurovascular status; surgical repair of hip fracture is traumatic because of bone and tissue injuries and can lead to complications, such as thrombophlebitis and fat or pulmonary embolism
  - Monitor the amount and type of wound drainage; drainage should be serosanguineous and should total no more than 200 mL over 3 days
  - Position the affected limb properly to prevent dislocation; use abduction if a prosthesis was inserted, but use a neutral position if another internal fixation device was inserted
  - Fit an overhead trapeze on the patient's bed so that they can use it to help lift themselves off the bed using the unaffected limb
  - Turn the patient on the nonoperative side as prescribed to facilitate circulation and recovery while easing tired muscles and relieving pressure; prop the operative limb with an abduction pillow if the patient has a prosthesis or with pillows if the patient has another internal fixation device
  - Teach the patient isometric quadriceps and gluteal-setting exercises to strengthen muscles
  - Encourage deep breathing and coughing every 2 hours, and use an incentive spirometer every 1 to 2 hours to prevent pulmonary complications
  - Auscultate all lung lobes for breath sounds, which should be clear
  - Check the color and amount of sputum, which should be clear
  - Monitor fluid intake and output and I.V. infusions; intake should be 3,000 mL daily; output should include 2,300 mL of urine and 300 to 700 mL of insensible water loss and perspiration
  - Provide a regular diet as prescribed, and monitor bowel sounds; a patient with good bowel sounds who is passing flatus can receive regular foods; nerve involvement from the hip may cause mild abdominal distention
  - Assess skin, and provide skin care to pressure areas (e.g., heels, back, sacrum, shoulders, and elbows)
  - Help the patient sit on the bed or in a chair on the first postoperative day; initially, weight-bearing activity is prohibited because it can cause excessive pressure on internal fixation devices; therefore, the patient must use a walker, which provides stability and allows ambulation with little or no weightbearing

- Make sure the hip isn't flexed more than 90 degrees for up to 2 months after surgery; during the first 10 postoperative days, even less flexion may be allowed
- Administer an opioid analgesic, or monitor the use of patient-controlled analgesia
- To prevent thrombophlebitis, administer an anticoagulant as ordered, and use external pneumatic compression devices and thigh high antiembolism stockings
- Perform dressing changes as needed using aseptic technique; the wound may be left uncovered after draining ceases
- Encourage the patient to perform foot and ankle exercises, including dorsiflexion and plantar flexion, to increase venous return and prevent thrombophlebitis
- Teach the patient about proper use of a walker and use of the prescribed amount of weightbearing

Gout

- Description
  - Gout is an inflammatory arthritis caused by uric acid and crystal deposits in the joints and other tissues that trigger an immune response
  - Gout results when uric acid crystallizes in blood or body fluids and the precipitate accumulates in connective tissue (tophi)
  - The disorder is characterized by red, swollen, and acutely painful joints; it mostly affects the feet, great toe, ankle, and midfoot
  - The patient may remain symptom-free for years between attacks
  - The first acute attack strikes suddenly and peaks quickly
  - Chronic polyarticular gout—the final, unremitting stage of the disease—is marked by persistent, painful polyarthritis
  - Causes of primary gout include decreased renal excretion of uric acid or oversecretion of uric acid; a genetic defect in purine metabolism (hyperuricemia); radical dieting practices that involve starvation; a diet high in red organ meats, seafood, or high-fructose corn syrup; and high alcohol consumption, especially of beer
  - Secondary gout is associated with certain drugs (such as thiazide diuretics and cyclosporine), diabetes mellitus, hypertension, leukopenia, myeloma, truncal obesity, polycythemia, renal disease, and hypercholesterolemia
  - Primary gout is more common in men than women and typically occurs between ages 30 and 60
  - Complications include renal calculi, atherosclerotic disease, cardiovascular lesions, and neuropathies
- Signs and symptoms
  - Symptoms of an acute attack appear suddenly and peak quickly; initially, one or a few joints are affected with such symptoms as pain, redness, tenderness, and warmth and inflammation at the affected joint; low-grade fever may also occur
  - Symptoms may subside quickly but tend to recur at irregular intervals; severe attacks can persist for days or weeks
  - In later stages of the disease after polyarticular gout has developed, polyarthritis develops in multiple joints, and subcutaneous tophi (urate crystal deposits) may occur
  - The skin over tophi may ulcerate and release a chalky white exudate or pus
- Diagnosis and treatment
  - Serum uric acid levels and WBC count are elevated during an acute gout attack; urine uric acid levels are chronically elevated in about 20% of patients
  - X-ray of the articular cartilage and subchondral bone shows evidence of chronic gout
  - Needle aspiration of synovial fluid shows needle-like intracellular crystals and an elevated WBC count
  - Treatment aims to bring acute attacks under control, reduce hyperuricemia, and prevent complications
  - Dietary restrictions include avoiding alcohol, eating purine-rich foods (such as anchovies, liver, and sardines) sparingly, and increasing fluid intake during acute attacks
  - Drug treatment includes the use of NSAIDs such as indomethacin (Indocin) for pain
  - Colchicine helps stop acute attacks
  - Corticosteroids may also be used
  - Allopurinol, febuxostat, probenecid, and sulfinpyrazone are used to treat chronic gout
- Nursing interventions
  - Institute bed rest during the initial phases of an acute attack, focusing on resting the affected joint
  - Use a bed cradle, if appropriate, to prevent irritation of and pressure on the affected area

- Administer prescribed drugs, including colchicine, within 24 hours of the onset of an acute attack
- Provide comfort measures and pain relief as needed
- If the patient can tolerate it, encourage liberal fluid intake
- Work with the patient to identify techniques and activities that promote rest and relaxation
- Provide dietary recommendations, review the patient's diet history for high-purine foods, help the patient select appropriate foods, and provide a low-purine diet
- Monitor the patient's serum uric acid levels and fluid balance, including intake and output
- Teach the patient and family about the disorder and its treatment, and provide support

Lower Back Pain

- Description
  - Lower back pain is pain that occurs in the lumbar region of the back
  - Lower back pain affects most of the population at some time
  - Most lower back pain is musculoskeletal; other common causes are degeneration and disk disease
  - Risk factors for lower back pain include obesity, poor body mechanics, lifting of heavy objects, and lack of exercise or physical activity
- Signs and symptoms
  - The patient reports lower back pain, which may radiate to one or both legs
  - Associated symptoms include impaired bladder and bowel function, paresthesia, and reduced motor function
- Diagnosis and treatment
  - Diagnosis is based on patient history, physical examination, and radiographic procedures, including X-rays, CT scan, MRI, myelogram, electromyogram, diskogram, and somatosensory evoked potentials
  - An NSAID and an analgesic are administered for pain, and muscle relaxants may be used to relieve muscle spasms
  - Epidural injections with a steroid may help decrease swelling and inflammation of spinal nerves
  - Short-term bed rest may be indicated initially
  - Physical therapy, ultrasound, heat or ice, whirlpool, and cognitive-behavioral therapy may be helpful
  - Surgical intervention may include discectomy, discotomy, laminectomy, and spinal fusion
- Preoperative nursing interventions
  - Help the patient achieve a comfortable position; elevate the head of the bed 30 degrees, and have the patient flex hips and knees slightly
  - Alternate the application of cold and heat, and administer an analgesic as indicated
  - Teach the patient the proper use of assistive devices
  - Demonstrate proper body mechanics to the patient
- Postoperative nursing interventions
  - Assess the patient's vital signs and level of pain; administer medications as ordered; teach the patient how to use patient-controlled analgesia if appropriate
  - Keep the head of the bed flat or elevated no more than 45 degrees for at least 24 hours after surgery; logroll the patient as indicated
  - Maintain activity restrictions
  - Assist the surgeon with the initial dressing change
  - Monitor the patient's intake and output
  - Assess the surgical wound and dressings; perform incision site care and dressing changes as appropriate
  - Monitor for drainage and bleeding
  - Monitor for cerebrospinal fluid leakage
  - Assess the patient's motor and neurologic function; compare the results with baseline findings

Osteoarthritis

- Description
  - Osteoarthritis is a noninflammatory joint disease characterized by degenerative changes in the articular cartilage; it primarily affects weight-bearing joints in the hips, knees, and vertebrae but may also affect the ankles, shoulders, wrists, fingers, and toes
  - Osteoarthritis affects more than 50 million American men and women, primarily those older than age 45
  - Osteoarthritis has been associated with aging, obesity, and wear and tear on the joints; however, a defective gene may account for many cases of idiopathic osteoarthritis

- Osteoarthritis may be *primary* (occurring with aging and possible genetic factors) or *secondary* (resulting from a joint injury, obesity, or a disease)
- Both types of osteoarthritis begin with the breakdown of the hyaline cartilage covering the ends of the bones on either side of the joint; the underlying bones become roughened, and bone cysts, fissures, or spurs develop on the bone surface; eventually, the joint space is lost as cartilage loss increases, and the joint ROM is progressively restricted
- Pain in the affected joints is caused by inflamed synovium, stretching of the joint capsule or ligaments, irritation of nerve endings in the periosteum, and muscle spasms
- Signs and symptoms
  - Joint stiffness and soreness may be accompanied by dull, aching pain that worsens with joint use and weightbearing; rest may relieve the pain
  - ROM is decreased, and crepitus may be felt with joint movement
  - Joints exhibit deformities, such as Heberden's nodes (bony outgrowths on the distal interphalangeal joints) and Bouchard's nodes (bony outgrowths on the proximal interphalangeal joints); the joints may also appear enlarged and edematous
  - Bone spurs may press on peripheral nerves, causing numbness or paralysis and hypoesthesia of the arms, forearms, hands, legs, and feet
  - Carpal tunnel syndrome and tarsal tunnel syndrome may result from pressure of bony growths on nerves
  - Gait analysis may show a discrepancy in leg length and joint alignments
- Diagnosis and treatment
  - Patient history, physical examination, X-rays, CT scan, MRI, arthrocentesis, arthrogram, and bone scan may be ordered; serologic studies, including complete blood count, erythrocyte sedimentation rate (ESR), creatinine level, mineral assays, and humoral tests for immunoglobulins, also may be performed
  - The patient may require support and stabilization of the joint, with a cane, crutches, a walker, braces, a cervical collar, or traction
  - Weight reduction is encouraged in an obese patient
  - Moist heat and paraffin dips are applied as needed; ice packs may also be used
  - Massage may be helpful
  - ROM exercises are performed for all joints, balancing rest with exercise
  - Properly fitted shoes are used to help maintain correct posture, decrease pressure on affected tissues, and increase ambulation
  - Medications such as salicylates, NSAIDs, acetaminophen, muscle relaxants, and intra-articular steroids may be prescribed to relieve soreness (systemic steroids aren't used to treat osteoarthritis because it isn't primarily an inflammatory disease)
  - Studies indicate that glucosamine and chondroitin may be useful in controlling symptoms and reducing functional impairment
  - Viscosupplementation—the injection of gellike substances into the affected joint—may be helpful
  - Surgery is considered when other treatments have failed; total or partial joint replacement, joint fusion (arthrodesis), or osteotomy may be performed
- Nursing interventions
  - Explain the proposed treatment regimen to the patient
  - Apply heat, cold, or other ordered treatments to the joint
  - Administer medications as prescribed
  - Consult a physical therapist about exercise and other treatments
  - Help the patient achieve a comfortable position, using pillows as needed, to promote rest
  - Teach the patient how to use an ambulatory aid; walkers, canes, and other aids decrease weight on the affected joints and help to minimize cartilage erosion; teach proper body mechanics to prevent injury
  - Encourage the patient to perform ADLs when possible to maintain muscle strength and joint ROM
  - Provide skin care to maintain skin integrity

Osteomyelitis

- Description
  - Osteomyelitis is an acute or a chronic infection of the bone or bone marrow that is hard to treat
    - The acute form may result from an infection in other tissues (hematogenic osteomyelitis) or from an open fracture with bacterial contamination

- ○ The chronic form may result from inadequate initial antimicrobial therapy or lack of response to treatment (relapse occurs when the patient's resistance is lowered)
  - The metaphyseal area in long bones is usually affected; the longer and larger the bone, the more susceptible it is to osteomyelitis; such bones include the femur, tibia, humerus, and vertebrae
  - Common pathogenic organisms are *Staphylococcus aureus* (which causes 90% of osteomyelitis), *Streptococcus pyogenes*, *Pseudomonas aeruginosa*, *Escherichia coli*, *Neisseria gonorrhoeae*, *Haemophilus influenzae*, and *Salmonella typhi*
  - Once the pathogens locate in the metaphysis, they grow and reproduce until they have formed a mass; leukocytes help wall off and localize the infection; bone cells in the area die, and purulent matter spreads along the bone, eventually penetrating through the tissues to the skin surface
- Signs and symptoms
  - The patient may complain of site pain and pressure; heat, edema, and tenderness may also be present
  - Associated systemic signs and symptoms include chills, fever, malaise, nausea, and tachycardia
  - The affected limb may be sore with use
  - An open, draining area may appear
- Diagnosis and treatment
  - Diagnosis may be based on patient history, bone scan, MRI, physical examination, X-rays of the involved bone, culture of the drainage, WBC count, and ESR
  - An antibiotic is administered I.V. in large doses after blood cultures are taken
  - Aspirin or acetaminophen is given to control fever and pain
  - Tetanus toxoid or antitoxin is given if the patient has an open wound
  - Hyperbaric oxygen treatments at twice the atmospheric pressure for 2 hours/day up to six times per week may be prescribed
  - After antibiotic therapy is completed, the bone is surgically scraped to clear away the dead bone and residue of infection
    - ○ Bone grafts may be used to aid bone healing and prevent fracture
    - ○ Tubes or catheters may be inserted to flush the site with an antibiotic to clear any residual organisms
    - ○ An external fixator may be placed above and below the osteomyelitic site to decrease the possibility of bone fracture
  - Surgery to drain infection may be necessary
  - Immobilization of the infected bone may be necessary using a cast, traction, or bed rest
- Nursing interventions
  - Monitor the type and amount of pain to determine the disease's status
  - Administer an antibiotic, an analgesic, or tetanus toxoid or antitoxin as prescribed
  - Administer I.V. fluids to maintain hydration
  - Perform neurovascular checks, and monitor vital signs
  - Use strict aseptic technique when required; the patient is more susceptible to additional infection or nosocomial infection
  - Help the patient achieve a comfortable position to relieve pressure on the affected tissues
  - Encourage the patient to perform ROM exercises for all unaffected tissues and joints to maintain strength
  - Teach the patient how to use an ambulatory aid (or arm sling)
  - Discuss concerns about the length and types of treatment
  - Provide and encourage diversionary activities to help the patient maintain a positive outlook

Osteoporosis

- Description
  - Osteoporosis is a systemic disease in which bone density and bone mass decrease because of a disturbance in the balance between bone resorption and bone deposition
  - Osteoporosis begins to develop after age 30 but progresses rapidly in postmenopausal women; 70% of women older than age 45 have osteoporosis
  - Causes of osteoporosis include menopausal decreases in estrogen, family history, immobility, insufficient intake of calcium and vitamin D, alcohol use, smoking, corticosteroid use, and caffeine intake
  - Patients with osteoporosis are susceptible to fractures (particularly of the femur, radius, and ulna) and compression or crush injuries of the vertebrae

- Signs and symptoms
  - Sometimes called a " silent disease" because the first sign may be a fracture
  - Pain may affect the lower back or thoracic spinal area
  - A loss of height may occur
  - Kyphosis, or dowager's hump, may be present
  - A minor twist or turn can cause a sudden fracture
  - Numbness or tingling in arms or legs may occur
- Diagnosis and treatment
  - Diagnosis is based on bone mineral density (BMD) testing, which results in a T-score for patients
  - Diagnosis may be based on patient history, physical examination, dual photon absorptiometry, and CT scans
  - Calcium intake is increased to 1,500 mg daily
  - Estrogen and progesterone are prescribed to restore hormonal balance
  - Calcitonin and bisphosphonates (etidronate and pamidronate) are prescribed to prevent bone resorption; alendronate, ibandronate, raloxifene, and risedronate are also used to treat osteoporosis
  - Back or neck supports are used to prevent stress fractures
  - Active exercises are encouraged to help retain calcium in the bones
- Nursing interventions
  - Monitor the amount and type of pain to determine its extent
  - Give an analgesic as prescribed to relieve pain and promote mobility
  - Teach the patient how to use an ambulatory aid to maintain mobility, and apply a neck or back support, if ordered
  - Teach the patient about dietary sources of calcium and calcium supplements; increased calcium intake decreases the risk of fractures
  - Refer the patient to a practitioner for possible estrogen replacement therapy (controversial)
  - Discuss methods of dressing to camouflage kyphosis
  - Discuss how to ensure a safe home environment to decrease the risk of falls, for example, by removing loose rugs and avoiding long, uncovered electrical cords
  - Encourage the patient to participate in active, weight-bearing exercises, such as walking and swimming, to maintain calcium in bones and preserve muscle strength
  - Encourage the patient to modify lifestyle choices by avoiding smoking, alcohol, caffeine, and carbonated beverages and increasing protein intake

Rhabdomyolysis

- Description
  - Rhabdomyolysis is the breakdown of muscle tissue and may cause myoglobinuria
  - Muscle tissue breakdown usually follows muscle trauma, especially a crush injury or lightening strike
  - The disorder may lead to renal failure if not treated
  - Causes of rhabdomyolysis, besides trauma, are excessive muscle activity (such as status epilepticus or severe dystonia), familial tendency, infection, medications (such as antihistamines, salicylates, fibric acid derivatives, HMG-CoA reductase inhibitors, neuroleptics, anesthetics, paralytic agents, corticosteroids, tricyclic antidepressants, and selective serotonin reuptake inhibitors), and sporadic strenuous exertion (e.g., running in a marathon)
- Signs and symptoms
  - Tenderness, swelling, and muscle weakness result from muscle trauma and pressure
  - Dark, reddish brown urine is caused by myoglobin release
- Diagnosis and treatment
  - Diagnosis is based on patient history that reveals myalgias or muscle pain; physical examination; elevated levels of serum myoglobin, creatine kinase, serum potassium, phosphate, and creatinine; and CT scan, MRI, and bone scintigraphy, which detect muscle necrosis
  - Treatment should focus on the underlying cause
  - I.V. crystalloids may be given to increase intravascular volume and glomerular filtration rate
  - Diuretics may be given
  - Dialysis may be required
  - Analgesics may be given for pain

- If compartment syndrome develops and venous pressure is greater than 25 mm Hg, immediate fasciotomy and debridement may be needed to relieve pressure and prevent tissue death
- Urine alkalinization and osmotic or loop diuretics may be implemented to prevent renal failure
- Nursing interventions
  - Administer I.V. fluids and diuretics to reduce nephrotoxicity
  - Monitor intake and output
  - Recommend exercise modification to prevent recurrence of rhadomyolysis

Tumors, Bone

- Description
  - Neoplasms of the musculoskeletal system are of various types, including osteogenic, chondrogenic, fibrogenic, and bone marrow cell tumors
  - Bone tumors may be primary or metastatic from primary cancers elsewhere in the body; metastatic bone tumors occur more commonly than primary bone tumors
  - Benign bone tumors include osteochondromas, bone cysts, osteoid osteomas, and fibromas; benign tumors are slow growing and encapsulated, present few signs and symptoms, and are rarely associated with mortality
  - Giant cell tumors may begin as benign tumors and remain that way for long periods; they have the potential to eventually become malignant
  - Primary malignant bone tumors are relatively rare; several types exist, including sarcomas (such as osteogenic sarcoma, chondrosarcoma, and fibrosarcoma), Ewing's sarcoma, and chordoma (see *Types of Primary Malignant Bone Tumors*, page 192)
  - Primary malignant bone tumors can be osseous (arising from the bony structure itself) or nonosseous (arising from hematopoietic, vascular, and neural tissues)
  - Osseous bone tumors include osteogenic sarcoma (most common), parosteal osteogenic sarcoma, chondrosarcoma (chondroblastic), and malignant giant cell tumor
  - Nonosseous bone tumors include Ewing's sarcoma, fibrosarcoma (fibroblastic), and chordoma
  - The exact causes of bone tumors are unknown, but they may be related to exposure to carcinogens, hereditary factors, and trauma
  - Bone cancers affect males and females equally; they occur more commonly in children and adolescents, although some types do occur in patients ages 35 to 60 years
  - The most common sites for tumors are the femur, tibia, and humerus
- Signs and symptoms
  - General symptoms include persistent, localized dull bone pain on weightbearing and at rest, unexplained weight loss, impaired mobility, and a history of pathologic fracture
  - Physical findings include swelling and tenderness at the affected site, a palpable bony or soft tissue mass, and an abnormal gait
- Diagnosis and treatment
  - Bone X-rays, radioisotope bone and computed tomography (CT) scans, and magnetic resonance imaging (MRI) all aid in diagnosis
  - Incision or aspiration biopsy confirms primary malignancy
  - Treatment depends on the type of tumor
- Nursing interventions
  - Encourage communication, and help the patient set realistic goals
  - Give prescribed I.V. infusions and medications; administer antinausea agents to minimize nausea
  - Provide small, frequent meals
  - Provide comfort measures to facilitate the administration of chemotherapy as indicated
  - Prepare the patient and family for possible surgery, including limb salvage and associated care
  - Offer support to the patient and family about the condition and effects of treatment, such as loss of part of a limb
  - Obtain blood specimens as ordered to evaluate for bone marrow suppression secondary to chemotherapy
  - Monitor vital signs and the neurovascular status of the affected extremity
  - Teach the patient and family about the disorder, diagnosis, prognosis, and treatment, including the need for surgery and possible follow-up chemotherapy
  - Teach about the use of assistive devices or prostheses and modifications, as needed
  - Provide support and encouragement, and refer the patient and family to support services as needed (Box 11-5)

Box 11-5: Types of Primary Malignant Bone Tumors

The chart below lists primary malignant bone tumors of both osseous and nonosseous origin, including their clinical features and treatment.

Type	Clinical features	Treatment
Osseous origin		
Chondrosarcoma	• Develops from cartilage • Dull pain; grows slowly but is locally recurrent and invasive • Occurs most commonly in pelvis, proximal femur, ribs, and shoulder girdle • Usually occurs in middle-age and older people, more common in males	• Hemipelvectomy, surgical resection (ribs) • Radiation (palliative) • Chemotherapy
Malignant giant cell tumor	• Arises from benign giant cell tumor • Found most commonly in long bones, especially in the knee area • Usually occurs in people ages 18 to 50	• Curettage • Total excision • Radiation for recurrent disease
Osteogenic sarcoma	• Osteoid tumor present in bone specimen • Tumor arises from bone-forming osteoblast and bone-digesting osteoclast. • Occurs most commonly in femur, but also in tibia and humerus; occasionally, in fibula, ileum, vertebra, or mandible • Acute pain and swelling and metastasizes quickly can result in death. • Usually occurs in teens and young adults in their 20s and occurs in males more than females	• Surgery (tumor resection, high thigh amputation, hemipelvectomy, interscapulothoracic surgery) • Chemotherapy
Parosteal osteogenic sarcoma	• Develops on surface of bone instead of interior • Progresses slowly • Occurs most commonly in distal femur, but also in tibia, humerus, and ulna • Usually occurs in people ages 30 to 40	• Surgery (tumor resection, possible amputation, interscapulothoracic surgery, hemipelvectomy) • Chemotherapy • Combination of the above
Nonosseous origin		
Chordoma	• Derived from embryonic remnants of notochord • Progresses slowly • Usually found at end of spinal column and in sphenooccipital, sacrococcygeal, and vertebral areas • Characterized by constipation and visual disturbances • Complicated tumors and they may reoccur after treatment and often show up in the original tumor spot • Usually occurs in people ages 50 to 60	• Surgical resection (often resulting in neural defects) • Radiation (palliative, or when surgery not applicable, as in occipital area)
Ewing's sarcoma	• Originates in bone marrow and invades shafts of long and flat bones • Usually affects lower extremities, most commonly femur, innominate bones, ribs, tibia, humerus, vertebra, and fibula; may metastasize to lungs • Pain increasingly severe and persistent • Usually occurs in children, teens, and young adults in their early 20s • Has a poor prognosis	• High-voltage radiation (tumor is radiosensitive) • Chemotherapy to slow growth • Amputation only if there's no evidence of metastasis
Fibrosarcoma	• Relatively rare • Originates in fibrous tissue of bone • Invades long or flat bones (femur, tibia, mandible) but also involves periosteum and overlying muscle • Nonspecific symptoms are gradual. Local tenderness with a mass sometimes palpable • Usually occurs in people ages 30 to 40	• Amputation • Radiation • Chemotherapy • Bone grafts (with low-grade fibrosarcoma)

Review Questions

Question 1. A patient in balanced suspension traction for a fractured femur needs to be repositioned toward the head of the bed. During repositioning, the nurse should:

A. maintain the same degree of traction tension.
B. place slight additional tension on the traction cord.
C. lift the traction and the patient during repositioning.
D. release the weights, and replace them immediately after positioning.

Correct answer: A Traction is used to reduce the fracture and must be maintained at all times, including during repositioning. Options B, C, and D are incorrect because it isn't appropriate to increase traction tension or release or lift the traction during repositioning.

Question 2. A patient undergoes cast placement for a fractured left radius. The nurse should suspect compartment syndrome if the patient experiences pain that:

A. radiates up the arm to the left scapula.
B. intensifies with the elevation of the left arm.
C. disappears with the flexion of the left arm.
D. increases with the arm in a dependent position.

Correct answer: B Pain is the most common symptom of compartment syndrome. Because the pain is the result of ischemia, elevating the limb reduces circulation, worsens the ischemia, and intensifies the pain. Options C and D are incorrect because these positions don't alter the pain of compartment syndrome. Option A is incorrect because the pain of compartment syndrome doesn't radiate up the arm to the scapula.

Question 3. A patient received a right hip prosthesis after a fall. In the immediate postoperative period, the nurse should:

A. maintain the leg in an adducted position.
B. maintain the leg in an abducted position.
C. maintain the leg in a neutral position.
D. maintain the leg with the hip flexed greater than 90 degrees.

Correct answer: B After receiving a hip prosthesis, the affected leg should be kept abducted. Adduction (Option A) may dislocate the hip. Option C would be correct if an internal fixation device was used. Option D is incorrect because the hip must not be flexed more than 90 degrees for the first 2 months and even less than that for the first 10 days.

Question 4. A 78-year-old patient has a history of osteoarthritis. Which signs and symptoms would the nurse document when performing a physical assessment?

A. Joint pain, crepitus, Heberden's nodes
B. Hot, inflamed joints; crepitus; joint pain
C. Tophi, enlarged joints, Bouchard's nodes
D. Swelling, joint pain, tenderness on palpation

Correct answer: A Signs and symptoms of osteoarthritis include joint pain, crepitus, Heberden's nodes, Bouchard's nodes, and enlarged joints. Joint pain occurs with movement and is relieved by rest. As the disease progresses, pain may also occur at rest. Heberden's nodes are bony growths that occur at the distal interphalangeal joints. Bouchard's nodes involve the proximal interphalangeal joints. Hot, inflamed joints (Option B) rarely occur with osteoarthritis. Tophi (Option C) are deposits of sodium urate crystals that occur with chronic gout, not osteoarthritis. Swelling, joint pain, and tenderness on palpation (Option D) occur with a sprain injury.

Question 5. The nurse is caring for an elderly female patient who has osteoporosis. When educating the patient, the nurse should include information about which major complication?

A. Bone fracture
B. Loss of estrogen
C. Scoliosis
D. Negative calcium balance

Correct answer: A Bone fracture is a major complication of osteoporosis that results when loss of calcium and phosphate increases the fragility of bones. Option B is incorrect because estrogen deficiencies result from menopause, not osteoporosis. Option D is wrong because calcium and vitamin D supplements may be used to support normal bone metabolism, but a negative calcium balance isn't a complication of osteoporosis. Option C is incorrect because, although the cause of scoliosis is unknown, it's not thought to be a complication of osteoporosis.

Question 6. The nurse would expect which of the following treatments to be ordered in the conservative treatment of a herniated nucleus?

A. Surgery
B. Spinal fusion
C. Bed rest, pain medication, and physiotherapy
D. Strenuous exercise, pain medication, and physiotherapy

Correct answer: C Conservative treatment of a herniated nucleus pulposus may include bed rest, pain medication, and physiotherapy. Aggressive, not conservative, treatment may include surgery (Option A), including spinal fusion (Option B). A regimen of strenuous exercise, pain medication, and physiotherapy (Option D) isn't recommended.

Question 7. A nurse is performing a physical assessment. Which areas will the nurse include in a neurovascular documentation?

A. Orientation, movement, pulses, and warmth
B. Capillary refill time, movement, pulses, and warmth
C. Orientation, pupillary response, temperature, and pulses
D. Respiratory pattern, orientation, pulses, and temperature

Correct answer: B A correct neurovascular assessment should include capillary refill time, movement, pulses, and warmth. Neurovascular assessment involves nerve and blood supply to an area. Orientation, pupillary response, temperature, and respiratory pattern (Options A, C, and D) aren't part of a neurovascular examination.

Question 8. A nurse is caring for a patient with a fracture. Which of the following findings should the nurse include in the documentation?

A. Tingling, coolness, and loss of pulses
B. Loss of sensation, redness, and coolness
C. Coolness, redness, and a new pain site
D. Discoloration, deformity, and pain at the site of injury

Correct answer: D Signs of a fracture may include discoloration, deformity, and pain at the site of injury.

Tingling, coolness (included in Options A, B, and C), and loss of pulses are signs of a vascular problem.

Question 9. The nurse expects which of the following diagnostic tests will be ordered in order to evaluate the presence of rhabdomyolysis?

A. Serum troponin
B. Bone biopsy
C. Serum myoglobin
D. Glycosylated hemoglobin serum

Correct answer: C A positive serum or urine myoglobin test indicates rhabdomyolysis. A glycosylated hemoglobin test (Option D) measures the amount of glycosylated hemoglobin in the blood and is used to monitor blood sugar. Serum troponin (Option A) is used to detect acute coronary syndrome. A bone biopsy (Option B) would be used to diagnose osteoporosis.

Question 10. The nurse knows which of the following may be a complication in a diabetic patient who has been placed in skeletal traction after a motor vehicle collision?

A. Osteoarthritis
B. Osteomyelitis
C. Osteoporosis
D. Osteosarcoma

Correct answer: B This patient has a significant risk of developing osteomyelitis secondary to the skeletal pin. Osteoarthritis (Option A) is a degenerative joint disease, osteoporosis (Option C) is a metabolic bone disorder, and osteosarcoma (Option D) is an aggressive form of bone cancer; none occur secondary to skeletal traction.

Selected References

American Academy of Orthopaedic Surgeons (AAOS). (2016). Biceps tendinitis. Retrieved from http://orthoinfo.aaos.org/topic.cfm?topic=a00026

Chordoma Foundation. (2017). Understanding chordoma. Retrieved from https://www.chordomafoundation.org/understanding-chordoma/

Ignatavicius, D, & Workman, L. (2016). *Medical-surgical nursing: Patient-centered collaborative care* (8th ed.). St. Louis, MO: Elsevier.

Jarvis, C. (2012). *Physical examination and health assessment* (6th ed.). St. Louis, MO: Elsevier.

Mayo Clinic. (2017). Knee bursitis. Retrieved from http://www.mayoclinic.org/diseases-conditions/knee-bursitis/symptoms-causes/dxc-20316555

Potter, P., Perry, A., Stokert, P., & Hall, A. (2017). *Fundamentals of nursing* (9th ed.). St. Louis, MO: Elsevier.

Chapter 12

Gastrointestinal Disorders

Introduction

- The gastrointestinal (GI), or digestive, system breaks down food and prepares it for absorption by the body's cells; nonabsorbable ingested substances pass through the system and are eliminated as solid waste
- Although not part of the alimentary canal, the liver, gallbladder, and pancreas are essential accessory components of the GI system

Nursing History

- The nurse asks the patient about the *chief complaint*
  - The patient with a GI problem may report a change in appetite, heartburn, nausea, pain, or vomiting
  - The patient may also report a change in bowel habits, such as constipation, diarrhea, or stool characteristics
- The nurse then asks the patient about the history of the *present illness*
  - Ask the patient about symptoms, including when it started, associated symptoms, location, radiation, intensity, duration, frequency, and precipitating and alleviating factors
  - Ask about the use of prescription and over-the-counter drugs, herbal remedies, and vitamin and nutritional supplements; ask about the use of laxatives
  - If the patient's chief complaint is diarrhea, inquire about recent travel abroad
  - Ask the patient about changes in appetite and in bowel habits (e.g., a change in the amount, appearance, or color of stool or the appearance of blood in it) and difficulty eating or chewing
- The nurse asks about *medical history*
  - Question the patient about other GI disorders, such as gallbladder disease, GI bleeding, inflammatory bowel disease, or ulcers
  - Also, ask about previous abdominal surgery or trauma
- The nurse then assesses the *family history*
  - Ask about a family history of diseases with a hereditary link, such as alcoholism, colon cancer, Crohn's disease, stomach ulcers, and ulcerative colitis
  - Also, question the patient about a family history of chronic diseases
- The nurse obtains a *social history*
  - Ask about work, exercise, diet, use of recreational drugs and alcohol, caffeine intake, and hobbies
  - Assess stress, support systems, and coping mechanisms
- Physical assessment
  - When assessing the abdomen, use this sequence: inspection, auscultation, percussion, and palpation; palpating or percussing the abdomen before you auscultate can change the character of the patient's bowel sounds and lead to an inaccurate assessment
  - The nurse begins with *inspection*
    - Observe the patient's general appearance, and note behavior
    - Inspect the skin for turgor, color, and texture; note abnormalities such as bruising, decreased axillary or pubic hair, edema, petechiae, scars, spider angiomas, and stretch marks
    - Observe the patient's head for color of the sclerae, sunken eyes, dentures, caries, lesions, breath odor, and tongue color, swelling, or dryness

- ○ Check the size and shape of the abdomen, noting distention, peristalsis, pulsations, contour, visible masses, and protrusions
- ○ Observe the rectal area for abnormalities
- The nurse continues by using *auscultation*
  - ○ Note the character and quality of bowel sounds in each quadrant
  - ○ Auscultate the abdomen for vascular sounds
- Then, the nurse *percusses* the abdomen
  - ○ Percuss the abdomen to detect the size and location of the abdominal organs
  - ○ Note the presence of air or fluid
- Next, the nurse uses *palpation*
  - ○ Palpate the abdomen to determine the size, shape, position, and tenderness of major abdominal organs and to detect masses and fluid accumulation
  - ○ Note abdominal muscle tone and tenderness
  - ○ Palpate the rectum, noting any abnormalities

Appendicitis

- Description
  - Appendicitis is an inflammation of the vermiform appendix; it results when mucosal ulceration triggers inflammation, which temporarily obstructs the appendix
  - In this disorder, bacteria multiply and inflammation and pressure increase, restricting blood flow and causing thrombus and abdominal pain
  - Causes include fecal mass (fecalith), foreign body obstruction, barium ingestion, neoplasm, stricture, and infection
  - Appendicitis is the most common major abdominal surgical disease; over a quarter million appendectomies are performed in the United States annually
  - If left untreated, it can be fatal; gangrene and perforation can develop within 36 hours with resulting peritonitis and sepsis
- Signs and symptoms
  - Appendicitis causes abdominal periumbilical pain that's initially generalized and then localizes in the right lower abdomen (McBurney's point)
  - The patient feels right lower quadrant and rebound tenderness and may continually adjust posture to relieve pain and exhibit guarding
  - The patient may display the Rovsing sign (pain in the right lower quadrant that occurs with palpation of left lower quadrant), psoas sign (abdominal pain that occurs when flexing the hip when pressure is applied to the knee), or obturator sign (abdominal pain that occurs when the hip is rotated)
  - A patient with a retrocele or pelvic appendix may not have abdominal or flank tenderness
  - Other signs and symptoms include anorexia, nausea, and vomiting, low-grade fever, and tachycardia
- Diagnosis and treatment
  - White blood cell (WBC) count may be elevated, with an increase in immature cells
  - Ultrasonography, magnetic resonance imaging (MRI), or CT of the abdomen can help diagnose a nonperforated appendix
  - Appendectomy is only effective treatment
- Nursing interventions
  - Place the patient in Fowler's position to minimize pain
  - Before surgery, administer analgesics judiciously because they may mask pain or perforation
  - Prepare the patient for appendectomy; initiate nothing-by-mouth status and establish I.V. access; administer I.V. fluids to prevent dehydration
  - After appendectomy, watch for surgical complications, including wound infection, intestinal obstruction, peritonitis, and abdominal abscess
  - Administer pain medication as needed
  - If the patient has developed peritonitis, administer antibiotics and maintain a nasogastric (NG) tube
  - Monitor the patient's vital signs closely
  - Increase the patient's activity and advance diet as tolerated

Cancer, Colorectal

- Description
  - Colorectal cancer is caused by a malignant tumor of the colon or rectum; it's the third most common site of new cancer diagnoses and the second leading cause of cancer-related deaths in both men and women
  - It almost always involves adenocarcinomas; about half are sessile lesions of rectosigmoid area; all others are polypoid lesions that begin as benign polyps and progress to malignancy
  - Tumors in the sigmoid and descending colon undergo circumferential growth and constrict the intestinal lumen
  - Tumors in the ascending colon are usually large at diagnosis and are palpable on physical examination
  - The disease progresses slowly; it has a better prognosis if it's detected early, before nodal involvement
  - Although the causes of colorectal cancer are unknown, risk factors include excessive intake of saturated fat; a history of ulcerative colitis, polyps, or inflammatory bowel disease; a family history of colon cancer; a low-fiber diet; and alcohol or tobacco use; those over age 50; diabetic patients have a higher risk
  - Being overweight or obese, especially with a larger waistline, increases the risk of colorectal cancer for all, but more so in males
  - Physical activity decreases the risk of colorectal cancer
  - Complications include partial or complete bowel obstruction and extension of the tumor into surrounding blood vessels, resulting in hemorrhage; perforation, abscess formation, peritonitis, sepsis, and death may occur
- Signs and symptoms
  - Signs and symptoms depend on the location of the tumor and the extent of the disease; they often don't develop until cancer is at an advanced stage
  - Early-stage right colon tumors typically don't cause signs and symptoms because stool is liquid in the right part of the colon
  - Left colon tumors cause abdominal pain, cramping, narrowed stools, constipation, and bright red blood in stools
  - The most common sign is a change in bowel habits, with passage of blood in the stool; black, tarry stools; cramping; straining; diarrhea; and constipation
  - Other signs and symptoms include unexplained anemia, fatigue, weight loss, and dull abdominal pain
  - The patient may have abdominal distention or visible or palpable masses as well as abdominal tenderness
  - Unintentional weight loss is common
- Diagnosis and treatment
  - Digital rectal examination can be used to detect suspicious rectal and perianal lesions but is no longer a stand-alone test as it only addresses the most distal colon and rectum
  - A fecal occult blood test completed on normally eliminated stool may be positive
  - Iron deficiency anemia may be present
  - Colonoscopy and biopsy confirm the diagnosis
  - A CT scan allows for staging; transrectal ultrasonography determines the extent of rectal lesions
  - Surgery is the primary treatment
    - ○ Resection or right hemicolectomy is the treatment for advanced disease; surgery may include resection of the terminal segment of the ileum, cecum, ascending colon, and right half of the transverse colon with corresponding mesentery
    - ○ Right colectomy includes the transverse colon and mesentery corresponding to midcolic vessels, or segmental resection of the transverse colon and associated midcolic vessels
    - ○ Abdominoperineal resection and permanent sigmoid colostomy may be performed
  - Chemotherapy and radiation therapy may also be used
- Nursing interventions
  - Provide physical and emotional support; allow the patient to verbalize feelings about diagnosis, condition, and discuss appropriate coping strategies
  - Give prescribed drugs, laxatives, enemas, and antibiotics preoperatively, as ordered
  - Prepare the patient for surgery; ensure patent I.V. access and administer I.V. fluids
  - After surgery, provide appropriate postoperative care
  - Monitor the patient's vital signs and fluid and electrolyte balance; be alert for signs of a leaking anastomosis, including fever and abdominal pain

- Advance the patient's diet as indicated, and provide adequate nutrition
- Before discharge, help the patient modify diet; encourage to avoid irritating foods, caffeine, and alcohol
- Teach the patient and family about the disorder, treatment, and follow-up care

Cancer, Esophageal

- Description
  - Two main types of esophageal cancer exist: adenocarcinoma and squamous cell carcinoma. Rarely, other types of carcinoma may start in the esophagus
  - Risk factors include chronic esophageal irritation such as occurs with gastroesophageal reflux disease (GERD), alcohol and tobacco use, chronic ingestion of hot liquids, and nutritional deficiencies
  - Cancer of the esophagus occurs more often in men than in women and more often in blacks than in whites; the incidence is much higher in other parts of the world, especially China and the Middle East
  - Tumors can spread through the esophageal mucosa and extend into the lymphatics, with possible mediastinal perforation and erosion of the great vessels
- Signs and symptoms
  - Esophageal obstruction causes dysphagia, initially with solid foods and eventually with liquids
  - Throat discomfort is common, along with a feeling of substernal pain or fullness, regurgitation of ingested food, and hiccups
  - Weight loss, vomiting, hiccoughs, chronic cough, and recurrent pneumonia may present
- Diagnosis and treatment
  - Endoscopy and biopsy confirm the diagnosis; CT and positron emission tomography (PET) scans help identify invasive disease and metastases
  - Treatment depends on the stage of disease at diagnosis; in early diagnosis, treatment aims to cure the disease; treatment in later stages is mainly palliative
  - Treatment options include combinations of surgery, chemotherapy, and radiation
  - Resection of the esophagus is possible, with a jejunal graft placed to provide esophageal continuity; a possible complication of this surgery is a leaking anastomosis
  - Palliative treatment seeks to keep the esophagus open through dilation, stent placement, and radiation or chemotherapy
- Nursing interventions
  - Preoperatively, optimize nutritional status, providing enteral or parenteral nutrition if necessary
  - Postoperative care is similar to other thoracic surgeries; place the patient in low Fowler's position to minimize gastric reflux and monitor for signs of aspiration
  - Monitor vital signs and cardiac rhythm; atrial fibrillation can occur due to the proximity of the heart and great vessels to the surgical area; administer antiarrhythmics as ordered
  - An NG tube may remain in place for several days; the nurse will maintain its patency and provide skin care and comfort measures
  - Advance diet and activity as indicated; provide adequate nutrition for wound healing
  - Educate the patient and family about the disease and treatment, and provide emotional support

Cancer, Gastric

- Description
  - Most gastric cancers are adenocarcinomas that can occur anywhere in the stomach; at the time of diagnosis, the tumor has usually infiltrated the surrounding mucosa and penetrated the wall of the stomach and adjacent organs and structures
  - The consumption of smoked, salted, and pickled foods seems to have an association with the development of gastric cancer
  - Other risk factors include chronic inflammation of the stomach, *Helicobacter pylori* infection and gastric ulcers, smoking, obesity, achlorhydria, and genetics
  - Most cases are discovered late in the disease process, resulting in a poor prognosis
  - Patients are usually diagnosed in their late 60s to 80s, but a noted increase starts at age 50; men have a higher incidence than women
  - Stomach cancer is most prevalent in most of Asia, Southern and Eastern Europe, and Central to South America. It is less common in Northern and Western Africa, South Central Asia, and North America

- Signs and symptoms
  - Early symptoms are nonspecific and include pain relieved by antacids
  - Symptoms of progressive disease include dyspepsia, a constant feeling of fullness, bloating after meals, weight loss, anorexia, nausea and vomiting, and abdominal pain
  - Ascites and hepatomegaly can be seen in advanced disease
  - Anemia is common
- Diagnosis and treatment
  - Endoscopy and biopsy confirm the diagnosis; barium studies, X-rays, and CT scans can further evaluate the extent of the tumor
  - Surgical excision is the treatment of choice for well-localized tumors; in more advanced disease, excision of the tumor may be palliative and relieve obstruction
  - Partial or total gastric resections can be performed; with a total gastrectomy, the GI tract is reconstructed by anastomosing the end of the jejunum to the end of the esophagus
  - Chemotherapy may follow surgical treatment
- Nursing interventions
  - Provide physical and emotional support; allow the patient to verbalize feelings about the condition, and discuss appropriate coping strategies
  - Give prescribed drugs, such as antacids, proton pump inhibitors and histamine-2 receptor antagonists
  - Prepare the patient for surgery; ensure patent I.V. access and administer I.V. fluids
  - After surgery, provide appropriate postoperative care
  - Monitor vital signs and fluid and electrolyte balance; be alert for signs of a leaking anastomosis, including fever and abdominal pain
  - Advance diet as indicated; be alert for signs of dumping syndrome and adjust diet to reduce these signs
  - Before discharge, help the patient modify diet; encourage avoidance of irritating foods, caffeine, and alcohol
  - Teach the patient and family about the disorder, treatment, and follow-up care

Cholecystitis

- Description
  - Cholecystitis is an acute or a chronic inflammation of the gallbladder; it's commonly associated with cholelithiasis (presence of gallstones)
  - In most cases, cholecystitis is caused by gallstones; bacterial infection plays a minor role in acute cholecystitis; secondary, bacterial infection occurs in approximately 50% of cases
- Signs and symptoms
  - Sharp abdominal pain may affect the right upper quadrant of the abdomen, especially after ingestion of fatty foods, and may be referred to the right shoulder area
  - Other GI effects include abdominal tenderness and muscle rigidity on palpation, eructation, flatulence, nausea, and vomiting
  - Fever may result from acute infection
  - Positive Murphy's sign (painful inspiration due to severe tenderness) may be present
  - Jaundice may occur if gallstones obstruct the common bile duct
- Diagnosis and treatment
  - Diagnosis is based on ultrasonography of the upper abdomen and oral cholecystography that shows an enlarged gallbladder and gallstones; cholecystitis with no stones may require cholescintigraphy
  - Percutaneous transhepatic cholangiography supports the diagnosis of obstructive jaundice and reveals calculi in the ducts
  - Levels of serum alkaline phosphate, lactate dehydrogenase, aspartate aminotransferase, cholesterol, and total bilirubin are elevated
  - The patient is placed on a low-fat diet
  - An anticholinergic, such as propantheline or dicyclomine (Bentyl), is given to decrease spasms of the common bile duct
  - An analgesic is prescribed for pain
  - An antibiotic may be given to prevent or treat infection
  - Chenodeoxycholic acid (Chenodal) or ursodeoxycholic acid (Actigall) may be administered to dissolve gallstones; it must be taken for 6 to 12 months to be effective
  - If pain persists, the gallbladder and gallstones are surgically removed by means of laparoscopic microsurgery or abdominal laparotomy; lithotripsy may also be performed to break up gallstones using ultrasonic waves

- Preoperative nursing interventions
  - Monitor the patient for abdominal pain in the right upper quadrant that may radiate to the right shoulder
  - Check the skin and conjunctivae for jaundice
- Postoperative nursing interventions
  - Monitor vital signs every 1 to 2 hours for 4 to 8 hours and then every 4 hours to detect fluid imbalances, hemorrhage, or shock
  - Monitor bowel sounds every 4 hours and bowel output to determine return of GI functions
  - Check the wound area for signs of bleeding and inflammation
  - Change the wound dressing as needed; the wound may be left uncovered if no drainage is present
  - Monitor drainage from the T tube, if present; a T tube is used if gallstones were in the common bile duct because it lets bile pass into the small intestine and decreases duct inflammation
  - Administer an opioid analgesic every 4 hours as needed and I.V. antibiotics every 6 to 8 hours as prescribed to maintain comfort and prevent infection
  - Make sure the patient maintains nothing-by-mouth status as prescribed, administer I.V. fluids (up to 3,000 mL daily) to maintain fluid balance, and also monitor fluid intake and output every 8 hours
  - Start giving the patient clear liquids and then progress to a regular diet as prescribed; fat restrictions may be lifted because gallbladder removal increases the patient's tolerance to fatty foods
  - Help the patient sit on the bed or in a chair and ambulate as prescribed to promote recovery from the surgery
  - Record pertinent data in the patient's chart for continuity of care

Cirrhosis of the Liver

- Description
  - Cirrhosis is a chronic, progressive disease that causes extensive degeneration and destruction of parenchymal liver cells; it's twice as common in men as in women, and most patients are between ages 40 and 60
  - Common types of cirrhosis include *micronodular* (Laënnec's), which is caused by excessive alcohol intake; *macronodular* (postnecrotic, toxin-induced), which is caused by chemicals, bacteria, and viruses; *biliary*, which is caused by irritating biliary products; *pigment*, which is caused by hemochromatosis; and *cardiac*, which is caused by right-sided heart failure and chronic liver disease
- Signs and symptoms
  - GI effects include anorexia, constipation or diarrhea, dull abdominal pain and heaviness, marked flatulence, nausea, vomiting, and weight loss
  - The liver may be enlarged and have nodules; jaundice and hepatic encephalopathy may occur
  - Hematologic effects may include anemia and thrombocytopenia
  - Fever and malaise may be present
  - Ascites, esophageal varices, and peripheral edema may occur
  - Skin lesions may include petechiae, purpura, and spider angiomas; dry skin and pruritus also may occur
  - Asterixis (liver flap, a hand-flapping tremor commonly seen in patients with hepatic coma), lethargy, mental changes, slurred speech, and peripheral neuropathies may occur
  - Endocrine effects may include gynecomastia and impotence in men and amenorrhea in women
- Diagnosis and treatment
  - Diagnosis is based on patient history (especially excessive alcohol intake or hepatitis), physical examination, liver biopsy and liver function studies, ultrasonography, CT scan, MRI, and serologic studies, including complete blood count (CBC), serum electrolyte levels, and prothrombin time (PT)
  - Paracentesis may be used to remove ascitic fluid
  - For intractable chronic ascites, a peritoneovenous shunt may be inserted to transfer ascitic fluid into the venous system for eventual excretion in the urine
  - A potassium-sparing diuretic is used to decrease ascites and peripheral edema
  - An antiemetic is used to reduce nausea and vomiting
  - Vitamin K is used to reduce bleeding tendencies stemming from hypothrombinemia
  - Lactulose is used to treat hepatic encephalopathy; lactulose decreases the pH of the colon, which inhibits the diffusion of ammonia from the colon into the blood
  - Bleeding esophageal varices are treated by administering vasopressin and a beta adrenergic blocker, performing endoscopic sclerosis, and inserting a Sengstaken-Blakemore tube or various surgical shunts (such as a portacaval shunt)

- Blood transfusions may be required for massive hemorrhage; I.V. therapy using colloid volume expanders or crystalloids may be given for volume expansion
  - The recommended diet is typically high in calories and has moderate- to high-protein, moderate- to low-fat, and low-sodium content; fluids are restricted; protein is restricted if encephalopathy develops
- Nursing interventions
  - Make sure the patient maintains bed rest; reposition him every 2 hours to help keep the skin intact and prevent pressure ulcers
  - Encourage active range-of-motion exercises, and use special mattresses to relieve pressure
  - Encourage deep breathing, and listen for breath sounds in all lung lobes
  - Observe closely for changes in behavior or personality, such as stupor, lethargy, hallucinations, or neuromuscular dysfunction
  - Administer an antiemetic as prescribed to control nausea and vomiting
  - Administer a diuretic as prescribed; weigh the patient daily, and measure fluid intake and output; note signs of hypokalemia
  - Measure abdominal girth and note changes
  - Check the patient's level of consciousness, neurologic status, and vital signs to detect encephalopathy or developing infection
  - Monitor the patient for bleeding by checking vomitus and stool for blood; apply pressure to injection sites to prevent bleeding
  - Monitor the results of laboratory tests and other studies; report abnormal findings to the practitioner
  - Consult the dietitian regarding a low-sodium, fluid-restricted diet; provide four to six small meals daily, including foods that the patient likes, when possible
  - Perform oral hygiene before meals and as needed to prevent stomatitis and remove characteristic fetid or ammonia-like mouth odor; have the patient use a soft toothbrush
  - Provide meticulous skin care to prevent excoriation; check for edema, jaundice, petechiae, pruritus, purpura, spider angiomas, and ulcerations
  - Tell the patient to avoid straining when turning, moving in bed, or defecating to lessen pressure on varices or hemorrhoids
  - Explain upcoming diagnostic tests or treatments as needed
  - Instruct the patient to avoid spicy or irritating foods, nonsteroidal anti-inflammatory drugs (NSAIDs), and aspirin
  - Discuss patient concerns about the disease and lifestyle or body image change; provide a psychological referral, if needed
  - Encourage the use of community agencies or services to help the patient control alcohol intake; stress the importance of abstaining from alcohol
  - Record all data in the patient's chart for continuity of care

Diverticular Disease

- Description
  - Diverticular disease is characterized by diverticula (bulging pouches) in the GI wall that push the mucosal lining through the surrounding muscle
  - There are two clinical forms: diverticulosis (diverticula are present but may cause only mild or no symptoms) and diverticulitis (diverticula are inflamed and may cause potentially fatal obstruction, infection, or hemorrhage)
  - The disorder results from high intraluminal pressure on an area of weakness in the GI wall, where blood vessels enter
  - Retained undigested food and bacteria accumulate in diverticular sac, cutting off the blood supply and leading to inflammation, perforation, abscess, peritonitis, obstruction, or hemorrhage
  - Causes are defects in the wall strength of the colon, diminished colonic motility and increased intraluminal pressure, and a low-fiber diet
- Signs and symptoms
  - In mild diverticulitis, moderate left lower abdominal pain, low-grade fever, and leukocytosis may occur; close proximity to urinary bladder may imitate urinary tract infection
  - In severe diverticulitis, abdominal rigidity from rupture of the diverticula, abscesses and peritonitis, left lower quadrant pain, high fever, chills, and hypotension from sepsis may occur

- In chronic diverticulitis, constipation, ribbon-like stools, intermittent diarrhea, abdominal distention resulting from intestinal obstruction, abdominal rigidity and pain, diminishing or absent bowel sounds, and nausea and vomiting secondary to intestinal obstruction may occur
- Diagnosis and treatment
  - Diagnosis may rely on patient history
  - The best test for diverticular disease is a CT scan with oral and IV contrast
  - A high-fiber diet may be recommended for the treatment of diverticulosis after pain has subsided
  - Antibiotics may be given to treat infection of the diverticula
  - Analgesics may be prescribed to control pain and to relax smooth muscle
  - Colon resection with removal of involved segments may be done to correct refractory cases; a temporary colostomy may be placed to drain abscess and to rest the colon
- Nursing interventions
  - Make sure the patient understands the importance of fiber in the diet
  - Advise the patient to relieve constipation with stool softeners or bulk-forming cathartics
  - Observe stools for frequency, color, and consistency
  - If bleeding of the diverticulum occurs, the patient may need angiography and placement of a catheter for infusing vasopressin
  - After surgery, watch for signs of infection and bleeding; encourage the patient to cough and breathe deeply
  - Teach the patient self-care for the ostomy as appropriate

Gastroesophageal Reflux Disease

- Description
  - GERD is the backflow of gastric contents or duodenal contents, or both, past the lower esophageal sphincter (LES) into the esophagus without associated belching or vomiting
  - The disorder occurs when the LES pressure is deficient or pressure in the stomach exceeds LES pressure
  - The degree of mucosal injury is based on the amount and concentration of refluxed gastric acid, proteolytic enzymes, and bile acids
  - Causes include anything that lowers LES pressure, such as alcohol, smoking, hiatal hernia, increased abdominal pressure with obesity or pregnancy, medications (such as morphine, diazepam, calcium channel blockers, meperidine, or anticholinergic), NG intubation for more than 4 days, and weakened esophageal sphincter
  - Patients with asthma are more likely to develop GERD
- Signs and symptoms
  - Burning pain in the epigastric area, possibly radiating to the arms and chest, results from reflux of gastric contents into the esophagus
  - Pain, usually after a meal or when lying down, occurs secondary to increased abdominal pressure, causing reflux
  - Feeling of fluid accumulation occurs in the throat without a sour or bitter taste because of hypersecretion of saliva
  - Gum irritation, dental cavities, and bad breath
  - Chronic sore throat, laryngitis, and chronic cough
- Diagnosis and treatment
  - Diagnosis is based on a patient history that reveals heartburn, physical examination, esophagoscopy, an upper GI series, ambulatory acid test, esophageal impedance testing, and an acid perfusion test
  - Abdominal pressure may be reduced by eating small, frequent meals and not eating before bedtime (see *Factors Affecting LES Pressure*, page 203)
  - Patient positioning may be helpful in reducing abdominal pressure and preventing reflux (e.g., sitting up during and after mealtimes or sleeping with the head of the bed elevated)
  - Antacids may help to neutralize the acidic content of the stomach
  - Histamine-2 receptor antagonists may be given to inhibit gastric acid secretion
  - Proton pump inhibitors may be prescribed to reduce gastric acidity on a short-term basis
  - Smoking cessation is recommended
- Nursing interventions
  - Teach the patient about the causes and symptoms of GERD
  - Tell the patient how to avoid reflux with an antireflux regimen that includes diet, weight loss, decreasing caffeine and alcohol intake, and antacids
  - Educate to elevate head of bed on blocks 6″ to 8″

Box 12-1: Factors Affecting LES Pressure

Various dietary and lifestyle factors can increase or decrease lower esophageal sphincter (LES) pressure. Take these factors into account when you plan the patient's treatment program.

Factors That Increase LES Pressure	Factors That Decrease LES Pressure
• Protein	• Fat
• Carbohydrates	• Whole milk
• Nonfat milk	• Orange juice
• Low-dose ethanol	• Tomatoes
	• Antiflatulent (simethicone)
	• Chocolate
	• High-dose ethanol
	• Cigarette smoking
	• Lying on the right or left side
	• Sitting
	• Caffeine

Gastrointestinal Bleeding

- Description
  - Acute GI bleeding can range from minor to severe
  - About 85% of GI bleeding involves the upper GI tract
  - Bleeding may be caused by a disrupted mucosal-epithelial barrier or by a ruptured artery or vein
  - Common conditions leading to GI bleeding include peptic ulcer disease, esophageal varices, diverticular disease, tumors, and ulcerative colitis
- Signs and symptoms
  - The patient may vomit blood or have coffee-ground vomitus
  - Stools may appear bloody, maroon-colored, or black and tarry
  - Abdominal cramping may occur
  - The patient with chronic bleeding may have symptoms of anemia
  - Signs of hypovolemic shock include cold, clammy skin, hypotension, reduced urine output, syncope, and tachycardia
- Diagnosis and treatment
  - Diagnosis is based on physical examination and patient history, including previous bleeding abnormalities, current medications, recent illnesses, and alcohol use
  - Colonoscopy and esophagogastroduodenoscopy can detect the source of the bleeding
  - Blood tests, such as CBC, coagulation studies, and liver function tests, are also helpful
  - CT scanning may assist with diagnosis of fistulae or bleeding from liver, gallbladder, or pancreas
  - Treatment depends on the location and cause of GI bleeding
  - Blood or blood component replacement may be indicated
  - An NG tube may be inserted and the stomach lavaged with room temperature fluid to remove blood and clots from the stomach
  - A Sengstaken-Blakemore tube may be indicated to apply direct pressure on bleeding esophageal varices
  - Bleeding blood vessels may be treated with cauterization or endoscopic injection sclerotherapy
  - A transjugular intrahepatic portosystemic shunt may be indicated to connect the portal and hepatic veins
  - Commonly administered drugs include antacids, histamine blockers, sucralfate, proton pump inhibitors, and antibiotics for the treatment of *H. pylori*; vasopressin may be administered to produce vasoconstriction
- Nursing interventions
  - Monitor vital signs and other hemodynamic parameters for early detection of bleeding and hypovolemic shock; monitor hourly intake and output; maintain nothing-by-mouth status until bleeding is controlled
  - Ensure patent airway
  - Initiate two large-bore I.V. lines for fluid, drug, and blood administration
  - Ensure patency and proper placement of the NG tube
  - If the patient has a Sengstaken-Blakemore tube, make sure it's properly positioned and secured; the balloon shouldn't be inflated for more than 72 hours because of the high risk of tissue damage; keep scissors at the bedside to cut the airway lumens for immediate tube removal should airway obstruction occur

- During vasopressin administration, continuously monitor electrocardiogram results and blood pressure
- Teach the patient how to prevent recurrence of GI bleeding by avoiding alcohol, aspirin, aspirin-containing products, and NSAIDs

Hepatitis

- Description
  - Hepatitis is an acute or a chronic inflammation of the liver
  - It's caused by viruses, bacteria, trauma, immune disorders, exposure to chemicals such as vinyl chloride and hydrocarbons, and toxins
  - Five major types of viral hepatitis exist: hepatitis A, B, C, D, and E (see *Characteristics of Viral Hepatitis*, page 205); of the 60,000 annual cases of viral hepatitis in the United States, about one half are hepatitis B; hepatitis G is a newly identified virus thought to be blood-borne, with transmission similar to that of hepatitis C
  - Hepatitis can be self-limiting or progress to scarring, cirrhosis, or liver cancer
- Signs and symptoms
  - The *prodromal* or *preicteric phase*, which lasts 1 to 2 days, can cause arthralgia, anorexia, aversion to cigarettes (among smokers), constipation or diarrhea, decreased senses of taste and smell, dislike of dietary protein, elevated serologic test results, headache, hepatomegaly, low-grade fever, lymphadenopathy, malaise, nausea, right upper quadrant pain or discomfort, splenomegaly, urticaria with or without rash, vomiting, and weight loss
  - The *clinical phase*, which lasts 1 to 2 weeks, may produce bilirubinuria, dark urine, fatigue, hepatomegaly, jaundice, light-colored stools, lymphadenopathy, pruritus, right upper quadrant tenderness, and weight loss
  - The *posticteric* or *recovery phase*, which averages 2 to 12 weeks, may result in easy fatigability, hepatomegaly, malaise, resolving jaundice (early in this phase), and resolving liver tenderness and enlargement
- Diagnosis and treatment
  - Diagnosis may rely on patient history; physical examination that reveals hepatomegaly, liver tenderness, and jaundice; serologic liver function tests (such as bilirubin and protein levels and PT); and antibody tests for surface or cellular antigens in serum (serologic assays for hepatitis G are being developed.)
  - Rest is prescribed, including bed rest if hepatomegaly is severe
  - Supplements of vitamins B, C, and K are administered
  - The recommended diet is high in calories and carbohydrates and has moderate to high protein and moderate fat
  - If the patient has hepatitis B, C, or D, antiviral therapy may be used for the treatment of chronic disease
- Nursing interventions
  - Use standard precautions to avoid spreading the disease and to protect the patient from other diseases
  - Balance rest and activity to reduce metabolic demands on the liver
  - Monitor the patient for changes in signs and symptoms—especially dark-colored urine, fatigue, fever, jaundice, and liver function—to assess the disease's status
  - Monitor fluid intake and output; correct fluid and electrolyte imbalances as prescribed
  - Administer immune serum globulin (ISG) as prescribed to modify the effects of hepatitis A and B in people who have been exposed
  - Consult a dietitian about the prescribed diet; discuss the patient's food preferences, and intervene to increase the patient's appetite and food retention to ensure adequate calorie and protein intake
  - Discuss the dangers of self-medication, and encourage the patient to use only prescribed medications; an inflamed liver can't metabolize drugs well, and some drugs—especially acetaminophen—may exacerbate inflammation
  - Follow preventive measures for hepatitis A: proper hand hygiene, good personal hygiene, environmental sanitation, screening and control of food handlers, enteric precautions, and ISG administration for exposure prophylaxis
  - Follow preventive measures for hepatitis B: proper hand hygiene, screening of blood donors for hepatitis B surface antigen, use of disposable needles and syringes, registration of carriers, passive immunization with ISG and hepatitis B immune globulin for exposure to mucous secretions or needlestick exposure, and active immunization with hepatitis B vaccine for high-risk populations such as health care providers
  - Follow the same preventive measures for hepatitis C as for hepatitis B

- Follow standard precautions for hepatitis A: use gloves and a gown if touching soiled or infective material (feces) is likely; place the patient who has poor personal hygiene in a private room, and follow precautions for 7 days after jaundice appears
- Follow standard precautions for hepatitis B: use gloves and a gown if touching soiled or infective materials (blood, body fluids, or feces if patient has GI bleeding) is likely
- Follow standard precautions for hepatitis C: use gloves and a gown if touching soiled or infective materials (blood or body fluids) is likely
- Provide a referral to a community nurse for continuity of care as needed

Box 12-2: Characteristics of Viral Hepatitis

Characteristic	Hepatitis A	Hepatitis B	Hepatitis C	Hepatitis D	Hepatitis E
Incubation period	15 to 45 days	28 to 180 days	15 to 160 days	28 to 180 days	14 to 63 days
Mode of transmission	Fecal-oral route	Parenteral (serum of infected persons); saliva, semen, and vaginal secretions	Parenteral (serum of infected persons)	Parenteral (serum of infected persons); saliva, semen, and vaginal secretions	Fecal-oral route
Sources of infection	Poor sanitation and personal hygiene; contaminated foods, milk, water, raw or steamed shellfish; persons with subclinical infections	Contaminated needles, syringes, blood products, and other instruments; sexual intercourse; kissing; asymptomatic carriers	Needles, syringes, blood and blood products	Contaminated needles, syringes, blood products, and other instruments; sexual intercourse; kissing; asymptomatic carriers	Poor sanitation, contaminated water
Virus in feces	3 to 4 weeks before jaundice	Degraded by enzymes, if present	Not identified in feces	Not applicable	Probably present in feces
Virus in serum	Briefly	Hepatitis B surface antigen (HBsAg) in serum through course of illness	Yes	Yes	Not applicable
Carrier state	No	Yes	Yes	Yes	Unknown
Prophylaxis	Immune serum globulin (ISG) within 2 weeks of exposure	Hepatitis B immune globulin (HBIG) or ISG within 2 weeks of exposure	Possible (some trials with immunoglobulin)	Avoidance of infection with hepatitis B (must be present for hepatitis D to develop)	Questionable protection with previous inoculation with immunoglobulin
Specific antigen in serum	Hepatitis A antigen	HBsAg, hepatitis B e antigen (HBeAg)	Hepatitis C virus	Hepatitis D virus	Not applicable
Specific antibody in serum	Anti–hepatitis A virus	HBsAg, antibody hepatitis B core antigen (HBcAg), anti–hepatitis E	Anti–hepatitis C virus	Anti–hepatitis D virus	Not applicable
Vaccine	Available	Available	None	None specifically for hepatitis D; vaccine for hepatitis B should be given	None
Prognosis	Complete recovery common; infection doesn't recur	Persistence in chronic or fulminant form is possible; possible precursor to a malignant liver tumor	Mild or severe and fulminant; many will have chronic infection	Increased mortality	Similar to hepatitis A except very severe in pregnant women

Large- and Small-Bowel Obstruction

- Description
  - Large-bowel obstruction can occur in the ascending, transverse, or descending colon, the rectum, or several areas simultaneously
  - Small-bowel obstruction can occur in any area of the duodenum, jejunum, or ileum or in several areas simultaneously
  - Small- and large-bowel obstructions may result from infection, tumor, or intestinal ulcerations with scar formation that leads to obstruction, volvulus, intussusception, adhesions, or paralytic ileus
  - Complications of small- and large-bowel obstruction include hypovolemic shock, peritonitis, rupture, septicemia, and death; strangulating obstruction with inadequate blood flow can progress to gangrene and infarction in less than 6 hours
- Signs and symptoms
  - Abdominal pain and distention may be mild to severe
  - Anorexia and nausea may be accompanied by severe vomiting with a fecal odor
  - Bowel sounds may be high pitched or absent
  - Constipation or obstipation may be present, or diarrhea may occur as liquid intestinal secretions and feces move around the obstruction; blood, mucus, or undigested food may appear in stool
  - Abdominal girth may increase due to distention
  - Vital sign changes may include fever and signs of shock, such as hypotension, tachycardia, and tachypnea
  - The patient may experience anxiety, dehydration, dry skin, fatigue, malaise, and weight loss
- Diagnosis and treatment
  - Diagnosis may require patient history, physical examination, abdominal X-rays (such as flat plate supine and upright of the abdomen, barium enema, and GI series), serologic studies, endoscopy, gastric analysis, stool examination, colonoscopy, and proctoscopy
  - Maintain nothing-by-mouth status, and administer I.V. therapy to restore fluid balance
  - An NG or intestinal tube is inserted to relieve abdominal distention and vomiting
  - An opioid analgesic is used to relieve pain
  - An antibiotic is administered to treat possible infection
  - Abdominal girth is measured every 2 to 4 hours
  - Bowel output is monitored, and stools are checked for occult blood
  - Surgery may be used to correct the obstruction; exploratory laparotomy can determine the cause, small- or large-bowel resection can remove diseased portions, ileostomy or colostomy may be done to permit waste discharge, and total ablation (removal) of the large and most of small intestine may be used if the obstruction is caused by mesenteric artery thrombosis
- Nursing interventions
  - Monitor vital signs, particularly noting signs of shock (increased pulse and respiratory rates and decreased blood pressure) and peritonitis or other infection (increased temperature)
  - Administer prescribed medications promptly to maintain therapeutic blood levels
  - Maintain I.V. therapy to ensure proper hydration because the patient must maintain nothing-by-mouth status
  - Monitor fluid intake and output (including vomitus and diarrhea) carefully; excessive fluid loss can lead to shock and dehydration
  - Monitor, measure, and record drainage from the NG or intestinal tube; check drainage for blood and odor, irrigate the tube as prescribed to maintain patency, and turn the patient as prescribed to facilitate tube passage to the obstruction site
  - Measure abdominal girth every 2 to 4 hours to assess distention
  - Auscultate and characterize bowel sounds; high-pitched sounds indicate anoxia resulting from marked distention or obstruction, whereas absent sounds indicate ileus or obstruction
  - Monitor eructation (a sign of continuing obstruction) or flatus passage (a sign of resolving obstruction)
  - Monitor the patient for abdominal pain or tenderness, noting its location; pain may be related to distention or inflammation
  - Encourage the patient to perform deep-breathing exercises every 2 hours; abdominal distention may elevate the diaphragm and decrease deep breathing
  - Prepare the patient for surgery, if indicated
  - Keep the patient and family apprised of the situation

Pancreatitis

- Description
  - Pancreatitis is an inflammation of the pancreas accompanied by the release of digestive enzymes into the gland, resulting in autodigestion of the organ
  - Pancreatitis may be acute or chronic
  - Causes of pancreatitis include alcohol abuse, trauma, infection, drug toxicity, high serum triglycerides, autoimmune responses, cystic fibrosis, and obstruction of the biliary tract
- Signs and symptoms
  - Pancreatitis is characterized by severe epigastric pain that worsens after meals and may radiate to the shoulder, substernal area, back, and flank
  - Fever and malaise may be present
  - The patient may experience abdominal tenderness and distention, nausea, and vomiting and may lie in a knee-chest or fetal position or lean forward for comfort
  - Bulky, fatty, foul-smelling stool may occur
  - Signs of hypovolemic shock may be present
- Diagnosis and treatment
  - Diagnosis is based on patient history, including alcohol intake and use of prescription and nonprescription drugs
  - Laboratory tests include increased serum amylase, aspartate aminotransferase, bilirubin, glucose, and lipase levels, increased WBC count, and decreased serum calcium levels
  - Imaging for diagnosis of pancreatitis includes endoscopic ultrasound, abdominal ultrasound, MRI, and CT. Cullen's sign (bruising of the subcutaneous tissue near the umbilicus) and Grey Turner's sign (bruising of the flanks of the abdomen) are positive
  - The patient maintains nothing-by-mouth status, and an NG tube is inserted; total parenteral nutrition may be indicated
  - I.V. fluids are administered, and electrolytes are replaced as indicated
  - An analgesic and an antibiotic may be prescribed; elevated glucose levels are controlled
  - Surgical intervention is used to treat the underlying cause, if appropriate
- Nursing interventions
  - Make sure the patient maintains nothing-by-mouth status during the acute phase; then, begin to introduce bland, low-fat, high-protein diet of small, frequent meals with restricted caffeine and gas-forming foods
  - Monitor for symptoms of calcium deficiency (such as tetany, cramps, carpopedal spasm, and seizures)
  - Provide mouth, nares, and skin care
  - Check the NG tube for patency and correct placement each shift
  - Monitor intake and output and vital signs, and obtain daily weights
  - Analgesia is controlled in a stepwise manner based on severity of pain. Tylenol or NSAIDs for mild to moderate pain, and opioids for more severe pain; Demerol (meperidine) is avoided. Advise the patient to avoid alcohol, caffeine, and spices
  - Explain the importance of a quiet, restful environment to conserve energy and decrease metabolic demands

Peptic Ulcer Disease

- Description
  - Peptic ulcer disease is characterized by ulcerations in the esophagus, stomach (gastric), or small intestine (duodenal); approximately 80% are duodenal
  - Peptic ulcer disease is caused by erosion of the lining cells of the stomach or duodenum; factors such as *H. pylori* infection and NSAIDs disrupt the normal mucosal defense, making the mucosa more susceptible to the effects of gastric acid
- Signs and symptoms
  - Gastric and duodenal ulcers have different signs and symptoms (see *Common Signs and Symptoms of Peptic Ulcer Disease*, page 209)
  - Other effects may include anorexia and eructation; dizziness, light-headedness, or syncope may correlate to blood loss

- The patient may have a family history of peptic ulcer disease, medication history of aspirin or other anti-inflammatory drug use, or a personal history of cigarette, alcohol, or caffeine use or of stressful conditions at home or on the job
- Diagnosis and treatment
  - Diagnosis may be based on patient history, physical examination, gastric endoscopy, barium test, upper GI series, gastric analysis, gastric cytology, serologic studies, testing for *H. pylori*, and stool tests for occult blood; a CBC is drawn to determine the presence of anemia
  - A proton pump inhibitor, such as esomeprazole (Nexium) or lansoprazole (Prevacid), may be used to suppress acid production by halting the mechanism that pumps acid into the stomach and are given before breakfast
  - A histamine blocker—such as famotidine (Pepcid), nizatidine (Axid), or ranitidine (Zantac)—is used to decrease gastric acid production; an antacid is also prescribed to neutralize hydrochloric acid
  - Sucralfate, a cytoprotective drug, may be prescribed; it works by forming a protective barrier over the ulcer's surface
  - Misoprostol (Cytotec), a synthetic prostaglandin analogue, may be prescribed to prevent ulcers from forming in patients who take high doses of an NSAID by protecting the gastric mucous; antibiotics may be prescribed to treat *H. pylori* infections; bismuth may also be used as adjunct therapy against *H. pylori*; histamine blockers may be prescribed to protect gastric mucosa in patients who take daily doses of NSAIDs
  - Stress reduction techniques are recommended to prevent development of a stress ulcer or worsening of peptic ulcers
  - Smoking cessation is recommended
  - If drug therapy is ineffective, surgical repair may include laser cauterization of a bleeding site, partial gastrectomy with gastroduodenostomy (Billroth I), partial gastrectomy with gastrojejunostomy (Billroth II), or vagotomy with pyloroplasty (rare)
- Nursing interventions
  - Administer prescribed medications
  - Help the patient identify and eliminate foods that cause distress
  - Teach the patient about the disease, its treatment, and stress reduction techniques, if needed
  - Encourage the patient to stop smoking to eliminate the effects of nicotine on ulcers
  - Provide postoperative care as needed
    - Verify placement and maintain patency of the NG tube
    - Make sure the patient maintains nothing-by-mouth status as prescribed; administer I.V. fluids to maintain fluid and electrolyte balance
    - To help control pain, encourage the patient to use patient-controlled analgesia, or administer an opioid analgesic every 3 to 4 hours
    - Measure abdominal girth to assess abdominal distention or ileus
    - Auscultate bowel sounds to detect the return of peristalsis
    - Help the patient perform deep-breathing exercises every 2 hours and use an incentive spirometer every 2 hours to prevent pulmonary complications; schedule while analgesia is most effective
    - Help the patient ambulate as prescribed
    - Take steps to avoid dumping syndrome (a rapid gastric emptying produced by a bolus of food, causing distention of the duodenum or jejunum)
    - Start giving the patient clear liquids when ordered; observe for nausea or vomiting, assess tolerance of intake, and increase to small, frequent meals
    - Monitor for flatus or bowel movements to determine bowel functions
    - Before discharge, teach the patient about rest, activity restrictions, diet, medications, smoking cessation, and stress control

Regional Enteritis and Ulcerative Colitis

- Description
  - *Regional enteritis*, also known as Crohn's disease, is an inflammatory disease of the small bowel that also may affect the large intestine; it typically begins in the ileum but can affect all areas of the small intestine and even the esophagus
  - *Ulcerative colitis* is a chronic inflammatory disease of the large intestine, commonly in the sigmoid and rectal areas

Box 12-3: Common Signs and Symptoms of Peptic Ulcer Disease

Symptom	Gastric Ulcer	Duodenal Ulcer
Pain type	Gnawing, burning, aching, heartburn	Gnawing, burning, cramping, heartburn at times
Duration	Constant unless relieved by food or drugs	Intermittent and relieved by food or drugs (steady pain may be related to a perforated ulcer of the posterior wall of the duodenum)
Site	Upper epigastrium with localization to left of umbilicus	Right epigastric area to right of umbilicus. Radiation of pain to right upper quadrant may be due to a perforated ulcer of the posterior wall of the duodenum.
Time of day	At night and when stomach is empty	At night and when duodenum is empty
Cause	Presence of hydrochloric acid in stomach	High acid content of chyme moving into duodenum
Periodicity	Recurs daily for a period of time, then disappears for months, only to recur	Recurs daily for a period of time, then disappears for months, only to recur
Nausea	Intermittent	Intermittent
Vomiting	Occasional (more often than with duodenal ulcers)	Occasional
Feeling of fullness	Present at times; eructation common	Present at times
Bleeding	Detected in vomitus, unless hemorrhage occurs	Detected in stools through stool guaiac tests, unless hemorrhage occurs

- Signs and symptoms
  - Regional enteritis and ulcerative colitis produce different signs and symptoms (see *Comparing Regional Enteritis and Ulcerative Colitis*, page 210)
  - The stool of a patient with ulcerative colitis may appear liquid, with blood, pus, and mucus; the patient with regional enteritis typically has diarrhea without visible blood
- Diagnosis and treatment
  - Regional enteritis and ulcerative colitis are diagnosed and managed similarly; regional enteritis is diagnosed by small bowel X-ray, barium study of the upper GI tract, barium enema, and intestinal biopsy; ulcerative colitis is diagnosed by biopsy with colonoscopy, barium enema, and abdominal X-ray
  - Tailored to the patient's specific needs, the diet typically restricts raw fruits and vegetables as well as fatty and spicy foods; debilitated patients may require total parenteral nutrition
  - An anticholinergic like dicyclomine (Bentyl) is used to manage intestinal spasms; an antidiarrheal to control diarrhea; an anti-inflammatory such as sulfasalazine to reduce inflammation; an antimicrobial to prevent infection; a corticosteroid to decrease inflammation; and an immunosuppressant to decrease antigen-antibody reactions
  - Surgery is indicated for fistula formation, intestinal obstruction, bowel perforation, hemorrhage, and intractable disease (if ulcerative colitis persists for more than 10 years, cancer may develop)
    - Intestinal resections may need to be performed repeatedly
    - Ileostomy is curative; ileorectal anastomosis may be performed
- Nursing interventions
  - Make sure the patient understands the purpose, therapeutic effects, and adverse effects of prescribed medications
  - Provide postoperative care for a patient undergoing surgery
  - Maintain patency of the NG tube, if present, by irrigating with normal saline solution every 2 hours as needed
  - Encourage the patient to use patient-controlled analgesia, or administer an opioid analgesic to relieve pain; administer a steroid to prevent adrenal insufficiency and an antibiotic to prevent infection
  - Monitor vital signs every 1 to 2 hours for 4 to 8 hours and then every 4 hours

- Make sure the patient maintains nothing-by-mouth status as prescribed; monitor I.V. fluids every 1 to 2 hours; up to 3,000 mL of fluid daily is needed
- Check wound sites for drainage and signs of inflammation, infection, and healing; use aseptic technique to prevent infection
- Monitor bowel sounds every 2 to 4 hours to detect the return of peristalsis or, possibly, ileus
- Monitor bowel output to determine return of bowel function
- Help the patient ambulate as prescribed
- Encourage the patient to perform deep-breathing exercises and use an incentive spirometer every 2 hours to prevent pulmonary complications
- Start giving the patient clear liquids when prescribed; the diet initially may be a low-residue one, gradually increasing to a regular diet as tolerated
- Provide care for a patient with an ileostomy or a colostomy (see *Comparing Colostomy and Ileostomy*, page 211)
  - Change bags if they start leaking to prevent skin excoriation; the patient may change bags on a regular schedule to prevent leaking
  - Make sure the opening of the bag around the stoma is no larger than 1/8″ (3 mm) to prevent skin excoriation
  - Refer the patient to an enterostomal nurse therapist for care of the stoma and colostomy and psychosocial adjustment
  - Provide opportunities for the patient to discuss feelings about the disease and its treatment
  - Teach the patient how to care for the incision or the colostomy or ileostomy
  - Refer the patient for continued nursing monitoring or assistance after discharge for continuity of care and support with new self-care procedures

Box 12-4: Comparing Regional Enteritis and Ulcerative Colitis

The following chart compares some key characteristics of regional enteritis (Crohn's disease) and ulcerative colitis.

Characteristic	Regional Enteritis	Ulcerative Colitis
Areas affected	All layers of the bowel in various areas of the bowel at the same time	Only the mucosal and submucosal layers
Lesion	"Skip" or discontinuous lesions; edematous, reddish-purple areas with granulomas (scarring)	Continuous, diffuse lesions that don't skip segments; ulcerations with erosion and bleeding
Incidence	Slightly more common in women than men, primarily between ages 20 and 50; more common in Jews and non-Whites	More common in women than men, primarily those between ages 20 and 40; more common in Jews and non-Whites
Cause	Unknown, but may be genetic or immunologic; may be exacerbated by stress	Unknown, but may be genetic, immunologic, or infectious
Signs and symptoms	• Abdominal distention • Anemia • Arthralgia • Cramping abdominal pain and tenderness • Dehydration and fluid and electrolyte imbalances • Flatulence • Low-grade fever • Nausea and vomiting • Three to four semisoft stools daily with no blood, except in patients with advanced disease. Some fat is present, and stools may be foul smelling • Weight loss	• Abdominal distention • Abdominal rigidity at times • Anemia • Bowel distention • Cramping abdominal pain, typically in lower left quadrant • Dehydration and fluid and electrolyte imbalances • Diarrhea (pronounced, 5 to 25 stools daily) with blood, mucus, and pus but no fat • Fever • Nausea and vomiting • Rectal bleeding • Weight loss
Diagnostic tests	• Barium enema • Proctosigmoidoscopy • Stool analysis for occult blood and culture • X-ray of small bowel	• Barium enema • Biopsy of rectal cells • Fiberoptic colonoscopy • Sigmoidoscopy • Stool analysis

Box 12-5: Comparing Colostomy and Ileostomy

Procedure	Type of Stool	Appliance and Bowel Regulation	Nursing Considerations
Single-barrel, or end, colostomy	Formed	Requires appliance until discharge becomes regulated; regulates bowel	Bowel is regulated through diet and irrigation (every 2 to 3 days).
Double-barrel and loop colostomy	Semiliquid, semiformed, proteolytic discharge	Requires appliance; doesn't regulate bowel	Stool is discharged from the proximal loop of the colostomy. Mucus may be discharged from a distal stoma. Loop colostomy has a plastic rod under the bowel to hold it to the outer abdominal wall; rubber tubing attached to the ends of the rod prevents it from being dislodged.
Conventional ileostomy	Semiliquid to liquid, frequent discharge of stool, proteolytic discharge	Requires appliance; doesn't regulate bowel	Ileostomy discharge may contain undigested food. Patient may become dehydrated from frequent discharges of semiliquid stool.
Continent ileostomy (Kock pouch)	Semiliquid to liquid, constant, proteolytic discharge	Doesn't require appliance or regulate bowel (ileostomy has one-way valve or nipple to prevent leakage)	Stoma is catheterized every 4 hours to empty Kock pouch.

Review Questions

Question 1. What lifestyle changes would be most beneficial for the nurse to teach to prevent gastrointestinal disease?

A. Exercise daily, drink plenty of water, and eat your daily serving of fruit with breakfast.
B. Stop smoking cigarettes, take a fiber laxative, and eat whatever you want every day.
C. Count calories, eat low-fat foods, and take a low dose of aspirin daily.
D. Eat a low-fat, high-fiber diet, drink alcohol not at all or in moderation, and lose weight.

Correct answer: D High-fiber, low-fat foods promote bowel health, decreasing or eliminating alcohol prevents damage to abdominal organs, and excess adipose tissue is a risk factor for many GI disorders. Smoking cessation, low-fat foods, drinking water, and daily exercise are beneficial to the body in many ways but are not specific to the GI system. Five or more servings of fruit or vegetables are recommended daily. Fiber laxatives help but are not meant to replace fiber from dietary sources. Daily aspirin is not recommended for gastrointestinal health.

Question 2. Which statement by the nurse is best for a patient with esophageal cancer?

A. Risk factors include GERD and alcohol and tobacco use.
B. People from Japan and China are more prone to esophageal cancer.
C. Blacks and women are patients most often seen with esophageal cancer.
D. Drinking cold beverages contributes to the risk of esophageal cancer.

Correct answer: A Risk factors for esophageal cancer include history of GERD, alcohol and tobacco use, being from the Middle East or China, being Black or male, chronic ingestion of hot beverages (Options B, C and D).

Question 3. Which statement by the patient recently diagnosed with early-stage right colon cancer indicates an understanding of the disease process?

A. "I would be better off if I had some lymph node involvement with my cancer…."
B. "Colon cancer grows quickly, so I do not have a lot of time to spend with my family…."
C. I put myself at risk for this cancer from eating all that high-fiber diet stuff…."
D. "I had no symptoms because of the location and early detection of my cancer…."

Correct answer: D Early-stage, right-sided colon cancer is usually asymptomatic. Early detection of slow-growing colon cancers, prior to nodal involvement, leads to better outcomes (Options A and B). High-fiber diets are protective of the bowel and are recommended to prevent colorectal cancer (Option C).

Question 4. Which interventions are best for a patient with cirrhosis of the liver?

A. Avoid stress to the patient by not teaching about tests that may need to be completed.
B. Check level of consciousness and neuro status to detect encephalopathy.
C. Anticipate that changes in patient behavior will occur and chart accordingly.
D. Ensure ample water is available to ensure the patient is fully hydrated.

Correct answer: B Encephalopathy is exhibited by a change in level of consciousness, a change in behavior, and altered neurological status and should be reported to provider immediately (Option C). Always prepare patients for upcoming testing necessary for diagnosis and treatment (Option B). Patients with cirrhosis of the liver are usually on fluid-restricted diets (Option D).

Question 5. When addressing the HPI of a patient, which is most appropriate for the nurse to assess?

A. Date of birth
B. Use of alcohol
C. When symptoms started
D. Other related health conditions

Correct answer: C History if presenting illness (HPI) addresses only information relevant to current symptoms. Alcohol use relates to social history (Option B), birth date relates to demographics (Option A), and other related health conditions fall under the medical history (option D).

Question 6. The newly admitted patient reports, "I have pain right under my right ribs and up in my right shoulder. It got worse after I had a burger, fries, and milk shake…." Which tests does the nurse anticipate for this patient?

A. Colonoscopy and coagulation studies
B. Pancreatic enzymes and CT
C. MRI and complete blood count
D. Ultrasound and hepatic panel

Correct answer: D Ultrasound and liver function are used to diagnose cholecystitis, which has classic symptoms of right upper quadrant pain with referred pain to the right shoulder and made worse with fatty foods. Colonoscopy and coagulation studies are ordered for gastrointestinal bleeding (Option A), and pancreatic enzymes with a CT (Option B) are used to diagnose pancreatitis. MRI and CBC are used in the diagnosis of appendicitis (Option C).

Question 7. Which of the following is correct when performing an abdominal assessment?

A. Check size and general shape of abdomen, palpate all quadrants, and percuss abdomen for air or fluid.
B. Inspect overall appearance, listen for bowel sounds, and tap fingers over abdomen to locate organs.
C. Percuss abdomen to find organs and masses, palpate abdominal muscle tone, and auscultate bowel sounds.
D. Palpate abdomen, auscultate vascular sounds, and inspect skin turgor, abdominal shape, and color of sclera.

Correct answer: B The order of assessing an abdomen is always inspect, auscultate, percuss, and palpate.

Question 8. When teaching a patient about GERD, which statement is the best?

A. A very full stomach holds the lower esophageal sphincter closed.
B. Smoking will not cause an increase in GERD symptoms.
C. It's acceptable to gain a little weight from eating more frequently.
D. Use gravity to keep stomach fluids from entering the esophagus.

Correct answer: D Gravity, from sitting up or having the head of the bed on 6" to 8" blocks, assists with keeping stomach contents in the stomach. A very full stomach will lower LES (Option A) and produce reflux. Smoking stimulates gastric secretion and lowers LES causing reflux (Option B). Excess weight is a contributor to GERD; teach that small, frequent meals should not contain more calories than the traditional three meals per day (Option C).

Question 9. Which statement by the patient indicates an understanding of diverticular disease?

A. "The high-fiber diet will help soften my stool because I should not strain when having a bowel movement…."
B. "Once I feel better, I will be able to eat cheeseburgers and fries for lunch at the counter with my friends every day…."

C. "I will need a colostomy in the future because there is no cure or treatment for this diverticulosis I have …."

D. "I am glad that I do not have to make any changes in my life and that this condition has no chance of killing me …."

Correct answer: A High-fiber diets help keep stool moving through the colon and make feces easier to pass; straining at stool causes increased pressure within the bowel that can cause diverticuli to form. Occasional cheeseburgers and fries may not cause problems; however, the nurse will want to be certain the patient understands the importance of a high-fiber diet (Option B). Lifestyle changes that can prevent the need for a colostomy include the high-fiber diet; antibiotics and analgesics can help with acute flares. However, diverticulitis can progress to inflammation, bowel perforation, peritonitis, bowel obstruction, abscesses, and death (Options C and D).

Question 10. Which intervention should the nurse anticipate for a patient with a bowel blockage?

A. Clear liquid diet
B. Fiber laxative and force fluids
C. Bed rest with bathroom privileges
D. Nasogastric tube insertion

Correct answer: D Nasogastric tubes are used for decompression. Options A and B are contraindicated since patients with bowel blockage are placed on NPO status. Option C is not necessary and ambulation may assist with peristalsis.

Selected References

American Academy of Allergy, Asthma & Immunology. (2017). Gastroesophageal reflux disease (GERD). Retrieved from http://www.aaaai.org/conditions-and-treatments/related-conditions/gastroesophageal-reflux-disease

American Cancer Society. (2017, April 6). What is colorectal cancer? Retrieved from https://www.cancer.org/cancer/colon-rectal-cancer/about/what-is-colorectal-cancer.html

American Cancer Society. (2017, February 4). What is cancer of the esophagus? Retrieved from https://www.cancer.org/cancer/esophagus-cancer/about/what-is-cancer-of-the-esophagus.html

American Cancer Society. (2016, February 10). About stomach cancer. Retrieved from https://www.cancer.org/cancer/stomach-cancer/about.html

Anand, B. S. (2017, January 29). Peptic ulcer disease. Retrieved from http://emedicine.medscape.com/article/181753-overview?pa=OL3aMB%2F4Xsb2DFor5HrclHlib9snPWZ%2F3wBJ4lsLbzNO7jYMUwKvc1WLU1scSLLTztVpOX3krW1EICnWlXZ3PON5lPYw%2FtQ7Z8WOOzpssmw%3D

Ansari, P. (2017, January). Intestinal obstruction. Retrieved from http://www.merckmanuals.com/professional/gastrointestinal-disorders/acute-abdomen-and-surgical-gastroenterology/intestinal-obstruction

Cerruli, M. A. (2016, March 21). Upper gastrointestinal bleeding. Retrieved from http://emedicine.medscape.com/article/187857-overview

Civan, J. M. (2016, January). Cirrhosis. Retrieved from https://www.merckmanuals.com/professional/hepatic-and-biliary-disorders/fibrosis-and-cirrhosis/cirrhosis

Crohn's and Colitis Foundation. (2017). What is Crohn's disease? Retrieved from http://www.crohnscolitisfoundation.org/what-are-crohns-and-colitis/what-is-crohns-disease/

Harvard Men's Health Watch. (2015, December 2). Diverticular disease of the colon. Retrieved from http://www.health.harvard.edu/diseases-and-conditions/diverticular-disease-of-the-colon

International Foundation for Functional Gastrointestinal Disorders. (2016, February 10). About GERD. Retrieved from http://www.aboutgerd.org

National Pancreatitis Foundation. (2017a). Acute pancreatitis. Retrieved from https://pancreasfoundation.org/patient-information/acute-pancreatitis/

National Pancreatitis Foundation. (2017b). Chronic pancreatitis. Retrieved from https://pancreasfoundation.org/patient-information/chronic-pancreatitis/

Nordqvist, C. (2017, April 25). Appendicitis: Signs, symptoms, and treatment. Retrieved from http://www.medicalnewstoday.com/articles/158806.php

Rabinowitz, S. S. (2015, October 29). Abdominal examination. Retrieved from http://emedicine.medscape.com/article/1909183-overview

Siddiqui, A. A. (2016, August). Cholecystitis. Retrieved from https://www.merckmanuals.com/professional/SearchResults?query=Cholecystitis&icd9=574.3%3b574.0%3b574.4%3b575.0%3b574.6%3b574.8%3b575.11%3b575.12%3b576.0

World Health Organization. (2016, July). What is hepatitis? Retrieved from http://www.who.int/features/qa/76/en/

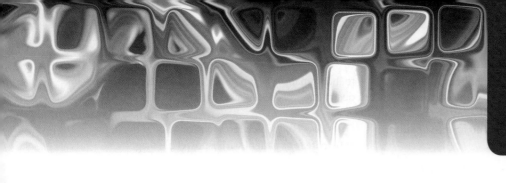

Chapter 13

Skin Disorders

Introduction

- The skin is the largest organ in the body
- It provides a barrier against pathogens, radiation, and trauma, regulates body temperature, stores water and fat, and is the site of vitamin D production
- Pressure receptors in the skin provide the sense of touch
- Nursing history
  - The nurse asks the patient about his *chief complaint*
    - The most common complaints concerning the integumentary system are itching, lesions, pigmentation abnormalities, and rashes
    - The patient may also have problems with changes in nail growth or color, hair loss, or increased growth or distribution of hair
  - The nurse then questions the patient about his *present illness*
    - Ask the patient about their symptom, including when it started, associated symptoms, location, radiation, intensity, duration, frequency, and precipitating and alleviating factors
    - Ask how and when skin changes occurred; ask if they have experienced any bleeding, drainage, or itching
    - Question the patient about any recent insect bites
    - Ask about the use of prescription and over-the-counter drugs (especially ointments, creams, or lotions), herbal remedies, and vitamin and nutritional supplements
  - The nurse asks about *medical history*
    - Question the patient about a history of skin, nail, or hair problems or changes
    - Ask about previous diseases or conditions
  - The nurse then assesses the *family history*
    - Ask about a family history of chronic skin infections, cancer, or other diseases
    - Question the patient about a family history of disorders of the hair or nails
    - Ask about a family history of other chronic diseases
  - The nurse obtains a *social history*
    - Ask about support systems, work, exercise, diet, use of recreational drugs, alcohol use, stress, hobbies, and coping mechanisms
    - Ask how much time the patient spends in the sun and whether protective clothing and sunscreen are worn
- Physical assessment
  - Nurse begins with *inspection*
    - Examine the patient's mucous membranes, hair, scalp, axillae, groin, palms, soles, and nails; note changes in pigmentation; note the color, size, shape, configuration, pattern of distribution, depth or height, texture, and location of any lesions (see *Differentiating Among Skin Lesions*, page 215)
    - Note the patient's level of hygiene, including any odors
  - Next, the nurse uses *palpation*
    - Palpate the skin and note texture, consistency, temperature, moisture, edema, and turgor
    - Note any areas of tenderness or lesions

Box 13-1: Differentiating Among Skin Lesions

These illustrations depict the most common primary skin lesions.

Primary Lesions

Bulla
Fluid-filled lesion more than 2 cm in diameter (also called a blister); occurs in patients with severe poison oak or ivy dermatitis, bullous pemphigoid, or second-degree burns

Comedo
Plugged, exfoliative pilosebaceous duct formed from sebum and keratin—for example, blackhead (open comedo) and whitehead (closed comedo)

Cyst
Semisolid or fluid-filled encapsulated mass extending deep into dermis—for example, acne

Macule
Flat, pigmented, circumscribed area less than 1 cm in diameter—for example, freckle or rash that occurs in patients with rubella

Nodule
Firm, raised lesion, 0.6 to 2 cm in diameter, which is deeper than a papule and extends into dermal layer—for example, intradermal nevus

Papule
Firm, inflammatory, raised lesion up to 1 cm in diameter that may be the same color as skin or pigmented—for example, acne papule and lichen planus

Patch
Flat, pigmented, circumscribed area more than 1 cm in diameter—for example, herald patch (pityriasis rosea)

Plaque
Circumscribed, solid, elevated lesion more than 1 cm in diameter that is elevated above skin surface and that occupies larger surface area in comparison with height, as occurs in psoriasis

Pustule
Raised, circumscribed lesion, usually less than 1 cm in diameter, that contains purulent material, making it a yellow-white color—for example, acne or impetiginous pustule and furuncle

Tumor
Elevated, solid lesion larger than 2 cm in diameter that extends into dermal and subcutaneous layers—for example, dermatofibroma

Vesicle
Raised, circumscribed, fluid-filled lesion less than 1 cm in diameter, as occurs in chickenpox or herpes simplex infection

Wheal
Raised, firm lesion with intense localized skin edema that varies in size, shape, and color (from pale pink to red) and that disappears in hours—for example, hives and insect bites

Basal and Squamous Cell Carcinoma

- Description
  - Basal cell carcinoma is an epidermal tumor predominantly found on exposed surfaces of the skin; tumors remain localized, and metastasis is rare
  - Basal cell carcinoma is a slow-growing, destructive skin tumor that usually occurs in people older than age 40; it's most prevalent in blonde, fair-skinned males and is the most common malignant tumor that affects Caucasians; chronic sun exposure is the most common cause
  - There are four types of basal cell carcinoma: nodular, superficial, morpheaform, and pigmented
  - Squamous cell carcinoma, an invasive tumor arising from keratinizing epidermal cells, has the potential for metastasis
  - Squamous cell carcinoma of the skin usually appears on sun-damaged skin but may arise from normal skin or preexisting lesions
  - Prognosis is good for basal cell carcinoma because tumors remain localized
  - Immunosuppressed patients have a higher incidence of both basal cell and squamous cell carcinoma

- Signs and symptoms
  - Basal cell carcinoma
    - A pearly papule, typically with telangiectasis, raised borders, and superficial ulceration, is characteristic of the nodular form
    - Superficial basal cell carcinoma appears as a well-demarcated erythematous scaly patch without ulceration, commonly on the trunk
    - A pale, yellow, or white flat or depressed scarlike plaque with indistinct borders suggests morpheaform basal cell carcinoma
    - Pigmented basal cell carcinoma appears as a pearly papule that contains melanin and looks blue, black, or brown in color
  - Squamous cell carcinoma
    - Squamous cell carcinoma appears as a red, crusted, scaly patch on the skin; a raised growth with a depressed center; or a firm, red-black nodule
    - It may also appear as sandpaper-like lesion
- Diagnosis and treatment
  - Basal and squamous cell carcinomas are diagnosed by their appearance; incisional or excisional biopsy and histologic study may help to determine the tumor type and histologic subtype
  - Treatment options include surgical excision, electrodesiccation and curettage, cryosurgery, radiation therapy, and Mohs' surgery
  - Interferon therapy and fluorouracil or imiquimod may also be used
- Nursing interventions
  - Monitor the skin after biopsy for bleeding
  - Explain to the patient which treatments he's receiving and answer all related questions
  - Encourage the patient to express feelings about changes in body image and a fear of dying; offer emotional support and encouragement
  - Provide postchemotherapy and postradiation nursing care to promote healing
  - Teach the patient and family members about wound care, protection from the sun, lifestyle modifications, skin examination, and the importance of follow-up examinations

Burns

- Description
  - A burn is a lesion caused by fire, friction or abrasion, heat, caustic substances, electricity, or radiation
  - Burn injury is the result of thermal energy causing tissue destruction from coagulation, protein denaturation, or ionization of cellular contents
  - Burns are classified by their depth and the amount of tissue damage (see *Burn Classification*, page 218)
  - Burns are also classified by the extent of the body surface area injured
  - Burns of less than 20% of total body surface area (TBSA) produce a primarily local response; burns of greater than 20% of TBSA produce both a local and a systemic response
  - Systemic responses include fluid and electrolyte shifts, hypovolemia, shock, and respiratory distress; complications include renal failure, immunologic compromise, and gastrointestinal (GI) bleeding
- Treatment in stage 1 (immediate or emergent stage)
  - Stage 1 begins when the patient is burned and continues until the patient's condition is stabilized and fluids have been replaced
  - The burn team implements lifesaving measures
    - A patent airway is established
    - Oxygen is supplied by nasal cannula or endotracheal tube
    - A patent large-bore I.V. line is established for fluid resuscitation, which is titrated to urine output (not burn size)
    - The extent and depth of burn area are determined
    - The patient is assessed for other injuries, including smoke inhalation that may require supportive pulmonary management
  - The severity of the burn is determined
    - The amount of body surface involved is determined by the rule of nines: head and neck (9%), arms (9% each), anterior trunk (18%), posterior trunk (18%), legs (18% each), and perineum (1%)
    - The specific body parts involved, such as the face and neck, are identified

- ○ The burn depth (partial- or full-thickness) is noted
- ○ The causative agent is identified as thermal, chemical, or electrical
- ○ The patient's age is documented because it alters body surface area estimates based on body proportions; the Lund-Browder classification is used to estimate body surface area burned in a pediatric patient
- Fluid and electrolyte balance is the chief concern for up to 48 hours after a major burn; the greatest fluid loss occurs in the first 12 hours; the larger the burned area, the greater the fluid loss
- Burns initially cause capillaries in the damaged area to dilate
  - ○ Increased hyperpermeability causes fluid to move out of cells into surrounding tissues; this fluid movement causes edema and vesiculation (blistering)
  - ○ Proteins, plasma, and electrolytes shift to the interstitial compartment; red blood cells remain in the vascular system, causing increased blood viscosity and false hematocrit elevation
- Burns also cause acute dehydration and poor renal perfusion
- Burn shock is a serious complication caused by decreased fluid volume
  - ○ Most burn-related deaths result from burn shock
  - ○ Signs and symptoms of burn shock include decreased urine output, tachycardia, hypotension, tachypnea with shallow respirations, and restlessness
- Treatment in stage 2 (intermediate or acute stage)
  - Stage 2 begins 48 to 72 hours after the burn injury
  - Circulatory overload is the chief concern as fluid shifts back into the cells from the interstitial areas, and the kidneys begin to excrete large volumes of urine (diuresis)
  - Vital signs, urine output, and level of consciousness must be monitored during this stage
  - Smoke inhalation damages the respiratory cilia and mucosa, decreases the amount of alveolar surfactant, and can cause atelectasis
    - ○ Breathing difficulties—especially in patients with burns in the upper chest, neck, and face—may occur immediately or may not occur for several hours
    - ○ Symptoms of smoke inhalation include hoarseness, productive cough, singed nasal hairs, agitation, tachypnea, flaring nostrils, retractions, and sooty septum
- Treatment in stage 3 (rehabilitation stage)
  - Stage 3 begins after the burn area is treated; prevention of infection is the chief concern, and the goal is to return the patient to a productive life
  - The patient may need to wear pressure therapy garments to decrease scarring and may need cosmetic surgery and psychological and vocational counseling
- Burn care
  - Burned areas may be left exposed (open to air) if the burn doesn't encircle the arm, trunk, or leg
  - An occlusive dressing may be applied (covered with a nonadhesive, water-permeable mesh gauze)
  - The burn may require primary excision or debridement (removal of necrotic or damaged tissue)
  - Skin grafting may be necessary
    - ○ Autograft is obtained from undamaged parts of the patient's body
    - ○ Homograft is obtained from a person other than the patient
    - ○ Xenograft is obtained from a different species such as a pig
    - ○ Isograft is obtained from an identical twin
- Nursing interventions
  - Maintain a patent airway and ongoing assessment of respiratory status
  - Monitor vital signs every 15 minutes to evaluate the effectiveness of fluid resuscitation and to detect secondary infections
  - Encourage coughing and deep breathing to promote lung expansion and adequate gas exchange
  - Establish an I.V. line to initiate fluid replacement with a colloid and crystalloid solution (lactated Ringer's solution) during the first 24 hours
  - Insert an indwelling urinary catheter to measure urine output and identify potential renal shutdown
  - If possible, weigh the patient on admission to obtain baseline data
  - Insert a nasogastric tube as ordered to decompress the stomach and prevent aspiration of stomach contents
  - If the patient hasn't had a booster shot within the past 5 years, administer tetanus toxoid; the patient may have an injury prone to tetanus
  - Administer an I.V. analgesic, such as morphine, to reduce discomfort

Box 13-2: Burn Classification

Characteristic	Superficial, Partial-Thickness (First-Degree) Burn	Deep, Partial-Thickness (Second-Degree) Burn	Full-Thickness (Third-Degree) Burn
Appearance	Dry with no blisters	Weeping, edematous blisters	Dry, leathery, and possibly edematous
Color	Pink	White to pink or red	White to charred
Comfort	Painful	Very painful	Little or no pain
Depth	Epidermis only	Epidermis, dermis, and possibly some subcutaneous tissue	Subcutaneous tissue and possibly fascia, muscle, and bone

- Administer an antibiotic as prescribed; the patient is more susceptible to infection because the skin's protective function is compromised
- Keep the patient warm; he may lose body heat through the burn area and may become hypothermic
- Use aseptic technique when assisting the patient in the whirlpool bath treatment(for debridement) and when changing dressings
- Apply the prescribed topical agent to prevent bacterial infections; be aware that silver nitrate produces stains, mafenide acetate (Sulfamylon) can cause temporary stinging and burning (analgesia may be needed before application), and silver sulfadiazine (Silvadene) maintains adequate hydration in a patient receiving sulfonamides
- Perform ROM exercises for affected areas, if possible, to maintain function
- Encourage the patient and family to discuss feelings and concerns

Lyme Disease

- Description
  - Lyme disease is an inflammatory, multisystemic disorder caused by the bacteria *Borrelia burgdorferi*, which is transmitted primarily by a deer tick bite; the disease is most common in the summer
  - Lyme disease causes many complications, such as arrhythmias, arthritis, cranial or peripheral neuropathies, encephalitis, meningitis, myocarditis, and pericarditis
- Signs and symptoms
  - Lyme disease may cause a distinctive, expanding skin lesion that is called *erythema chronicum migrans* (bull's-eye rash), is warm to the touch, and has an intense red border
    - The rash appears 3 to 30 days after the tick bite
    - Common lesion sites are the groin, buttocks, axillae, trunk, upper arms, and legs
  - Lyme disease occurs in three stages
    - Stage 1 begins with a tick bite and *erythema chronicum migrans*, followed by chills, fatigue, fever, sore throat, and stiff neck—these signs and symptoms may be mistaken for meningitis; the classic bull's-eye skin lesion begins as a small papule at the site of the bite and gradually enlarges into a round or oval ring with central clearing
    - Stage II is characterized by neurologic effects, such as Bell's palsy, arthritis in the large joints, and cardiac effects, such as arrhythmias or heart block; this is also called the disseminated phase and can occur months to years after the tick bite
    - Stage III, the chronic phase, is characterized by recurrent exacerbations of arthritis, usually of the knees, for up to 3 years after the appearance of the rash
- Diagnosis and treatment
  - A two-part blood test is the standard for diagnosis; the first part uses an enzyme immunoassay, and if this is negative, no further testing is recommended, but if results are positive and then the second step is completed, it is an immunoblot test
  - It is only considered a positive result when both tests are positive
  - Serologic tests don't always confirm the diagnosis—especially in the early stages before the body produces antibodies or seropositive for *B. burgdorferi*

- Mild anemia along with elevated aspartate aminotransferase levels, erythrocyte sedimentation rate, serum immunoglobulin M levels, and white blood cell count support the diagnosis
  - A lumbar puncture may be ordered if Lyme disease involves the central nervous system
  - As soon as the diagnosis is made, the patient is treated with oral doxycycline, amoxicillin, or cefuroxime for 10 to 21 days
  - Patients in stages II and III are treated with I.V. or I.M. penicillin or ceftriaxone
  - Symptom management for pain, sleep disturbances, and depression should also be addressed
- Nursing interventions
  - Plan care to provide adequate rest
  - Monitor vital signs to evaluate the patient's response to treatment
  - Use a cardiac monitor or electrocardiogram to determine cardiac involvement
  - Check for neurologic signs to assess neurologic involvement
  - Promote the patient's comfort with position changes and skin care
  - Educate the patient about the disease, including measures to prevent and avoid exposure to ticks; also, explain that if he finds a tick on his body, he should grasp it with tweezers and pull it straight out
  - Encourage the patient to discuss feelings about the disease
  - Report infections to the Centers for Disease Control and Prevention

Malignant Melanoma

- Description
  - Malignant melanoma is a neoplasm derived from dermal or epidermal cells; it's the leading cause of death from skin cancer
  - Prognosis is related to the thickness of the tumor and where it is in the body at the time of diagnosis
  - Exposure to sunlight and tanning bed use increase the risk of malignant melanoma; fair-skinned, blonde- or red-haired people are at greater relative risk than persons with darker pigmentation; genetic predisposition may contribute to the development of melanoma
  - Melanoma originates in normal skin or an existing mole and metastasizes to other areas of the body; common sites are the back, legs, between the toes, scalp, back of the hands, face, and neck
  - The 5-year survival rate is poor when the lesion is more than 1.5 mm thick or regional lymph nodes are involved
- Signs and symptoms
  - Signs of melanoma include a change in borders, color, size, or shape of a preexisting skin lesion or an irregular, flat or slightly elevated lesion with hues of tan, black, white, or blue
  - A nodular melanoma is spherical and may resemble a blood blister; its color is blue-black
  - The lesion may produce local soreness and may be accompanied by pruritus, oozing, bleeding, or crusting
- Diagnosis and treatment
  - An excisional skin biopsy shows cytology positive for malignant melanoma
  - Diagnostic studies may include chest X-ray, a gallium scan, bone scan, magnetic resonance imaging, and computed tomography scans of the head, chest, and abdomen to evaluate possible metastases
  - Treatment depends on lesion thickness; initial treatment includes a wide excision of the lesion and involved lymph nodes in the vicinity of the tumor; skin grafting may follow
  - There are no dependable, curative, systemic treatments for malignant melanoma; most treatments are aimed at slowing progression and relieving symptoms
  - A chemotherapeutic agent may be directly infused into the lesion, or a combination of direct infusion and systemic chemotherapeutic treatment may be used
  - Administration of interferon and interleukin-2 may achieve temporary remission
  - Radiation therapy may be used for palliative effects and to improve quality of life
- Nursing interventions
  - Medicate for discomfort, especially if a wide excision is necessary
  - Teach the patient about the disease, including prevention measures, such as decreasing exposure to ultraviolet rays, using sunscreen, avoiding tanning booths, and performing a monthly self-examination, during which time they should check all skin lesions for changes
  - Answer the patient's questions to decrease anxiety
  - Identify resources and support systems to help the patient cope
  - Encourage the patient to express feelings about the disease

Psoriasis

- Description
  - Psoriasis is a chronic, noninfectious inflammatory skin disease; it occurs in up to 3% of the population
  - It is a chronic autoimmune disease and has been proven to be a highly heritable condition
  - The disease is most often diagnosed in people ages 15 to 35 and has a tendency to improve and recur periodically
  - Common triggers are infections, smoking, obesity, skin trauma, consumption of alcohol, stress, and certain medications
  - Psoriatic arthritis may develop as a complication
- Signs and symptoms
  - Psoriasis is characterized by reddish papules and plaques covered with silvery scales; scaly patches form from the buildup of living and dead skin
  - Skin patches are dry and may be pruritic; the patient's nails may be pitted, discolored, and crumbling
  - Lesions appear bilaterally and may range from mild to severe; the scalp, face, elbows, knees, lower back, and genitalia are most often affected
- Diagnosis and treatment
  - Diagnosis is based on a thorough skin assessment and occasionally a biopsy
  - Current treatment options make clear or nearly clear skin a realistic goal
  - Topical treatments include coal tar products, steroidal and nonsteroidal anti-inflammatory ointments, retinoids, and medicated shampoos
  - Systemic treatments include, cyclosporine, oral retinoid, methotrexate, and PDE4 inhibitors
  - Biologic agents that may be used include infliximab (Remicade), adalimumab (Humira), secukinumab (Cosentyx), ustekinumab (Stelara), and etanercept (Enbrel)
  - Ultraviolet A or B light treatments may also be effective
- Nursing interventions
  - Teach the patient about the disease; help identify disease triggers and work with the patient to modify those triggers
  - Discuss treatment options and the need for consistency and compliance to achieve optimal results
  - Teach the patient about the possible need for frequent and prolonged bathing to soften and remove scales, followed by application of prescribed creams or ointments
  - Discuss establishing a skin care program, even when the disease isn't in the acute phase
  - Provide emotional support to the patient experiencing body image concerns or depression related to this chronic disease
  - Provide treatment options to relieve itching and pain

Review Questions

Question 1. The nurse is teaching a patient diagnosed with basal cell carcinoma. The most common cause of basal cell carcinoma is:

A. immunosuppression.
B. radiation exposure.
C. sun exposure.
D. burns.

Correct answer: C Sun exposure is the best known and most common cause of basal cell carcinoma. Immunosuppression (Option A), radiation (Option B), and burns (Option D) are less common causes.

Question 2. A patient received burns to his entire back and left arm. Using the rule of nines, the nurse can calculate that he has sustained burns on what percentage of his body?

A. 9%
B. 18%
C. 27%
D. 36%

Correct answer: C According to the rule of nines, each of the posterior and anterior trunks and legs makes up 18% of the total body surface, each of the arms makes up 9%, the head and neck make up 9%, and the perineum makes up 1%. In this case, the patient received burns to his back (18%) and one arm (9%), totaling 27% of his body.

Question 3. A patient is admitted to a burn intensive care unit with extensive full-thickness burns. The nurse is most concerned about the patient's:

A. fluid and electrolyte status.
B. risk of infection.
C. body image.
D. level of pain.

Correct answer: A During the early phase of burn care, the nurse is most concerned with fluid resuscitation and electrolyte balance, to correct large-volume fluid loss through the damaged skin. Infection (Option B), body image (Option C), and pain (Option D) are significant areas of concern but are less urgent than fluid status.

Question 4. A patient undergoes a biopsy to confirm a diagnosis of skin cancer. Immediately following the procedure, the nurse should observe the site for:

A. infection.
B. dehiscence.
C. hemorrhage.
D. swelling.

Correct answer: C The nurse's main concern following a skin biopsy procedure is bleeding. Infection (Option A) is a later possible consequence of a biopsy. Dehiscence (Option B) is more likely in larger wounds such as surgical wounds of the abdomen or thorax. Swelling (Option D) is a normal reaction associated with any event that traumatizes the skin.

Question 5. The nurse is caring for a patient with malignant melanoma. The nurse explains that the first and most important treatment for malignant melanoma is:

A. chemotherapy.
B. immunotherapy.
C. radiation therapy.
D. wide excision.

Correct answer: D Wide excision is the primary treatment for malignant melanoma and removes the entire lesion and determines the level and staging. Chemotherapy (Option A) may be used after the melanoma is excised. Immunotherapy (Option B) is experimental. Radiation therapy (Option C) is palliative.

Question 6. A 19-year-old patient comes to the clinic with dark red lesions on her hands, wrist, and waistline. She has scratched several of the lesions so that they are open and bleeding. The nurse instructs the patient to try pressing on the itchy lesions. What is the rationale for this intervention?

A. Pressing the skin spreads the beneficial microorganisms.
B. Pressing is suggested before scratching.
C. Pressing the skin promotes breaks in the skin.
D. Pressing the skin stimulates nerve endings.

Correct answer: D Pressing the skin stimulates nerve endings and can reduce the sensation of itching. Pressing the skin (Option A) doesn't spread microorganisms; instead, scratching the skin opens portals of entry for harmful bacteria. Scratching (Option B) isn't recommended at all. Pressing the skin doesn't promote breaks in the skin (Option C).

Question 7. A patient arrives at the office of his physician complaining of a rash. The nurse assesses the patient and notes several palpable, elevated masses, each about 0.5 cm in diameter. What term would the nurse use to accurately describe these masses?

A. Erosions
B. Macules
C. Papules
D. Vesicles

Correct answer: C Papules are firm, palpable raised lesions of up to 0.6 cm in diameter. Erosions (Option A) are characterized as a loss of some or all of the epidermal layer. Macules (Option B) are nonpalpable, flat changes in skin color. Vesicles (Option D) are fluid-filled lesions.

Question 8. A patient has thick, discolored nails with splintered hemorrhages, easily separated from the nail bed. There are also "ice pick" pits and ridges. The nurse explains to the patient that these findings are most closely associated with:

A. paronychia.
B. psoriasis.
C. seborrhea.
D. scabies.

Correct answer: B Psoriasis, a chronic skin disorder with an unknown cause, can result in these characteristic changes in the nails. A paronychia (Option A) is a bacterial infection of the nail bed. Seborrhea (Option C), also called cradle cap, is a chronic inflammatory dermatitis that typically affects the scalp. Scabies (Option D) are mites that burrow under the skin, generally between the webbing of the fingers and toes.

Question 9. After the initial phase of a burn injury, the primary focus of a patient's cure is:

A. enhancing self-esteem.
B. promoting hygiene.
C. reducing anxiety.
D. preventing infection.

Correct answer: D Because the body's protective barrier is damaged and the immune system is compromised, preventing infection is the primary goal. Enhancing self-esteem (Option A), promoting hygiene (Option B), and reducing anxiety (Option C) are important, but they're not the primary focus of treatment.

Question 10. Which patient is at greatest risk for impaired wound healing after surgery?

A. A 65-year-old patient with hypertension
B. A 60-year-old patient who is slightly overweight
C. A 78-year-old patient in general good health
D. A 75-year-old patient with poorly controlled diabetes mellitus

Correct answer: D Poorly controlled diabetes is a serious risk factor for impaired wound healing. Other factors that delay wound healing include advanced age, inadequate blood supply, nutritional deficiencies, and obesity. Hypertension (Option A), being slightly overweight (Option B), and being older but in generally good health (Option C) aren't as serious risk factors in wound healing.

Selected References

Burn triage and treatment—Thermal injuries. (n.d.). Retrieved from chemm.nlm.nih.gov/burns.htm

Casey, G. (2016, April). Disorders of the skin. *Kai Tiaki Nursing New Zealand*, 22, 20–24. Retrieved from www.ebscohost.com

Kanchan, T., Geriani, D., & Savithry, K. S. (2014, July 28). Curling's ulcer- Have these stress ulcers gone extinct? *Burns*, 41, 196–202. Retrieved from http://dx.doi.org/10.1016/j.burns.2014.06.019

Kottner, J., & Surber, C. (2016, September). Skin care in nursing: A critical discussion of nursing practice and research. *International Journal of Nursing Studies*, 61, 20–28. Retrieved from http://dx.doi.org/10.1016/J.IJNURSTU.2016.05.002

Lavrentieva, A. (2015, April 17). Critical care of burn patients. New approaches to old problems. *Burns*, 42(1), 13–19. Retrieved from http://dx.doi.org/10.1016/J.BURNS;2015.04.009

Lyme disease. (2017). Retrieved from www.cdc.gov

Miraglia, C. M. (2016, August 4). A review of the centers for disease control and prevention's guidelines for the clinical laboratory diagnosis of lyme disease. *Journal of Chiropractic Medicine*, 15(4), 272–280. Retrieved from http://dx.doi.org/10.1016/j.jcm.2016.08.003

Onselen, J. V. (2015). Working together to manage common skin conditions. *British Journal of Nursing*, 24, 1052–1053. Retrieved from www.ebscohost.com

Pearson, S. (2015). Lyme disease: Cause, symptoms, prevention, and treatment. *Nurse Prescribing*, 13(2), 88–93. Retrieved from www.ebscohost.com

Psoriasis. (n.d.). Retrieved from www.aad.org

Screening for skin cancer: Recommendation statement. (2016). Retrieved from www.aafp.org/afp

Chapter 14

Endocrine Disorders

Introduction

- The endocrine system plays a significant role in human growth, metabolism, and environmental adaptation
- Along with the nervous system, the endocrine system provides a communication system for the body
- By releasing hormones from various ductless glands, the endocrine system carefully regulates many physiologic functions
- Nursing history
  - The nurse asks the patient about his *chief complaint*
    - A patient with an endocrine disorder may report abnormalities of fatigue, mental status changes, polydipsia, polyuria, weakness, and weight change
    - The patient with an endocrine disorder may also report problems of sexual maturity and function
  - The nurse then questions the patient about his *present illness*
    - Ask the patient about his symptom, including when it started, associated symptoms, location, radiation, intensity, duration, frequency, and precipitating and alleviating factors
    - Ask about the use of prescription and over-the-counter drugs, herbal remedies, and vitamin and nutritional supplements
  - The nurse asks about *medical history*
    - Question the patient about other endocrine disorders, such as diabetes mellitus, Addison's disease (AD), and Cushing's disease; height and weight problems; sexual problems; and thyroid disease
    - Ask the female patient about past reproductive problems and use of oral contraceptives and hormones; also ask whether she's premenopausal or postmenopausal
  - The nurse then assesses the *family history*
    - Ask about a family history of endocrine disorders, such as diabetes mellitus and thyroid disorders
    - Question the patient about his cultural background and heredity
  - The nurse obtains a *social history*
    - Ask about work, exercise, diet, use of recreational drugs, alcohol use, and hobbies
    - Also ask about stress, support systems, and coping mechanisms
- Physical assessment
  - The nurse begins with *inspection*
    - Observe the patient's general appearance and development, height, weight, posture, body build, proportionality of body parts, and distribution of body fat and hair
    - Note affect, speech, level of consciousness, orientation, appropriateness of behavior, grooming and dress, and activity level
    - Assess overall skin color, turgor, and moisture and, for areas of abnormal pigmentation, note any bruising, lesions, petechiae, or striae
    - Assess the face for erythematous areas, noting facial expression, shape, and symmetry of the eyes; also note abnormal lid closure, eyeball protrusion, and periorbital edema, if present
    - Inspect the tongue for color, size, lesions, tremor, and positioning
    - Inspect the neck area for symmetry
    - Evaluate the overall size, shape, and symmetry of the chest, noting any deformities, especially around the nipples
    - Check for truncal obesity, supraclavicular fat pads, and buffalo hump

○ Inspect the external genitalia for normal development

○ Inspect the arms and legs for tremors, muscle development and strength, symmetry, color, hair distribution, and edema

○ Examine the feet, noting size, deformities, lesions, marks from shoes and socks, maceration, dryness, or fissures

- Next, the nurse uses *palpation*
  ○ Palpate the thyroid gland for size, symmetry, and shape; note any nodules or irregularities
  ○ Palpate the testes for size, symmetry, and shape; note any nodules or deformities
- Then, the nurse uses *auscultation*
  ○ Auscultate the thyroid gland to identify systolic bruits
  ○ Auscultate the heart, noting heart rhythm disturbances that may occur in endocrine disorders

Addison's Disease

- Description
  - The adrenal cortex produces *cortisol*, a glucocorticoid, which controls glucose metabolism and is needed for a normal stress response; *aldosterone*, a mineralocorticoid, regulates sodium and potassium levels and thereby influences fluid balance and acid-base balance; and *androgens* contribute to growth and development in both sexes
  - AD is chronic adrenocortical insufficiency, which is rare but has a high morbidity and mortality with the lack of or delayed treatment. AD is classified as primary insufficiency, secondary insufficiency, or acute adrenal crisis. Primary insufficiency commonly occurs between 30 and 50 years of age, affects women more than men, and results from low levels of cortisol and aldosterone. In Western countries, it is most commonly caused by autoimmune destruction of the adrenal cortex, whereas tuberculosis is the main culprit in developing countries
  - Other causes of primary adrenal insufficiency include diseases such as sarcoidosis and histoplasmosis, metastatic disease (rarely), radiation therapy, sudden withdrawal of steroid therapy, surgical removal of both adrenal glands, and human immunodeficiency virus (HIV) infection
  - Secondary adrenal insufficiency stems from inadequate pituitary secretion of corticotropin (ACTH)
  - Acute adrenal crisis is life-threatening and results from a serious lack of cortisol, which can occur in adrenal hemorrhage or thrombosis; from medications, such as ketoconazole, phenytoin (Dilantin), and rifampin; from rapid withdrawal of long-term steroid therapy; or in stressful situations (infection, trauma, surgery, emotional, or psychological stress)
  - Lack of cortisol diminishes gluconeogenesis, decreases liver glycogen, and increases the sensitivity of peripheral tissues to insulin
  - Lack of aldosterone decreases the kidney's ability to retain sodium, which contributes to hypovolemia, and causes potassium reabsorption
  - Low levels of androgens affect libido, menstrual cycles, and hair distribution
- Signs and symptoms
  - Almost all patients complain of fatigue, progressive muscle weakness, poor appetite, and weight loss
  - The skin and mucous membranes may appear bronze from increased levels of melanocyte-stimulating hormone, and with chronic adrenal insufficiency, some patients have vitiligo
  - Patients may crave salt and present with signs of dehydration, hyperkalemia, hypoglycemia, hyponatremia, and loss of axillary, extremity, and pubic hair. Male patients may complain of impotence and decreased libido; females may have amenorrhea
  - In adrenal crisis, patients will present with confusion to being comatose; have abdominal or flank pain, nausea, vomiting, high fever, hypoglycemia, and hyponatremia; and exhibit signs of vascular collapse (shock) and acute kidney injury (AKI)
- Diagnosis and treatment
  - Laboratory tests may show low levels of plasma and urine cortisol and elevated levels of plasma corticotropin as well as hyperkalemia, hyponatremia, hypoglycemia, and metabolic acidosis. If hypovolemic, blood urea nitrogen (BUN), creatinine, hemoglobin, and hematocrit levels will be increased
  - In a rapid corticotropin test (cosyntropin test), plasma cortisol levels remain low
  - Other diagnostic procedures such as computed tomography (CT) scans, CXR, EKG, and tests for tuberculosis, if suspected, may be ordered

- Treatment consists of replacing cortisol with glucocorticoids such as prednisone (Deltasone), which is given in two daily doses (usually on arising and at 6 p.m.) to mimic the body's diurnal variations; doses must be increased during periods of stress. Mineralocorticoid replacement is done with fludrocortisone (Florinef), which is given daily
  - Treatment also includes the prevention of acute adrenal crisis. In the event of a crisis, patients require immediate IV normal saline to restore fluid balance, IV cortisol replacement with high doses of hydrocortisone sodium succinate (Cortef) or dexamethasone (Decadron), IV pressors, NGT to prevent aspiration, bed rest, decreased environmental stimuli, and frequent monitoring of labs, vital signs, and their overall condition
- Nursing interventions
  - Monitor the patient's daily weight, glucose and electrolyte levels, vital signs, cardiac rhythm, intake and output, and renal function to determine the effectiveness of treatment and to watch for signs and symptoms of adrenal crisis
  - Ensure strict adherence to the steroid replacement schedule to prevent crisis
  - Decrease environmental stressors as much as possible
  - Educate and prepare the patient for the diagnostic procedures
  - Teach the patient and family about the disease and its treatment (the dosage, purpose, frequency and effects of steroid replacement therapy, the significance of never omitting a medication dose, notifying the practitioner for any illness [cold, flu, etc.] so dosage adjustments can be made, the need for consistent follow-up care/management, and the need to wear a medical identification bracelet)
  - Teach the patient to avoid undue stress and to seek learning stress management techniques, if needed, to prevent an adrenal crisis
  - Teach the patient and family the signs/symptoms of an adrenal crisis and to seek help immediately from a practitioner. If a glucocorticoid injection kit is prescribed to be carried in case of an emergency, ensure they know how to use it

Cushing's Syndrome

- Description
  - Cushing's syndrome is hyperfunction of the adrenal cortex caused by an overabundance of cortisol
  - It is classified as corticotropin (ACTH) dependent (80% of cases) or independent (20%)
    - With ACTH-dependent Cushing's syndrome, the pituitary's excessive secretion of ACTH results in cortical hyperfunction; 65% to 70% of these cases are related to a pituitary adenoma
    - With ACTH-independent Cushing's syndrome, high levels of cortisol are independent of corticotropin regulation; 18% to 20% of cases are caused by an adrenal cortex adenoma or carcinoma. The majority of ACTH-independent Cushing's syndrome cases are due to long-term glucocorticoid (such as prednisone) administration to treat a nonendocrine disorder
  - For patients with this disorder, excessive cortisol leads to excessive glucose production and interferes with the cells' ability to use insulin; sodium retention, potassium excretion, and protein breakdown occur; body fat is redistributed from the arms and legs to the face, shoulders, trunk, and abdomen; and the immune system becomes less effective at preventing infection
- Signs and symptoms
  - Muscle weakness and atrophy may be accompanied by fat deposits on the trunk, abdomen, over the upper back ("buffalo hump"), and face ("moon face")
  - Skin changes may include acne, bruising, facial flushing, hyperpigmentation, striae, thinning of the skin, and hirsutism (fine, downy hair on the face and upper body)
  - Erectile dysfunction or decreased libido may occur in men; menstrual irregularities, in women
  - Other clinical manifestations may include arrhythmias, edema, hypertension, hyperglycemia, polyuria, hypokalemia, emotional lability, psychosis, GI disturbances, headaches, infection, osteoporosis, pathological fractures (vertebral, rib, long bone), and weight gain/obesity
- Diagnosis and treatment
  - The low-dose dexamethasone suppression test, 24-hour urine-free cortisol test, and late-night salivary cortisol level test are standard screening tests for Cushing's syndrome. Low-dose dexamethasone does not suppress the plasma cortisol levels, urine cortisol levels are elevated three to four times above normal, and high levels of cortisol are noted in late-night salivary test for patients with Cushing's syndrome

- Laboratory tests may show coagulopathies, leukocytosis, hyperglycemia, hypokalemia, hypernatremia, and increased aldosterone and cortisol levels. CT scan or magnetic resonance imaging (MRI) may show a pituitary or adrenal tumor
- The goal of treatment is to restore normal cortisol levels by addressing the primary cause
  - For a pituitary tumor, a transsphenoidal microadenomectomy is recommended; for failed pituitary surgeries or a suspected pituitary tumor, pituitary gland irradiation is used
  - For adrenal cortex adenoma or carcinoma, unilateral or bilateral adrenalectomy is required. For pituitary destruction and after bilateral adrenalectomy, the patient requires lifelong corticosteroid replacement. The patient will require hormone placement therapy for signs/symptoms of hypopituitarism. Lifelong mineralocorticoid replacement is also required for patients who have undergone a bilateral adrenalectomy
- If surgery is contraindicated, delayed or unsuccessful, drug therapy is used to decrease cortisol levels. For ACTH-dependent Cushing's syndrome, pasireotide (Signifor) is given to inhibit ACTH secretion, which thereby decreases cortisol levels. Drugs used to control adrenal cortisol secretion are ketoconazole (Nizoral) and metyrapone (Metopirone). Ketoconazole is the most commonly used in the United States; patients must be closely monitored for hepatotoxicity. For patients with an adrenal carcinoma or as an adjunct to therapy, an adrenolytic agent, mitotane (Lysodren), may be used. Mifepristone (Korlym) has been used to block glucocorticoid receptors to control hyperglycemia with type 2 diabetic patients and those who have failed surgeries
- Nursing interventions
  - Teach the patient and family about the disorder, diagnostic procedures, treatment, medications, surgery and/or radiation (as required). Encourage wearing a medical alert bracelet, utilizing effective coping strategies, and seeking ongoing follow-up care from a practitioner
  - Administer replacement medication as prescribed, and be familiar with its adverse effects
  - Encourage the patient to express concerns about altered body image and offer emotional support
  - Protect the patient from injury related to osteoporosis and abnormal fat distribution by maintaining a safe environment, teaching to the proper use of a walker or cane, encouraging the use of well-fitting shoes or slippers, and attending to complaints of lower back pain or joint pain
  - Encourage a high-protein, high-potassium, high-calcium, low-carbohydrate, low-sodium diet
  - Protect the patient from injury related to easy bruising and protein wasting by avoiding unnecessary venipunctures, using paper tape for dressing changes, avoiding overinflation of the blood pressure cuff, keeping the skin clean and dry, and using a waffle mattress, a water mattress, or an air bed for a patient with skin breakdown
  - Provide care related to limited mobility and muscle weakness resulting from protein catabolism by planning rest periods, encouraging range-of-motion exercises or daily muscle-strengthening exercises, and referring the patient for physical therapy, if needed
  - Protect the patient from infection related to decreased immune function by using strict aseptic technique (when appropriate), encouraging hand hygiene, and discouraging ill family members from visiting the patient. Offer age-appropriate vaccinations such as influenza, H. zoster, and pneumococcal vaccines
  - Provide postoperative care after adrenalectomy, including monitoring vital signs frequently, ensuring adequate pain relief and fluid intake and output, and monitoring for and preventing complications of hypoglycemia, atelectasis, hemorrhage, deep vein thrombosis, atelectasis, and adrenal crisis. For patients requiring transsphenoidal surgery, provide pain relief and frequent mouth care, keep the head of the bed elevated 30 degrees to decrease swelling, avoid activities that would increase intracranial pressure, monitor for and be prepared to care for signs/symptoms of bleeding, diabetes insipidus, hypopituitarism, and cerebrospinal fluid leak

Diabetes Insipidus and Syndrome of Inappropriate Antidiuretic Hormone

- Description
  - Vasopressin is natural antidiuretic hormone (ADH) that is produced by the hypothalamus and secreted by the posterior pituitary. ADH controls water reabsorption by the kidney. Diabetes insipidus (DI) is a deficiency of ADH, resulting in excessive diuresis, which can potentially cause severe dehydration, if not treated. *Central diabetes insipidus* results from the disruption of the normal production, storage, and/or

release of ADH. *Nephrogenic diabetes insipidus* results when the renal tubules do not respond to ADH, also known as vasopressin

- Syndrome of inappropriate antidiuretic hormone (SIADH) is caused by the release of excessive ADH, resulting in water retention (see *Comparing Diabetes Insipidus and SIADH*, pages 227–228)
- Nursing interventions
  - Educate and support the patient during the water deprivation test
  - Assess the patient's hydration status and monitor for signs and symptoms of fluid volume overload (FVO) and/or fluid volume deficit (FVD). Assess electrolytes, BUN/creatinine, and hemoglobin/hematocrit results. Maintain strict intake and output; monitor urinary color and specific gravity, daily weights, and vital signs. Notify the practitioner for noted complications
  - Administer prescribed medications and/or fluid therapies as ordered
  - Provide oral and skin care, and reposition the patient frequently to prevent skin breakdown
  - Conserve energy for a patient with DI who is up often during the night to void or drink; encourage short naps to prevent sleep deprivation
  - Protect the patient from injury related to fatigue, weakness, dehydration, or confusion by providing a safe environment, encouraging a weak patient to request assistance in walking to and from the bathroom, teaching a patient to sit up gradually to prevent dizziness resulting from orthostatic hypotension, and instituting seizure precautions for a patient with severe hyponatremia
  - Teach the patient and family to recognize the signs/symptoms of diabetes insipidus and SIADH, FVO, and FVD and the need to maintain follow-up appointments after discharge to determine the maintenance and effectiveness of therapy
  - Teach the patient about the dosage, purpose, action, effect, and side effects of all prescribed medications, and encourage wearing a medical alert bracelet

Box 14-1: Comparing Diabetes Insipidus and SIADH

This chart summarizes the major characteristics of central and nephrogenic diabetes insipidus and syndrome of inappropriate antidiuretic hormone (SIADH).

Characteristic	Central Diabetes Insipidus	Nephrogenic Diabetes Insipidus	SIADH
Cause	• Head trauma or surgery • Pituitary or hypothalamic tumor • Intracerebral occlusion or infection	• Systemic diseases involving the kidney, such as multiple myeloma, sickle cell anemia, and Sjögren's syndrome • Polycystic kidney disease • Pyelonephritis • Medications such as lithium and demeclocycline • Genetics (X-linked recessive gene) • Chronic hypercalcemia • Chronic hypokalemia	• Central nervous system disorders, such as head trauma, infection, cerebral hemorrhage, cerebrovascular accidents (CVA), or tumor • Pharmacologic agents, including chemotherapeutic agents, opiates, barbiturates, phenothiazines, tricyclic antidepressants, and Ecstasy • Pulmonary disorders and treatment, such as pneumonia, pneumothorax, atelectasis, chronic obstructive pulmonary disease (COPD), and positive-pressure ventilation • Neoplasms
Pathophysiology	• Loss of vasopressin-producing cells, causing deficiency in antidiuretic hormone (ADH) synthesis or release; deficiency in ADH, resulting in an inability to conserve water, leading to extreme polyuria and polydipsia	• Inability of the nephrons to respond to ADH, causing extreme polyuria and polydipsia	• Inappropriate release of ADH, causing dilutional hyponatremia, leading to cellular swelling and water retention

(continued)

Box 14-1: Comparing Diabetes Insipidus and SIADH (continued)

Characteristic	Central Diabetes Insipidus	Nephrogenic Diabetes Insipidus	SIADH
Signs and symptoms	• Polyuria with urine output of 5 to 15 L daily • Polydipsia, especially a desire for cold fluids • Marked dehydration, as evidenced by dry mucous membranes, dry skin, decreased skin turgor weight loss, decreased alertness, tachycardia, hypotension, postural hypotension • Anorexia and epigastric fullness • Nocturia and related fatigue from interrupted sleep	• Same as for central diabetes insipidus	• Excessive or inappropriate water retention (FVO): tachycardia, edema, shortness of breath, crackles in lungs • Weight gain, decreased urinary output, dark amber urine • Initially, malaise, anorexia, headaches, nausea, and vomiting • Later, confusion, irritability, seizures, and coma from severe hyponatremia
Diagnostic test results	• High serum osmolality, usually above 300 mOsm/kg of water • Low urine osmolarity, usually <200 mOsm/kg of water; low urine-specific gravity of <1.005 • Increased creatinine and blood urea nitrogen (BUN) levels, hypernatremia (Na+ > 145 mEq/L), elevated hemoglobin/hematocrit resulting from dehydration • Positive response to water deprivation test: urine output decreases and specific gravity increases after vasopressin administration • MRI to assess the hypothalamus and pituitary gland for tumors, etc.	• Same as for central diabetes insipidus, except that plasma vasopressin levels are elevated in relation to plasma osmolality, and there is no response to exogenous vasopressin administration	• Low serum osmolality • High urine osmolality • Low serum sodium level <135 mEq/L • High urine sodium level, usually over 20 mEq/L • Decreased to normal creatinine and BUN levels • Elevated serum ADH levels • Negative response to water deprivation test: urine output increases and specific gravity decreases
Treatments	• Replacement vasopressin therapy with oral, intranasal, or I.V. desmopressin acetate (DDAVP) • Correction of dehydration and electrolyte imbalances	• A thiazide diuretic to deplete sodium and increase renal water reabsorption • Potassium-sparing diuretic such as amiloride hydrochloride (Midamor) • Nonsteroidal antiinflammatory agents (NASIDs) such as indomethacin (Indocin) • Restriction of salt and protein intake	• Restriction of water intake to 1 qt (0.9 L) daily • Loop diuretics to decrease fluid volume • *For emergent care*: infusions of 3% sodium chloride to replace sodium • *For acute care*: demeclocycline to reverse hyperosmolarity • Vasopressin receptor antagonists such as tolvaptan (Samsca) or conivaptan (Vaprisol) for dilutional hyponatremia

Diabetes Mellitus

- Description
  - Diabetes mellitus is a chronic systemic disease that results from insulin deficiency, insulin resistance, or both, which makes insulin unavailable to cells; the discrepancy between the amount of insulin available to tissues and the amount needed leads to impaired carbohydrate, protein, and fat metabolism. It's the most common endocrine disorder and the seventh leading cause of death in the United States. Four general classifications are recognized:
  - *Prediabetes* is when the fasting blood glucose is greater than 100 mg/dL and less than 126 mg/dL, the hemoglobin A_{1C} ranges from 5.7% to 6.4%, or glucose levels are outside the normal range (140 to 199 mg/dL) following a glucose tolerance test
  - *Type 1 diabetes mellitus* (T1DM), previously insulin-dependent (IDDM) or juvenile-onset diabetes mellitus, is an absolute deficiency of insulin secretion. It may be hereditary, or due to toxic chemicals, histocompatibility antigens, some viruses, or abnormal antibodies that attack the islet of Langerhans cells
  - *Type 2 diabetes mellitus* (T2DM), previously non–insulin-dependent (NIDDM) or adult-onset diabetes mellitus, starts with insulin resistance (cells do not properly use insulin) and later results from defects in insulin secretion as beta cell function decreases over time. It accounts for 90% to 95% of diabetic patients
  - *Gestational diabetes mellitus* is glucose intolerance during pregnancy and is most common in obese females and those with a family history of diabetes mellitus. It usually disappears after delivery but 5% to 10% may develop into T1DM or T2DM
  - Other types of diabetes mellitus can be linked either to a disorder (such as an endocrinopathy, a genetic syndrome, an insulin receptor disorder, or an infection) or to the use of a drug or a chemical (such as a corticosteroid, epinephrine, furosemide, glucagon, lithium, or phenytoin)
  - Many complications and premature death are associated with diabetes mellitus; hence, early detection and constant surveillance and therapy are paramount
    - Macrovascular changes increase the risk of heart disease, accelerate atherosclerotic disease, and cause cerebrovascular accidents (CVA), hypertension, and peripheral vascular disease
    - Microvascular changes thicken capillary basement membranes and cause changes in the vessels of the nerves, kidneys, and eyes (glaucoma, retinopathy, cataracts, and corneal disease). Diabetes mellitus is the top cause of blindness and kidney failure
    - Motor and sensory neuropathies may result in weakness, hyperesthesia, hypoesthesia, and pain; autonomic neuropathy generally occurs after many years and may cause cardiac abnormalities, diabetic diarrhea, gastroparesis, impotence, and urinary retention. Of patients with diabetes mellitus, 60% to 70% suffer with nervous system damages, and diabetes is attributable to 60% of nontraumatic lower limb amputations. Infections can result from accumulation of serum glucose in the skin and poorly functioning white blood cells
- Signs and symptoms
  - The classic signs and symptoms are polydipsia, polyphagia, polyuria, and weight loss
  - Other effects may include fatigue, somnolence, and recurrent infections
- Diagnosis and treatment
  - Diagnosis may be based on symptoms of diabetes mellitus and a casual plasma glucose level greater than 200 mg/dL, an 8-hour fasting plasma glucose level greater than 126 mg/dL, or a 2-hour postload glucose level greater than 200 mg/dL during an oral glucose tolerance test; testing must be confirmed on a subsequent day
  - Hemoglobin A_{1C} levels reflect the plasma glucose level during the past 2 to 3 months (less than 7% reflects good control and decreases complications, whereas greater than or equal to 8% indicates poor glycemic control)
  - The first goal of treatment is to maintain a normal blood glucose level through compliance with oral antidiabetic or insulin therapy, diet control, weight control, physical activity, and education (see *Treatments for Diabetes Mellitus*, pages 232–233)
  - The second goal of treatment is to prevent or delay the complications
    - A decrease in A_{1C} by 1% will reduce microvascular changes by 40%
    - Losing weight and increasing physical activity in prediabetes can delay diabetes, and bringing blood glucose levels to normal decreases the risk for heart disease and stroke

○ Strict glycemic control, controlling hypertension and dyslipidemia, and smoking cessation are necessary to prevent retinopathy, nephropathy, and neuropathy. Hypoglycemia (insulin shock) is a condition in which the blood glucose level falls below the level required to sustain homeostasis (usually less than or equal to 70 mg/dL); it may result from too little food, too much insulin or oral antidiabetic agents, or too much exercise and can cause permanent neurologic damage or rebound hyperglycemia

   ○ Onset occurs in minutes to hours, but most often before meals, especially if meals are delayed or snacks omitted

   ○ Initially, patients may experience sweating, weakness, fatigue, tremor, tachycardia, palpitations, headache, light-headedness, hunger, anxiety, irritability, or inappropriate behavior

   ○ They may also have a blood glucose level less than or equal to 70 mg/dL; pallor; cool, moist skin; confusion; hallucinations; blurred vision; nausea; vomiting; and, in extreme cases, seizures, coma, or death

○ Hypoglycemia is treated with 15 g of carbohydrates (4 oz apple juice, 4 oz regular soda, three glucose tablets, 5 to 6 hard candies, or 1 tbsp honey) if the patient is awake; if the patient is unconscious, treatment is an I.V. bolus of 50% dextrose solution, or 1 mg glucagon given subcutaneously or I.M.; the patient requires follow-up glucose monitoring in 15 minutes after treatment, and retreatment, if necessary. Once the hypoglycemia is reversed, the patient needs to eat a regular meal or snack to prevent repeated hypoglycemia. If the meal is more than one hour from the hypoglycemic episode, a snack of 15 gm carbohydrates (CHO) and 1 oz protein should be eaten. The cause should be identified. If the patient required glucagon to be given, follow-up oral or I.V. glucose is required

○ Hyperglycemia is a condition in which the blood glucose level exceeds 140 mg/dL

   ○ When blood glucose exceeds 180 mg/dL, glucose is excreted in urine along with large amounts of water and electrolytes. Without treatment, excessive thirst, hunger, dehydration, and ketosis also occur

   ○ Hyperglycemia is treated with short-acting insulin, CHO restriction, and exercise to lower blood glucose levels

○ Diabetic ketoacidosis (DKA) affects T1DM patients and results from too little insulin, which prevents glucose from entering cells and causes it to accumulate in the blood

   ○ DKA is treated with regular I.V. insulin, I.V. fluids to supplement intravascular volume, potassium replacement, and sodium bicarbonate if the pH is less than 6.9

○ Hyperosmolar hyperglycemic nonketotic syndrome (HHNS) is associated with T2DM patients and resembles DKA, but ketoacidosis doesn't occur because the pancreas secretes enough insulin to inhibit lipolysis (see *Understanding the Difference Between DKA and HHNS*, page 233)

   ○ HHNS can be precipitated by infection, myocardial infarction (MI), stroke, pancreatitis, a severe burn treated with a high concentration of sugar, stress, or therapy with thiazide diuretic, a mannitol steroid, phenytoin, or total parenteral nutrition

   ○ It occurs most frequently in persons ages 50 to 70 who have no history of diabetes as well as in those with mild type 2 diabetes

   ○ It's treated with insulin, I.V. fluids with half-normal saline solution or normal saline solution, and potassium replacement when urine output is adequate

● Nursing interventions

  ● Protect the patient from infection and injury related to circulatory compromise and possible nerve impairment. Educate the patient and family to check the feet daily, to avoid heating pads, and to exercise caution when near open fires because burns are more difficult to treat in diabetic patients

  ● Apply lanolin to the feet and ankles after hygiene and carefully dry the patient's feet, especially between the toes. Encourage the use of cotton socks to reduce moisture, and suggest wearing high-quality, well-fitting shoes with pressure-absorbing insoles

  ● Have the patient's toenails clipped by a podiatrist

  ● Discuss causes of an aching, burning, or numbness sensation in the feet, legs, or hands and the importance of glucose control to prevent further damage

  ● Provide foot cradles to prevent contact with bed linens for a patient in severe pain

  ● Encourage exercise as tolerated, which helps to relieve pain, improve muscle strength, and prevent atrophy. Instruct the patient about the medications that may be ordered for peripheral neuropathy such as gabapentin (Neurontin) or pregabalin (Lyrica)

- Inform the patient and family of routine skin care and treatment of minor injuries; discuss which injuries and/or wounds should be reported to a practitioner
- Diabetic foot ulcers require a multidisciplinary team approach and consistent follow-up
- Care during DKA or HHNS:
  - Treat fluid loss caused by hyperglycemia by infusing I.V. isotonic (normal) or hypotonic (half-normal) saline solution
  - Administer IV insulin as ordered
  - When blood glucose level falls below 200 mg/dL, administer I.V. dextrose 5% in water to prevent hypoglycemia
  - Closely monitor serum glucose levels, hourly urine output, and key laboratory results such as serum electrolyte levels, arterial pH, serum bicarbonate, BUN, and creatinine to assess treatment effects and prevent complications
  - Monitor potassium level and replace potassium as needed
- Encourage the patient to obtain and maintain good nutritional habits
  - Obtain a diet history, and note the impact of lifestyle, literacy, and culture on food intake
  - Instruct the patient and family how to count carbohydrate intake, the significance of portion control, making healthy food choices, and eating on a consistent time schedule to prevent hypoglycemia. Encourage the overweight and obese patient to lose weight
  - Explain the importance of exercise and a balanced diet
  - Instruct the patient and family that glucose levels are best checked 30 minutes before eating
  - Encourage attending a class with a registered dietician and seeking consistent follow-up
- Teach the patient and family about the disease, complications, and treatment in focused, short, culturally appropriate sessions encouraging self-care and efficacy
  - Ensure the patient and family are able to perform blood glucose self-testing and are knowledgeable of the significance of self-monitoring on a routine, consistent basis. Have the patient and family verbalize the signs/symptoms, causes, treatment, and complications of hyperglycemia and hypoglycemia
  - For patients who require insulin:
    - Make sure the patient and family know the differences in the type of insulin(s) ordered; how to adjust insulin doses for changes in diet, exercise, and stress level; how to safely store supplies and needs during travel. Have the patient or a family member demonstrate the technique for drawing up and administering insulin utilizing proper site rotation
    - For patients requiring an insulin infusion pump, specific detailed education is needed for starting, maintaining, and adjusting the device and dosages, and routine site care
  - Educate the patient and the family about care during illness—monitor blood glucose levels more frequently, increase fluid intake, and not to stop taking the antidiabetic medication without consulting with the practitioner
- Help the patient to establish a physical activity plan—90 to 150 minutes or more of physical activity per week of moderate-intensity aerobic physical activity 3 days/week, but no more than 2 consecutive days without exercise. Encourage the patient to decrease extended amounts of sedentary time. Exercise can improve A_{1C} in 6 to 12 months in patients with T2DM
- For patients with gastroparesis, provide psychological support and encourage the patient to stop smoking and ingesting alcohol; administer prescribed drugs such as metoclopramide hydrochloride (Reglan) to promote gastric emptying; avoid GLP-1 analogues and amylin analogues; and teach the patient to modify the diet by decreasing fatty, spicy, acidic, and roughage-laden foods, which enhance symptoms, and to eat small, frequent meals. Antiemetics may be required if the patient suffers from nausea and vomiting
- Encourage annual eye exams to prevent retinopathy. For those with advanced visual problems, laser photocoagulation can decrease severe vision loss by 50% to 60%. For patients with retinopathy, encourage independence, provide a safe environment, and elicit the support of community agencies
- Encourage the patient to keep vaccinations up to date and to wear a medical alert bracelet/necklace. Encourage and/or set up diabetic education with trained diabetic educators
- Provide care for a patient with diabetes who has a sexual dysfunction related to neuropathy by encouraging the expression of feelings, exploring options such as a penile prosthesis, and recommending professional counseling as needed
- Promote healthy coping behaviors to improve quality of life, and beware of cognitive and behavioral manifestations of depression, which may require counseling and further follow-up

Box 14-2: Treatments for Diabetes Mellitus

A patient with diabetes mellitus commonly follows a regimen that requires medications (an oral antidiabetic or insulin), diet, and physical activity.

Oral antidiabetics

An oral antidiabetic may be prescribed alone or in combination with another drug and/or insulin for a patient with type 2 diabetes mellitus.

Agents that stimulate insulin release are sulfonylureas and meglitinides.

- A *sulfonylurea* works by stimulating the pancreas to release insulin. Examples are acetohexamide (Dymelor), chlorpropamide (Diabinese), glimepiride (Amaryl), glipizide (Glucotrol), glyburide (Glynase), tolazamide (Tolinase), and tolbutamide (Orinase)
- *Meglitinide analogs* stimulate beta cells to produce insulin in the presence of glucose after eating. Medications in this category are repaglinide (Prandin) and nateglinide (Starlix)

Agents that reduce insulin resistance are biguanides and thiazolidinediones.

- *Biguanides* work by reducing the production of glucose in the liver, making the tissues more sensitive to insulin, and reducing the amount of sugar absorbed by the intestines and may cause hypoglycemia. The most common biguanide is metformin (Glucotrol). Metformin is not for patients with severe renal insufficiency and is a contraindication for IV contrast dye
- *Thiazolidinediones*, such as pioglitazone (Actos) and rosiglitazone (Avandia), increase insulin sensitivity by acting on fat, muscle, and liver cells to increase glucose utilization and decrease glucose production. Thiazolidinediones potentiate the risk of heart failure and edema
  - *Alpha-glucosidase inhibitors* reduce glucose levels by interfering with glucose absorption in the small intestine and have no direct effect on insulin secretion and sensitivity; they should be taken before meals. When used alone, these drugs don't cause hypoglycemia; examples are acarbose (Precose) and miglitol (Glyset)
  - *Amylin analogues*, such as pramlintide (Symlin), are used with T1DM and T2DM patients because they delay gastric emptying and decrease postprandial glucagon to lower blood glucose levels
  - *Incretin therapy* is useful in T2DM patients not well managed with metformin alone and exists in two categories: DPP-4 inhibitors and GLP-1 receptor agonists
- *Dipeptidyl peptidase-4 inhibitors (gliptins/DPP-4 inhibitors)* are oral agents that improve glucose control by blocking the DPP-4 enzyme. Hence, the GLP-1 hormone increases, thereby potentiating insulin secretion and suppressing glucagon release. Sitagliptin (Januvia), alogliptin (Nesina), anagliptin (Suiny), linagliptin (Tradjenta), saxagliptin (Onglyza), teneligliptin (Tenelia), and vildagliptin (Galvus) are in this drug classification
- *Glucagon-like peptide analogues (GLP-1 agonists)* such as exenatide (Byetta), liraglutide (Victoza), lixisenatide (Lyxumia), dulaglutide (Trulicity), and albiglutide (Tanzeum) *are given subcutaneously* and activate GLP-1 receptors on pancreatic beta cells to lower glucose levels, delay gastric emptying, and promote weight loss
  - *Sodium glucose cotransporter 2 inhibitors (SGLT-2 inhibitors)* block reabsorption of glucose in the kidney. This drug classification includes canagliflozin (Invokana), dapagliflozin (Forxiga), and empagliflozin (Jardiance)

Unless combined with insulin, the agents that should not cause hypoglycemia are thiazolidinediones, DDP-4 inhibitors, GLP-1 agonists, SGLT-2 inhibitors, and alpha-glucosidase inhibitors.

Insulin

Insulin therapy may be prescribed for T1DM, T2DM uncontrolled with oral agents, and other patients experiencing hyperglycemia.

Regular insulin is *short-acting*, with an onset of 30 to 60 minutes, a peak of 2 to 4 hours, and a duration of 6 to 10 hours; use of this insulin increases the chance of hypoglycemia if given three to four times per day due to action overlap.

Lispro (Humalog) and aspart (NovoLog) are *rapid-acting* insulins with an onset of 5 to 15 minutes, a peak of 1 to 2 hours, and a duration of 3 to 6 hours. Rapid-acting insulins should be held if the patient is NPO or unable to tolerate food or caloric intake.

NPH (Novolin N/Humulin N) insulin is an *intermediate-acting* therapy with an onset of 1 to 2 hours, produces peak action in 4 to 12 hours, and produces effects for 14 to 24 hours.

Glargine (Lantus) and detemir (Levemir) insulins are *basal* insulins. They have an onset of 1 to 2 hours, have no peak effectiveness period, and last 20 to 24 hours. Basal insulins are administered daily and should be given regardless of nutritional intake and not held if glucose levels are within normal levels. If the patient is hospitalized, to maintain glucose management, basal insulin should be given according to the patient's home schedule.

A basal bolus insulin regimen is the preferred approach to glucose control because it mimics normal physiology. The bolus dose is prandial/mealtime insulin based on CHO ingestion. Correction dose insulin is not synonymous with sliding scale insulin (SSI). Correction dose insulin is given based on the patient's glucose level 30 minutes before mealtime. An SSI regimen alone provides inadequate glucose control.

(continued)

Box 14-2: Treatments for Diabetes Mellitus (continued)

An insulin pump may be used to deliver rapid-acting insulin to meet both basal and bolus needs; the pump can be implanted under the skin or worn externally.

Concentrated insulins such as Humulin R U-500 and insulin glargine U-200 or U-300 are available for patients who are severely insulin resistant. Concentrated glargine insulins are routinely given via prefilled pens. U-500 insulin is to be administered with its own U-500 syringe.

Diet

Diet therapy is individualized based on metabolic, nutritional, and lifestyle requirements. Emphasis is placed on achieving glucose (A_{1C}), lipid (low-density lipoprotein [LDL] cholesterol), and blood pressure control by focusing on the quantity of intake, the timing of meals and snacks, and their nutritional content. Fat intake should focus on fat quality more than fat quantity; saturated and trans fatty acids should be minimized while monosaturated and polyunsaturated fat encouraged. Protein intake should be 10% to 20% of total calories depending on the patient's medical condition. Lean meats, fish, eggs, beans, peas, soy products, nuts, and seeds are preferable over red meats. Fiber intake of 14 g/1,000 calories daily is recommended with sodium intake limited to 2,000 to 2,300 mg daily. Monitoring the amount of carbohydrates ingested and ensuring a consistent intake are crucial to improving glycemic control, preventing hypoglycemia, promoting weight loss for overweight and obese patients, and positively impacting hypertension and lipid levels. Carbohydrates from fruits, vegetables, legumes, and low-fat milk are encouraged. For those patients who wish to drink alcohol (ETOH), it should be limited to one drink per day for females and two for males, consumed with food, counted as carbohydrate intake, and its effects on the blood glucose levels monitored.

Physical activity

Exercise lowers blood glucose levels, maintains normal cholesterol levels, helps blood vessels perform more effectively, and may reduce the amount of insulin needed. Therefore, the patient should follow a consistent exercise program, engaging in activity when glucose levels are high. (Carbohydrate intake must be increased if the patient exercises when glucose levels are low or strenuous activity is planned.)

Box 14-3: Understanding the Difference Between DKA and HHNS

Diabetic ketoacidosis (DKA) and hyperosmolar hyperglycemic nonketotic syndrome (HHNS), both acute complications associated with diabetes, share some similarities, including changes in level of consciousness and extreme volume depletion, but they're two distinct conditions. The following chart helps determine which condition your patient is experiencing.

	Associated with	Onset	Symptoms
DKA	Type 1 diabetes mellitus	Rapid	• Hyperventilation (Kussmaul's respirations) • Acetone breath odor • Blood glucose level above normal (200 to 800 mg/dL) • Mild hyponatremia • Positive or large serum ketones • Serum osmolality slightly elevated • Hyperkalemia initially, then hypokalemia • Metabolic acidosis
HHNS	Type 2 diabetes mellitus	Slow	• Slightly rapid respirations • No breath odor • Blood glucose level markedly elevated (above 600 mg/dL) • Hypernatremia • Negative or small serum ketones • Serum osmolality markedly elevated • Normal serum potassium • Lack of acidosis

Hyperparathyroidism

- Description
  - Hyperparathyroidism is characterized by excessive uncontrolled secretion of parathyroid hormone (PTH), one of the two major hormones that modulates calcium and phosphate homeostasis. PTH is necessary for the formation of active vitamin D, which stimulates intestinal absorption of calcium; acts on bone to release calcium; and acts on the kidney to foster calcium uptake and eliminate phosphorus
  - Hyperparathyroidism is classified as primary or secondary
    - In primary hyperparathyroidism, inappropriately high PTH secretion results in hypercalcemia from an adenoma, hyperplasia, or malignancy
    - In secondary hyperparathyroidism, the parathyroid glands respond appropriately to a reduced level of extracellular calcium. PTH concentrations rise causing increased intestinal absorption of calcium and removal of calcium from the bones. The most common cause is chronic kidney disease (CKD); other causes include decreased intestinal absorption or insufficient consumption of vitamin D or calcium and genetic disorders
  - Primary hyperparathyroidism can occur at any age, but the majority of cases occur in the elderly with 90% being women, probably because the increase in bone resorption that follows menopause unmasks parathyroid gland hyperactivity. Patients who have had neck radiation therapy and those who have taken lithium for bipolar disorder are also prone to its development
  - Complications may include osteoporosis, long bone or rib fractures, renal calculi development, cardiac arrhythmias, hypertension, cholelithiasis, and pancreatitis
  - Hypercalcemic crisis can occur with extreme elevations of serum calcium levels and can result in life-threatening neurologic, cardiovascular, and renal complications
- Signs and symptoms
  - Some patients may be asymptomatic or have vague symptoms. Clinical manifestations result from hypercalcemia. Renal signs/symptoms include polyuria and thirst, a history of recurring nephrolithiasis, and hypercalciuria. Osteoporosis contributes to pathologic fractures. GI symptoms include abdominal pain, anorexia, nausea, vomiting, pancreatitis, or peptic ulcer development. Patients may also complain of muscle weakness, cardiac arrhythmias, and personality changes, lethargy, depression, confusion, and cognitive dysfunction
  - Laboratory findings show persistently elevated serum PTH and calcium levels, elevated urine calcium levels, and decreased serum phosphorus levels
  - Bone densitometry (DXA scan) shows diffuse bone demineralization, bone cysts, outer cortical bone loss, and subperiosteal erosion of the phalanges
  - Sestamibi imaging, ultrasonography, CT scan, and MRI help identify enlargement and abnormally functioning areas
- Diagnosis and treatment
  - The recommended treatment for symptomatic primary hyperparathyroidism is the surgical removal of the abnormal parathyroid tissue. The patient can live normally with half of one functioning parathyroid gland. In some cases, autotransplantation of the parathyroid gland is done in the nondominant lower arm to prevent hypoparathyroidism after surgery
  - For secondary disease, the goal is to correct the underlying cause of the parathyroid hypertrophy
  - For patients who are unable or choose not to undergo surgery, there are no available medications specifically for asymptomatic primary hyperparathyroidism. For symptomatic hypercalcemia, hydration with IV saline followed by loop diuretics such as furosemide (Lasix) can help decrease serum calcium levels in patients without renal failure. Calcimimetics such as cinacalcet hydrochloride (Sensipar) are used to decrease calcium and PTH levels. To reduce bone turnover and maintain bone density, bisphosphonates such as alendronate sodium (Fosamax) are used
- Nursing interventions
  - Teach the patient and family about the disease and its treatment. Encourage the patient to stay well hydrated, participate in regular exercise activities, avoid smoking and immobilization, restrict dietary calcium intake (e.g., dairy products, broccoli, calcium-containing antacids), and undergo regular follow-up tests and procedures

- For patients with secondary hyperparathyroidism, teach the patient to restrict foods high in phosphates and the dosage, frequency, and action of phosphate binders and vitamin D supplements
- Prepare the patient for surgery, if indicated, and provide emotional support
- Monitor the patient's serum potassium, calcium, phosphate, magnesium, and BUN/creatinine levels
- Watch for hypercalcemic crisis; be prepared to administer calcitonin, IV normal saline, and loop diuretics
- Postoperatively, patients may remain for a night or be sent home after a few hours depending on their age, health status, and surgical complications. Patients should be positioned with the head of the bed elevated or using 2 to 3 pillows to diminish edema formation
- Observe for signs of hypocalcemia (numbness and tingling around the mouth and in the extremities, tetany, and laryngeal spasms) and be prepared to administer high doses of calcium and vitamin D
- Before discharge, teach the patient the signs and symptoms of complications (airway restriction, hypocalcemia, infection, bleeding) and appropriate actions to take and how to care for the surgical site; review activity restrictions, pain management, and the importance of follow-up care—including laboratory testing—to evaluate the effectiveness of therapy

Hyperthyroidism

- Description
  - Hyperthyroidism is the excessive production of thyroid hormone resulting in a hypermetabolic state
  - Severe hyperthyroidism can precipitate a thyroid storm or crisis, which is a rare life-threatening emergency; the crisis can be triggered by salicylates, minor trauma, or stress such as surgery, infection, pregnancy, and DKA. Without treatment, there is a 90% mortality rate
  - Hyperthyroidism can be caused by an autoimmune disorder known as Graves' disease, which is the most common, toxic multinodular goiter or toxic adenoma (which is rare) in which the growths make too much thyroid hormone. Hyperthyroidism can also result from discontinuation or noncompliance with antithyroid medications, excessive iodine intake, painless thyroiditis that is triggered by childbirth, and medications such as lithium or amiodarone
  - Signs and symptoms vary with the cause and severity of the disease (see *Signs and Symptoms of Hyperthyroidism*, page 237)
    - Graves' disease commonly occurs in the third or fourth decade of life, is more common in women than in men, and has a familial predisposition. It may cause extrathyroidal symptoms and goiter
    - Toxic multinodular goiter generally occurs in people older than 50, in those who live in iodine deficit areas, and is more common in females than males
- Diagnosis and treatment
  - Laboratory tests show increased levels of thyroid hormones (triiodothyronine [T_3] and thyroxine [T_4]), decreased thyroid-stimulating hormone (TSH) level, and hyperglycemia resulting from impaired insulin secretion
  - Thyroid scan shows increased uptake of radioactive iodine
  - Electrocardiography (ECG) may show sinus tachycardia, atrial fibrillation, or other arrhythmias depending on the severity of the disease and the patient's past medical history
  - The principal goal of treatment is to normalize thyroid hormone levels, thereby preventing a thyroid storm
    - Antithyroid medications are used to decrease morbidity and prevent complications. They are used as a bridge before radioactive iodine or surgery and are used as long-term therapy in the elderly or those patients with cardiac disease. Methimazole (Tapazole) and propylthiouracil (PTU) are slow-acting drugs that block thyroid hormone synthesis and typically produce improvement after 2 to 4 weeks of therapy. The optimal duration of antithyroid medication therapy is a titrated regimen for 12 to 18 months; those with Graves' disease may go into remission. Neither medication is considered safe in pregnancy due to their teratogenic effects
    - As an adjunct to control the sympathetic nervous system's effect on the cardiac system, a beta adrenergic blocker such as propranolol (Inderal) may be used especially in older patients, patients with a heart rate greater than 90, and those with known cardiovascular disease
    - Surgery (subtotal/total thyroidectomy) is reserved for patients with a very large gland, those who cannot tolerate or who are noncompliant with other treatments, those who have thyroid cancer, those with

Graves' disease who wish to become pregnant, and those with recurrent symptoms after medical therapy. Before surgery, the patient receives antithyroid medication to reduce hormone levels and saturated solution of potassium iodide (SSKI) to decrease gland vascularity. The most common complications of a thyroidectomy are injury to the parathyroid glands and/or the recurrent laryngeal nerve. If the patient is at risk for developing hypoparathyroidism after the surgery, calcium and vitamin D preparations are administered preoperatively

- ○ Radioactive iodine therapy (I131) is the treatment of choice for toxic multinodular goiter and toxic adenoma; dosing is based on the patient's symptoms. It's contraindicated during pregnancy, breastfeeding, those who wish to become pregnant in 4 to 6 months, or coexisting or suspected thyroid cancer. Many patients who receive radioactive iodine become euthyroid or hypothyroid requiring lifelong levothyroxine (Synthroid) treatment

- Nursing interventions
  - Obtain baseline serum lab results (T3, T4, TSH, liver function tests, BMP, CBC w/differential) for diagnostic purposes. Monitor for changes to determine the effectiveness of treatment, to prevent complications, and to assess for the occurrence of side effects from antithyroid medications, especially propylthiouracil (PTU), which can result in liver toxicity
  - If the patient has atrial fibrillation, the patient is generally anticoagulated to prevent thrombosis. Follow coagulation lab results as appropriate and teach the patient and family about risks of bleeding
  - Maintain normal fluid and electrolyte balance to prevent arrhythmias and dehydration
  - Tell the patient to avoid caffeine, sugary foods and drinks, and energy bars, which stimulate the sympathetic nervous system. Soy, seafood, and high-iodine foods should also be avoided. The patient should not smoke
  - Provide a high-calorie, high-protein diet through several small, well-balanced meals and snacks
  - Balance rest and activities to conserve the patient's energy to decrease metabolism needs
  - Provide patient and family education about the signs and symptoms of the disease and thyroid storm; the purpose, dosing, and frequency of all prescribed medications; the need for long-term follow-up; and wearing a medical alert bracelet. Teach them to inform their provider of jaundice, dark urine, abdominal pain, nausea, fatigue, rash, and pharyngitis (possible side effects of agranulocytosis or hepatic toxicity from antithyroid medications). Teach them to identify and modulate environmental stressors to prevent thyroid storm and seek medical attention immediately for a fever
  - For women of child-bearing age who desire pregnancy, advocate counseling to assist in their decision-making relative to available treatments
  - If the patient has exophthalmos, administer artificial tears or ointment, and encourage the use of sunglasses for comfort and to protect the eyes from corneal ulcerations. Provide education and emotional support for patients who may receive corticosteroids and orbital radiotherapy for Graves' ophthalmopathy
  - If the patient has diaphoresis, keep the skin dry with powders that contain cornstarch, and frequently change bed linens
  - If the patient undergoes I131 ablation therapy, provide radiation safety education to the patient and close family members. If precautions cannot be followed, an alternative treatment is needed. Ensure a pregnancy test is done on women of child-bearing age before radioactive iodine therapy commences
  - If the patient undergoes a thyroidectomy, keep the bed in Fowler's position to promote venous return from the head; assess for signs of respiratory distress and vocal changes; keep a tracheotomy tray at the bedside; monitor for signs of hemorrhage; monitor serum calcium levels and assess for hypocalcemia (such as tingling and numbness of the extremities, muscle twitching, laryngeal spasm, and positive Chvostek's sign [inducing spasm or twitching of the mouth, nose, and eye by sharply tapping over the facial nerve] and Trousseau's sign [inducing carpopedal spasm by occluding blood flow to the arm with a blood pressure cuff]), which may occur if the parathyroid glands are damaged; keep calcium gluconate available for emergency I.V. administration; and assess for signs of thyroid storm
  - In the event of a thyroid crisis, patients require ICU monitoring and care. Use a cooling blanket and administer acetaminophen (Tylenol) to achieve a normal temperature; establish a cool, calm, dim environment; encourage the use of relaxation techniques; be prepared to administer antithyroid drugs, steroids, beta adrenergic blockers, inorganic iodine, and IV fluids; and provide respiratory support as needed. Progress should be noted in 24 to 48 hours

Box 14-4: Signs and Symptoms of Hyperthyroidism

Graves' disease (signs and symptoms of hypermetabolism and sympathetic nervous system overactivity)

- Brittle hair and friable nails
- Emotional lability, anxiety, irritability, and insomnia
- Fatigue
- Heat intolerance
- Increased respiratory rate and shortness of breath
- Increased sweating
- Loss of pubic hair in women; premature graying in men
- Muscle weakness and atrophy
- Hyperreflexia and hyperkinesis
- Tachycardia with palpitations
- Hypertension
- Tremor
- Warm, moist skin
- Weight loss despite normal or increased appetite
- Polyuria and/or nocturia
- Menstrual disorders
- Gynecomastia and/or erectile dysfunction
- Hyperdefecation (not diarrhea)
- Dysphagia due to the goiter
- New-onset atrial fibrillation (more common in the elderly)
- Cardiac failure

Graves' disease (extrathyroid signs and symptoms; worse in smokers)

- Exophthalmos, diplopia, photophobia, compressive optic neuropathy, exposure keratopathy
- Eyelid lag or a slowed movement of the lid in relation to the eyeball
- Periorbital edema
- Pretibial myxedema that produces raised, thickened skin that may be hyperpigmented, itchy, and well demarcated from normal skin; lesions that appear plaquelike or nodular
- Staring with decreased blinking
- Goiter

Thyroid storm or crisis

- Fever (temperature greater than 38.5°C (101.3°F) that can progress to above 41°C (105.8°F) usually precedes thyroid storm
- Hypertension with widening pulse pressure; hypotension, if shock
- Severe tachycardia and other cardiac arrhythmias such as atrial fibrillation and ventricular tachycardia
- Anxiety and restlessness, which can progress to delirium, seizures, and coma
- Chest pain
- Profuse sweating
- Heat intolerance
- Dehydration
- Respiratory distress
- Vomiting and diarrhea
- Multiple organ failure, which will result in death

Hypoparathyroidism

- Description
  - Hypoparathyroidism occurs when the parathyroid glands do not secrete enough PTH, or the bones and kidneys do not respond to the PTH, resulting in decreased serum calcium levels and elevated phosphorus levels
  - It can be acute or chronic and is classified as idiopathic, acquired, or reversible
  - Hypoparathyroidism, a rare condition, commonly results from inadvertent removal of the parathyroid glands during thyroidectomy. Other causes include congenital/genetic disorders, autoimmune disorders, radiation to the neck, neoplasms, hypomagnesemia, and trauma

- The disorder affects men and women equally
- Complications include cardiac arrhythmias, heart failure, cataracts, bone deformities, and seizures
- Signs and symptoms
  - Because parathyroid glands primarily regulate calcium balance, neuromuscular signs and symptoms range from numbness and tingling (paresthesia) around the mouth or in the extremities to severe cramps and muscle spasms (tetany). The patient may experience wheezing, difficulty breathing, and voice changes due to bronchospasm, laryngeal spasm, and carpopedal spasm (Trousseau's sign) and progress to seizure activity, although rare
  - Positive Chvostek's and Trousseau's signs indicate latent tetany. Trousseau's sign is more indicative of hypocalcemia as Chvostek's sign has been absent in 1/3 of patients with hypocalcemia
  - Other signs and symptoms of the disorder include dry hair, coarse skin, brittle nails, anxiety, irritability, confusion, delirium, mood swings, and EKG changes
- Diagnosis and treatment
  - Increased serum phosphate and decreased serum calcium levels (7.5 mg/dL or less) indicate hypoparathyroidism. There may be EKG changes; urine results may indicate hypercalciuria. Magnesium levels are checked to rule out it being the cause
  - CT scan may show frontal lobe and basal ganglia calcifications
  - X-rays show increased bone density and bone malformation in chronic hypoparathyroidism
  - Therapy aims to increase serum calcium levels to between 9 and 10 mg/dL and to eliminate symptoms
  - A diet high in calcium (dairy products, breakfast cereals, fortified orange juice, and green, leafy vegetables) and low in phosphorus (carbonated soft drinks, eggs, and meat) is prescribed
  - Calcium supplements and vitamin D (calcitriol or ergocalciferol [Calciferol]) are given. In the case of abnormal magnesium levels causing hypoparathyroidism, magnesium levels are normalized. For patients with chronic hypoparathyroidism uncontrolled with calcium and activated vitamin D supplementation, recombinant human parathyroid hormone (1-84) [rhPTH(1-84)] is given parenterally (studies are ongoing to determine its long-term safety)
- Nursing interventions
  - Teach the patient and family about the disease, prescribed medications, high-calcium low-phosphorus diet, the importance of wearing a medical alert bracelet, and receiving lifelong follow-up care to determine the effectiveness of therapy. Provide emotional support
  - Assess the patient for signs/symptoms of hypocalcemia and be prepared to administer IV calcium gluconate, if needed
  - Monitor serum electrolyte levels, especially serum calcium, phosphorus, and magnesium levels
  - Administer calcium supplements and activated vitamin D as ordered, and/or magnesium supplements, if needed

Hypothyroidism

- Description
  - Hypothyroidism is the inadequate production of thyroid hormone resulting in decreased cognitive processes and hypometabolism. Severe hypothyroidism is also known as myxedema
  - Hypothyroidism is more prevalent in Caucasians and Mexican Americans, females more than males, and the incidence increases with age
  - Primary hypothyroidism is caused by thyroid gland dysfunction, while secondary hypothyroidism results from an insufficient secretion of TSH by the pituitary gland, or inadequate release of TSH by the hypothalamus
  - Unrecognized and untreated congenital hypothyroidism, known as cretinism, results in permanent mental and physical retardation
  - Myxedema coma or crisis is a rare, life-threatening clinical situation secondary to long-standing, undiagnosed or untreated hypothyroidism that requires immediate medical attention
  - Hypothyroidism may be caused by worsening of a preexisting hypothyroid condition; insufficient thyroid hormone replacement therapy after hyperthyroidism treatment; pituitary gland dysfunction due to infection, surgery, trauma, or tumor; autoimmune disease; dietary iodine deficiency; and drugs (such as lithium and amiodarone)

- Signs and symptoms
  - Clinical manifestations are dependent on the severity of the hormone deficiency and the acuteness of its development
  - Vital sign measurements may reveal weak pulses, bradycardia, decreased respiratory rate with shallow inspirations, hypotension, and hypothermia
  - Hoarseness, impaired hearing, slowed speech, and slowed movements
  - Sacral or peripheral nonpitting edema periorbital edema; a puffy face, hands, and tongue; and adventitious breath sounds
  - Other effects may include intolerance to cold; dry, coarse skin; fatigue and weakness; cognitive dysfunction, lethargy, apathy, and depression; menstrual irregularities and decreased libido; alopecia; brittle nails, anorexia, constipation, and weight gain (not morbid obesity); muscle cramps and joint pain
  - If untreated, the patient will exhibit signs of myxedema coma, which includes stupor or coma, ascites (rare), hypercapnia, hypoglycemia, hyponatremia, hypothermia, pericardial effusion, and cardiogenic shock
- Diagnosis and treatment
  - Diagnostic tests may include measurement of serum TSH, T_3, and T_4, and free T_4 levels; T_3 resin uptake test; and radioisotope thyroid uptake test
  - Laboratory studies may show a decreased serum T_4 level, a decreased blood glucose level, decreased plasma osmolality, a decreased TSH level (with a pituitary or hypothalamic defect) or an increased TSH level (with a thyroid defect), hyponatremia, hyperlipidemia, and lactic acidosis
  - The primary treatment is lifelong replacement of the deficient hormone to achieve a euthyroid state. Synthetic levothyroxine sodium (Synthroid) is the preferred thyroid hormone replacement and typically relieves symptoms in 2 to 3 days.
  - If myxedema coma develops, immediate I.V. administration of a corticosteroid, glucose, and levothyroxine sodium can reverse this life-threatening condition.
- Nursing interventions
  - Administer replacement therapy as prescribed
  - Avoid sedating the patient, which may further decrease respirations
  - Recognize that slower metabolism may slow drug absorption and excretion
  - Provide frequent skin care to prevent breakdown and decrease the risk of infection
  - Administer fluids as prescribed; correct imbalances without causing fluid overload
  - Monitor fluid intake and output, and weigh the patient daily to check for fluid retention
  - If the patient has hypothermia, increase body temperature gradually by using warm blankets or increasing the room temperature. Do not use a warming blanket, which could potentiate shock
  - Encourage coughing and deep breathing, and administer oxygen as prescribed
  - Gradually increase their activities as their metabolism is restored to normal.
  - Educate the patient and family about the disease and its treatment, the importance of wearing a medical alert bracelet, and the need for consistent lifelong follow-up. Ensure their understanding of the name, purpose, effects, food and drug interactions with the replacement therapy, and the importance of taking it on an empty stomach either early in the morning before breakfast or at bedtime
  - For patients in myxedema coma, maintain a patent airway and be prepared to administer oxygen and provide ventilator support; provide close monitoring of vital signs, ABGs, daily weights, neuro and cardiac status, electrolytes, glucose levels, and I&O. Provide I.V. fluid, electrolyte, and thyroid hormone replacement until the patient begins to recover

Pheochromocytoma

- Description
  - Pheochromocytoma is a tumor that usually originates from the chromaffin cells of the adrenal medulla in 80% to 85% of patients. In a minority of patients, it can occur in the extra-adrenal tissue located in or near the aorta, liver, bladder, or other organs; malignancy is seen more with this tumor type
  - Pheochromocytoma can occur at any age, but its peak incidence is from ages 40 to 60. It affects men and women equally and has a 40% genetic association

- Signs and symptoms
  - The type and severity of signs and symptoms depends on the relative proportions of epinephrine, norepinephrine, or dopamine secreted. In 40% of patients, the classical signs and symptoms are headaches, diaphoresis, palpitations, and hypertension that may be intermittent or persistent
  - Other signs and symptoms may include tremors, flushing, nervousness, and hyperglycemia
  - Forty-five percent of patients present with the paroxysmal form of pheochromocytoma, which is typically characterized by acute, unpredictable attacks that last from seconds to several hours, with symptoms typically beginning abruptly and subsiding slowly. The patient becomes extremely anxious, tremulous, and weak and may have other symptoms, such as tachycardia, nausea, vomiting, diarrhea, abdominal pain, visual disturbances, dizziness, and a feeling of impending doom
  - Severe hypertension can cause serious, life-threatening complications, such as angina, cardiac arrhythmias, myocarditis, dissecting aneurysm, heart failure, stroke, and acute renal failure
- Diagnosis and treatment
  - Pheochromocytoma is suspected in the patient with signs of sympathetic nervous system overactivity such as hypertension, headache, excessive sweating, hypermetabolism, and hyperglycemia
  - Increased urine and plasma levels of catecholamines and metanephrine, a catecholamine metabolite, are the most direct and conclusive tests for overactivity of the adrenal medulla. Urinary vanillylmandelic acid (VMA) and serum chromogranin A (CgA), a tumor marker, may also be ordered
  - If urine and plasma tests of catecholamines are inconclusive, a clonidine suppression test can identify excess catecholamine release that bypasses normal storage and release mechanisms, a characteristic of pheochromocytoma
  - Imaging studies such as CT scanning, MRI, and radiotracing imagery can localize the pheochromocytomas and determine whether the patient has more than one tumor
  - Initial treatment aims to reduce blood pressure to normal levels with phenoxybenzamine (Dibenzyline), an alpha adrenergic blocking agent, being the most common first-line therapy. Other alpha adrenergic and calcium channel blockers may also be used. Beta blockers are to be used only after alpha blockade agents are in use to prevent pulmonary edema
  - If the blood pressure is still not controlled, catecholamine synthesis inhibitors such as metyrosine (Demser) may be used, but side effects can be disabling with long-term use
  - Glucose levels and hemoglobin A_{1C} are monitored. Hyperglycemia is appropriately treated with oral hypoglycemic agents and/or insulin
  - The definitive treatment for pheochromocytoma is surgical removal of the tumor via laparoscopic adrenalectomy unless malignancy is suspected, in which an open approach is required
  - A patient who has undergone bilateral adrenalectomy requires corticosteroid replacement
  - Postoperatively, the patient's blood pressure and catecholamine levels should return to normal; if not, the patient should be evaluated for retention of pheochromocytoma tissue
- Nursing interventions
  - Preoperatively, the goals are to normalize the patient's heart rate and blood pressure and restore intravascular volume. Thus, close monitoring of the patient's pulse and blood pressure is crucial
  - Teach the patient and family about the disease, including signs/symptoms, medications, the importance of hydration before surgery, and how to monitor the patient's pulse and blood pressure at home
  - Administer antihypertensive medications as ordered. Ensure the patient is well hydrated and has a liberal salt intake to prevent severe hypotension after tumor removal
  - Postoperatively, cardiac monitoring for arrhythmias and close monitoring of the patient's blood pressure for severe fluctuations are recommended. Manipulation of the tumor during surgical excision may cause the release of stored epinephrine and norepinephrine, with marked increases in blood pressure and heart rate changes. Tumor excision will result in lowered catecholamine levels causing hypotension, which may necessitate vasopressor therapy and fluid replacement therapy
  - Administer corticosteroids as ordered to prevent adrenal insufficiency
  - Monitor for hypoglycemia and treat accordingly
  - Collect blood and urine samples for catecholamine and metabolite testing to evaluate complete tumor removal
  - Provide emotional support to the patient and family, who may fear repeated attacks
  - Before discharge, educate the patient/family on the signs/symptoms to watch for recurrence, medications, and importance of follow-up care

Review Questions

Question 1. A 28-year-old woman is scheduled for a glucose tolerance test. She asks the nurse what results indicate diabetes mellitus. The nurse should respond that the minimum parameter for indication of diabetes mellitus is a 2-hour blood glucose level greater than:

A. 120 mg/dL.
B. 150 mg/dL.
C. 200 mg/dL.
D. 250 mg/dL.

Correct answer: C A glucose tolerance test indicates a diagnosis of diabetes mellitus when the 2-hour blood glucose level is greater than 200 mg/dL. Confirmation occurs when at least one subsequent result is greater than 200 mg/dL. Options A and B are incorrect because they're below the minimum parameter; Option D is incorrect because it's above the minimum parameter.

Question 2. A patient is diagnosed with hyperthyroidism. The nurse should expect clinical signs and symptoms similar to:

A. Addison's disease.
B. benzodiazepine overdose.
C. hypovolemic shock.
D. sympathetic nervous system stimulation.

Correct answer: D Hyperthyroidism is a hypermetabolic state characterized by such signs and symptoms as anxiety, increased blood pressure, and tachycardia—all seen in sympathetic nervous system stimulation. Symptoms of Addison's disease (Option A), benzodiazepine overdose (Option B), and hypovolemic shock (Option C) are more similar to a hypometabolic state.

Question 3. A patient with thyroid cancer undergoes a thyroidectomy. After surgery, the patient develops peripheral numbness and tingling and muscle twitching and spasms. The nurse should expect to administer:

A. a barbiturate.
B. a thyroid supplement.
C. an antispasmodic.
D. I.V. calcium gluconate.

Correct answer: D Damage to the parathyroid glands during thyroidectomy can cause hyposecretion of parathyroid hormone, leading to calcium deficiency. Symptoms of calcium deficiency include muscle spasms, numbness, and tingling. Treatment includes immediate I.V. administration of calcium gluconate. A barbiturate (Option A) isn't indicated. Thyroid supplementation (Option B) is necessary following

thyroidectomy but isn't specifically related to the identified problem. An antispasmodic (Option C) doesn't treat the problem.

Question 4. A patient with intractable asthma develops Cushing's syndrome. Development of this complication can most likely be attributed to long-term or excessive use of:

A. cromolyn (Intal).
B. metaproterenol (Alupent).
C. prednisone.
D. theophylline.

Correct answer: C Cushing's syndrome results from long-term or excessive use of a glucocorticoid such as prednisone. Cromolyn (Option A), metaproterenol (Option B), and theophylline (Option D) don't cause Cushing's syndrome.

Question 5. Which nursing diagnosis is most likely for a patient with an acute episode of diabetes insipidus?

A. Deficient fluid volume
B. Imbalanced nutrition: more than body requirements
C. Impaired gas exchange
D. Ineffective tissue perfusion: cardiopulmonary

Correct answer: A Diabetes insipidus causes a pronounced loss of intravascular volume; therefore, the most prominent risk to the patient is deficient fluid volume. The patient is at risk for imbalanced nutrition, impaired gas exchange, and ineffective tissue perfusion (Options B, C, and D), but these risks stem from the deficient fluid volume.

Question 6. A patient presents with diaphoresis, palpitations, jitters, and tachycardia approximately 1½ hours after taking his regular morning insulin. Which treatment option is appropriate for this patient?

A. Blood glucose level monitoring and carbohydrate administration
B. Nitroglycerin administration and ECG
C. Pulse oximetry monitoring and oxygen therapy
D. Salt restriction, diuretic administration, and paracentesis

Correct answer: A The patient is experiencing signs and symptoms of hypoglycemia. It's appropriate to monitor his blood glucose level and administer carbohydrates to increase his blood glucose level. Nitroglycerin administration and ECG (Option B) are treatments for MI. Monitoring the patient's pulse oximetry and providing oxygen therapy (Option C) won't increase the patient's blood glucose level. Salt restriction, diuretic administration, and paracentesis (Option D) are treatments for ascites.

Question 7. When teaching a newly diagnosed diabetic patient about diet and exercise, the nurse should teach the patient how to:

A. manage caloric goals, diet, and physical activity.
B. manage fluids, proteins, and electrolytes.
C. reduce calorie intake before exercising.
D. use fiber laxatives and bulk-forming agents.

Correct answer: A Diabetic patients must be taught to manage caloric goals, diet, and physical activity. Managing fluids, proteins, and electrolytes (Option B) is important for a patient with acute renal failure. The diabetic patient may need additional calories—not reduced calories (Option C)—before exercising. Fiber laxatives and bulk-forming agents (Option D) are treatments for constipation.

Question 8. A 52-year-old patient reports weight gain and fatigue. On assessment, her vital signs are a blood pressure of 120/74 mm Hg, a pulse rate of 52 beats/minute, a respiratory rate of 20 breaths/minute, and a temperature of 98°F (36.7°C). Laboratory results show low T_4 and T_3 levels. The nurse knows these signs and symptoms are associated with which condition?

A. Hyperthyroidism
B. Hypocalcemia
C. Hypokalemia
D. Hypothyroidism

Correct answer: D Weight gain, fatigue, and a slow pulse rate, along with decreased levels of T_3 and T_4—thyroid hormones that affect growth and development as well as metabolic rate—indicate hypothyroidism. Hyperthyroidism (Option A) results in increased levels of the T_3 and T_4. Hypocalcemia (Option B) is defined as a low-calcium level and results in tetany. Hypokalemia (Option C) is defined as a low-potassium level.

Question 9. A patient is admitted with a diagnosis of hyperparathyroidism. Which of the following signs would the nurse expect to find?

A. Bulging eyes
B. Renal calculi
C. Weight gain
D. Weight loss

Correct answer: B Hyperparathyroidism is overproduction of parathyroid hormone, characterized by bone calcification or renal calculi. Bulging eyes (Option A) and weight loss (Option D) are signs of hyperthyroidism, and weight gain (Option C) is a sign of hypothyroidism.

Question 10. A 37-year-old patient complains of muscle weakness, anorexia, and darkening of his skin. The nurse reviews his laboratory data and notes findings of low serum sodium and high serum potassium levels. The nurse recognizes that these signs and symptoms are associated with which condition?

A. Addison's disease
B. Cushing's syndrome
C. Diabetes insipidus
D. Thyroid storm

Correct answer: A The clinical picture of Addison's disease includes muscle weakness, anorexia, darkening of the skin's pigmentation, and low-sodium and high-potassium levels. Cushing's syndrome (Option B) causes obesity, "buffalo hump," "moon face," and thin extremities. Signs of diabetes insipidus (Option C) include excretion of large volumes of dilute urine, leading to hypernatremia and dehydration. Thyroid storm (Option D) can occur with severe hyperthyroidism.

Selected References

Pheochromocytoma

Galati, S., Said, M., Gospin, R., Babic, N., Brown, K., Geer, E. B., … Inabnet, W. B. (2015). The Mount Sinai clinical pathway for management of pheochromocytoma. *Endocrine Practice*, 21(4), 368–382.

Gaujoux, S., Lentschener, C., & Dousset, B. (2015). Letter to the Editor: Per-operative hemodynamic instability in normotensive patients with incidentally discovered pheochromocytomas. *Journal of Clinical Endocrinology and Metabolism*, 100(4), 417–421.

Grossman, A. B. (2017). *Pheochromocytoma. Merck manual professional version*. Kenilworth, NJ: Merck Sharp & Dohme, Corp.

Lenders, J. W., Duh, Q. Y., Eisenhofer, G., Gimenez-Roqueplo, A. P., Grebe, S. K., Murad, M. H., … Young, W. F. (2014). Pheochromocytoma and paraganglioma: An Endocrine Society clinical practice guideline. *Journal of Clinical Endocrinology and Metabolism*, 99(6), 1915–1942.

Livingstone, M., Duttchen, K., Thompson, J., Sunderani, Z., Hawboldt, G., Rose, M. S., & Pasieka, J. (2015). Hemodynamic stability during pheochromocytoma resection: Lessons learned over the last two decades. *Annals of Surgical Oncology*, 22, 4175–4180.

Lyubimova, N. V., Churikova, T. K., & Kushlinskii, N. E. (2016). Chromogranin as a biochemical marker of neuroendocrine tumors. *Bulletin of Experimental Biology and Medicine*, 160(5), 657–660.

Mamoojee, Y., Arham, M., Elsaify, W., & Nag, S. (2016). Lesson of the month 2: Catecholamine-induced cardiomyopathy—Pitfalls in diagnosis and medical management. *Clinical Medicine, 16*(2), 201–203.

Morley-Smith, A. C., & Lyon, A. B. (2016). Stressing the importance of cardiac assessment in pheochromocytoma. *Journal of the American College of Cardiology, 67*(20), 2375–2377.

Mosby, Inc. (2017). *Mosby's dictionary of medicine, nursing and health professions* (10th ed., pp. 1384–1385). St. Louis, MO: Mosby.

Mula-Abed, W. S., Ahmed, R., Ramadhan, F. A., Al-Kindi, M. K., Al-Busaidi, N. B., Al-Muslahi, H. N., & Al-Lamki, M. A. (2015). A rare case of adrenal pheochromocytoma with unusual clinical and biochemical presentation: A case report and literature review. *Oman Medical Journal, 30*(5), 382–390.

Ramachandran, R., & Rewari, V. (2017). Current perioperative management of pheochromocytomas. *Indian Journal of Urology, 33*(1), 19–25.

Soltani, A., Pourian, M., & Davani, B. M. (2016). Does this patient have pheochromocytoma? A systematic review of clinical signs and symptoms. *Journal of Diabetes Metabolic Disorders, 15*(6).

Wang, W., Li, P., Wang, Y., Wang, Y., Zhiyong, M., Wang, G., … Zhou, H. (2015). Effectiveness and safety of laparoscopic adrenalectomy of large pheochromocytoma: A prospective, nonrandomized, controlled study. *American Journal of Surgery, 210*(2), 230–235.

Zawadzka-Leska, S. K., Radziszewski, M., Malec, K., Stadnik, A., & Ambroziak, U. (2016). Predictive value of chromogranin A in a diagnosis towards pheochromocytoma in adrenal incidentaloma. *Acta Endocrinologica, 12*(4), 437–442.

Parathyroid

2017 AORN Guidelines for Perioperative Practice.

(2016). Hypoparathyroidism. https://medlineplus.gov/ency/article/000385.htm

(2017). Before and after parathyroid surgery. Division of Surgical Oncology: Endocrine surgery. www.mcw.edu/Surgical-Oncology/MP/Endocrine-Surgery/Before-After-Surgery/Parathyroid.htm

Barbieri, I., Baumnamm, J., Casal, M. C., Gurevich, A., Pancirova, J., Paulia, K., & Riemann, A. (2015). An overview of nurses' management of secondary hyperparathyoidism: How is Europe doing? *Journal of Renal Care, 41*(3), 202–210.

Bredenkamp, J. K. (2016). *Parathyroidectomy.* Retrieved from http://www.medicinenet.com/parathyroidectomy/page6.htm

Cavallaro, G., Iorio, O., Centanni, M., Porta, N., Iossa, A., Garagno, L., … Silecchia, G. (2015). Parathyroid reimplantation in forearm subcutaneous tissue during thyroidectomy: A simple and effective way to avoid hypoparathyroidism. *World Journal of Surgery, 39*, 1936–1942.

Delgado, A. (2016). Hyperparathyroidism. Healthline Reference Library.

Fraser, M., & Brannigan, D. (2015). Adherence to phosphate binders: Improving patient engagement. *Journal of Renal Nursing, 7*(4), 168–175.

Gupta, A. (2015a). *Primary hyperparathyroidism: Management.* Joanna Briggs Institute (JBI7781).

Gupta, A. (2015b). *Secondary hyperparathyroidism: Management.* Joanna Briggs Institute (JBI7796).

Hallock, A. (2017). Osteoporosis in patients with CKD: A diagnostic dilemma. *Nephrology Nursing Journal, 44*(1), 13–17.

Kim, L., Harris, E. H., & Krause, M. W. (2017). Hyperparathyroidism. *MedScape.* Retrieved from http://emedicine.medscape.com/article/127351-overview

Kitada, M., Yasuda, S., Nana, T., Ishibashi, K., Hayashi, S., & Okazaki, S. (2016). Surgical treatment for mediastinal parathyroid adenoma causing primary hyperparathyroidism. *Journal of Cardiothoracic Surgery, 11*(44), 1–4.

McGowan, J. A., & Hillar, K. (2017). Hyperparathyroidism and hypoparathyroidism. In *Magill's medical guide (online edition).*

Norman, J. (2016). *Hypoparathyroidism.* Retrieved from https://www.endocrineweb.com/conditions/hypoparathyroidism

Parathyroid gland removal. (2016). *MedlinePlus medical encyclopedia.* Retrieved from https://medlineplus.gov/ency/article/002931.htm

Rodriguez, M., Goodman, W. G., Liakopoulos, V., Messa, P., Wiecek, A., & Cunnginham, J. (2015). The use of calcimimetics for the treatment of secondary hyperparathyroidism: A 10 year evidence review. *Seminars in Dialysis, 28*(5), 497–505.

Salen, P. N. (2016). Hyperparathyroidism in emergency medicine medication. *MedScape.* Retrieved from http://emedicine.medscape.com/article/766906-medication#5

Sharata, A., Kelly, T. L., Rozenfeld, Y., Hammill, C. W., Schuman, E., Carlisle, J. R., & Aliabadi-Wahle, S. (2017). Management of primary hyperparathyroidism: Can we do better? *The American Surgeon, 83*(1), 64–70.

Smith, J. C. (2015). *Parathyroidectomy.* Retrieved from http://emedicine.medscape.com/article/1829698-overview

Shoback, D. (2017). Hypoparathyroidism. National Organization for Rare Disorders.

Van Bussel, B. C., & Koopmans, R. P. (2016). *Trousseau's sign at the emergency department.* BMI Publishing Group.

Walsh, J., Gittoes, N., & Selby, P. (2016). Emergency management of acute hypercalcemia is adult patients. *Endocrine Connections, 5*(5).

Diabetes Insipidus/SIADH

Bichet, D. G. (2017). *Treatment of nephrogenic diabetes insipidus.* Retrieved from https://www.uptodate.com/contents/treatment-of-nephrogenic-diabetes-insipidus

Grant, P., Ayuk, J., Bouloux, P. M., Cohen, M., Cranston, I. O., Murray, R. D., … Grossman, A. (2015). The diagnosis and management of inpatient hyponatremia and SIADH. *European Journal of Clinical Investigation, 45*(8), 888–894.

Khardori, R. (2017). *Diabetes insipidus.* Retrieved from http://emedicine.medscape.com/article/117648-overview

Thomas, C. P. (2016). *Syndrome of inappropriate antidiuretic hormone secretion.* Retrieved from http://emedicine.medscape.com/article/246650-overview

Retrieved from https://medlineplus.gov/ency/article/000511.htm

Addison's Disease

Bornstein, S. R., Allolio, B., Arlt, W., Barthel, A., Don-Wauchope, A., Hammer, G. D., … Torpy, D. J. (2016). Diagnosis and treatment of primary adrenal insufficiency: An Endocrine Society clinical practice guideline. *Journal of Clinical Endocrinology and Metabolism, 101*(2), 364–389.

Burton, C., Cottrell, E., & Edwards, J. (2015). Addison's disease: Identification and management. *British Journal of General Practice, 65*(638), 488–490.

Griffing, G. T. (2017). *Addison's disease.* Retrieved from http://emedicine.medscape.com/article/116467-overview

Mosby, Inc. (2017). *Mosby's dictionary of medicine, nursing & health professions* (10th ed., pp. 1384–1385). St. Louis, MO: Mosby.

Nieman, L. K. (2017). *Adrenal insufficiency*. Retrieved from www.uptodate.com

Nieman, L. K., Biller, B. M., Findling, J. W., Murad, M. H., Newell-Price, J., Savage M. O., & Tabarin A. (2015). Treatment of Cushing's syndrome: An Endocrine Society clinical practice guideline. *Journal of Clinical Endocrinology and Metabolism, 100*(8), 2807–2831.

Cushing's Syndrome

Nieman, L. K. (2015a). *Establishing the diagnosis of Cushing's syndrome*. Retrieved from www.uptodate.com

Nieman, L. K. (2015b). *Overview of the treatment of Cushing's syndrome*. Retrieved from www.uptodate.com

Neiman, L. K. (2015c). *Primary therapy of Cushing's disease: Transsphenoidal surgery and pituitary irradiation*. Retrieved from www.uptodate.com

Nieman, L. K. (2016). *Medical therapy of hypercortisolism (Cushing's syndrome)*. Retrieved from www.uptodate.com

Nieman, L. K. (2017a). *Causes and pathophysiology of Cushing's syndrome*. Retrieved from www.uptodate.com

Nieman, L. K. (2017b). *Epidemiology and clinical manifestations of Cushing's syndrome*. Retrieved from www.uptodate.com

Nieman, L. K. (2017c). *Patient education: Cushing's syndrome treatment (Beyond the Basics)*. Retrieved from www.uptodate.com

Nguyen, H. C. T. (2015). *Endogenous Cushing syndrome*. Retrieved from http://emedicine.medscape.com/article/2233083-overview#a2

Thyroid

Alexander, P., et al. (2017). 2017 guidelines of the American Thyroid Association for the diagnosis and management of thyroid disease during pregnancy and the postpartum. *Thyroid, 27*(3).

Chen, Z. (2016). *Hyperthyroidism: Treatment*. Joanna Briggs Institute (JBI7647).

Chu, W. H. (2015). *Hypothyroidism: Management*. Joanna Briggs Institute (JBI7698).

Felcilda-Reynaldo, R. F., & Kenneally, M. (2016). Antithyroid drugs for hyperthyroidism. *Medsurg Nursing, 25*(1), 50–54.

Fong, E. (2015). *Graves' ophthalmopathy: Treatment*. Joanna Briggs Institute (JBI7646).

Geer, M., Potter, D. M., & Ulrich, H. (2015). Alternative schedules of levothyroxine administration. *American Journal of Health-System Pharmacy, 72*, 373–377.

Jonklaas, J., Bianco, A. C., Bauer, A. J., Burman, K. D., Cappola, A. R., Celi, F. S., … Sawka, A. M. (2014). Guidelines for the treatment of hypothyroidism: Prepared by the American Thyroid Association Task Force on thyroid hormone replacement. *Thyroid, 24*(12), 1670–1751.

Hackethal, V., & Barclay, L. (2017). *ATA issues revised guidelines on thyroid disease in pregnancy*. Retrieved from http://www.medscape.org/viewarticle/875165

Huang, S. M., Miao, W. T., Lin, C. F., Sun, H. S., & Chow, N. H. (2015). Effectiveness and mechanism of preoperative Lugol's solution for reducing thyroid blood flow in patients with euthyroid Graves' disease. *World Journal of Surgery, 40*(3), 505–509.

Kravets, I. (2016). Hyperthyroidism: Diagnosis and treatment. *American Family Physician, 93*(5), 363–370.

Misra, M. (2016). *Thyroid storm*. Retrieved from www.medscape.com/article/925147

Ross, D. S. (2015a). *Diagnosis of hyperthyroidism*. Retrieved from www.uptodate.com

Ross, D. S. (2015b). *Myxedema coma*. Retrieved from www.uptodate.com

Ross, D. S. (2016). *Overview of the clinical manifestations of hyperthyroidism in adults*. Retrieved from www.uptodate.com

Ross, D. S. (2017). *Treatment of primary hypothyroidism in adults*. Retrieved from www.uptodate.com

Ross, D. S., & Sugg, S. L. (2016). *Surgical management of hyperthyroidism*. Retrieved from www.uptodate.com

Ross, D. S., Burch, H. B., Cooper, D. S., Greenlee, M. C., Laurberg, P., Maia, A. L., … Walter, M. A. (2016). 2016 American Thyroid Association Guidelines for diagnosis and management of hyperthyroidism and other causes of thyrotoxicosis. *Thyroid, 26*(10), 1343–1421.

Orlander, P. R. (2016). *Toxic nodular goiter*. Retrieved from www.medscape.com/article/120497

Schreiber, M. L. (2017). Thyroid storm. *Medsurg Nursing, 26*(2), 143–145.

Surks, M. (2016). *Clinical manifestations of hypothyroidism*. Retrieved from www.uptodate.com

Yeung, S. J. (2017). *Graves disease*. Retrieved from www.medscape.com/article/120619

Diabetes Mellitus

Academy of Nutrition and Dietetics. (2015). *Diabetes type 1 and type 2 evidenced-based nutrition practice guideline*. Chicago, IL: Author.

Bellman, S. (2016). *Type 2 diabetes management: The role of incretins*. Joanna Briggs Institute (JBI8487).

Camilleri, M. (2015). *Treatment of gastroparesis*. Retrieved from www.uptodate.com

Delahanty, L. M., & McCulloch, D. K. (2017a). *Nutritional considerations in Type 1 diabetes mellitus*. Retrieved from www.uptodate.com

Delahanty, L. M., & McCulloch, D. K. (2017b). *Nutritional considerations in Type 2 diabetes mellitus*. Retrieved from www.uptodate.com

Freeland, B. (2016). Hyperglycemia in the hospital setting. *Medsurg Nursing, 25*(6), 393–396.

Khalil, H. (2016a). *Diabetes: Foot care (older people)*. Joanna Briggs Institute (JBI8864).

Khalil, H. (2016b). *Diabetes (non-hospitalized patient): Self-management education*. Joanna Briggs Institute (JBI304).

Khalil, H. (2016c). *Diabetes mellitus: Clinician information*. Joanna Briggs Institute (JBI63).

Li, Y. (2017a). *Diabetes (older people): Restricted diets*. Joanna Briggs Institute (JBI8877).

Li, Y. (2017b). *Diabetes (Older people): Vision loss*. Joanna Briggs Institute (JBI8863).

Li, Y. (2017c). *Diabetes: Visual impairment prevention*. Joanna Briggs Institute (JBI633).

Lizarondo, L. (2015). *Hypoglycemia in diabetes: Management*. Joanna Briggs Institute (JBI529).

Lizarondo, L. (2016a). *Diabetes (Type 2): Blood glucose management*. Joanna Briggs Institute (JBI4527).

Lizarondo, L. (2016b). *Hypoglycemia in diabetes: Management*. Joanna Briggs Institute (JBI7209).

McCulloch, D. K. (2017a). *Clinical presentation and diagnosis of diabetes mellitus in adults*. Retrieved from www.uptodate.com

McCulloch, D. K. (2017b). *General principles of insulin therapy in diabetes mellitus.* Retrieved from www.uptodate.com

McCulloch, D. K. (2017c). *Overview of medical care in adults with diabetes mellitus.* Retrieved from www.uptodate.com

Pietrangelo, A. (2017). Diabetes by the numbers: Facts, statistics, and you. Healthline Media.

Service, F. J., Cryer, P. E., & Vella, A. (2017). *Hypoglycemia in adults: Clinical manifestations, definitions, and causes.* Retrieved from www.uptodate.com

Slade, D. (2017). *Diabetes (hospital patients): Perioperative management.* Joanna Briggs Institute (JBI7646).

Slade, S. (2015). *Diabetes (type 2): Dietary management.* Joanna Briggs Institute (JBI3732).

Stephenson, M. (2016). *Diabetes (type 2): Education.* Joanna Briggs Institute (JBI1607).

Xue, Y. (2014). *Diabetes: Nephropathy and foot disease management.* Joanna Briggs Institute (JBI635).

Chapter 15

Renal and Urinary Tract Disorders

Introduction

- The urinary system forms and stores urine, regulates body fluids and electrolytes, and controls urine elimination
- Urinary tract infections (UTIs) and obstructions may cause permanent loss of renal function
- Acute and chronic renal failures are both serious and potentially life-threatening conditions
  - In a patient with *renal impairment* or *diminished renal reserve*, the healthier kidney compensates for the impaired kidney and continues to clear metabolic waste unless it meets with increased demand or unusual stress; as a result, the patient is asymptomatic, and specific concentration and dilution tests are needed to detect reduced renal function
  - In a patient with *renal insufficiency*, compensation begins to fail and metabolic wastes build up; the degree of insufficiency can be mild, moderate, or severe and is measured by the decreasing glomerular filtration rate (GFR)
  - In a patient with *end-stage renal disease*, the kidneys can't perform their normal homeostatic functions or meet normal body demands
    - Excess nitrogenous wastes build up in the blood
    - Fluid, electrolyte, and acid-base abnormalities occur
    - Dialysis or kidney transplantation is necessary to sustain life
- Nursing history
  - The nurse asks the patient about the *chief complaint*
    - A patient with a renal or urinary tract disorder may be experiencing output changes, such as polyuria, oliguria, or anuria
    - The patient may also see changes in voiding pattern, such as hesitancy, frequency, urgency, nocturia, or incontinence; urine color changes; or pain
  - The nurse then questions the patient about his *present illness*
    - Ask the patient about his symptom, including when it started, associated symptoms, location, radiation, intensity, duration, frequency, precipitating, aggravating, and alleviating factors
    - Ask about the use of prescription and over-the-counter drugs, herbal remedies, and vitamin and nutritional supplements
    - Ask about the use of any nonpharmacological interventions such as heat, ice, or meditation that the patient has used and if they were effective
  - The nurse asks about *medical history*
    - Question the patient about other renal and urinary disorders, such as UTIs, kidney trauma, renal cancers, and kidney stones
    - Ask about a history of other chronic illnesses that may affect the renal system, such as diabetes mellitus or hypertension
  - The nurse then assesses the *family history*
    - Ask about a family history of chronic illnesses that can affect the renal system, such as hypertension, diabetes mellitus, coronary artery disease, vascular disease, or hyperlipidemia

○ Determine whether the family history suggests a genetic predisposition to certain renal diseases such as polycystic kidney disease (PKD)
- The nurse obtains a *social history*
  ○ Ask about work, exercise, diet, use of recreational drugs and alcohol, and hobbies
  ○ Also ask about stress, support systems, and coping mechanisms
- Physical assessment
  - Nurse begins with *inspection*
    ○ Observe the patient's overall appearance; note his mental status and behavior
    ○ Examine his skin for color, turgor, intactness, edema, and texture
    ○ Inspect his abdomen for size and shape, noting any abnormal markings
  - Next, the nurse uses *palpation*
    ○ Palpate the bladder for distention
    ○ Note any areas of tenderness
  - Then, the nurse uses *percussion*
    ○ Percuss for costovertebral tenderness
    ○ Percuss the bladder to elicit tympany or dullness
  - The nurse then uses *auscultation*
    ○ Listen for renal artery bruits
    ○ Note any bruits over the aorta, iliac, and femoral arteries

Acute Kidney Injury

- Description
  - Acute kidney injury is a sudden and almost complete loss of kidney function characterized by rising levels of blood urea nitrogen (BUN) and serum creatinine and an inability of the kidneys to regulate fluid and electrolyte balance; it occurs over several hours to several days
  - Acute kidney injury may be reversible—or it may lead to death
  - *Prerenal failure*, or prerenal azotemia, occurs when blood flow to the kidneys is disrupted, which causes ischemia and nephron damage
    ○ It can result from a condition that decreases blood flow and kidney perfusion, such as hypovolemia, hemorrhage, dehydration, or burns; a condition that decreases cardiac output, such as a myocardial infarction (MI), congestive heart failure (CHF), or an arrhythmia; vascular failure related to sepsis, anaphylaxis, or severe acidosis; or an occlusion that obstructs renal arteries
    ○ It generally can be reversed by treating the cause and restoring normal intravascular volume
  - *Intrarenal failure* occurs when the renal parenchyma is damaged; when this occurs, the kidneys can't concentrate urine or excrete nitrogenous wastes
    ○ Intrarenal failure can be caused by nephron damage resulting from acute tubular necrosis, acute glomerulonephritis, or a related disorder or from exposure to a nephrotoxic drug or chemical, such as certain antibiotics, an antineoplastic, a fluorinated anesthetic, a heavy metal, or a radiographic contrast dye
    ○ Other causes include trauma, neoplasms, hypertension, small vessel thrombosis, systemic lupus erythematosus, toxemia of pregnancy, and hypercalcemia
    ○ Genetic disorders such as PKD
    ○ Intrarenal failure can usually be reversed
  - *Postrenal failure*, or postrenal azotemia, occurs when urine flow from the collecting ducts in the kidney to the external urethral orifice is obstructed or when venous blood flow from the kidney is obstructed
    ○ Renal calculi, tumors, clots, benign prostatic hyperplasia, strictures, trauma, bilateral renal vein thrombosis, and congenital malformation can all cause urinary obstruction
    ○ Bladder obstruction can block the outflow of urine
    ○ Postrenal failure is usually reversible
  - Acute kidney injury can lead to hyperkalemia and severe metabolic acidosis and can cause uremia that compromises the immune system
- Signs and symptoms
  - Acute kidney injury typically progresses through three phases: an oliguric or anuric phase, a diuretic phase, and a recovery phase; signs and symptoms vary from phase to phase
  - The oliguric phase produces a BUN level of 25 to 30 mg/dL, a serum creatinine level of 1.5 to 2 mg, sudden oliguria (urine output less than 400 mL daily) or anuria (rare), and reduced GFR

- The diuretic phase causes a gradual return of renal function; normal or high urine output (1 to 5 L daily); potentially life-threatening loss of sodium, potassium, and magnesium; and increased azotemia (elevated BUN and serum creatinine levels)
- The recovery phase is associated with decreasing BUN and serum creatinine levels; it continues until normal renal tubular function is established
- High-output renal failure, a type of acute nonoliguric renal failure, occasionally occurs; it commonly results from the use of a nephrotoxic antibiotics such as aminoglycosides (gentamicin), beta-lactams (penicillin and cephalosporins), sulfonamides, and vancomycin
  - Although symptoms of acute kidney injury may develop, fluid overload generally isn't a problem
  - If high-output renal failure is recognized early, and the antibiotic is discontinued, normal renal function gradually returns
- Diagnosis and treatment
  - Diagnosis of acute kidney injury is based on patient history and abnormal laboratory findings (see *Understanding Acute Renal Failure*, page 249), assessment of fluid balance, preexisting disorders, precipitating events, and current health status
  - Other diagnostic tests may include abdominal X-ray, ultrasonography, or computed tomography (CT), excretory urography or cystoscopy with retrograde pyelography, renal angiography, and renal biopsy
  - Laboratory tests include serum creatinine and BUN levels (the normal ratio of BUN to creatinine ranges from 10:1 to 15:1), electrolyte and hemoglobin levels, hematocrit, urinalysis, and creatinine clearance; laboratory changes can help differentiate among prerenal, intrarenal, and postrenal acute renal failure (ARF)
    - With prerenal acute kidney injury, the BUN-creatinine ratio is greater than 15:1; urine specific gravity and osmolarity are increased, and the urine sodium level is decreased
    - With intrarenal acute kidney injury, urine specific gravity and osmolarity fall to levels similar to those in serum or plasma, and the urine sodium level may exceed 30 mEq/L
    - With postrenal acute kidney injury, urine osmolarity and sodium levels may be normal; if the condition isn't quickly diagnosed and treated, the patient may develop urinary system changes similar to those of intrarenal ARF
  - Treatment aims to identify and eliminate or control the underlying cause, restore normal fluid and electrolyte balance, and prevent uremic complications while the kidneys repair themselves
  - Reduced intravascular volume is treated early with aggressive fluid therapy to restore urine output and prevent acute tubular necrosis
    - A therapeutic fluid challenge (500 mL over 30 minutes) may be used to differentiate prerenal from intrarenal causes of oliguria
    - If urine output improves after the fluid challenge, I.V. fluids are continued at a rate that maintains adequate hourly urine volume
    - If the fluid challenge is unsuccessful, a diuretic—such as mannitol (Osmitrol), bumetanide (Bumex), furosemide (Lasix), or ethacrynic acid (Edecrin)—may be used to restore urine output
  - A patient with hypervolemia and fluid overload, hyperkalemia, metabolic acidosis, severe hyponatremia, encephalopathy, or pericarditis may require dialysis (see *Comparing Types of Dialysis*, page 250)
  - Hyperkalemia is aggressively treated with I.V. hypertonic glucose and insulin, which causes extracellular potassium to move into cells. Oral or rectal administration of the cationexchange resin sodium polystyrene sulfonate (Kayexalate) causes an exchange of sodium for potassium ions in the gastrointestinal (GI) tract. Dialysis can be used to maintain normal potassium levels when these interventions fail.
  - Hyperkalemic patients with electrocardiogram changes such as elevated T waves are commonly treated with I.V. calcium gluconate to prevent arrhythmias
  - Hypotension is commonly treated with volume replacement, although a vasopressor may be needed
  - Hypertension is treated with restriction of fluid intake to prevent fluid overload, restriction of dietary sodium, and antihypertensive therapy
  - Severe metabolic acidosis can be treated with IV infusion of sodium bicarbonate if the patient is not in fluid overload
  - Diet therapy helps manage ARF; the recommended diet is high in calories and carbohydrates, is low in potassium, and may restrict protein (depending on the degree of azotemia and the frequency of dialysis); protein in the diet must provide essential amino acids while minimizing the degree of nitrogenous waste products
- Nursing interventions
  - Monitor for signs of acute kidney injury and its complications
  - Monitor fluid intake and output, weigh the patient daily, and administer fluids carefully; monitor electrolyte levels, and maintain proper electrolyte balance

- Prevent infection by frequently washing your hands; using aseptic technique with incisions, wound care, and care of I.V. and central venous catheters; assisting the patient with hygiene, including oral hygiene; frequently turning and positioning him; encouraging deep breathing, coughing, and ambulation (if possible); and avoiding use of an indwelling urinary catheter
- Monitor the patient for signs of infection, such as fever, local redness, swelling, heat, drainage, and elevated white blood cell (WBC) count; watch for signs and symptoms of pericarditis, including pleuritic chest pain, tachycardia, and pericardial friction rub
- Provide a diet high in calories and low in potassium, protein, and sodium
- Monitor the patient's response to medications; because many drugs are excreted by the kidneys, the type of drug, dosage, or administration interval may need to be adjusted, based on the patient's renal function (as evidenced by GFR and other indicators)
- Teach the patient and family the reasons for interventions and the importance of infection prevention measures; because the patient may be acutely ill and have a decreased level of consciousness, information should be given verbally (briefly) and in writing
- Encourage the patient and family to express their concerns

Box 15-1: Understanding Acute Renal Failure

The pathophysiologic processes of acute renal failure (ARF) determine the patient's signs, symptoms, and laboratory test result changes.

Pathophysiologic process	Signs and symptoms	Laboratory test results
Inability to excrete nitrogenous wastes	• Nausea, vomiting, GI bleeding • Drowsiness, confusion, delirium, coma • Pericarditis • Asterixis	• Elevated blood urea nitrogen • Elevated creatinine
Decreased urine volume	• Edema, heart failure, pulmonary edema, interstitial infiltrates in lungs • Hypertension	• In prerenal ARF, increased urine specific gravity and osmolarity and decreased urine sodium level • In intrarenal ARF, decreased urine specific gravity and osmolarity and increased urine sodium level • In postrenal ARF, possibly normal urine osmolarity and urine sodium level
Inability to regulate electrolytes	• Electrocardiogram (ECG) changes (peaked, tentlike T waves, widened QRS complex, and arrhythmias); neuromuscular changes (weakness and paralysis) • Dyspnea, edema, anasarca, increased jugular vein distention, crackles • Thirst, dry mouth, weakness, tachycardia, hypotension, decreased skin turgor (diuretic phase) • Weakness, paralysis, constipation, paralytic ileus, hypoventilation, prominent U waves on ECG (diuretic phase) • Muscle weakness, hypoventilation, hypotension, flushing • Tremors, seizures	• Hyperkalemia • Hypernatremia • Hyponatremia • Hypokalemia • Hypermagnesemia • Hyperphosphatemia and hypocalcemia
Inability to maintain acid-base balance	• Hyperventilation, Kussmaul's respirations, weakness	• Metabolic acidosis (decreased pH and bicarbonate levels)
Uremic syndrome	• Early manifestations: anorexia, nausea, vomiting • Later manifestations: bleeding, uremic pneumonitis, pericarditis, colitis, pericardial effusion • Other manifestations: increased susceptibility to infection; dry, itchy skin	• Altered platelet function, anemia

Box 15-2: Comparing Types of Dialysis

Peritoneal dialysis, hemodialysis, and continuous renal replacement therapy (CRRT) may be used to treat acute renal failure (ARF). They vary in several ways.

Selection criteria

Peritoneal dialysis typically is used for patients with cardiovascular instability because it doesn't have the same effect on cardiac output as hemodialysis. It also may be used for patients with recent cerebral bleeding, GI bleeding, or blood dyscrasias because it requires no heparinization.

Hemodialysis is more appropriate for patients who have had recent abdominal surgery or who have abdominal adhesions because these conditions interfere with the clearance ability of the peritoneal membrane used as the dialyzable surface in peritoneal dialysis. Hemodialysis also is more commonly used for patients with severe catabolism, fluid overload, or hyperkalemia because it removes wastes and fluids more rapidly than peritoneal dialysis.

CRRT may be used for critically ill patients with ARF who can't tolerate hemodialysis or peritoneal dialysis because of hemodynamic instability. CRRT is used 24 hours per day, over several days, to slowly remove fluid and solutes.

Advantages and disadvantages

Hemodialysis is a complex procedure that requires expensive equipment and skilled personnel. Consequently, it may not be available in a convenient location. Peritoneal dialysis is less complex and less expensive and is available in a wider variety of settings. Home dialysis is possible with both procedures, but peritoneal dialysis is less expensive and requires a shorter training period.

Peritoneal dialysis allows the patient to be more independent, promotes more steady blood chemistry levels, and permits the patient to eat a less-restricted diet. Techniques developed by Popovich in the late 1970s, along with Tenckhoff's development of a permanent peritoneal catheter, have contributed to the increased use of peritoneal dialysis in patients with chronic renal failure.

CRRT removes fluid and solutes slowly, making it more suitable for critically ill patients with unstable conditions. However, it requires a highly trained staff. Types of CRRT include continuous arteriovenous hemofiltration, continuous venovenous hemofiltration, continuous arteriovenous hemodialysis, and continuous venovenous hemodialysis.

Types of peritoneal dialysis

Continuous ambulatory peritoneal dialysis (CAPD) can be performed independently by the patient in any location and frees him from dependence on a machine or dialysis center. With CAPD, dialysis fluid is continuously present in the peritoneum but is drained and replaced with fresh fluid three to five times per day based on the patient's clearance needs. This technique closely resembles normal renal function, avoiding extreme shifts in blood chemistries and fluid that occur with hemodialysis.

In *continuous cyclic peritoneal dialysis* (CCPD), a cycling machine performs frequent exchanges while the patient sleeps. After the last exchange in the morning, fresh dialysate is left in the peritoneum until nighttime. CCPD generally is performed 6 or 7 days a week.

With *intermittent peritoneal dialysis* (IPD), frequent fluid changes are performed over 8 to 10 hours, 3 to 5 days a week. Dialysate isn't left in the peritoneum between dialysis periods. Although IPD can be done manually by a trained nurse, an automated cycling machine is commonly used. IPD is performed in a hospital, dialysis center, or at home, usually at night.

Chronic Kidney Disease

- Description
  - Chronic kidney disease (CKD) is a slow, insidious, irreversible deterioration in renal function
  - It typically progresses through four stages:
    - Reduced renal reserve: GFR of 60% to 89% of normal
    - Renal insufficiency: GFR of 30% to 59% of normal
    - Renal failure: GFR of 15% to 29% of normal
    - End-stage renal disease: GFR less than 15% of normal
  - Diseases that contribute to CKD include diabetes, gout, and hypertensive nephropathies, chronic glomerulonephritis, pyelonephritis, urinary tract obstruction, PKD, renal cell carcinoma, renovascular disease, lupus nephritis, multiple myeloma, amyloidosis, chronic hypercalcemia and hypokalemia, renal tuberculosis, and sarcoidosis

- CKD begins with a functional loss of nephrons that is asymptomatic, except for decreased urinary creatinine clearance; creatinine clearance normally ranges from 85 to 135 mL/minute; in patients with mild renal failure, it ranges from 50 to 84 mL/minute; in patients with moderate renal failure, from 10 to 49 mL/minute; and in patients with severe renal failure, 10 mL/minute or less
- Next, renal insufficiency occurs as more nephrons cease to function; insufficiency may be mild, moderate, or severe
  - At first, the patient experiences no physical limitations in daily activity, although laboratory changes—such as azotemia, anemia, and loss of the ability to concentrate urine—are detectable
  - As renal deterioration continues, the kidneys' ability to function under stress (e.g., during dehydration, salt depletion, or heart failure) is impaired; renal insufficiency may progress to renal failure during periods of stress
  - Once renal failure develops, the patient must limit daily activities; he'll eventually develop overt signs of renal failure and uremia, beginning with fluid, electrolyte, and metabolic abnormalities (including azotemia, anemia, metabolic acidosis, hypertension, and hypocalcemia)
  - End-stage renal disease occurs when most of the nephrons have been irreversibly damaged; the GFR falls below 100 mL/minute, and the patient requires long-term dialysis or kidney transplantation
- Signs and symptoms
  - CKD is usually discovered during routine blood or urine tests. Most patients are asymptomatic until CKD becomes severe.
  - Altered fluid, electrolyte, and acid-base balances may include dehydration (early) or overhydration (later in the disease), hypocalcemia and hyperkalemia, and metabolic acidosis (as evidenced by low arterial blood pH and decreased bicarbonate levels)
  - Skin changes may include gray-bronze or yellow skin color related to uremia or pallor related to anemia, dry skin, uremic frost (white, dustlike deposits of urea and phosphate crystals on the face, nose, forehead, and upper trunk), pruritus, excoriations, ecchymosis, purpura, or infections; related changes may include thin, brittle nails and a whitened proximal section with a darker distal edge and nail ridges
  - Cardiovascular effects may include hypertension, acceleration of atherosclerosis, increased risk of MI and stroke, left ventricular hypertrophy, heart failure, pericarditis (which may cause a fever and pericardial friction rub and, rarely, chest pain and hypotension), pericardial effusion (which causes disappearance of any friction rub and appearance of a paradoxical pulse), cardiac tamponade (which causes hypotension, muffled heart sounds, narrowed pulse pressure, weak peripheral pulses, and bulging neck veins), peripheral edema, life-threatening cardiac arrhythmias, and cardiac arrest
  - Respiratory effects may include dyspnea, a thick, tenacious sputum, and a depressed cough reflex, which increase the risk of pulmonary infections and complications; Kussmaul's respirations; uremic breath odor; increased incidence of infections, including tuberculosis; pulmonary edema; pleural effusion; and uremic pneumonitis
  - Hematologic effects may include normochromic, normocytic anemia (which causes fatigue, weakness, pallor, exertional dyspnea, and intolerance of activity and cold), platelet dysfunction (which causes prolonged bleeding time, clotting abnormalities, easy bruising, purpura, and bleeding from mucous membranes and other body parts), and changes in the immune system and granulocytic function (which decrease cellular and humoral immunity and the inflammatory response)
  - GI effects may include a metallic or ammonia-like taste in the mouth, stomatitis, ammonia or fishy breath odor, an increased incidence of oral infections and tooth decay, anorexia (especially for high-protein foods), nausea, vomiting, GI bleeding, increased gastric acid production, diarrhea or constipation, fecal impaction, and an increased incidence of diverticulosis
  - Urinary symptoms include nocturia and polyuria
  - The patient may develop hepatitis (see *Chapter 12, Gastrointestinal Disorders*, for information about this disease)
  - Metabolic dysfunction may include carbohydrate intolerance (with abnormal glucose clearance), accumulation of end products of protein metabolism (which causes lethargy, headache, fatigue, irritability, and depression), and hyperlipidemia
  - Central nervous system effects may include decreased attention span, memory problems, inability to think clearly (progressing to actual confusion), flattened affect, insomnia, depression, irritability, lability, stupor, coma, and seizures

- Peripheral nervous system effects may include peripheral neuropathies (numbness, tingling, or pain of the feet and hands, weakness of the feet, and atrophy of leg muscles), footdrop, loss of motor function, and "burning feet" syndrome (swelling, redness, and extreme tenderness of the soles and dorsum of the feet)
- Autonomic nervous system effects may include loss of the ability to compensate for a change in blood pressure through reflex tachycardia or bradycardia, which leads to poor blood pressure control
- Musculoskeletal effects may include impaired physical mobility, loss of muscle mass and muscle strength, osteomalacia, osteoporosis, and osteitis fibrosa cystica
- Reproductive effects may include impotence in men, amenorrhea and infertility in women, and markedly decreased libido in both sexes
- Diagnosis and treatment
  - Laboratory tests, X-rays, and other diagnostic tests for CKD are the same as those for AKI; renal biopsy establishes the percentage of functioning nephrons
  - Urine albumin-creatinine ratio (ACR) is used to measure the degree to which large molecules like protein and blood are not filtered out in the kidneys. GFR measures the volume of blood being filtered each minute. Creatinine is a product of muscle metabolism, and if kidney function is decreased, creatinine is increased in the blood.
  - Treatment has several goals: to preserve current renal function and prevent or delay further deterioration of function by managing risk factors, to prevent and treat symptoms of uremia, to postpone or eliminate the need for long-term dialysis or kidney transplantation, and to promote comfort and improve the patient's quality of life
  - Most patients with CKD can be managed successfully with diet and fluid therapy; long-term dialysis or kidney transplantation is unnecessary until the GFR falls to 10% to 15% of the normal rate
  - Strict adherence to a low-protein diet can delay progression to end-stage renal disease
    - A high-protein load causes the kidneys to dilate from increased blood flow and increased GFR in an attempt to clear the by-products of protein metabolism; this increased vasodilation accelerates the deterioration of renal function
    - For adult patients, a protein intake of about 50 g daily appears to have a therapeutic effect without contributing to malnutrition; most of the protein must be of high biological value to supply sufficient essential amino acids; protein of low biological value increases the waste load to the kidneys
  - Depending on the stage of the disease and on fluid and electrolyte alterations, fluid intake may need to be restricted
    - If urine output is decreased, and fluid overload becomes a problem, fluid intake typically is restricted to the previous day's urine output plus 500 mL for insensible loss
    - If excessive fluid is lost—for example, because of fever, vomiting, or diarrhea—fluid requirements may increase
  - Sodium, potassium, and phosphorus also may be restricted
    - Sodium restriction may be warranted if the patient develops hypertension, edema, or heart failure
    - Dietary potassium generally isn't restricted if the urine output exceeds 1,000 mL daily; it's restricted if the serum potassium level exceeds 5.5 mEq/L
  - Supplements of B-complex vitamins, folic acid, and vitamin C may be needed to compensate for deficiencies that result from a restrictive diet or dialysis; iron and zinc supplements also may be prescribed
  - Once long-term dialysis begins, a more liberal protein intake is allowed, and the fluid intake is controlled to allow a weight gain of 2 to 2.5 lb (0.9 to 1.1 kg) between dialysis treatments
  - Despite anorexia, nausea, and taste changes, the patient must consume sufficient calories to prevent catabolism and muscle breakdown
  - Disturbances in calcium metabolism may be managed with calcium supplements, dietary restriction of phosphorus, and phosphate binders, such as aluminum hydroxide gels (Amphojel), which are given at mealtimes; a patient receiving hemodialysis may receive calcium carbonate instead of a phosphate binder, which can exacerbate bone disease and promote faulty mineralization
  - When end-stage renal disease develops, and diet, fluid restrictions, and drugs are no longer effective, the patient may undergo long-term dialysis (peritoneal dialysis or hemodialysis) or kidney transplantation; peritoneal dialysis and hemodialysis achieve the same results but in different ways
- Nursing interventions
  - Monitor physiologic changes and fluid and electrolyte changes
  - Consult the dietitian about ways to ensure that the patient consumes sufficient calories while adhering to dietary restrictions

- Teach the patient how to relieve uremic skin symptoms; dry, itchy skin contributes to discomfort, irritability, restlessness, and frustration, and scratching increases the risk of infection
  - Use tepid water and avoid soap (hot water and soap can worsen dryness and itching); use emollients, creams, and bath oils liberally to control dryness
  - Administer antihistamines and antipruritics as needed to control itching
  - Keep the patient's nails clean and trimmed short to reduce the risk of infection from scratching; tell the patient to use a soft washcloth, not fingernails, to scratch
  - Keep the patient's hair clean and moisturized but avoid frequent shampooing to prevent dryness
- Teach the patient how to perform oral care; decreased salivary flow and fluid restrictions can contribute to problems in the oral mucosa
  - Encourage frequent and gentle brushing with a soft toothbrush to decrease oral bacteria, prevent stomatitis, improve taste, and eliminate mouth odors
  - Encourage the patient to use mouthwash and to suck on hard candy to treat dry mouth, alleviate thirst, and improve taste
- Educate the patient how to prevent constipation by encouraging increased intake of dietary fiber, use of stool softeners, and increased activity; advise him to avoid laxatives that contain magnesium because of the risk of magnesium toxicity
- Help the patient increase mobility and activity as tolerated—for example, help him plan activities to avoid fatigue, teach him how to use ambulatory aids, and refer him to a physical therapist if needed
- Help prevent pulmonary complications by teaching the patient how to cough and deep-breathe exercises, and use an incentive spirometer to prevent atelectasis and infection and by preventing and treating fluid overload
- Educate the patient and family about the disease, its complications, and measures that can prevent further renal deterioration; refer the patient to the National Kidney Foundation
- Encourage patient and family to express their concerns
- Make sure the following areas are discussed with the patient and family: monitoring of fluid intake and output; signs of fluid overload and common electrolyte imbalances; therapeutic and adverse effects of prescribed drugs; methods of promoting skin integrity; methods of preventing infection, pulmonary complications, hyperkalemia, constipation, and fecal impaction; importance of controlling blood pressure; methods of maintaining mobility; need for phosphate binders to prevent bone disease; need for dietary modifications; advantages and disadvantages of peritoneal dialysis and hemodialysis; and home dialysis

Glomerulonephritis

- Description
  - Glomerulonephritis is an inflammation of the glomeruli
  - Acute glomerulonephritis follows a streptococcal infection of the respiratory tract or, less commonly, a skin infection, such as impetigo, immunoglobulin A nephropathy (Berger's disease), or lipid nephrosis; most people fully recover, but others may progress to CKD
  - Chronic glomerulonephritis is a slowly progressive disease that results in sclerosis, scarring, and, eventually, renal failure
- Signs and symptoms
  - The patient with acute glomerulonephritis may experience sudden onset of azotemia, dyspnea, edema, fatigue, hematuria, mild to severe hypertension, oliguria, proteinuria, and RBC casts in urine
  - Chronic glomerulonephritis develops insidiously and without symptoms, typically over many years; when it becomes suddenly aggressive, the patient may have edema and hypertension; in later stages, the patient may complain of nausea, vomiting, pruritus, dyspnea, malaise, fatigue, and mild to severe edema
- Diagnosis and treatment
  - Urinalysis typically reveals proteinuria, hematuria, WBCs, and casts
  - A 24-hour urine sample shows low creatinine clearance and impaired glomerular filtration
  - Blood studies reveal rising BUN and serum creatinine levels in those with advanced renal insufficiency as well as a decrease in hemoglobin levels
  - Renal biopsy can confirm the diagnosis and identify underlying disease
  - Elevated antistreptolysin-O titers, elevated streptozyme and anti-Dnase B titers, and low serum complement levels verify recent streptococcal infection

- Treatment depends on the cause and is mainly supportive; the goals are to correct fluid overload, hypertension, and uremia
  - ○ Antibiotics are given to treat streptococcal infections
  - ○ Antihypertensives are given to control hypertension
  - ○ Diuretics may be given to reduce fluid overload
  - ○ Sodium, potassium, protein, and fluid restrictions may be instituted
  - ○ Dialysis may be necessary to correct fluid and electrolyte imbalances
  - ○ Dialysis or kidney transplantation for chronic glomerulonephritis may be needed
- Nursing interventions
  - Check vital signs and electrolyte levels, monitor fluid intake and output and daily weight, assess renal function daily through serum creatinine and BUN levels and urine creatinine clearance, and watch for signs of ARF, including oliguria, azotemia, and acidosis
  - Consult the dietitian to provide a diet high in calories and low in protein, sodium, potassium, and fluids
  - Provide bed rest during the acute period of the disease
  - Provide emotional support for the patient and family; if the patient is receiving dialysis, explain the procedure
  - Teach the patient to report signs and symptoms of infection to the practitioner and the importance of follow-up examinations
  - Explain any dietary restrictions to the patient and family

Nephrotic Syndrome

- Description
  - Nephrotic syndrome is a type of kidney injury characterized by increased glomerular permeability, marked proteinuria, hypoalbuminemia, and edema
  - Prognosis varies depending on the underlying cause; some forms progress to end-stage renal failure
  - Nephrotic syndrome can result from many intrinsic renal and systemic diseases that cause glomerular damage; causes include glomerulonephritis; certain neoplastic diseases such as multiple myeloma; bronchogenic, breast, and colon cancer; lymphomas; leukemias; circulatory diseases; and diabetes mellitus
- Signs and symptoms
  - Edema is the major manifestation; it's typically soft and pitting and commonly occurs around the eyes, in dependent areas, and on the abdomen
  - Other signs and symptoms include weight gain, protein malnutrition, dyspnea, orthostatic hypotension, hypovolemia, hypertension, hyperlipidemia, ascites, pleural effusion, irritability, thromboembolism, malaise, AKI, and decreased urination
- Diagnosis and treatment
  - Proteinuria that exceeds 3.5 g/day is a hallmark of the disorder
  - Urinalysis reveals an increased number of hyaline, granular, waxy, fatty casts, oval fat bodies, and consistent, heavy proteinuria (levels greater than 30 mg/dL for 24 hours)
  - Serum cholesterol, phospholipid, and triglyceride levels are elevated, and the serum albumin level is decreased
  - A needle biopsy of the kidney can confirm the diagnosis
  - Treatment focuses on treating the underlying disease state responsible for proteinuria and relieving symptoms
  - Drug treatment includes diuretics, angiotensin-converting enzyme inhibitors, antithrombotic medications such as warfarin (Coumadin) or heparin, and antilipid agents; the patient should also follow a high-protein, low-sodium diet
- Nursing interventions
  - Teach the patient and family about the disease and its treatment; provide support
  - Weigh the patient and measure his abdominal girth daily
  - Monitor the patient's fluid and electrolyte status
  - Administer medications as ordered, and note the patient's response
  - Provide a low-cholesterol, no-added-salt diet with adequate protein; if appropriate, encourage the patient to consume foods high in potassium

- Obtain urine specimens for testing to evaluate the degree of proteinuria
- Teach the patient about follow-up care, and tell him to report any exacerbation of his symptoms

Neurogenic Bladder

- Description
  - Neurogenic bladder refers to all types of bladder dysfunction caused by an interruption of normal bladder innervation (see *Types of Neurogenic Bladder*, page 256)
  - Subsequent complications include incontinence, residual urine retention, UTI, stone formation, and renal failure
  - A neurogenic bladder may be described as spastic (resulting from an upper motor neuron lesion) causing an overactive bladder or flaccid (resulting from a lower motor neuron lesion) causing an underactive bladder
  - Neurogenic bladder may result from an acute infectious disease, Alzheimer's disease, birth defects of the spinal cord such as spinal bifida, brain or spinal cord tumors, cerebral palsy, encephalitis, multiple sclerosis, Parkinson's disease, spinal cord injury, stroke, chronic alcoholism, distant effects of cancer such as primary oat cell carcinoma of the lung, heavy metal toxicity, herpes zoster, long-term diabetes, vitamin B_{12} deficiency, syphilis, and nerve damage from surgery or herniated disk/spinal stenosis
- Signs and symptoms
- An underactive bladder causes full bladder with leakage, inability to tell when bladder is full, decreased anal sphincter tone, difficulty starting the flow of urine, and urinary retention
- An overactive bladder causes frequency, urgency, increased anal sphincter tone, urinary retention, and loss of bladder control
- Other signs and symptoms may include altered micturition, hydronephrosis, incontinence, and vesicoureteral reflux (passage of urine from the bladder back into a ureter)
  - The patient may also have symptoms of a UTI or kidney stones
- Diagnosis and treatment
  - Voiding cystourethrography evaluates bladder neck function, vesicoureteral reflux, and continence
  - Urodynamic studies—which consist of cystometry, uroflowmetry, urethral pressure profiles, and sphincter electromyography—help evaluate how urine is stored in the bladder, how well the bladder empties, and how quickly urine moves out of the bladder during voiding
  - Techniques for bladder elimination include Valsalva's maneuver, Kegel exercises, indwelling urinary catheter insertion, intermittent self-catheterization, and Crede's maneuver (pressing on the suprapubic area with a downward motion to express urine from the bladder)
  - Drug therapy may include terazosin (Hytrin), doxazosin (Cardura), bethanechol (Urecholine), and phenoxybenzamine (Dibenzyline) to facilitate bladder emptying and propantheline (Pro-Banthine), flavoxate (Urispas), dicyclomine (Bentyl), imipramine (Tofranil), and pseudoephedrine (Sudafed) to aid urine storage
  - When conservative treatment fails, surgery may be used to correct the structural impairment through transurethral resection of the bladder neck, urethral dilation, external sphincterotomy, sling surgery, or urinary diversion surgery creating a stoma; implantation of an artificial urinary sphincter may be necessary if permanent incontinence follows surgery, electrical device implanted near the bladder nerves to stimulate bladder muscles
- Nursing interventions
  - Use strict aseptic technique during insertion and maintenance of an indwelling urinary catheter; don't interrupt the closed drainage system for any reason; keep the drainage bag below the level of the bladder
  - Assess the patient for signs and symptoms of infection
  - Educate the patient to report signs and symptoms of infection and how to prevent UTI; encourage him to increase his fluid intake
  - Educate dietary measures to prevent kidney stone formation
  - Keep the patient as mobile as possible; perform range-of-motion exercises, if necessary
  - Educate the patient on Crede's maneuver, Kegel exercises, and intermittent self-catheterization
  - If a urinary diversion procedure is to be performed, arrange for consultation with an enterostomal therapist
  - Encourage patient and family to express their concerns

Box 15-3: Types of Neurogenic Bladder

Different types of neurogenic bladder have varied causes as summarized below.

Neural lesion	Type	Cause
Upper motor	Uninhibited	• Lack of voluntary control in infancy • Multiple sclerosis
	Reflex or automatic	• Spinal cord transection • Cord tumors • Multiple sclerosis
Lower motor	Autonomous	• Sacral cord trauma • Tumors • Herniated disk • Abdominal surgery with transection of pelvic parasympathetic nerves
	Motor paralysis	• Lesions at levels S2, S3, S4 • Poliomyelitis • Trauma • Tumors
	Sensory paralysis	• Posterior lumbar nerve roots • Diabetes mellitus • Tabes dorsalis

Urinary Calculi

- Description
  - Urinary calculi (stones) are the most common urologic problem in adults; *nephrolithiasis* is the presence of calculi in the renal parenchyma, *urolithiasis* is the presence of calculi in the urinary tract, and *ureterolithiasis* is the presence of calculi in the ureters
  - Calculi vary in size, from the size of a grain of sand to the size of a baseball; they're more common in men than in women, more common in hot summer months, and often recur
  - Urinary calculi vary in type and composition (see *Types of Urinary Calculi,* page 259)
  - Urinary calculi may be caused by infection, urinary retention, urinary stasis, immobility, dehydration, sedentary lifestyle, or persistently low urine output
  - The exact mechanism of stone formation is unknown; it may be related to changes in urine pH, volume depletion, or use of diuretics or other drugs
  - Calculi formed in the kidney may pass into the ureter, occlude the flow of urine, and cause urine to back flow into the kidney; this can lead to ureteral spasm, hematuria, urinary stasis, UTI, impaired renal function, and, eventually, hydronephrosis (kidney enlargement)
- Signs and symptoms
  - Symptoms vary with the location of the calculi and the presence of obstruction, infection, and edema
  - Small or large nonobstructing stones in the renal calyces or renal pelvis may cause no symptoms
  - Obstructing stones in the renal calyces or renal pelvis can cause recurrent infection, flank pain (described as a sudden, constant, intense, deep, dull ache) that radiates into the testicles or vulvar region, hematuria, and hydronephrosis; pyelonephritis and gram-negative septicemia may occur. The patient will have severe nausea with or without vomiting
  - Renal calculi that pass into the ureter or become lodged at the ureteropelvic junction result in mild to severe, colicky pain in the lumbar area that does not radiate to the groin; microscopic or gross hematuria occurs. There is dysuria and diarrhea
  - Extremely small renal calculi may pass through the urinary system without causing noticeable symptoms

- Bladder calculi usually cause irritation and inflammation or, if they obstruct the urethra, urine retention and urinary obstruction
- Costovertebral tenderness commonly accompany colicky pain
- Diagnosis and treatment
  - The diagnosis is often made by clinical symptoms and diagnostic tests are used to confirm diagnosis
  - Abdominal CT without contrast.
  - Abdominal X-ray or KUB X-ray of the kidneys, bladder, and ureters can detect calculi; renal ultrasound; IVP (urography); retrograde pyelography
  - Other diagnostic tests may include urinalysis and urine culture; CBC with differential, serum electrolytes, serum calcium, phosphorus, creatinine, uric acid, and electrolyte levels; urine pH; and tests for hypercalciuria, hyperuricuria, urinary oxalate, citrate, and cystine (using a 24-hour urine specimen)
  - Because the causes and treatment of urinary calculi are based on their chemical composition, recovered stones are usually analyzed
  - The main goals of treatment are to relieve pain, prevent nephron destruction, eliminate calculi, and prevent recurrence
    - Opioids, such as morphine sulfate, oxycodone/APAP (Percocet), hydrocodone/APAP (Norco), and hydromorphone (Dilaudid). NSAIDs such as ketorolac (Toradol). Antispasmodics such as oxybutynin (Ditropan) are used to control urinary spasms; antiemetics such as metoclopramide (Reglan), promethazine (Phenergan), and ondansetron (Zofran) are used when pain is accompanied by nausea and vomiting
    - Nephron destruction is prevented by controlling infection and by removing obstructions to urine flow to prevent backflow; urosepsis (septicemia related to UTI) is prevented with prophylactic antibiotic therapy
    - Because almost 90% of urinary calculi pass spontaneously, calculi that aren't causing renal damage, obstruction, or infection are left in place for several months in the hope that they'll pass spontaneously
    - Depending on the underlying causes and chemical composition of the calculi, dietary modifications and drug therapy may be used to help prevent recurrence; a fluid intake of 3 to 4 qt (3 to 4 L) daily is recommended, regardless of the type of calculi
  - Procedures to remove renal calculi include extracorporeal shockwave lithotripsy, ureteroscopic stone removal, and percutaneous nephrolithotomy
    - Extracorporeal shockwave lithotripsy is the most commonly used procedure to treat urinary calculi
      - In this procedure, ultrasonic shock waves pulverize the calculi into many small fragments that pass through the urinary tract over several months
      - The procedure has reduced the need for surgery and endoscopy to treat urinary calculi
    - Percutaneous nephrolithotomy is used for removing large or inaccessible stones
      - A nephroscope is inserted through an incision to the kidney, where the stone is removed
      - Ultrasound may be needed to break up larger stones
    - Stent placement or open nephrostomy
    - Ureteroscopic stone removal may be used for stones in the ureters
      - A fiberoptic ureteroscope is passed through the urethra and bladder into the ureters
      - The calculi is then removed or treated with shock waves
- Nursing interventions
  - Promote comfort for the patient with renal calculi
    - Administer opioid analgesics, antispasmodics, and antiemetics, as prescribed
    - Give hot baths or apply warm, moist packs to promote relaxation
    - Administer 3 to 4 qt (3 to 4 L) of fluids daily to help calculi passage; use I.V. fluids if the patient can't tolerate oral fluids
    - Encourage the patient to participate in usual activities and to ambulate frequently; these actions promote calculi passage
  - Prevent urinary obstruction and infection
    - Teach the patient the importance of monitoring urine output for changes in voiding pattern or amount and for cloudiness, foul odor, and blood

○ Tell the patient to promptly report signs of UTI and flank, lumbar, and abdominal pain to the practitioner

○ Teach the patient the importance of completing the full course of antibiotic therapy and the need to maintain fluid intake at 2 to 3 qt (2 to 3 L) daily to promote dilution and rapid drug excretion

○ Encourage the patient to increase daily fluid intake to 3 qt (3 L) or more to promote urine flow, dilute crystalloids in the urine, and prevent precipitation of crystalloids into stones

○ Encourage the patient with calcium-containing calculi to increase fluid intake 2 to 4 hours after meals, during heavy physical activity and dehydration, and at night; urine is more likely to be saturated with calcium at these times

● Prevent urinary calculi from recurring

  ○ Encourage increased fluid intake to prevent urinary stasis and calculi development

  ○ Instruct the patient to strain the urine to recover the calculi

  ○ Teach the patient about predisposing factors, such as dehydration, low urine output, prolonged immobilization, and UTI

  ○ Teach the patient with phosphate or uric acid stones how to monitor urine pH and alkalinize or acidify his urine

  ○ Provide instructions about diet and prescribed drugs for a patient with calcium calculi

    ○ Reduce dietary intake of calcium and vitamin D, which prevents parathyroid hormone production

    ○ Restrict sodium intake to reduce intestinal absorption of calcium

    ○ Limit refined carbohydrates and animal protein to decrease hypercalciuria

    ○ Encourage the intake of high-fiber foods to help bind calcium

    ○ Suggest the use of orthophosphates to decrease the incidence of recurrent calculi formation in patients with hypercalciuria

    ○ Administer thiazide diuretics, as prescribed, to increase calcium reabsorption in the kidneys and reduce calcium excretion

    ○ Administer sodium cellulose phosphate, which binds calcium in the intestinal tract, to lower the urinary calcium level

  ○ If the patient has phosphate calculi, provide instructions about diet and prescribed drugs

    ○ Because phosphate stones develop in alkaline urine, encourage the intake of ascorbic acid, cranberry and prune juices, plums, meats, eggs, and fish to maintain acid urine

    ○ Use an aluminum hydroxide gel, which combines with excess phosphorus and increases phosphorus excretion through the intestines

  ○ If the patient has oxalate calculi, provide instructions about diet and prescribed drugs

    ○ Restrict the intake of oxalate-rich foods and drinks, including apples, asparagus, beans, beer, chocolate, citrus fruits, colas, cranberries, grapes, green leafy vegetables (such as spinach and cabbage), instant coffee, peanut butter, peanuts, rhubarb, and tea

    ○ Make sure the patient's urine remains diluted to prevent more calculi from developing

    ○ Administer an antacid that contains aluminum to help bind oxalate and prevent urinary excretion

  ○ If the patient has uric acid calculi, provide instructions about diet and prescribed drugs

    ○ Recommend a low-purine diet that avoids fish (including shellfish), red wine, and rich foods, such as organ meats and foods with heavy sauces

    ○ If the patient has gout, restrict dietary intake of protein

    ○ Because uric acid stones are less likely to form in alkaline urine, encourage the use of sodium bicarbonate or sodium citrate solutions to maintain alkaline urine

  ○ If the patient has struvite calculi, provide instructions about diet and prescribed drugs

    ○ Make sure that the patient receives prompt treatment for UTIs and that measures are taken to reduce the incidence of infection

    ○ Administer acetohydroxamic acid to inhibit the chemical reaction caused by bacteria, which may help prevent struvite calculi

  ○ If the patient has cystine calculi, provide instructions about diet and prescribed drugs

    ○ Restrict dietary protein intake, and encourage the use of measures to alkalinize the urine

    ○ Use penicillamine to reduce cystine in the urine

Box 15-4: Types of Urinary Calculi

Different types of calculi vary in chemical content, incidence, and predisposing factors.

Calculi and description	Predisposing factors
Calcium calculi Formed from calcium oxalate, calcium phosphate, or both and account for 80% to 90% of all urinary calculi	• Immobility • Hyperthyroidism • Myeloproliferative disease • Renal tubular acidosis • Hyperuricemia • Increased dietary intake of milk, alkali products (such as antacids), and vitamin D • Prolonged use of steroids
Oxalate calculi Formed from oxalate and are the second most common type of calculi	• High intake of grains • Inflammatory bowel disease • Small-bowel resection • Ileostomy • Vitamin A deficiency
Uric acid calculi Formed from uric acid and account for 5% to 10% of calculi in the United States	• Hyperuricemia • Gout • High dietary intake of purine-rich foods, such as herring, sardines, organ meats, and yeast
Struvite (staghorn) calculi Formed from magnesium ammonium phosphate and account for 1% to 4% of urinary calculi	• Chronic urinary tract infections caused by urea-splitting bacteria, such as *Proteus*, *Pseudomonas*, *Klebsiella*, and *Staphylococcus*
Cystine calculi Formed from cystine and account for 1% to 4% of urinary calculi	• Genetic defect in the renal transport of cystine
Xanthine calculi Formed from xanthine and are rare	• Hereditary condition that causes xanthine oxidase deficiency

Urinary Tract Infection

- Description
  - *Urinary tract infection* is a general term used to describe infections of the upper or lower urinary tract; upper UTIs affect the kidneys, whereas lower UTIs affect the urinary bladder (cystitis) and urethra (urethritis)
  - UTIs are the most common bacterial infections in all patients and are a significant source of morbidity; they're more common in women than in men, and they increase in frequency with age
  - Factors that increase the risk of developing a UTI include female sex, increased sexual activity, pregnancy, structural and functional urinary tract abnormalities (such as strictures), obstructed urine flow, impaired bladder innervation, urinary stasis, incomplete bladder emptying, chronic health problems that alter renal tissue structure and function, urinary tract instrumentation (such as bladder catheterization and cystoscopy), and age
  - UTIs in men and women typically develop as an ascending infection from the urethra; other pathways for infection—such as hematogenous spread, lymphatic spread, and direct extension from other organs—are rare
  - A shorter urethra and its anatomic closeness to the vagina and rectum predispose women to ascending UTIs; besides anatomic differences that help protect men against UTIs, prostatic fluid provides an antibacterial effect
  - Infection of the kidney by bacteria usually occurs secondary to ascending infection from the bladder; infection commonly results from ureterovesical reflux in which an incompetent valve allows urine to flow back into the ureters during voiding

- Gram-negative bacteria (typically *E. coli*) cause most bacterial UTIs; gram-negative and gram-positive bacteria (typically different strains of Staphylococcus) may occasionally cause pyelonephritis (an infectious inflammation of the renal pelvis, tubules, and interstitial tissue that can be acute or chronic and may affect one or both kidneys)
  - Acute pyelonephritis is seldom associated with permanent renal damage
  - Chronic pyelonephritis is commonly associated with structural abnormalities and other conditions (such as calculi and diabetes) that contribute to repeated infection; it's more likely than acute pyelonephritis to cause permanent kidney damage and dysfunction from repeated inflammation and scarring
- Signs and symptoms
  - Symptoms of UTIs vary; some UTIs are asymptomatic and are diagnosed when routine urine testing detects bacteriuria
  - Cystitis commonly causes urinary frequency, urinary urgency, and dysuria (pain and burning on urination); it also may produce microscopic to gross hematuria, urinary tenesmus (persistent desire to urinate small amounts), suprapubic and bladder spasms, and cloudy, foul-smelling urine, and pelvic pain in women.
  - Acute pyelonephritis typically manifests with an abrupt onset of shaking chills and moderate to high fever (101.3° to 104° F [38.5° to 40° C]), tachycardia, flank pain, malaise, nausea, vomiting, and costovertebral angle tenderness
    - These signs and symptoms may be accompanied by symptoms of lower urinary tract involvement (dysuria and urinary frequency and urgency)
    - Chills, fever, and signs of toxicity (such as falling blood pressure, tachycardia, and skin color changes) suggest deeper infection of the kidney
  - Chronic pyelonephritis develops slowly and may progress to chronic renal failure
- Diagnosis and treatment
  - Diagnosis is usually based on the initial clinical presentation
  - Urine culture may reveal at least 10^5 (100,000) colonies of bacteria per milliliter from a clean-catch midstream or catheterized urine specimen
    - Urinalysis shows WBCs, casts, bacteria, and, possibly, red blood cells
    - Suprapubic needle aspiration of the bladder (if done) shows bacteria in the specimen
  - Patients with recurrent or complicated UTIs may undergo additional diagnostic studies—such as abdominal ultrasonography, excretory urography, cystography, cystoscopy with retrograde pyelography and voiding urography, and abdominal CT—to rule out calculi or structural abnormalities of the urinary tract as the cause of recurrent infections
  - Treatment of UTI and acute pyelonephritis has two goals: sterilizing the urine with antibacterial, antimicrobial, or urinary antiseptic drug therapy and identifying any illness or urinary tract abnormality that may be contributing to the infection
  - Increased urine output dilutes the urine, which relieves urethral irritation and burning; a continual urine flow also discourages urinary stasis and organism growth
  - Acute UTI symptoms may be relieved temporarily with urinary analgesics (such as a phenazopyridine, anticholinergics, or antispasmodics)
- Nursing interventions
  - If the patient has a lower UTI, administer antimicrobials, urinary analgesics, or antispasmodics, as prescribed; increase fluid intake up to 3 qt (3 L) daily to help dilute the urine; and give the patient a warm sitz bath two or three times a day for 10 to 20 minutes to relieve local symptoms
  - If the patient has pyelonephritis, administer antimicrobials, analgesics, antipyretics, and antiemetics, as prescribed, and maintain adequate fluid intake and output
  - Emphasize to the patient the importance of taking antimicrobial medication for the full course of therapy, even if symptoms improve
  - Teach the patient how to prevent urinary stasis by drinking 2 to 3 qt (2 to 3 L) of fluid daily, voiding every 2 to 3 hours, and emptying the bladder completely
  - Stress to the patient the importance of emptying the bladder as soon as the urge to urinate occurs; delayed urination encourages UTI by promoting urinary stasis
  - Encourage women whose UTIs are related to sexual activity to empty their bladders before and after sexual intercourse
  - Teach female patients how to reduce the number of pathogens in the perineal area by wiping from front to back after urination or defecation and cleaning the perineal and perianal area after each bowel movement

Review Questions

Question 1. The nurse is providing postprocedure care for a patient who underwent extracorporeal shockwave lithotripsy for the treatment of renal calculi. The nurse should instruct the patient to:

A. limit oral fluid intake for 1 to 2 weeks.
B. report the presence of fine, sandlike particles in the urine.
C. notify the practitioner about fever and chills.
D. report bright pink urine within 24 hours after the procedure.

Correct answer: C The patient should report fever and chills. Option A is incorrect because, unless contraindicated, the patient should be instructed to drink large quantities of fluid each day to flush the kidneys. Option B is incorrect because sandlike debris is normal due to residual stone products. Option D is incorrect because hematuria is common after lithotripsy.

Question 2. The nurse is planning a teaching session for a female patient who had a UTI. Which point should the nurse include?

A. Limit fluid intake to reduce the need to urinate.
B. Take the prescribed antibiotic until symptoms subside.
C. Urinating after intercourse can decrease the risk of UTI.
D. Wear only nylon underwear to reduce the chance of irritation.

Correct answer: C Urinating after intercourse can help prevent the spread of fecal bacteria to the bladder. The flow of urine flushes bacteria from the urethra. Option A is incorrect because women should be instructed to drink 2 to 3 qt (2 to 3 L) of fluid a day to dilute the urine and reduce irritation on the bladder mucosa. Option B is incorrect because the patient must take the full amount of antibiotics prescribed for her UTI, despite the improvement in her symptoms. Option D is incorrect because women should wear cotton underwear, not nylon, to reduce the chance of irritation.

Question 3. The nurse is caring for a patient with acute kidney injury. The nurse should expect hypertonic glucose, insulin infusions, and sodium bicarbonate to be used to treat:

A. hypernatremia.
B. hypokalemia.
C. hyponatremia.
D. hyperkalemia.

Correct answer: D Hyperkalemia is a common complication of acute kidney injury. It's life-threatening if immediate action isn't taken to reverse it. The administration of glucose and regular insulin infusions, with sodium bicarbonate if necessary, can temporarily prevent cardiac arrest by moving potassium into the cells and temporarily reducing serum potassium levels. Hypernatremia (Option A), hypokalemia (Option B), and hypercalcemia (Option C) don't usually occur with acute renal failure and aren't treated with glucose, insulin, or sodium bicarbonate.

Question 4. The nurse is teaching a patient with chronic kidney disease which foods to avoid. It would be most accurate for the nurse to teach the patient to avoid foods high in:

A. honey.
B. milk.
C. spinach.
D. steak.

Correct answer: D Proteins such as steak are typically restricted in patients with chronic kidney disease because of their metabolites. Carbohydrates such as honey and milk (Options A and B) and iron (Option C) aren't restricted.

Question 5. A patient with acute kidney injury is being assessed to determine whether the cause is prerenal, renal, or postrenal. If the cause is prerenal, which condition most likely caused it?

A. Sepsis
B. Renal carcinoma
C. Ureterolithiasis
D. Aminoglycoside toxicity

Correct answer: A Sepsis can lead to vascular collapse, which can cause the organs to receive inadequate perfusion. This can lead to prerenal failure. Renal carcinoma (Option B) and aminoglycoside toxicity (Option D) are renal causes, and ureterolithiasis (Option C) is a postrenal cause.

Question 6. A 35-year-old woman develops nephrotic syndrome. A nurse is educating the patient before discharge. Which statement indicates that the patient needs further education?

A. "I can prop my feet on a pillow to help with the swelling in my ankles."
B. "I can expect that my protein in my blood to be low because it is coming out in my urine."
C. "I am to take the cholesterol medication that I have been started on until my physician says it's ok to stop."
D. "It is ok to drink orange juice whenever I want."

Correct answer: C Hemolytic streptococci are common in throat infections and can cause an immune reaction that results in glomerular damage. Because of this, the patient should seek early treatment for respiratory infections. Avoiding physical activity (Option A) may promote urination, but it won't prevent the recurrence of glomerulonephritis. Straining all urine (Option B) helps identify renal calculi that have passed through the urine. Daily monitoring of urine specific gravity (Option D) helps assess hydration status, but it won't help prevent glomerulonephritis.

Question 7. A patient diagnosed with chronic kidney disease is told he must start hemodialysis. During patient teaching, the nurse should instruct the patient to:

A. follow a high-potassium diet.
B. strictly follow the hemodialysis schedule.
C. eat food high in dairy such as cheese and ice cream
D. use alcohol to clean the skin because of integumentary changes.

Correct answer: B To prevent life-threatening complications, the patient must strictly follow the hemodialysis schedule. The patient should follow a low-potassium diet—not a high-potassium diet (Option A)—because potassium levels increase in chronic renal failure. Patients with CKD are unable to clear phosphorus. As a result, they can develop hyperphosphatemia and should avoid foods high in phosphorus (Option C). The patient shouldn't use alcohol to clean the skin (Option D) because it would further dry out his skin.

Question 8. A 15-year-old patient has just been diagnosed with strep throat. How long should the patient be monitored for acute glomerulonephritis?

A. 3 days
B. 7 days
C. 2 weeks
D. 2 months

Correct answer: C Circulating immune complexes may become trapped in the glomeruli and cause inflammation for up to 14 days. Options A, B, and D are incorrect.

Question 9. During a health history, which statement by a patient indicates a risk of renal calculi?

A. "I've been drinking a lot of cola and soft drinks lately."
B. "I've been jogging more than usual."
C. "I've had more stress since we adopted a child last year."
D. "I am really bad about staying hydrated."

Correct answer: D Kidney stones can be caused by a buildup of minerals in the urine. Dehydration can cause these minerals to collect and form a stone. Cola and soft drinks (Option A) don't contain ingredients that would increase the risk of renal calculi. Jogging (Option B) and increased stress (Option C) aren't considered risk factors for renal calculi formation.

Question 10. Diuretics are ordered for a patient. What would be the best time of day for the nurse to schedule this medication?

A. Evening
B. At bedtime
C. Morning
D. Noon

Correct answer: C. Giving a diuretic in the morning allows it to work throughout the day. Giving a diuretic in the evening (Option A) or at noon (Option D) wouldn't provide this advantage. Giving a diuretic at nighttime (Option B) would cause the patient to get up frequently to go to the bathroom, interrupting sleep and increasing their risk for falls.

Selected References

National Institute of Diabetes and Digestive and Kidney Diseases. (2017). *Bladder infections in adults.* Retrieved from https://www.niddk.nih.gov/health-information/urologic-diseases/bladder-infection-uti-in-adults. Accessed March 27, 2017.

Brusch, J. L., Bavaro, M. F., Cunha, B. A., & Tessier, J. M. (2016, August 15). Cystitis in females: treatment and management. Retrieved on March 27, 2017 from http://emedicine.medscape.com/article/233101-treatment

Chirag, D., & Schwartz, B. F. (2016, December 3) Nephrolithiasis. Retrieved on March 27, 2017 from http://emedicine.medscape.com/article/437096-treatment

Cohen, E. P., & Batuman, V. (2016, December 24). Nephrotic syndrome. *Medscape.* Retrieved March 27, 2017 from http://emedicine.medscape.com/article/244631-overview

Curhan, G. C., Aronson, M. D., & Preminger, G. M. (2017). Diagnosis and acute management of suspected nephrolithiasis in adults. In S. Goldfarb, & M. P. O'Leary (Eds.), *UpToDate.* Wolters Kluwer. Retrieved from www.uptodate.com

Druml, W., Lenz, K., & Lagger, A. N. (2015). Our paper 20 years later: from acute renal failure to acute kidney injury—The metamorphosis of a syndrome. *Intensive Care Medicine, 41,* 1941–1949. doi:10.1007/s00134-015-3989-5.

Gill, B. C., Vasavada, S. P., Firoozi, F., & Rackley, R. R. (2017, March 9). Neurogenic bladder. Retrieved on March 27, 2017 from http://emedicine.medscape.com/article/453539-overview

Herbert, L. A., & Parikh, S. V. (2017). Differential diagnosis and evaluation of glomerular disease. In R. J. Glassock (Ed.), *UpToDate*. Wolters Kluwer. Retrieved from www.uptodate.com

Hooten, T. M., & Gupta, K. (2017). Acute uncomplicated cystitis and pyelonephritis in women. In S. B. Calderwood (Ed.), *UpToDate*. Wolters Kluwer. Retrieved from www.uptodate.com

Kelepouris, E., & Rovin, B. H. (2017). Overview of heavy proteinuria and the nephrotic syndrome. In R. J. Glassock (Ed.), *UpToDate*. Wolters Kluwer. Retrieved from www.uptodate.com

Palevsky, P. M. (2017). Definition and staging criteria of acute kidney injury (acute renal failure). In G. C. Curhan (Ed.), *UpToDate*. Wolters Kluwer. Retrieved from www.uptodate.com

Parmer, M. S., & Batuman, V. (2016, August 4). *Acute glomerulonephritis*. Retrieved March 27, 2017 from http://emedicine.medscape.com/article/239278-overview

Rosenberg, M. (2017). Overview of the management of chronic kidney disease in adults. In G. C. Curhan (Ed.), *UpToDate*. Wolters Kluwer. Retrieved from www.uptodate.com

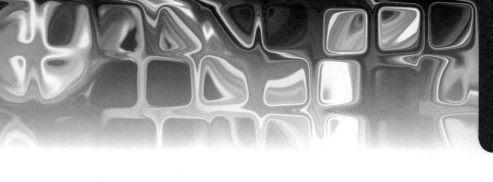

Chapter 16

Reproductive System Disorders

Introduction

- The chief function of the reproductive system is procreation and the manufacture of sex hormones
- Alterations in the reproductive system affect the ability to procreate and alter human social and emotional health
- Nursing history
  - The nurse asks the patient about the *chief complaint*
    - The female with a reproductive disorder may be experiencing pain, vaginal discharge, abnormal uterine bleeding, pruritus, or infertility
    - The male with a reproductive disorder may be experiencing penile discharge, impotence, infertility, or scrotal or inguinal masses, pain, or tenderness
  - The nurse then questions the patient about the *present illness*
    - Ask the patient about symptoms, including when they started, associated symptoms, location, radiation, intensity, duration, frequency, and precipitating and alleviating factors
    - Ask about the use of prescription and over-the-counter drugs; herbal remedies; vitamin and nutritional supplements, including oral contraceptives and hormones; and use of any alternative therapies
  - The nurse asks about the *medical history*
    - Question the female patient about her reproductive history, endocrine disorders, human immunodeficiency virus (HIV) status, infection or cancer of the reproductive organs, and sexually transmitted disease (STD)
    - Question the male patient about his medical history, including diabetes, hypertension, mumps, HIV status, STD, endocrine disorders, and infection or cancer of the reproductive organs
  - The nurse then assesses the *family history*
    - Ask about a family history of diabetes and hypertension
    - Also question the patient about a family history of cancer of the reproductive organs, diethylstilbestrol exposure, and other reproductive disorders
  - The nurse obtains a *social history*
    - Ask about work, exercise, diet, use of recreational drugs and alcohol, and hobbies
    - Also ask about stress, support systems, and coping mechanisms
    - Then, question the patient about the use of birth control, safe sex practices, sexual preference, number of sexual partners, and satisfaction
- Physical assessment
  - The nurse begins with *inspection*
    - Observe the patient's general appearance, noting behaviors, and mental status
    - Inspect the external genitalia and pubic hair, noting any swelling, lumps, discharge, rashes, lesions, lice, or odors
    - Observe the size and shape of the breasts, noting any nipple discharge
    - Inspect the female patient's internal genitalia using a speculum
    - Assess the male patient for inguinal and femoral hernias during Valsalva's maneuver and while coughing

- Next, the nurse uses *palpation*
  - ○ Palpate the external genitalia, noting any areas of swelling, tenderness, or hardness
  - ○ Palpate the breasts for lumps and nipple discharge
  - ○ Palpate the male patient's scrotal sac, noting the size and shape of the testicles and the presence of masses or tenderness
  - ○ If the patient is a male, palpate the inguinal area and check for hernias

Benign Prostatic Hyperplasia

- Description
  - Benign prostatic hyperplasia (BPH) is prostate gland enlargement; about 50% of men older than age 50 and 75% of men older than age 70 have symptoms of such enlargement
  - The cause is unknown but may be linked to hormonal changes
  - As the prostate enlarges, the urethral opening narrows and obstructs or interferes with urine flow, causing urine retention or incomplete emptying; eventually, the ureters and kidneys dilate, and urinary tract infections (UTIs) result from urinary stasis
  - Progressive bladder distention may cause a pouch to form in the bladder that retains urine when the rest of the bladder empties
- Signs and symptoms
  - Signs and symptoms include urinary frequency; nocturia; smaller, less-forceful urine stream; urinary hesitancy; dribbling after urination; bladder distention; cystitis; and acute urine retention
  - Hematuria, bladder calculi, impaired renal function, fatigue, nausea, vomiting, anorexia, and abdominal discomfort also may occur
- Diagnosis and treatment
  - Digital rectal examination can detect the enlarged lateral lobes of the prostate; cystoscopy and hematologic and kidney function studies may be performed; prostate-specific antigen (PSA) can help to rule out prostatic carcinoma; and postvoid residual urine test and transrectal ultrasonography may also be performed
  - Conservative treatment may include finasteride (Proscar) to decrease the size of the prostate and alpha-adrenergic blockers, such as prazosin (Minipress), doxazosin (Cardura), tamsulosin (Flomax), and terazosin (Hytrin), to relax the muscles and promote urination
  - For acute cases, a urologist may insert a urinary catheter; a stylet may be needed to pass through the obstruction, or a suprapubic cystostomy (incision and catheter placement in the bladder through the abdomen wall) may be needed
  - When a urinary obstruction is present, prostatectomy (surgical removal of soft tissue from the prostate) by one of four techniques is commonly performed (see *Types of prostatectomies*, page 267)
  - Newer treatments include laser therapy and intraurethral stents
  - Other minimally invasive surgical techniques include:
    - ○ Transurethral needle ablation (TUNA) radiofrequency energy produces localized heat to burn away well-defined regions of the prostate, thereby improving urine flow with less risk
    - ○ Transurethral microwave treatment (TUMT) to destroy portions of the prostate with heat
- Preoperative nursing interventions
  - Explain the surgical procedure, perioperative experience, and expected postoperative course to help decrease the patient's anxiety
  - Allow the patient to discuss fears and concerns about postoperative urinary incontinence and impotence but assure him that they aren't common after prostate surgery, only after radical perineal resection
- Postoperative nursing interventions
  - Evaluate the patient's pain and response to analgesia
    - ○ Explain to the patient that after transurethral resection of the prostate (TURP), bladder spasms are typical; explain to him that the sensation of needing to void is normal and that avoiding straining may decrease the frequency and intensity of bladder spasms
    - ○ Observe and maintain the patency of the three-way irrigation system; clots can obstruct the system and cause pain and bladder spasms; if clots form, increase the flow of saline solution to dilute the urine and allow the clots to flow out

○ Check for pain at the incision site, penile inflammation at the catheter site, and pain in the flank area caused by UTI

○ Administer opioids for pain as prescribed

● Monitor the patient for potential complications

○ Watch for hemorrhage and shock, which can occur postoperatively because the prostate is a highly vascular gland

○ Check urinary drainage, which initially should be reddish pink with a few small clots and then lighter pink during the first 24 hours after surgery; bright red drainage with clots indicates arterial bleeding and typically requires surgical intervention

○ Check for hemodynamic alterations (such as tachycardia, increased respiratory rate, and decreased blood pressure) and other signs of hemorrhage, including restlessness, pallor, and cold, clammy skin

○ Monitor the patient's fluid and electrolyte status

○ Make sure that the catheter drains well; catheter obstruction by clots can cause prostatic capsule or bladder distention and hemorrhage

○ Assess the patient for bladder distention by palpating for a rounded swelling above the pubis

○ Using aseptic technique, perform manual irrigation when needed with 50 mL of sterile normal saline solution to remove clots

○ Carefully record the intake of irrigating solution and the output of urine and irrigating solution

○ Observe the patient for signs of cerebral edema, such as confusion and agitation; water intoxication can result when the irrigating solution is absorbed into the vascular system during surgery

○ Check for and take precautions to prevent wound infection, UTI, and epididymitis

○ Use aseptic technique when performing catheter care and changing dressings and irrigation solution containers

○ Avoid taking rectal temperatures and administering enemas to prevent trauma to the operative area

○ Monitor the patient for signs of infection, such as fever, redness, swelling, and drainage from the incision site

○ Change wet dressings frequently to prevent skin maceration

○ After a suprapubic, perineal, or retropubic prostatectomy, monitor the patient for and take steps to prevent deep vein thrombosis (DVT) and pulmonary embolism

○ Monitor the patient for postoperative respiratory complications

● Assess urinary continence after the catheter is removed

○ Monitor urine output, and observe the patient for urine retention

○ Explain that incontinence is normal after prostate surgery, that it's transient and will gradually improve, except after radical perineal surgery

○ Encourage perineal exercises and voluntary interruption of the urine stream to expedite the return of bladder control

● Prepare the patient for discharge

○ Encourage the patient to discuss his feelings about sexual activity

○ Discuss with the surgeon when the patient can resume sexual activity (usually within 3 to 8 weeks)

○ Advise the patient about retrograde ejaculation to the bladder (urine may appear milky)

○ Refer a patient who has had a radical prostatectomy for counseling because physiologic impotence may occur

○ Tell the patient to avoid prolonged sitting, vigorous exercise, heavy lifting, and straining to decrease pressure on the operative area and help prevent bleeding

○ Discuss ways to avoid constipation; provide dietary suggestions to promote soft stools and enhance wound healing

○ Advise the patient to drink 2½ qt (2.5 L) of fluid daily to keep stools soft and prevent urinary stasis and UTI (unless contraindicated); discourage the intake of caffeine-containing beverages, which can irritate the urinary system; and encourage decreased fluid intake in the evening to minimize nocturia

○ Alert a patient who has undergone TURP about the possibility of secondary hemorrhage 2 weeks after the operation

○ Instruct the patient to call the surgeon immediately if bleeding, decreased urinary stream, or signs of infection develop

Box 16-1: Types of Prostatectomies

Four types of prostatectomy may be used to treat BPH.

Transurethral resection of the prostate

Transurethral resection of the prostate (TURP) is the most common surgical procedure for treating BPH. The urologist passes an endoscopic instrument directly through the urethra to visualize the prostate without making an incision. Then the urologist removes the medial lobe of the gland in small pieces, leaving behind the prostatic capsule. After removing the prostate tissue, the urologist inserts a large, three-way indwelling urinary catheter with a 30-ml balloon to continuously irrigate the bladder and keep it free from clots. Traction may be placed briefly on the catheter to facilitate hemostasis at the operative site. However, prolonged traction can cause tissue necrosis.

The traction and balloon pressure cause transient postoperative bladder spasms and a continual urge to void. Postoperative complications include hemorrhage, clot retention, bladder perforation during surgery, catheter displacement, UTI, and water intoxication related to continuous bladder irrigation.

Suprapubic prostatectomy

Suprapubic prostatectomy is performed when a large mass of tissue must be removed. After making an abdominal incision, the urologist removes the prostate through the bladder. Then a suprapubic catheter, indwelling urinary catheter, and sometimes a surgical drain are put in place, and the bladder is irrigated continuously for the first 24 hours after surgery to remove clots. The suprapubic catheter is removed 3 to 4 days after surgery; the indwelling urinary catheter remains in place until the suprapubic catheter site heals.

Suprapubic prostatectomy can produce the same complications as TURP as well as complications related to abdominal surgery.

Perineal prostatectomy

Perineal prostatectomy, which is commonly performed while treating prostate cancer, removes prostate tissue through an incision made between the rectum and the scrotum. If cancer is confirmed, adjacent tissue also may be removed in a procedure called radical perineal resection. An indwelling urinary catheter and sometimes a surgical drain are put in place.

The chief postoperative complication is wound infection because of the incision's location. Urinary incontinence and impotence can result from radical perineal resection.

Retropubic prostatectomy

Retropubic prostatectomy takes an abdominal approach to excising a large prostate gland high in the pelvis. The bladder is retracted, and the prostate is removed through an incision in the prostatic capsule. An indwelling urinary catheter is put in place.

Postoperative complications are the same as for suprapubic prostatectomy.

Breast Cancer

- Description
  - Breast cancer is the most common cancer in women and the second leading cause of cancer deaths in women; it affects one of eight women in the United States, and its incidence increases with age; 1% of all breast cancer occurs in men
  - The cause of breast cancer is unknown, but risk factors include a family history of breast cancer, inherited gene factors BRCA1 and BRCA2, obesity, diabetes, exposure to ionizing radiation or chemical carcinogens, nulliparity, no full-term pregnancies, use of estrogen replacement therapy for menopausal symptoms, a high-fat diet, 2 to 5 alcoholic drinks daily and the onset of menarche before age 12, menopause after age 55, and first pregnancy after age 30
  - The lifetime risk of breast cancer for women with BRCA1 mutation is 50% to 85%, compared with a risk of 11% for women without this gene mutation
  - The prognosis depends on the type of cancer and the stage of the disease at the time of treatment; early detection and treatment result in a more favorable prognosis
  - Breast cancer commonly begins as atypical cells, progresses to ductal or lobular carcinoma in situ, and then enters an invasive stage; in the invasive stage, the cancer can spread quickly to regional lymph nodes and the systemic circulation
  - Common metastatic sites include the lungs, bone, liver, brain, pelvis, and abdomen

- Signs and symptoms
  - A small, nontender, palpable, movable mass in the breast is an early sign of breast cancer, although it may go undetected until later signs develop; the common site for such a mass is the upper outer quadrant of the breast (tail of Spence)
  - Late signs of breast cancer include skin dimpling or puckering (Peau d'Orange), skin color changes over the lesion, nipple retraction, breast contour changes, serous or bloody nipple discharge, palpable axillary or other lymph nodes, breast asymmetry, erythema, ridging, and a prominent venous pattern
  - Inflammatory carcinoma is a rare form of breast cancer that produces a tender, enlarged, reddened, hot breast; in advanced cases, the breast may become ulcerated, infected, and necrotic
- Diagnosis and treatment
  - About 90% of breast cancers are discovered by breast self-examination (BSE); BSE and annual breast examination by a health care professional may detect early disease; however, micrometastases may have disseminated by the time the tumor is palpable
  - The American Cancer Society guidelines state that women over age 40 should have a mammogram annually and a clinical examination at least annually and all women should perform BSE monthly
  - Mammography can detect early lesions before they're palpable; digital mammogram with computer-assisted detection (CAD), ultrasonography, magnetic resonance imaging (MRI), and positron emission tomography also may be used
  - The diagnosis of breast cancer is made by fine-needle aspiration and excisional biopsy of the tumor; the biopsied tissue is analyzed to determine whether the tumor is hormone-dependent, a factor that influences treatment
    - Newer biopsy techniques include stereotactic core biopsy, minimally invasive breast biopsy, and advanced breast biopsy instrument
    - Ductal lavage may also be performed to detect malignant cells
    - Sentinel lymph node mapping, in which a radioactive substance or blue dye is injected around the biopsy site, may be performed before surgery; the sentinel node (the one most likely to contain malignant cells) is the one that contains the most radioactivity and blue dye, which then will be biopsied
  - Treatment depends on the tumor's histopathology and aggressiveness, hormonal factors (the patient's menopausal status and the tumor's hormone dependency), extent of disease, and the patient's overall health and treatment preferences
  - Surgery is the primary treatment for breast cancer; breast reconstruction surgery may be performed immediately after surgery or later (see *Types of breast surgery*, page 270); laser ablation is an alternative to lumpectomy in women with tumors that are smaller than ¾" (2 cm)
  - Radiation therapy is the primary treatment for patients who can't tolerate anesthesia or surgery or who have inflammatory carcinoma:
    - Primary radiation therapy with "boost" to the tumor site (application of additional radiation by external beam or placement of iridium needles in the former tumor site) may be used in early stages of breast cancer as a supplement to surgery and primary radiation
    - Radiation therapy to the breast and lymph nodes followed by "boost" to the tumor site is used after breast-preserving surgery (such as lumpectomy, quadrantectomy, and simple mastectomy)
  - Adjuvant chemotherapy is recommended after primary treatment and typically involves a combination of doxorubicin (Doxil), cyclophosphamide (Cytoxan), paclitaxel (Abraxane), methotrexate (Trexall, Rasuvo), tamoxifen (Nolvadex), and fluorouracil (Floururacil); metastatic breast cancer is usually treated with fluorouracil (Floururacil), paclitaxel (Abraxane), or docetaxel (Taxotere), capecitabine (Xeloda), vinorelbine (Navelbine), or gemcitabine (Gemzar)
  - Hormone therapy or surgery is indicated for patients with hormone-dependent breast cancer; antiestrogen drugs such as tamoxifen (Nolvadex) may be prescribed, and adrenalectomy, oophorectomy, or hypophysectomy may be considered
  - Monoclonal antibodies such as trastuzumab (Herceptin) may be used to treat metastatic breast cancer in women who have an excess amount of breast cancer cell antigen HER2
  - Bone marrow or blood stem cell transplantation may be used to restore stem cells
- Nursing interventions for a patient with early breast cancer
  - Assess the patient's and family's understanding of the disease, diagnostic tests, and treatments, and intervene accordingly
  - Encourage the patient to discuss her fears and concerns about the disease, diagnostic tests, treatments, and sexuality; clarify misconceptions, and be aware that breast cancer treatment can change the patient's body image and self-concept

- Evaluate the patient's support systems, and refer her to clergy members, home health care services, hospices, or support groups (such as Reach to Recovery, a group of volunteers who provide emotional and educational support during the preoperative and postoperative periods)
- Nursing interventions for a patient undergoing mastectomy
  - Monitor the patient for complications of general anesthesia and surgery, such as hemorrhage, wound infection, and altered respiratory status
    - During the initial postoperative period, frequently check the dressing and JP (Jackson Pratt) drains for excessive bleeding
    - Check the patency of the drains, and empty drains when half full to maintain suction and prevent fluid accumulation; drains are typically removed after 3 to 5 days
    - Use strict aseptic technique for dressing changes
    - Encourage the patient to perform deep-breathing and coughing exercises; administer analgesics to prevent respiratory splinting
    - Evaluate the patient's nutritional status, and promote adequate nutritional intake to foster wound healing
  - Evaluate the patient's level of pain and response to analgesia and comfort measures
    - Promote comfort by elevating the head of the bed and positioning the patient on the unaffected side supported by pillows (lying on the affected side can cause severe pain)
    - Position the affected arm on pillows to provide support and enhance circulation
    - Encourage the patient to use her unaffected arm to help change position or get out of bed
  - Monitor the patient for lymphedema, and take steps to prevent it
    - Never perform blood pressure readings, venipuncture, or injections on the affected arm
    - Check for edema in the affected arm; diuretics may be prescribed in the acute phase, and an elastic sleeve may be used during the chronic phase
    - Elevate, massage, and exercise the affected arm to improve circulation and prevent edema; teach the patient to do this at home
    - Teach the patient other techniques for preventing lymphedema, such as avoiding sun exposure, applying cream several times a day, using a thimble while sewing, using gloves while cleaning or gardening, wearing medical identification at all times, avoiding restrictive jewelry and clothing, not carrying heavy objects with the affected arm, and elevating the arm above the right atrium to promote circulatory and lymphatic flow
  - Teach the patient arm exercises to prevent muscle shortening, stiffening, and contracture and to preserve muscle tone
  - Encourage early and frequent ambulation; help the patient from her unaffected side, and help her maintain posture
  - Provide rest periods between activities to avoid tiring the patient
  - Prepare the patient for discharge by providing verbal and written instructions about pain medications, activity restrictions, arm exercises, lymphedema prevention, follow-up treatments, referrals to postdischarge support services, and information about prostheses; also provide an opportunity to discuss the effect of surgery on sexuality
- Nursing interventions for a patient receiving chemotherapy after a mastectomy
  - Monitor for and teach the patient about the adverse effects and toxicity of chemotherapeutic agents (see *Nursing implications in oncology care*, pages 341–347)
  - Follow guidelines for handling chemotherapeutic agents to prevent personal risks associated with repeated exposure to these drugs
  - Monitor the patient for adverse effects of hormone therapy such as fluid retention
- Nursing interventions for a patient receiving breast-preserving surgery and radiation therapy
  - Follow postoperative nursing interventions for a patient undergoing mastectomy
  - Monitor the patient for complications of radiation therapy, such as nausea, dyspepsia, esophagitis, transient pneumonitis, cough, fatigue, depression, and altered skin integrity at the surgical site and iridium needle site
  - Provide emotional support to the patient and family during "boost" therapy with an internal interstitial implant because radiation precautions require a private room and restricted visitation while the implant is in place (about 2 days) because of gamma ray emissions
- Nursing interventions for a patient with advanced breast cancer
  - Develop an individualized plan of care based on the patient's treatment: radiation therapy, chemotherapy, hormone therapy, oophorectomy, adrenalectomy, or hypophysectomy
  - Evaluate the patient's pain and response to pain-control and comfort measures; inform the practitioner and other health care team members if pain-control measures are ineffective

- Promote comfort by positioning the patient, applying heat or cold, using massage, providing pillows and a firm mattress, and teaching the patient relaxation techniques and guided imagery
- Promote adequate nutritional intake, particularly protein
  - Collaborate with the dietitian to improve nutrition; assess the need for supplements
  - Administer antiemetics as prescribed, and provide meticulous oral hygiene to improve the patient's ability and desire to eat
- Prevent alterations in skin integrity
  - Observe the patient's skin and mucous membranes for signs of impaired skin integrity; radiation therapy, chemotherapy, inadequate nutrition, and impaired mobility can lead to skin breakdown and mucous membrane irritation
  - Provide oral and skin care; applying lip gloss or petroleum jelly to the lips may be helpful
  - Promote activity and position changes to prevent prolonged pressure and tissue necrosis
  - Ensure adequate nutrition

Cervical Cancer

- Description
  - Cervical cancer is one of the most common cancers of the female reproductive system; it's most common in women between ages 30 and 50 and among Black, Hispanic, and Native American women
  - The most important risk factor for cervical cancer is infection with human papillomavirus (HPV); 90% of all cervical cancers are attributed to certain HPV types (HPV strain #16 and #18)
  - Risk factors include first intercourse at a young age, multiple male sex partners, long-term cigarette smoking, a weakened immune system, HIV infection, use of oral contraceptives for longer than 5 years, and having given birth to three or more children
  - About 95% of cervical cancers are squamous cell carcinomas, which affect the epidermal layer of the cervix; the precursor of this type of carcinoma is called dysplasia or cervical intraepithelial neoplasia
  - About 5% of cervical cancers are adenocarcinomas, which arise from the mucus-producing gland cells of the cervix; these cancers have no precursor
  - Cervical cancer is categorized according to the extent of the primary tumor, lymph node involvement, and metastasis
  - The prognosis depends on the stage of the disease and the treatment required; cure rates are as high as 100% in the early stages
- Signs and symptoms
  - Early stages of cervical cancer are asymptomatic
  - Later stages may cause vaginal discharge (leukorrhea) that gradually increases in amount and changes from watery to dark and foul smelling; irregular vaginal bleeding or spotting between menstrual periods or after menopause may occur; spotting or bleeding may occur after intercourse, douching, or bowel movements
  - Advanced invasive disease is associated with chronic infections, ulcers, pelvic pressure or pain, or abscesses at the tumor site; severe back and leg pain; anorexia; and anemia

---

Box 16-2: Types of Breast Surgery

Several surgical options are available for a patient with breast cancer.

- *Lumpectomy* or *tumorectomy* (simple excision of the tumor along with a margin of normal tissue) is used to treat early disease.
- *Quadrantectomy* (resection of the involved breast quadrant and dissection of axillary lymph nodes) also may be used to treat early disease.
- *Simple mastectomy* (removal of the main breast structure) may be performed for early disease or palliation in advanced, ulcerative disease. It doesn't remove the overlying skin, axillary nodes, and underlying muscles.
- *Modified radical mastectomy* (removal of the entire breast, some overlying skin and adjacent soft tissue, axillary lymph nodes, and the pectoralis major muscle) is the most common surgery for early disease.
- *Radical mastectomy* (removal of the entire breast, both pectoral muscles, and axillary nodes) is rarely used since the advent of less disfiguring procedures.

- Diagnosis and treatment
  - The Papanicolaou (Pap) test is used to screen for cervical cancer
  - If cervical neoplasia or cancer is detected on a Pap test, then colposcopy, punch biopsy, or endocervical curettage may be performed; lymphangiography, computed tomography (CT), and MRI also may be performed
  - The treatment of cervical cancer depends on the patient's health and age and the presence of other complications
  - Dysplasia and noninvasive cervical cancer (carcinoma in situ) may be removed by cryotherapy, carbon dioxide laser therapy, or conization (removal of a cone-shaped section of the cervix); these procedures maintain fertility but require frequent follow-up to detect recurrence
  - Noninvasive cervical cancer may be treated with a simple hysterectomy (removal of the cervix and uterus) in women who don't want future pregnancies
  - Invasive cervical cancer may be treated by radiation therapy, radical surgery, or chemotherapy (see *Treatments for invasive cervical cancer*, page 272)
- Nursing interventions for a patient with early cervical cancer
  - Assess the patient's and family's understanding of the disease, diagnostic tests, and treatments, and intervene accordingly
  - Allow the patient to discuss fears and concerns about the disease, diagnostic tests, treatments, and sexuality; clarify misconceptions and be aware that cervical cancer can change the patient's body image and self-concept
  - Evaluate the patient's support systems, and make referrals to clergy members, home health care services, hospices, or support groups as needed
- Nursing interventions for a patient undergoing cryotherapy, carbon dioxide laser therapy, or cervical conization
  - During the immediate postoperative period, monitor the patient for complications of anesthesia—typically a local anesthesia—and hemorrhage
  - Before discharge, provide verbal and written instructions about activity restrictions, and tell the patient to avoid using tampons and douching and to watch for and report increased vaginal bleeding or discharge and fever
- Nursing interventions for a patient undergoing hysterectomy
  - Monitor the patient for complications after general anesthesia and major abdominal surgery—and take steps to prevent them
    - ○ Monitor the patient for hemorrhage by assessing vital signs, wound drainage, and vaginal drainage; she may have surgical drains connected to a JP (Jackson Pratt) Drain.
    - ○ Initiate leg exercises and early ambulation to prevent venous stasis and thrombophlebitis
    - ○ Monitor bowel sounds and encourage early ambulation to expedite the return of bowel function; a nasogastric tube may be in place for the first 24 hours after surgery
    - ○ Observe the patient for altered urinary elimination; because the surgery is performed near the bladder, it can cause nerve damage and trauma to the ureter and bladder
  - Assess the patient's pain and response to analgesia
    - ○ If possible, administer analgesics using patient-controlled analgesia
    - ○ Ensure adequate pain relief, which encourages the patient to perform leg exercises, deep-breathing and coughing exercises, and early ambulation
  - Provide written and oral discharge instructions, and instruct the patient to take showers instead of baths to prevent vaginal inflammation and infection; explain activity restrictions; encourage her to avoid sitting for prolonged periods, lifting and straining until the first postoperative checkup, and intercourse for 4 to 6 weeks; instruct her to notify the practitioner if vaginal discharge, bleeding, or fever develop; and teach her about the therapeutic and adverse effects and dosing schedule of prescribed medications
- Nursing interventions for a patient undergoing radiation therapy
  - Assess the patient's comfort level and response to analgesia; administer opioids at regularly scheduled intervals
    - ○ Position the patient for comfort, using pillows for support; strict bed rest in the supine position is maintained while the implant is in place

○ Advise the patient that cell destruction by radiation causes foul-smelling vaginal discharge; minimize these effects with meticulous perineal care, a room deodorizer, and reassurance that the discharge is a temporary result of treatment

● Monitor the patient for local and systemic complications of radiation therapy
● Promote adequate nutritional and fluid intake to maintain skin integrity, promote tissue healing, and prevent urinary complications
● Follow the facility's radiation precautions; provide emotional support to a patient who feels isolated because of restricted visitation
● Prepare the patient for discharge by providing verbal and written instructions about medications, wound care, activity restrictions (including sexual activity), and follow-up appointments; also advise her that she must douche twice daily as prescribed, that vaginal drainage and bleeding should diminish gradually over 1 to 3 months, and that she should contact the practitioner if fever, increased pain, increased drainage, or altered urinary or bowel elimination occurs

● Nursing interventions for a patient undergoing pelvic exenteration
  ● Implement the same preoperative and postoperative nursing interventions as for a patient undergoing hysterectomy
  ● Be sensitive to the fact that this procedure exacts a tremendous physical, psychosocial, and emotional toll on the patient and requires a multidisciplinary approach to patient care, involving an enterostomal therapist, a social worker, and a dietitian
  ● Refer the patient for support to help her cope with the resulting changes in lifestyle, body image, and sexuality

● Nursing interventions for a patient whose ovaries have been removed or undergoing radiation therapy
  ● A premenopausal woman whose ovaries have been removed or irradiated will experience menopause
  ● Discuss the physiologic changes of menopause and self-care practices to promote optimal health and a feeling of well-being; recommend regular exercise, calcium and vitamin D and B-complex supplements, a calcium-rich diet, vaginal lubricants, and hormone therapy (controversial) to relieve various menopausal symptoms

---

Box 16-3: Treatments for Invasive Cervical Cancer

Radiation therapy, radical surgery, or chemotherapy may be used to treat invasive cervical cancer.

Radiation therapy

Radiation therapy, which uses whole pelvic irradiation and intracavitary implants, causes ovarian function to cease. Before treatment, the patient follows a low-residue diet, receives enemas, and has an indwelling urinary catheter inserted to prevent bowel and bladder distention. These procedures allow more room for the implant and may protect the bowel and bladder from radiation. Complications of radiation therapy include nausea, vomiting, diarrhea, malaise, fever, hemorrhage, cystitis, proctitis, phlebitis, vesicovaginal fistulas, and ureterovaginal fistulas.

Surgery

Radical hysterectomy removes the uterus and proximal vagina through an abdominal incision. Pelvic lymph node dissection may be performed for stage I and early stage II disease; a salpingo-oophorectomy also may be performed. Surgical drains are placed below the incision site to drain excess fluid. An indwelling urinary catheter is placed preoperatively to prevent bladder trauma during surgery and to allow for postoperative urine drainage. (In the immediate postoperative period, the bladder may be atonic.)

Pelvic exenteration is used for advanced or recurrent cervical cancer confined to the pelvis. Total exenteration removes the bladder, rectosigmoid, and all reproductive organs and nodes. The bladder and sigmoid may be preserved if disease isn't evident in these structures.

For either type of surgery, complications include abdominal distention, paralytic ileus, thrombophlebitis, wound infection, atelectasis, and other complications of general anesthesia and major abdominal surgery.

Chemotherapy

Chemotherapy commonly includes fluorouracil, ifosfamide, and cisplatin alone or in combination to treat metastatic or nonresectable disease.

Endometrial Cancer

- Description
  - Endometrial cancer is one of the most commonly diagnosed gynecologic cancers
  - Risk factors include early menarche, late menopause, infertility, extended use of tamoxifen or unopposed estrogens, obesity, diabetes, advancing age, high-fat diet, history of breast and ovarian cancers, previous pelvic radiation, and family history
  - Most endometrial cancers are adenocarcinomas and are slow to grow and metastasize; common sites for metastasis are the lungs, liver, and bone
- Signs and symptoms
  - The woman may report abnormal vaginal bleeding, especially after menopause
  - Difficult or painful urination, pain during intercourse, and pelvic pain may also occur
  - In advanced cases, lymph node enlargement, pleural effusion, abdominal masses, or ascites may be present
- Diagnosis and treatment
  - Diagnosis is based on a physical examination and history
  - Other diagnostic tools include transvaginal ultrasound, endometrial biopsy, CA-125 blood test, CT scan, MRI, cystoscopy, and Pap test
  - The primary treatment for endometrial cancer is hysterectomy; a bilateral salpingo-oophorectomy may also be performed
  - Progesterone therapy may be indicated for patients with recurrent disease
  - Women with metastatic disease may receive combination chemotherapy that may include doxorubicin (Adriamycin), cisplatin (platinol), paclitaxel (abraxane), etoposide (toposar), and dactinomycin (cosmegen)
  - Radiation therapy may be indicated before, after, or instead of surgery in some women; radioactive implants may be used
- Nursing interventions
  - Assess the patient's and family's understanding of the disease, diagnostic tests, and treatments, and intervene accordingly
  - Provide analgesics and comfort measures as needed
  - Encourage the patient to discuss feelings regarding self-esteem and body image disturbance
- Nursing interventions for a patient undergoing other treatments
  - Provide care related to abdominal hysterectomy and bilateral salpingo-oophorectomy and pelvic radiation therapy (see *Cervical cancer*, page 270)
  - Provide care related to systemic chemotherapy (see *Nursing implications in oncology care*, pages 341–347)

Endometriosis

- Description
  - Endometriosis is a benign condition in which the endometrial cells that normally line the uterus are dispersed throughout the pelvis; the most common ectopic tissue sites are the ovaries, fallopian tubes, uterosacral ligaments, cul-de-sac of Douglas, pelvic peritoneum, rectovaginal septum, and cervix
  - The misplaced endometrial cells respond to normal ovarian hormone stimulation; during menstruation, the ectopic endometrial tissue grows, becomes secretory, and bleeds, which causes pressure and inflammation at the involved site and creates fibrosis, adhesions, and cysts
  - Endometriosis may result from the transfer of endometrial cells by blood flow, lymphatic flow, or retrograde menstrual flow or from autoimmune or congenital factors
  - Risk factors for endometriosis include family history, delayed childbearing, retroflexed uterus, use of an intrauterine device (IUD), polymenorrhea, hypermenorrhea, menstrual periods that last longer than 5 days, spotting, and being of Asian descent
  - Endometriosis can occur in any woman of childbearing age but usually begins between ages 30 and 40; it's responsible for 30% to 45% of female infertility
- Signs and symptoms
  - The chief symptom of endometriosis is painful menstruation (dysmenorrhea) or menstrual cramps
  - Many women with advanced disease are asymptomatic; the disease is discovered when they undergo testing related to infertility

- Other symptoms of endometriosis include dyspareunia, painful defecation, rectal pressure, and abnormal uterine bleeding (menstrual cycles of less than 27 days; menses that last longer than 7 days)
- The pelvic examination may reveal bluish lesions on the labia, perineal area, cervix, or vaginal wall; tender nodules in the posterior vaginal fornix of the vagina, along the uterosacral ligaments, and along the cul-de-sac; adnexal thickening and nodules; tender, enlarged, and fixed ovaries; and a fixed, retroverted uterus that's painful when moved
- Diagnosis and treatment
  - The diagnosis of endometriosis is determined by patient history and physical examination; biopsy—using laparoscopy—of the endometrial tissue is required to confirm the diagnosis
  - Vaginal ultrasonography, complete blood count, cultures and blood tests for STDs, Pap test, urinalysis, and a pregnancy test may be performed
  - Treatment of endometriosis depends on the patient's age, symptoms, stage of disease, and desire to have children
  - Drugs may be used to treat endometriosis (see *Drug therapy for endometriosis*, page 275)
  - Laparoscopy, under general anesthesia, may be used to diagnose and treat endometriosis; after inserting a scope into the peritoneal cavity through a small abdominal incision, the surgeon insufflates carbon dioxide into the abdominal cavity to separate the intestines from the pelvic organs and to improve visualization; after determining the extent of the disease, the surgeon uses fulguration or laser surgery to treat lesions and adhesions
  - Women with severe, symptomatic, painful endometriosis may decide to undergo bilateral salpingo-oophorectomy and total abdominal hysterectomy; laser surgery may also be used
  - In some women, endometriosis may disappear without treatment; in others, pregnancy causes remission of the disease
- Nursing interventions
  - Teach the patient about reproductive anatomy and physiology, the disease, and the medications used to treat it
  - Teach the patient about activities that may promote comfort and help relieve symptoms: regular exercise, sexual excitement and orgasm, increased intake of natural diuretics (such as watermelons, cranberry juice, peaches, and asparagus), decreased intake of salt and high-sodium foods, increased intake of iron-rich foods, application of heat to the pelvic area and lower back, relaxation techniques, and guided imagery
  - Allow the patient to discuss feelings about how the disease affects her lifestyle, body image, and self-concept
  - Provide additional emotional support to a patient who is infertile; also refer the patient for infertility testing and counseling
  - Provide postoperative care for a patient undergoing laparoscopy; monitor her for complications of general anesthesia and hemorrhage, and provide verbal and written discharge instructions to ensure that she understands self-care measures and follow-up treatment
    - Teach the patient and family about wound care
    - Advise the patient to expect several days of gaslike pain in the abdomen and referred shoulder pain from carbon dioxide insufflation; recommend analgesics, local heat application, and a light diet to enhance comfort
    - Inform the patient about pain medications, activity restrictions (including sexual activity), and follow-up treatment
  - Provide postoperative care for a patient undergoing hysterectomy, oophorectomy, or bilateral salpingectomy; this care is the same as that for a patient with cervical cancer who undergoes these procedures (see *Cervical cancer*, page 270)

Erectile Dysfunction

- Description
  - Erectile dysfunction is the inability to attain or maintain penile erection long enough to complete intercourse
  - The disorder is classified as primary or secondary
    - In *primary impotence*, the patient never achieves sufficient erection
    - In *secondary impotence*, the patient has achieved erection and completed intercourse in the past
    - In most cases, erectile dysfunction has an organic cause, such as vascular insufficiency or veno-occlusive dysfunction

Box 16-4: **Drug Therapy for Endometriosis**

Various types of drugs are prescribed to manage endometriosis.

- Analgesics, nonsteroidal anti-inflammatory drugs, and diuretics are prescribed to relieve pain, inflammation, and fluid retention.
- Oral contraceptives interrupt ovulation and produce endometrial atrophy, thereby decreasing endometrial flow in the peritoneal cavity. Their adverse effects include nausea, vomiting, weight gain, depression, fatigue, breast tenderness, and recurrent vaginitis.
- Danazol, a synthetic androgen, may be prescribed for 6 months to suppress ovarian activity and cause ectopic endometrial atrophy. The most effective drug for endometriosis, danazol, relieves pain in about 90% of patients. Because endometriosis recurs in 5% to 20% of patients, repeated 6-month courses of therapy may be needed. Adverse effects include acne, decreased breast size, voice deepening, depression, hirsutism, hot flashes, oily skin, vaginal dryness, and weight gain.
- Nasally administered nafarelin (Synarel), a gonadotropin-releasing hormone (GnRH) agonist, creates a reversible "pharmacologic oophorectomy" to control ectopic endometrial activity. Nafarelin causes fewer adverse effects than danazol; nafarelin's adverse effects may include depression, hot flashes, insomnia, and vaginal dryness.
- Medroxyprogesterone, a progestin, reduces dysmenorrhea and pelvic pain. Adverse effects include breakthrough bleeding, emotional lability, blood clots, myocardial infarction, pulmonary embolism, nausea, vomiting, depression, headache, and fatigue.
- Leuprolide (Lupron) and goserelin (Zoladex), GnRH agonists, block the production and release of luteinizing hormone and follicle-stimulating hormone, thereby reducing estrogen production and leading to decreased pelvic pain and shrinking of endometrial implants. Treatment is limited to 6 months because long-term use can cause bone loss. Common adverse effects may mimic symptoms of menopause, including hot flashes, vaginal dryness, decreased libido, headache, and mood swings.

- Other causes include certain medications, such as antihypertensives and diuretics, and alcohol and drug abuse
  - Some cases may be psychogenic
  - All age groups may be affected, although the incidence increases with age
- Signs and symptoms
  - Onset may occur suddenly, or the patient may experience a gradual decline in sexual function
  - A history of medical disorders, drug therapy, or psychological trauma may accompany the disorder
- Diagnosis and treatment
  - Laboratory findings may include a decrease in serum testosterone levels
  - Glycosylated hemoglobin level may be elevated, indicating uncontrolled diabetes mellitus
  - Urinalysis results may be abnormal, indicating kidney damage or diabetes mellitus
  - Lipid profiles may be increased, indicating atherosclerosis
  - Blood glucose levels may be increased, a sign of diabetes mellitus
  - Serum creatinine levels may be elevated, resulting from kidney damage
  - PSA results help rule out prostate cancer
  - Ultrasonography evaluates vascular function; angiography evaluates vasoocclusive disease
  - Direct injection of alprostadil (Caverject) into the corpora evaluates the quality of erection
  - Nocturnal penile tumescence testing helps distinguish psychogenic impotence from organic impotence
  - For erectile dysfunction that stems from an organic cause, treatment aims to correct the underlying cause
  - For dysfunction that results from a psychogenic cause, psychological counseling and sex therapy may help
  - An external vacuum device may allow the patient to achieve a temporary erection
  - Phosphodiesterase type 5 (PDE5) inhibitors, such as sildenafil (Viagra) , vardenafil (Levitra), and tadalafil (Cialis) are the first line of drug treatment
  - The patient may benefit from a surgically inserted inflatable or semirigid penile prosthesis
- Nursing interventions
  - Teach the patient and partner about the disorder and treatment options
  - Encourage the patient to discuss concerns, and provide support; include the patient's partner in your care
  - Assist with measures to determine a possible underlying organic cause
  - Provide postoperative care after penile prosthesis surgery; monitor the patient for bleeding, swelling, and infection
  - Teach the patient to avoid alcohol before engaging in sexual activity; teach about the proper use of medications to treat erectile dysfunction
  - Refer the patient to a practitioner, nurse, psychologist, social worker, or counselor trained in sex therapy as needed

Ovarian Cancer

- Description
  - Ovarian cancer is the most common fatal gynecologic cancer and the fifth leading cause of cancer death in women; principal sources include the epithelial cells (serous, mucous, or endometrial cells), germ cells (in cases of teratoma or dysgerminoma), mesenchymal cells (in cases of fibroma, lymphoma, or sarcoma), and gonadal stroma (granulosa, theca, Sertoli's, or Leydig's cells)
  - Although unconfirmed, risk factors for ovarian cancer may include nulliparity; infertility or history of difficulty becoming pregnant; family history; previous breast, endometrial, or colon cancer; exposure to environmental carcinogens; lack of breastfeeding; use of fertility drugs; or use of talcum powder in the genital area
  - Ovarian cancer can occur at any age but is most common between ages 50 and 60
  - The 5-year survival rate for stage I ovarian cancer is 85% to 90%; stage II, 0% to 70%; and stages III and IV, 17% to 39%
- Signs and symptoms
  - Ovarian cancer typically doesn't produce any signs or symptoms until the advanced stages of the disease
  - It should be suspected in women with irregular menses, early menopause, uterine bleeding before puberty or after menopause, or other signs of endocrine dysfunction, such as infertility and masculinization
  - GI signs and symptoms—such as abdominal discomfort and a feeling of fullness, abdominal distention, nausea, vomiting, dyspepsia, flatulence, and constipation—may occur as the tumor enlarges
  - Ovarian enlargement (or palpable ovaries before menarche or after menopause) suggests ovarian cancer
  - Other signs and symptoms include urinary frequency and weight loss
- Diagnosis and treatment
  - No early screening tests exist for ovarian cancer
  - Because the ovaries are located deep in the abdomen, pelvic examination may not detect early disease; diagnosis is made after biopsy of the tumor, during exploratory laparotomy
  - CA-125 is a tumor marker specific to epithelial ovarian cancer; significantly elevated CA-125 levels are usually found in patients with ovarian cancer
  - Other diagnostic tools include transvaginal ultrasonography (TVUS), urine estrogen levels, pregnanediol levels, CT scan, MRI, and pelvic X-rays
  - Treatment depends on the cancer's stage, which is determined during exploratory laparotomy; during this procedure, a total abdominal hysterectomy and bilateral salpingo-oophorectomy are performed to remove as much of the tumor as possible along with affected lymph nodes and other peritoneal structures
  - Radiation therapy or chemotherapy is usually recommended with surgery, for all stages of the disease
    - ○ Radiation therapy techniques include external pelvic irradiation or intraperitoneal instillation of radioactive phosphorus
    - ○ Combination chemotherapy commonly consists of carboplatin and paclitaxel
  - Patients may undergo a "second-look" laparotomy after treatment of the early stages to detect persistent disease
  - Treatment of advanced ovarian cancer is usually palliative
- Nursing interventions for a patient with early ovarian cancer
  - Assess the patient's and family's understanding of the disease, diagnostic tests, and treatments, and intervene accordingly
  - Encourage the patient to discuss fears and concerns; be aware that treatment for ovarian cancer can change the patient's body image and self-concept and that the diagnosis may come at a time of life when the patient is experiencing difficulty with the physical and sociocultural aspects of aging
  - Evaluate the patient's support systems, and refer her to clergy members, home health care services, hospices, or support groups as needed
- Nursing interventions for a patient with advanced ovarian cancer
  - Administer analgesics, as indicated
  - Position and support the patient to promote comfort; also apply heat or cold, massage painful areas, use pillows, and teach the patient relaxation techniques and guided imagery
- Nursing interventions for a patient with early or advanced ovarian cancer
  - Promote adequate nutritional intake by collaborating with the dietitian to determine what type of food the patient should eat, how much, and how often; assessing the need for supplements; administering antiemetics as prescribed; and providing meticulous oral hygiene to improve the patient's ability and desire to eat

- Prevent alterations in skin integrity
  - ○ Observe the patient's skin and mucous membranes for signs of impaired skin integrity; radiation therapy, chemotherapy, inadequate nutrition, and impaired mobility can increase the risk of skin breakdown and mucous membrane irritation
  - ○ Provide oral hygiene and skin care to prevent stomatitis and skin breakdown
  - ○ Promote activity and position changes to prevent prolonged pressure and tissue necrosis
- Nursing interventions for a patient receiving intraperitoneal chemotherapy
  - Intervene as appropriate for systemic chemotherapy (see *Nursing implications in oncology care,* pages 341–347), and perform interventions specific to intraperitoneal chemotherapy
  - Warm the drug, which typically is given in 2 L of normal saline solution, to body temperature, and infuse it by gravity as rapidly as tolerated; to improve flow, check for kinks in the tubing or catheter obstruction, and encourage the patient to gently turn from side to side
  - Gently irrigate the catheter with normal saline solution; use an I.V. infusion to promote flow as long as the catheter is patent
  - After instillation, clamp the tubing and let the solution remain in the peritoneal cavity for 4 hours (the dwell time)
  - Unclamp the drainage tubing after the dwell time to let fluid drain out of the peritoneum; facilitate drainage by aspiration, frequent changes in patient position, Valsalva's maneuver, and application of mild pressure to the abdomen
  - After drainage is completed, flush the catheter first with preservative-free saline solution and then with heparinized saline, and remove the needle from the port; the drainage may be sent to the laboratory for analysis
  - Monitor the patient for fluid and electrolyte imbalances related to chemotherapy-induced nephrotoxicity and intraperitoneal fluid infusion
    - ○ Administer I.V. fluid supplemented with potassium and magnesium on the evening before treatment, as prescribed
    - ○ Measure fluid intake and output, and notify the practitioner if the 4-hour urine output falls below 240 mL
    - ○ Monitor electrolyte levels daily
  - Monitor the patient for infection, and take steps to prevent it by using strict aseptic technique when handling the peritoneal access device and checking for local erythema, fever, and other signs of sepsis or peritonitis
  - Check for alterations in respiratory status; keep the head of the bed elevated, and make sure that oxygen is nearby
  - Watch for complications resulting from a detached or obstructed catheter; if severe pain occurs, stop the infusion and obtain X-rays to confirm catheter migration into the peritoneal cavity
  - Promote comfort by administering antiemetics, pain medications, and sedatives as needed; also provide extra blankets because the patient may feel chilled during the procedure as a result of the instilled fluids
  - Prepare the patient for discharge by providing verbal and written instructions about pain medications, adverse effects of chemotherapy, catheter care, activity restrictions, and follow-up treatment
- Nursing interventions for a patient undergoing other treatments
  - Provide care related to abdominal hysterectomy and bilateral salpingo-oophorectomy and pelvic radiation therapy (see *Cervical cancer,* page 270)
  - Provide care related to systemic chemotherapy (see *Nursing implications in oncology care,* pages 341–347)

Pelvic Inflammatory Disease

- Description
  - Pelvic inflammatory disease (PID) refers to any acute, subacute, recurrent, or chronic infection of the oviducts and ovaries with adjacent tissue involvement
  - PID includes inflammation of the cervix (cervicitis), uterus (endometritis), fallopian tubes (salpingitis), and ovaries (oophoritis)
  - The inflammation may extend to connective tissue that lies between the broad ligaments (parametritis)
  - PID is typically caused by bacteria—usually gonorrheal and chlamydial organisms—but it may also result from a virus
  - Normally, the cervical mucus and cervicovaginal flora serve as a protective barrier; when this barrier is altered or destroyed—for instance, from sexual activity or instrumentation—bacteria can enter the vagina and cervix and ascend and enter the uterine cavity, causing inflammation of various structures; retrograde menstrual flow may help promote the ascent of such organisms

- Risk factors for PID include multiple sexual partners, a history of STIs, uterine infection after pregnancy, and IUD insertion
- Complications include infertility, septicemia, pulmonary embolus, peritonitis, and shock
- Signs and symptoms
  - PID may be asymptomatic; if signs and symptoms do occur, they may include low-grade fever, malaise, lower abdominal pain that worsens with intercourse, irregular vaginal bleeding, and purulent vaginal discharge
  - Other signs and symptoms include pain during cervical examination and possibly a palpable adnexal mass
- Diagnosis and treatment
  - Culture and sensitivity testing and Gram stain of endocervix or cul-de-sac secretions show the causative agent; urethral and rectal secretions can also show the causative agent
  - The patient's C-reactive protein level, white blood cell count, and erythrocyte sedimentation rate are elevated
  - TVUS may show the presence of thickened, fluid-filled fallopian tubes
  - CT scan may show complex tubo-ovarian abscesses, and MRI may show images of soft tissue; these tests are useful not only for establishing the diagnosis of PID but also for detecting other processes responsible for symptoms
  - Diagnostic laparoscopy identifies cul-de-sac fluid, tubal distention, and masses in a pelvic abscess
  - Treatment aims to eradicate the underlying infection with antibiotics
  - Laparoscopy allows for drainage of pelvic abscesses, pelvic lavage, or lysis of adhesions
  - If the patient develops a ruptured pelvic abscess—a life-threatening situation—she may require a total hysterectomy with bilateral salpingo-oophorectomy
- Nursing interventions
  - Teach the patient about the disorder, including treatment options and how to prevent future infections
  - Administer prescribed antibiotics and analgesics; if I.V. antibiotics are ordered, initiate I.V. access and ensure its patency
  - Provide frequent perineal care; inspect the patient's perineal pads, noting the color and characteristics of drainage
  - Use meticulous hand hygiene technique
  - Encourage the patient to discuss feelings about condition and sexuality; offering emotional support
  - Help patient to develop effective coping strategies
  - Palpate the patient's abdomen for pain and tenderness, noting any distention or rigidity; auscultate bowel sounds for changes
  - Be alert for signs of peritonitis
  - Prepare the patient and family for possible surgery if an abscess develops or ruptures
  - Provide appropriate postoperative care
  - Before discharge, teach the patient to report any fever, increased vaginal discharge, or increases in pelvic pain to her practitioner
  - Emphasize the importance of completing the full course of antibiotics to ensure complete eradication of the infection

Prostate Cancer

- Description
  - Prostate cancer is the second leading cause of cancer death in men in the United States and the most common type of cancer overall, the most common type in African-American men, and the second most common type in American men older than age 50
  - Risk factors for prostate cancer include advancing age; North American, African, Australia and Northwestern European descent; a high-fat diet; physical inactivity; and a family history
  - Adenocarcinoma is the type of tumor found in prostate cancer
  - Common metastatic sites are the brain, lungs, bone, and lymph nodes
- Signs and symptoms
  - Early prostate cancer is asymptomatic; in about 50% of patients, the disease is in the advanced stages or has metastasized by the time it's discovered
  - As the disease progresses and the size of the neoplasm increases, urinary obstruction occurs, thereby producing dysuria, urinary frequency, blood in the ejaculate, urine retention, decreased size and force of the urinary stream, and hematuria
  - Signs and symptoms of metastasis include hip pain, backache, rectal or perineal discomfort, anemia, nausea, weight loss, weakness, shortness of breath, and edema

- Diagnosis and treatment
  - A firm nodule felt on digital rectal examination suggests prostate cancer; a biopsy of surgically removed tissue can confirm the diagnosis
  - Other helpful diagnostic tests include serum acid phosphatase, PSA, and testosterone levels; bone scans to detect metastasis; and kidney function tests
  - Treatment is based on the patient's age, overall health, symptoms, stage of the disease, and survival prognosis
  - Radical perineal prostatectomy is the standard surgical procedure for patients with potentially curable disease; bilateral orchiectomy is commonly performed along with prostatectomy
  - Curative radiation therapy may be indicated if the patient is in the early stages of prostate cancer; this treatment may preserve sexual functioning
  - Palliative measures are indicated for patients with advanced tumors or signs of metastasis (see *Palliative treatments for prostate cancer*, page 280)
- Nursing interventions
  - Assess the patient's and family's understanding of the disease, diagnostic tests, and treatments and intervene accordingly
  - Encourage the patient to discuss fears and concerns
  - Evaluate the patient's support systems and refer to clergy members, home health care services, hospices, or support groups as needed
  - Evaluate the patient's response to pain control; notify the practitioner if pain-control measures are ineffective
  - Promote comfort by applying heat or ice, massaging painful areas, providing pillows and a firm mattress, and teaching the patient to use relaxation techniques and guided imagery
  - Monitor the patient for complications of radiation therapy, such as systemic adverse reactions (including nausea, vomiting, headache, skin reactions, fatigue, and malaise) and transitory proctitis and cystitis
  - Monitor the patient for complications of chemotherapy (see *Nursing implications in oncology care*, pages 341–347); handle chemotherapeutic agents according to federal safety guidelines
  - Promote adequate nutritional intake by collaborating with the dietitian to determine what types of food the patient should eat, how much, and how often; assessing the need for supplements; administering antiemetics as prescribed; and providing meticulous oral hygiene to improve the patient's ability and desire to eat
  - Prevent alterations in skin integrity by observing the patient's skin and mucous membranes for signs of impaired skin integrity; radiation therapy, chemotherapy, inadequate nutrition, and impaired mobility can predispose the patient to skin breakdown and mucous membrane irritation
    - Provide oral hygiene and skin care to prevent stomatitis and skin breakdown
    - Promote activity and position changes to prevent prolonged pressure and tissue necrosis
  - Maintain adequate urinary elimination
    - Determine the patient's urinary elimination pattern
    - Monitor patient for urine retention; record the frequency and amount of urine output, and assess for urinary urgency, dysuria, and suprapubic distention
    - Facilitate bladder emptying
      - Ensure adequate fluid intake, and encourage the patient to urinate when feels the urge.
      - Help the patient to a normal position for voiding when possible, and unless contraindicated, use Valsalva's maneuver to initiate urine flow
      - Administer cholinergics, as prescribed, to stimulate bladder contraction
      - Determine whether the patient needs intermittent or indwelling urinary catheterization
  - Assess the patient's potential for injury, and take safety precautions; bone metastasis, pain, weakness, and peripheral neuropathy may predispose the patient to falls or other injuries
  - Prepare the patient for discharge
    - Provide sexual counseling, emotional support, and self-catheterization and catheter care instructions as needed
    - Teach the patient exercises to strengthen the perineal muscles
    - Caution the patient to avoid taking rectal temperatures and to allow suppositories to reach room temperature before inserting them into the rectum
    - Provide referrals for home health care and other services as needed
    - Provide verbal and written instructions about prescribed medications, activity restrictions, diet, and follow-up care

Box 16-5: Palliative Treatments for Prostate Cancer

Several palliative treatments may be used for a patient with advanced or metastatic prostate cancer.

- Radiation therapy may be used for patients with late-stage disease. Because it alters cell growth and reproduction through ionization, it affects cancerous—and healthy—cells.
- Suppressive hormone therapy may be used to decrease tumor size and relieve pain because prostatic adenocarcinomas are hormone dependent. Suppression may be achieved by orchiectomy or administration of drugs, such as luteinizing hormone–releasing hormone analogs, antiandrogens, and other androgen-suppressing drugs (such as diethylstilbestrol).
- Chemotherapy may slow the disease process and provide palliative relief. It directly interferes with the biochemistry of the cancer cells, altering their growth, metabolism, and reproduction.
- Cryosurgery, which freezes the target tissue, is another palliative measure used for locally recurrent disease.
- Repeated transurethral resections of the prostate may be needed to maintain urine flow. Eventually, permanent urinary or suprapubic catheterization may be needed.
- Corticosteroids and neurosurgery may relieve pain by interrupting pain receptors in the spinal cord.

Sexually Transmitted Diseases

- Description
  - STDs are the most common infections in the United States; acquired immunodeficiency syndrome (AIDS), herpes, gonorrhea, and hepatitis are considered epidemic (see *Chapter 17, Immune system disorders,* for details on AIDS)
  - These contagious diseases are usually transmitted through intimate sexual contact with an infected person; some are transmitted to an infant during pregnancy or childbirth
  - People younger than age 25, those with multiple sex partners, and those with a history of STDs are at higher risk for infection; the incidence of STDs is higher among prostitutes and people having sexual contact with prostitutes, drug abusers, or prison inmates
  - Morbidity and mortality depend on the type and stage of STD; many STDs are easy to treat when detected early
  - STDs can be prevented by educating the public, identifying and treating partners and contacts of infected people, and identifying and treating symptomatic or asymptomatic infected patients; barrier methods of contraception, such as a condom and a diaphragm with spermicide, reduce the risk of certain infections
  - More than 21 diseases are classified as STDs; they're caused by bacteria, viruses, protozoans, fungi, and ectoparasites
- Signs and symptoms
  - The chief signs of STDs are vaginitis, recurrent vaginitis, epididymitis, lower abdominal pain, pharyngitis, prostatitis, and skin or mucous membrane lesions
  - Many STDs are asymptomatic, especially in women; by the time the STD is detected, the woman may have severe complications, such as PID, infertility, ectopic pregnancy, or chronic pelvic pain
- Diagnosis and treatment
  - The diagnosis of a specific STD is made by physical examination, patient history, and laboratory tests to determine the causative organism
  - Treatment is based on the specific causative organism; treatment guidelines for each STD are available from the Centers for Disease Control and Prevention (CDC) (see *Sexually transmitted diseases,* page 282)
  - The CDC recommends that specific resources be available for patients with STDs: medical evaluation and treatment facilities for patients with HIV infection; hospitalization facilities for patients with complicated STDs, such as PID and disseminated gonococcal infection; referrals for medical, pediatric, infectious disease, dermatologic, and gynecologic-obstetric services; family planning services; and substance abuse treatment programs
- Nursing interventions
  - Develop a therapeutic relationship with the patient that fosters trust and preserves the patient's dignity; ensure privacy and confidentiality, and avoid judging the patient's lifestyle or making assumptions about sexual preference

- Provide emotional support, and encourage the patient to discuss feelings; the patient may be anxious and fearful and may experience altered self-esteem and self-image
- Teach the patient about the STD and its treatment
  - Discuss disease transmission, signs and symptoms, the length of the infectious period, infection prevention, and cure (if the STD can be cured)
  - Discuss the health consequences of improper treatment, and emphasize that the patient's partner is also at risk
  - Clarify common misconceptions and promote understanding of healthful sexual practices
    - Inform the patient that washing his hands and genital area before and after sexual contact doesn't prevent STDs
    - Encourage the patient to urinate after intercourse
    - Advise women to avoid douching because it can alter the normal vaginal flora
    - Tell the patient that condoms and a diaphragm with spermicide may provide some protection against certain STDs, but IUDs and birth control pills don't
  - Encourage a sexually active patient who has multiple partners and no STD symptoms to have an STD examination twice a year
  - Tell the patient to seek immediate treatment if STD symptoms develop
  - Inform the patient that treatment doesn't provide immunity from the same or a different STD
  - Advise the patient to abstain from sexual activity until the posttreatment follow-up verifies a cure
  - Discuss modifications of sexual activity to prevent recurrence: reducing the number of sex partners, avoiding partners who have multiple partners, and questioning partners about their STD history
- Teach the patient about the prescribed medication and its dosing schedule and adverse effects; stress the importance of completing the medication regimen, even if symptoms disappear; advise the patient to return if adverse reaction develops so that another medication can be prescribed
- Teach the patient about lesion care, including soaking in a tub two to three times a day, keeping lesions clean and dry between baths, wearing cotton underwear, avoiding panty hose and restrictive clothing, and avoiding creams, lotions, and ointments except those specifically prescribed
- Refer the patient to other social and health services as needed
- Report the STD according to local health department or state health board requirements

Testicular Cancer

- Description
  - Testicular cancer is the most common type of cancer in men between ages 15 and 35; it's the third leading cause of death in these men but has an overall cure rate of 95% when detected early
  - Although the cause of testicular cancer is unknown, incidence is higher in men with cryptorchidism; the disease is also associated with scrotal trauma, heredity, infection, hormonal abnormalities, and orchiopexy (surgical repair of undescended testis)
  - Testicular tumors are histologically classified as seminomas or nonseminomas
    - Seminomas typically are localized and highly sensitive to radiation therapy; the prognosis is good with early treatment
    - Nonseminomas are faster growing and more diffuse; they require more aggressive treatment with surgery and chemotherapy
  - Educating men to perform testicular self-examination facilitates earlier detection and intervention; however, many patients don't seek treatment for 3 to 6 months after detecting a tumor
- Signs and symptoms
  - Most patients with testicular cancer report unilateral testicular enlargement, a "dragging" sensation in the lower abdomen, and heaviness in the scrotum; 70% to 90% of patients don't report pain as an early symptom
  - A patient with a palpable tumor that doesn't transluminate may have testicular cancer
  - A patient with metastasis to retroperitoneal lymph nodes may report lower back pain, lymphadenopathy, fatigue, weight loss, and anorexia; the next most common site of metastasis is the lungs
  - The patient also may experience breast enlargement and tenderness

Box 16-6: Sexually Transmitted Diseases

Name and Organism	Possible Signs and Symptoms	Treatment	Special Considerations
Chlamydia *Chlamydia trachomatis*	• Purulent discharge • *Males*: burning on urination and symptoms of epididymitis • *Females*: usually asymptomatic	Doxycycline (Vibramycin) or azithromycin (Zithromax)	• All sexual contacts must be treated. • Potential complications in females are pelvic inflammatory disease (PID), infertility, and spontaneous abortion; in males, urethritis, epididymitis, and prostatitis. • Patient should take medication as prescribed, follow up in 7 to 10 days, and abstain from sexual activity until treatment is completed.
Genital herpes, herpes simplex type 2	• *Females*: purulent vaginal discharge • Multiple vesicles on the genital area, buttocks, or thighs • Painful dysuria • Fever • Headache • Malaise	Famciclovir (Famvir), valacyclovir or acyclovir (Zovirax), topical anesthetic ointment	• Warm baths and mild analgesics may relieve pain. • Patient should avoid sexual activity during the prodromal stage and during outbreaks until all lesions have dried up. • Many patients have recurrences every 2 to 3 months; local hyperesthesias may occur 24 hours before the outbreak of lesions.
Gonorrhea *Neisseria gonorrhoeae*	• Purulent discharge • Dysuria • Urinary frequency	Ceftriaxone (Rocephin) plus azithromycin (Zithromax) or doxycycline (Vibramycin)	• All sexual contacts must be treated. • Potential complications in females are PID, sterility, and ectopic pregnancy; in males, prostatitis, urethritis, epididymitis, and sterility. • Patient should take medication as prescribed, follow up in 7 to 10 days, and abstain from sexual activity until treatment is completed.
Human papillomavirus (HPV)	• Pink-gray soft lesions, singularly or in clusters	Podophyllin 10% to 25% or imiquimod to lesions; cryosurgery	• Patient should receive frequent Papanicolaou tests. • HPV has an 80% chance of recurrence. • HPV is the most common cause of cervical cancer.
Syphilis *Treponema pallidum*	• Chancre on genitalia, mouth, lips, or rectum • Fever • Lymphadenopathy • Positive results for Venereal Disease Research Laboratories test, fluorescent treponemal antibodies test, and rapid plasma reagin test	Penicillin	• Syphilis may be characterized as primary, secondary, or tertiary. • All sexual contacts must be treated. • Patient should take medication as prescribed, follow up in 7 to 10 days, and abstain from sexual activity until treatment is completed.
Trichomoniasis *Trichomonas vaginalis*	• *Males*: urethritis or penile lesions; usually asymptomatic • *Females*: frothy vaginal discharge with erythema and pruritus; may be asymptomatic	Metronidazole (Flagyl)	• All sexual contacts must be treated. • Complications in females include recurrent infections and salpingitis. • Patient should take medication as prescribed, follow up in 7 to 10 days, and abstain from sexual activity until treatment is completed. • Patients should avoid alcohol during treatment and for at least 3 days after its completion.

- Diagnosis and treatment
  - Diagnosis of suspected testicular cancer is based on the patient's symptoms and history, testicular examination, urine estrogen and testosterone levels, scrotal illumination, and scrotal ultrasonography; radioimmunoassay studies, which measure antigens produced by malignant cells, aid in diagnosis
  - Excretory urography may be used to evaluate renal function and structure; chest X-ray, CT, and MRI are used to evaluate metastasis
  - The histologic diagnosis is made by inguinal orchiectomy; testicular biopsy isn't done because it can promote the spread of tumor cells
  - Testicular cancer is treated with radiation therapy, chemotherapy, and surgery; one, two, or all three of these treatments may be used, depending on the stage of the disease and the type of tumor (see *Treatment for testicular cancer*, page 284)
- Nursing interventions for a patient in the early stages of testicular cancer
  - Assess the patient's and family's understanding of the disease, diagnostic tests, and treatments, and intervene accordingly
  - Encourage the patient to discuss his fears and concerns; clarify misconceptions, and be aware that orchiectomy can change the patient's body image and self-concept; discuss the possibility of joining a sperm bank if sterility is a concern
- Nursing interventions for a patient undergoing orchiectomy
  - Monitor the patient for complications of anesthesia and hemorrhage immediately after surgery
  - Prepare the patient for discharge
    - Teach the patient and family about wound care at home
    - Provide verbal and written instructions about pain medications, activity restrictions (including sexual activity), and follow-up care
- Nursing interventions for a patient undergoing retroperitoneal lymph node dissection
  - Observe the patient for postoperative complications, such as hemorrhage, fluid and electrolyte imbalances, atelectasis, paralytic ileus, DVT, and wound infection
  - Monitor hemodynamics and fluid and electrolyte status
  - Initiate leg and breathing exercises and early ambulation to prevent circulatory, respiratory, and GI complications
  - Assess the patient's pain and response to analgesia; patient-controlled analgesia is an effective way of administering opioids
  - Prepare the patient for discharge
    - Provide verbal and written instructions about pain medications, activity restrictions, and follow-up care
    - Tell the patient to avoid lifting and straining until after returning to the practitioner for 6-week postoperative visit
    - Inform the patient that sexual activity generally can be resumed in 4 to 6 weeks
- Nursing interventions for a patient receiving chemotherapy
  - Be fully knowledgeable about the prescribed chemotherapeutic agents, including their administration protocols, therapeutic and adverse effects, and specific nursing considerations; handle chemotherapeutic agents according to federal safety guidelines
  - Monitor and treat the patient for complications of chemotherapy (see *Nursing implications in oncology care*, pages 341–347)
  - Prepare the patient for discharge
    - Provide verbal and written instructions about pain medications, wound care, activity restrictions (including sexual activity), and follow-up care
    - Make sure the patient understands how to manage the adverse effects of chemotherapy
    - Teach the patient how to perform testicular self-examination; patients who have had testicular cancer are at higher risk for developing another tumor than those who haven't had the disease
    - Tell the patient about the need for follow-up visits; recurrence is most common in the first year after treatment
- Nursing interventions for a patient receiving radiation therapy
  - Observe the patient for complications of treatment; common systemic adverse reactions include nausea, vomiting, headache, skin reactions, fatigue, and malaise
  - Check for alterations in skin integrity

Box 16-7: **Treatment for Testicular Cancer**

Testicular cancer may be treated with radiation therapy, chemotherapy, surgery, or any combination of these.

Radiation therapy

Radiation therapy is primarily used to treat pure seminomas after surgery because these tumors are highly sensitive to radiation. It also may be indicated for patients who are poor candidates for surgery or who don't respond to chemotherapy. To preserve fertility, the unaffected testis is shielded to prevent irradiation.

Chemotherapy

When used with surgery, chemotherapy has provided the most effective treatment of nonseminoma tumors. Cisplatin commonly is used to treat testicular cancer in combination with bleomycin, etoposide, vinblastine, ifosfamide, and cyclophosphamide.

Surgery

Unilateral radical orchiectomy is performed through an inguinal incision. It typically is a 1-day surgical procedure performed under local or spinal anesthesia, depending on the patient's health status. It may be the only surgery needed for patients with stage I and II seminomas who also undergo postoperative radiation therapy.

Orchiectomy and *retroperitoneal lymph node dissection* (RPLND) are used to treat stage II and III disease. Because RPLND is major abdominal surgery, it poses all the associated risks and potential complications. Therefore, the patient is monitored closely after surgery. RPLND typically is performed after the staging orchiectomy and intensive chemotherapy. A unilateral (modified) RPLND is performed, unless regional metastasis is present. After full RPLND, orgasm and libido remain intact, but the patient is sterile.

Uterine Leiomyomas

- Description
  - Uterine leiomyomas—also known as *myomas*, *fibromyomas*, or *fibroids*—are the most common benign uterine tumors; they're malignant in less than 0.1% of patients
  - The tumors, composed of smooth muscle, usually occur in the uterine corpus, although they may appear on the cervix or on the round or broad ligament
  - Classified according to location, these tumors may be located within the uterine wall (intramural) or protrude into the endometrial cavity (submucous) or from the serosal surface of the uterus (subserous)
  - The tumors are typically firm and surrounded by a pseudocapsule composed of compressed but otherwise normal uterine myometrium
  - Uterine leiomyomas may cause the uterine cavity to become larger, increasing the endometrial surface area, which can increase uterine bleeding
  - Tumor size varies greatly; possible regulators of leiomyoma growth include several growth factors (including epidermal growth factor) as well as steroid hormones, such as estrogen and progesterone
  - Although the cause of uterine leiomyomas is unknown, they may be correlated with estrogen stimulation; the tumors typically arise after menarche and regress after menopause, implicating estrogen as a promoter of leiomyoma growth
  - Uterine leiomyomas affect three times as many black women as white women; they may occur at any age but are most common in women ages 40 to 50
  - Complications include spontaneous abortion, preterm labor, anemia secondary to excessive bleeding, infection, infertility, and bowel obstruction; the tumors may also mask signs of endometrial or ovarian cancer
- Signs and symptoms
  - This disorder commonly causes no symptoms
  - If signs and symptoms do occur, they may include a history of abnormal menstrual bleeding, urinary frequency, or incontinence; abdominal cramping during menstruation; pelvic pressure; and lower back pain
  - A physical examination may reveal abdominal distention; palpable firm, smooth nodules; or mobile, painless masses
- Diagnosis and treatment
  - Blood tests may show anemia from abnormal bleeding, which may support the diagnosis
  - Ultrasonography allows an accurate assessment of the dimension, number, and location of tumors; MRI may reveal calcified fibroids

- Hysterosalpingography may detect myomas
- Fractional dilation and curettage helps to rule out cervical and uterine cancers
- Laparoscopy helps to rule out other pelvic diseases and disorders
- An endometrial biopsy may rule out endometrial cancer in patients who have abnormal uterine bleeding and are older than age 35
- Treatment is conservative for asymptomatic myomas, with the patient undergoing pelvic examination and ultrasonography every 3 to 6 months if the size remains stable
- Progestins, such as norethindrone or medroxyprogesterone, reduce overall uterine size; a combination of oral contraceptives prevents the development of new myomas
- A luteinizing hormone–releasing hormone, such as nafarelin, goserelin, and leuprolide, induces abrupt artificial menopause to promote atrophy of myomas
- Iron supplements, as indicated, treat anemia
- Nonsteroidal anti-inflammatory drugs provide pain relief
- Surgical measures include abdominal, laparoscopic, or hysteroscopic myomectomy
- Endometrial ablation treats small submucosal myomas
- Uterine artery embolization (a radiologic procedure) blocks the uterine arteries using small pieces of polyvinylchloride
- Magnetic resonance–guided focused ultrasonography surgery causes coagulative necrosis of myomas
- Severe cases of the disorder may require hysterectomy
- Nursing interventions
  - Teach the patient and family about the diagnosis and treatments, including medications, surgery, and uterine artery embolization if indicated; explain that myomas typically regress after menopause
  - Administer iron supplements and blood transfusions as ordered for a patient with severe anemia from excessive bleeding
  - Encourage frequent rest periods if the patient experiences fatigue related to anemia
  - Give goserelin subcutaneously, leuprolide I.M., and nafarelin by nasal spray, as ordered
  - Encourage the patient to use prescribed pain medications as ordered for pain relief
  - Encourage the patient to verbalize her feelings, questions, and concerns about the disease and its effects on her lifestyle; provide clear explanations, and answer any questions
  - Reinforce the patient's self-esteem
  - Urge the patient to participate in self-care activities and decision making to foster a sense of control
  - Reassure the patient that she won't experience premature menopause if her ovaries are left intact
  - Prepare the patient physically and psychologically for surgery as indicated
  - Provide preoperative and postoperative care as appropriate
  - Teach about the importance of regular gynecologic examinations, including pelvic evaluations and ultrasonography for newly diagnosed symptomatic or excessively large myomas; laboratory testing, such as hemoglobin levels and hematocrit for excessive uterine bleeding; and monitoring once uterine size and symptoms stabilize

Review Questions

Question 1. Which patient has the highest risk of ovarian cancer?

A. A 30-year-old woman taking an oral contraceptive
B. A 45-year-old woman who has never been pregnant
C. A 40-year-old woman with three children
D. A 36-year-old woman who had her first child at age 22

Correct answer: B The incidence of ovarian cancer increases in women who have never been pregnant, are older than age 40, are infertile, or have menstrual irregularities. Other risk factors include a family history of breast, bowel, or endometrial cancer. The risk of ovarian cancer hasn't been linked to oral contraceptives (Option A), multiple births (Option C), or having a first child at a young age (Option D).

Question 2. A patient with a small, in situ breast nodule asks the nurse about her treatment options. Which treatments would be considered for this patient?

A. Lumpectomy and radiation
B. Partial mastectomy and radiation
C. Partial mastectomy and chemotherapy
D. Total mastectomy and chemotherapy

Correct answer: A Treatment for breast cancer depends on the disease stage and type, the patient's age and menopausal status, and the disfiguring effects of the surgery. For this patient, lumpectomy is the most likely option. Lumpectomy involves a small incision with removal of the surrounding tissue and, possibly, the nearby lymph nodes. The patient usually undergoes radiation therapy afterward. With partial mastectomy (Options B and C), the tumor is removed along with a wedge of normal tissue, skin, and possibly axillary lymph nodes. With a total (simple) mastectomy (Option D), the entire breast is removed.

Question 3. The nurse is assessing a male patient with syphilis. Which symptom most likely prompted him to seek medical attention?

A. Rashes on the palms of the hands and soles of the feet
B. Cauliflower-like warts on the penis
C. Painful red papules on the shaft of the penis
D. Foul-smelling discharge from the penis

Correct answer: A Rash on the palms of the hands and soles of the feet is a sign of the secondary stage of syphilis. Signs and symptoms of gonorrhea (Option D) in men include purulent, foul-smelling drainage from the penis and painful urination. Cauliflower-like warts on the penis (Option B) are a sign of human papillomavirus. Painful red papules on the shaft of the penis (Option C) may be a sign of the first stage of genital herpes.

Question 4. The nurse is speaking to a group of women about early detection of breast cancer. The average age of the women in the group is 47. Following the American Cancer Society guidelines, the nurse should recommend that the women:

A. perform BSE annually.
B. have a mammogram annually.
C. have a hormonal receptor assay annually.
D. have a practitioner conduct a clinical examination every 2 years.

Correct answer: B The American Cancer Society guidelines state "Women older than age 40 should have a mammogram annually and a clinical examination at least annually; all women should perform breast self-examination monthly." Option A is incorrect because women should perform BSE monthly. The hormonal receptor assay (Option C) is done on a known breast tumor to determine whether the tumor is estrogen dependent or progesterone dependent. Option D is incorrect because women older than age 40 should have an annual clinical examination.

Question 5. The nurse is teaching a male patient to perform monthly testicular self-examinations. What is the appropriate point to make?

A. Testicular cancer is highly curable.
B. Testicular cancer is difficult to diagnose.
C. Testicular cancer is the number one cause of cancer deaths in men.
D. Testicular cancer is more common in older men.

Correct answer: A Testicular cancer is highly curable, particularly when it's treated in its early stage. Option B is incorrect because self-examination allows early detection and facilitates the early initiation of treatment. Option C is incorrect because the highest mortality rates from cancer among men are in men with lung cancer. Option D is incorrect because testicular cancer is found more commonly in younger men.

Question 6. On a follow-up visit after having a vaginal hysterectomy, a 32-year-old patient has swelling and pain in the left calf. Which complication does this suggest?

A. Hematoma
B. Hypovolemia
C. Infection
D. Thrombus

Correct answer: D Swelling and pain in one or both calves, especially after surgery, highly symptomatic of thrombus. An elevated temperature and decreased hematocrit (Option A) are signs of hematoma, a delayed complication of abdominal and vaginal hysterectomy. Signs of hypovolemia (option B) include increased hematocrit and hemoglobin values. Although elevated temperature is a classic sign of infection (Option C), a decreased hematocrit isn't.

Question 7. An annual Pap test is most important in patients:

A. with a history of recurrent candidiasis.
B. who became pregnant before age 20.
C. infected with HPV.
D. who have used oral contraceptives for a short time.

Correct answer: C Cervical cancer is attributed to HPV in 90% of cases. Recurrent candidiasis (Option A), becoming pregnant before age 20 (Option B), and using oral contraceptives for a short time (Option D) don't increase the risk of cervical cancer.

Question 8. When planning to teach an adolescent female patient about PID, which of the following statements should the nurse include?

A. "Good hygiene practices prevent the development of PID."
B. "The use of hormonal contraceptives decreases the risk of PID."
C. "PID can lead to long-term complications of the reproductive tract."
D. "Infants born to adolescents with PID are at risk for birth defects."

Correct answer: C Long-term complications of PID include abscess formation in the fallopian tubes and adhesion formation, which can lead to an increased risk of ectopic pregnancy or infertility. Good hygiene practices don't prevent PID (Option A), and using hormonal contraceptives doesn't decrease the risk (Option B), although some forms of contraception—such as the male or female condom—do help to decrease the incidence. An infant born to an adolescent with PID isn't at greater risk for birth defects (Option D).

Question 9. Nocturia and urinary hesitancy in the absence of any observable cause suggests which condition?

A. Endometriosis
B. Benign prostatic hyperplasia (BPH)
C. Prostatitis
D. Renal calculi

Correct answer: B Nocturia, urinary hesitancy, weak urinary stream, terminal dribbling, and urgent need to void are signs of BPH. Prostatitis (option C) can cause pain or discomfort in the perineal area. Endometriosis (Option A) can cause pain low in the abdomen, deep in the pelvis, or in the rectal or sacrococcygeal area, depending on the location of the ectopic tissue. Renal calculi (Option D) typically produce flank pain.

Question 10. Which statement should the nurse include when teaching a patient newly diagnosed with testicular cancer?

A. "Testicular cancer isn't responsive to chemotherapy, but it's highly curative with surgery."
B. "Radiation therapy is never used so that the unaffected testicle can remain healthy."
C. "Testicular self-examination is still important because having testicular cancer increases the risk of developing a second tumor."
D. "Taking testosterone after orchiectomy prevents changes in appearance and sexual function."

Correct answer: C Because a history of a testicular malignancy puts the patient at increased risk for a second tumor, testicular self-examination becomes critical to improving the chances of early detection. Patients who have evidence of metastasis after irradiation receive chemotherapy (Option A). Radiation therapy is used on the retroperitoneal lymph nodes (Option B). Testosterone typically is not needed because the unaffected testis usually produces sufficient hormone (Option D).

Selected References

American Cancer Society (2017). Human Papillomavirus (HPV). Retrieved from: https://www.cancer.org/cancer/cancer-causes/infectious-agents/hpv.html

American Cancer Society (2017b). Key statistics for prostate cancer. Retrieved from: https://www.cancer.org/cancer/prostate-cancer/about/key-statistics.html

American Cancer Society (2017c). What is ovarian cancer. Retrieved from: https://www.cancer.org/cancer/ovarian-cancer/about/what-is-ovarian-cancer.html

Centers for Disease Control and Prevention (2017). Sexually transmitted diseases (STDs). Retrieved from: https://www.cdc.gov/STD

Karch, A. M. (2017). Focus on nursing pharmacology (7th ed.). Philadelphia, PA: Lippincott Williams & Wilkins.

Smeltzer, S. C., & Bare, B. G. (2014). Brunner & Suddarth's textbook of medical-surgical nursing (13th ed.). Philadelphia, PA: Lippincott Williams & Wilkins.

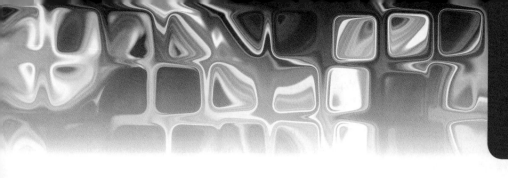

Chapter 17

Immune System Disorders

Introduction

- The immune system is a complex organization of highly specialized cells and tissue that protect the body from various foreign organisms
- The bone marrow and thymus manufacture the immune cells, which work together with lymphoid tissue to destroy foreign organisms that enter the body; B lymphocytes and T lymphocytes are the primary cells of the immune system
- Nursing history
  - The nurse asks the patient about the *chief complaint*
    - The patient with an immunologic disorder reports vague signs and symptoms, such as lack of energy, light-headedness, frequent infections or bruising, and slow wound healing
    - Unexplained joint pain, fever, and rashes
  - The nurse then questions the patient about his *present illness*
    - Ask the patient about the symptom, including when it started, associated symptoms, location, radiation, intensity, duration, frequency, and precipitating and alleviating factors
    - Ask about the use of prescription and over-the-counter (OTC) drugs, herbal remedies, vitamin and nutritional supplements, and alternative therapies
  - The nurse asks about the *medical history*
    - Question the patient about changes in overall health, allergies, childhood diseases, recurrent infections, and immunizations
    - Ask about unexplained rashes, visual disturbances, fever, and changes in elimination patterns
    - Question the patient about a history of immune disorders
    - Ask the female patient about changes in menstrual patterns
  - The nurse then assesses the *family history*
    - Ask about a family history of immune disorders
    - Also ask about a family history of recurrent infections, allergies, and cancer
  - The nurse obtains a *social history*
    - Ask about work, exercise, diet, use of recreational drugs and alcohol, and hobbies
    - Also ask about stress, support systems, and coping mechanisms
    - Question the patient about exposure to chemicals and pathogens
- Physical assessment
  - The nurse begins with *inspection*
    - Inspect the patient's appearance and note signs of acute and chronic illness, pain, fatigue, and malnutrition
    - Observe the patient's movements, posture, gait, coordination, balance, range of motion (ROM), and strength
    - Inspect the skin, noting color, rashes, and lesions and evaluate skin integrity
    - Note hair growth, including texture, distribution, color, and amount
    - Check the nose for evidence of chronic allergies; observe mucous membranes for ulcers, patches, and plaques; and observe the eyes for redness, infection, and hydration

- o Inspect the extremities for blanching, cyanosis, pallor, edema, and reddening
- o Assess level of consciousness and mental status, noting behavior, emotional stability, and cognition
- Next, the nurse performs *palpation* and *percussion*
  - o Take the patient's vital signs
  - o Feel the lymph nodes, noting any enlargement or tenderness
  - o Palpate and percuss various organs, noting enlargement, inflammation, masses, or tenderness
  - o Assess musculoskeletal integrity and ROM, particularly in the hands, wrists, and knees
  - o Palpate the joints to detect nodules, swelling, tenderness, and pain
- Then the nurse performs *auscultation*
  - o Listen to the lungs, noting abnormal breath sounds
  - o Auscultate the heart, listening for abnormal sounds, rhythm, and rate
  - o Listen for bowel sounds in all abdominal quadrants

The Immune Response

- General information
  - The primary function of the immune system is to protect the body against pathogenic microorganisms and malignant cells
  - The immune response is a complex sequence of events triggered by a stimulus (antigen) and culminating in the elimination of the foreign substance; the process requires the differentiation of intrinsic organisms from foreign organisms
    - o Antigens (immunogens) are any substances recognized as foreign that stimulate an immune response; viruses, bacteria, fungi, and parasites are antigens
    - o Antibodies (immunoglobulins) are proteins that are formed in response to exposure to an antigen
  - The following factors can decrease the immune response: genetics, age extremes, protein-calorie malnutrition, vitamin or mineral deficiency, certain drugs, radiation, and stress
- Natural immunity
  - Natural, innate immunity is the body's first line of defense against invading pathogens; this nonspecific mechanism can differentiate intrinsic from foreign organisms but can't identify the specific pathogen
  - Types of natural immunity include *physical barriers*, such as intact skin and mucous membranes; *chemical barriers*, such as gastric acidity and enzymes in the saliva; and *inflammation*, which is the sequence of vascular and cellular responses to tissue injury and immunologic stimuli (see *Chapter 6, Disruptions in Homeostasis*, for details)
- Acquired immunity
  - Adaptive, acquired immunity is the body's second line of defense; it's gained through exposure to pathogens, distinguishes intrinsic from foreign organisms, identifies the specific pathogen, and responds to previously encountered pathogens
  - Four types of acquired immunity exist
    - o *Passive immunity* occurs when antibodies, such as immunoglobulin, of an infectious agent are supplied to the host's body, providing temporary immunity; antibodies may be obtained by injection, or they may be transferred from mother to neonate
    - o *Active immunity* results from direct exposure to an antigen by immunization (such as by tetanus toxoid) or exposure to disease
    - o *Humoral immunity*, primarily mediated by B cells, is the body's ability to respond to antigens by forming specific antibodies; the term humoral indicates that immunity is transferable by serum
    - o *Cell-mediated immunity* is primarily mediated by T cells and macrophages, which are responsible for antigen destruction and delayed hypersensitivity; unlike humoral immunity, cell-mediated immunity isn't readily transferred to another person by serum
- Hypersensitivity and allergic reactions
  - Hypersensitivity and allergic reactions are destructive immune responses that occur after reexposure to an antigen; they can produce various symptoms within minutes to several days
  - Hypersensitivity reactions may be humoral or cell mediated (see *Types of Hypersensitivity*, page 290)

Box 17-1: Types of Hypersensitivity

The following chart summarizes the four major types of hypersensitivity.

Type and Description	Effects	Common Causes
Type I (immediate type) Humoral hypersensitivity mediated by immunoglobulin (Ig) E antibodies	• Local reactions, such as allergic rhinitis and urticaria • Systemic, life-threatening (anaphylactic) reactions that can lead to respiratory distress and shock	• Hay fever, drugs, and foods (local reactions) • Penicillin allergy and insect stings (systemic reactions) • Diagnostic agents
Type II (tissue specific) Humoral hypersensitivity (cytotoxic or cytolytic reaction) mediated by IgG or IgM antibodies; cell specific	• Inflammation, phagocytosis, and cell breakdown through complement system activation	• Blood transfusion reaction • Hemolytic disease of the newborn
Type III (immune complex mediated) Humoral hypersensitivity (immune complex reaction) mediated by IgG or IgM antibodies; tissue versus cell specific	• Itching and discomfort at the injection site (early) • Lymphadenopathy, fever, urticaria, and joint pain (late)	• Drugs such as penicillin • Serum sickness, caused by injection of bovine or equine serum antitoxin, renal damage, and vasculitis
Type IV (delayed type; cell mediated) Cell-mediated hypersensitivity (T-cell–mediated reaction)	• Delayed response caused by direct or indirect antigen destruction	• Poison ivy • Graft rejection • Tuberculin reaction • Latex allergy

Acquired Immunodeficiency Syndrome

- Description
  - Acquired immunodeficiency syndrome (AIDS) is caused by a retrovirus called human immunodeficiency virus (HIV) that attacks the immune system and causes a progressive compromise of the immune system
  - AIDS is the final stage of an HIV infection and occurs when HIV is left untreated. Without treatment, the patient's immune system becomes so compromised that they can no longer fight infections and the patient usually dies from opportunistic infections or cancers. There is no cure
  - The Centers for Disease Control (CDC) have developed a classification method that covers the spectrum of the progression of HIV infection (see *Classification system for HIV Infection and Expanded AIDS Surveillance Case Definition for Adolescents and Adults*, page 293)
  - AIDS is caused by infection with HIV type 1 (HIV-1) or HIV type 2 (HIV-2); HIV is a retrovirus that selectively infects cells with a CD4+ surface marker, usually T_4 lymphocytes
  - HIV is transmitted primarily through sexual intercourse, during which blood, semen, vaginal, and anal secretions are shared
  - HIV can be transmitted through contaminated blood that enters the body by way of parenteral or percutaneous routes or by way of mucous membranes or open wounds; such transmission can result from sharing or accidental injection with a contaminated needle, transfusion of contaminated blood, or perinatal transfer in the womb, during birth, or through breast milk
  - HIV cannot be transmitted through saliva, tears, sweat, feces, urine, sharing food, hugging, shaking hands, etc.
  - HIV infection reduces cell-mediated immunity by destroying T_4 lymphocytes
    - ○ This decreases the ratio of helper T cells to suppressor T cells, which normally is 2:1 (CD4+: CD8+ ratio)
    - ○ It also increases the patient's susceptibility to opportunistic infections and certain cancers
  - HIV infection also affects humoral immunity by producing more nonspecific antibodies that are ineffective and by altering the function of monocytes and macrophages; these cells may be responsible for transporting the virus to other organs, such as the brain and lungs

- Signs and symptoms
  - HIV infection may be asymptomatic or cause a mononucleosis-like syndrome associated with seroconversion; symptoms include fever, headache, sore throat, mouth sores, rash, myalgia/arthralgia, diarrhea, weight loss, malaise, and swollen lymph nodes and last about 2 weeks (see *AIDS Indicator Diseases*, pages 294–295)
    - Persistent generalized lymphadenopathy at two or more extrainguinal sites may persist for more than 3 months in the absence of concurrent illness
    - The infected patient also may display signs of opportunistic infections and other diseases
  - HIV can produce central nervous system effects
    - AIDS dementia complex, also called HIV encephalopathy, causes cognitive changes, such as confusion, impaired concentration, and memory loss; motor disturbances, such as ataxia, leg weakness, and diminished fine motor movements; and behavioral changes, such as apathy, depression, reduced spontaneity, social withdrawal, anxiety, agitation, and personality changes
    - Atypical aseptic meningitis causes headache, fever, and signs of meningeal infection
    - Vacuolar myelopathy (spinal cord degeneration) may produce leg weakness, incontinence, and ataxia
  - HIV wasting syndrome may occur as a complication of advanced HIV infection; it's associated with involuntary weight loss of more than 10% of body weight and diarrhea, recurrent or sustained fevers, and chronic weakness for more than 1 month in the absence of a causative illness, such as cancer or tuberculosis
- Diagnosis and treatment
  - The enzyme-linked immunosorbent assay (ELISA) detects the presence of HIV-1 antibodies; if a patient's blood has a positive reaction on two ELISA tests, the Western blot test is used to confirm the results
  - The Western blot test detects the presence of HIV antibodies and determines their type
  - HIV infection is characterized by a progressive decline of the CD4+ T-cell count over months to years
  - A CD4+ T-cell count of less than 200 cells/μL is diagnostic of AIDS and indicates that the patient is at risk for an opportunistic infection
  - Polymerase chain reaction may detect viral genetic material (HIV ribonucleic acid [HIV RNA]) in patients for whom antibodies haven't yet developed
  - Other laboratory tests may include hematocrit (below 30%, indicating anemia), white blood cell (WBC) count (below 2,500/cm^3, indicating leukopenia), the ratio of helper T cells to suppressor T cells (decreased to 1:2), and platelet count (below 100,000/mm^3)
  - Because many opportunistic infections are reactivations of previous infections, the patient may also be tested for syphilis, hepatitis B, tuberculosis, and toxoplasmosis
  - Drug therapy for HIV infection includes six types of antiretrovirals
    - Protease inhibitors, such as ritonavir (Norvir), indinavir (Crixivan), nelfinavir (Viracept), fosamprenavir (Lexiva), and saquinavir (Invirase)
    - Nucleoside and nucleotide reverse transcriptase inhibitors, such as zidovudine (Retrovir), didanosine (Videx), lamivudine (Epivir), abacavir (Ziagen), and tenofovir (Viread)
    - Nonnucleoside reverse transcriptase inhibitors, such as nevirapine (Viramune), efavirenz (Sustiva), and etravirine (Intelence)
    - Integrase inhibitors such as raltegravir (Isentress), elvitegravir (EVG), and dolutegravir (Tivicay)
    - CCR5 coreceptor antagonist such as maraviroc (Selzentry) and enfuvirtide (Fuzeon)
    - Fusion inhibitors, such as enfuvirtide, which interfere with the virus' ability to fuse with the cellular membrane, thereby blocking entry into the host cell
    - These antiretrovirals are used in various combinations to inhibit HIV viral replication; this is called highly active antiretroviral therapy HAART
    - Treatment protocols combine two or more drugs in an effort to gain the maximum benefit with the fewest adverse reactions
    - Combination therapy helps to inhibit the production of resistant, mutant strains
    - Combination agents that combine two or three drugs in one dose are available and help improve compliance
  - Different treatments are required for AIDS indicator diseases (see *AIDS Indicator Diseases*, pages 294–295)
- Nursing interventions
  - Provide respiratory care
  - Encourage activity, as tolerated, to prevent fatigue and dyspnea
    - Administer medications, as prescribed, to relieve symptoms and prevent or treat infection
    - Monitor vital signs and laboratory values (arterial blood gas levels, oxygen saturation by pulse oximetry, sputum cultures, CD4+ count, and complete blood count [CBC]) to determine the effectiveness of treatment

- ○ Provide pulmonary hygiene (including cough and deep-breathing exercises every 2 hours), splinting while coughing, and suctioning to prevent atelectasis and clear airway secretions; maintain adequate hydration to thin mucus secretions
- ○ Provide throat lozenges and warm saline gargles to soothe an irritated throat and mouth ulcers
- ○ Administer antitussives and expectorants, as prescribed, for cough
- ○ If appropriate, help the patient to decrease or stop smoking
- Perform gastrointestinal (GI) care
  - ○ Monitor fluid intake and output, weight, urine specific gravity, serum electrolyte levels, and skin turgor to evaluate hydration
  - ○ Obtain stool cultures to identify enteric pathogens
  - ○ Encourage the patient to drink at least 3 qt (3 L) of fluid daily; administer I.V. therapy, as prescribed, to maintain hydration
  - ○ Administer antibiotics and antivirals to treat infectious diarrhea and antidiarrhea medications to lessen the severity of diarrhea
- Promote good nutrition
  - ○ Offer small, frequent meals to reduce fatigue
  - ○ Engage the patient in menu planning, and invite the patient's family and friends to meals to encourage eating
    - ○ Allowing the patient to include personal food preferences gives the patient some control over the diet
    - ○ Eating with others may improve appetite
  - ○ Encourage the patient to eat meals sitting up and out of bed; sitting up aids digestion and decreases the risk of aspiration
  - ○ Provide a low-residue, high-protein, high-potassium, high-calorie, lactose-free diet to minimize diarrhea and maximize caloric, electrolyte, and fluid intake
  - ○ Use oral dietary supplements, such as Vivonex T.E.N.; initiate and monitor tube feedings or total parenteral nutrition as prescribed
  - ○ Administer appetite stimulants such as megestrol acetate (Megace) as ordered
  - ○ Avoid serving rare meats and raw vegetables, which may harbor living microbes
  - ○ Monitor daily weight and laboratory values—including serum protein, albumin, blood urea nitrogen, hemoglobin, and serum electrolyte levels and hematocrit—to evaluate nutrition
  - ○ Provide mouth care, using viscous oral lidocaine (Xylocaine) before meals to relieve mouth, pharyngeal, and esophageal pain; use saline rinses after meals to prevent exacerbation of infection
- Perform skin care
  - ○ Use pressure-relieving devices (convoluted foam mattress, pressure mattress, or pressure pads), and turn the patient every 2 hours to prevent skin deterioration caused by pressure and inadequate circulation
  - ○ Apply A + D Original Ointment or other skin barrier to the perianal area to prevent further maceration of the anal mucosa
  - ○ Maintain wound and skin precautions to prevent further spread of infection
- Prevent and control infection
  - ○ Restrict the patient's contact with visitors, staff members, and other patients who have infections, such as colds or flu
  - ○ Make sure that staff members and visitors adhere to hand hygiene procedures before approaching the patient
  - ○ Use reverse isolation if the patient is immunocompromised
  - ○ Consider moving the patient to a private room and leaving equipment—such as a thermometer, blood pressure cuff, and stethoscope—in the room to minimize pathogen exposure
  - ○ Follow standard precautions to reduce pathogen transfer
  - ○ Inspect the skin, I.V. sites, vascular access devices, and invasive cardiovascular monitoring lines; loss of skin integrity is a potential source of infection
  - ○ Monitor antimicrobial therapies; antibiotics can increase the likelihood of superinfection and the development of resistant organisms
  - ○ Encourage and maintain adequate nutritional intake, which promotes healing and prevents infection
- Provide neuropsychiatric care
  - ○ Encourage the patient to discuss emotional issues; mood swings may be related to an inability to cope with the illness
  - ○ Identify resources for patient and family support
  - ○ Use reminder devices, such as pictures and appointment books, to help orient the patient
  - ○ Arrange for continuity of caregivers, and avoid frequent room changes to prevent patient confusion
  - ○ Consult occupational and physical therapists; the patient may need special devices, such as a cane or walker, and physical therapy to maintain or prevent further loss of function

- Promote health maintenance
  - ○ Teach the patient, family, significant others, and caregivers about the diagnosis, treatments, modes of transmission, and symptoms to report
  - ○ Explain medications to the patient, including dose, frequency, and adverse effects; reinforce the importance of compliance to help suppress the virus and to prevent the development of drug-resistant strains
  - ○ Discuss the importance of avoiding high-risk behaviors and reducing the risk of transmission to others
  - ○ Make appropriate referrals—for example, for home care, pain management, legal services, support groups, financial support, and hospice care

Box 17-2: Classification System for HIV Infection and Expanded AIDS Surveillance Case Definition for Adolescents and Adults

Diagnostic categories

As of January 1, 1993, people with acquired immunodeficiency syndrome (AIDS) indicator conditions (clinical category C) and those in categories A3 or B3 were considered to have AIDS.

CD4+ T-cell and Clinical Categories	Clinical Category A: Asymptomatic, Acute (Primary) HIV or PGL	Clinical Category B: Symptomatic not (A) or (C) Conditions	Clinical Category C: AIDS Indicator Conditions
≥ 500/μL	A1	B1	C1
200 to 499/μL	A2	B2	C2
<200/μL AIDS indicator T-cell count	A3	B3	C3

Clinical category A

Includes one or more of the following in an adult or adolescent with confirmed human immunodeficiency virus (HIV) infection and without conditions in clinical categories B and C:
- Asymptomatic HIV infection
- Persistent generalized lymphadenopathy
- Acute (primary) HIV infection with accompanying illness or history of acute HIV infection

Clinical category B

Examples of conditions in clinical category B include, but aren't limited to:
- Bacillary angiomatosis
- Candidiasis, oropharyngeal (thrush) or vulvovaginal (persistent, frequent, or poorly responsive to therapy)
- Cervical dysplasia (moderate or severe) or cervical carcinoma in situ
- Constitutional symptoms, such as fever (101.3°F [38.5°C]) or diarrhea exceeding 1 month in duration
- Hairy leukoplakia, oral

- Herpes zoster (shingles), involving at least two distinct episodes or more than one dermatome
- Idiopathic thrombocytopenic purpura
- Listeriosis
- Pelvic inflammatory disease, particularly if complicated by tuboovarian abscess
- Peripheral neuropathy

Clinical category C

Examples of conditions in adults and adolescents include:
- Candidiasis of bronchi, trachea, lungs, or esophagus
- Cervical cancer, invasive
- Coccidioidomycosis, disseminated or extrapulmonary
- Cryptococcosis, extrapulmonary
- Cryptosporidiosis, chronic intestinal (exceeding 1 month's duration)
- Cytomegalovirus disease (other than liver, spleen, or lymph nodes)
- Cytomegalovirus retinitis (with loss of vision)
- Encephalopathy, HIV related

- Herpes simplex: chronic ulcers (exceeding 1 month's duration) or bronchitis, pneumonitis, or esophagitis
- Histoplasmosis, disseminated or extrapulmonary
- Isosporidiosis, chronic intestinal (exceeding 1 month's duration)
- Kaposi's sarcoma
- Lymphoma, Burkitt's (or equivalent term); immunoblastic (or equivalent term); primary, of brain
- *Mycobacterium avium complex* or *Mycobacterium kansasii*, disseminated or extrapulmonary
- *Mycobacterium tuberculosis*, any site (pulmonary or extrapulmonary)
- *Mycobacterium*, other species or unidentified species, disseminated or extrapulmonary
- *Pneumocystis jiroveci* pneumonia
- Pneumonia, recurrent
- Progressive multifocal leukoencephalopathy
- *Salmonella* septicemia, recurrent
- Toxoplasmosis of brain
- Wasting syndrome due to HIV

Adapted from Centers for Disease Control and Prevention, U.S. Department of Health and Human Services (1992). 1993 revised classification system for HIV infection and expanded surveillance case definition for AIDS among adolescents and adults. *MMWR Recommendations and Reports, 41*(RR-17), 1–19). Atlanta, GA: Centers for Disease Control and Prevention.

Box 17-3: AIDS Indicator Diseases

The following chart summarizes the clinical signs and symptoms and treatments of major indicator diseases of acquired immunodeficiency syndrome (AIDS).

Disease	Clinical Signs and Symptoms	Treatments
Viral infections		
Cytomegalovirus retinitis	• Floaters • Blurred vision • Decreased vision that may lead to blindness	• I.V. ganciclovir (Cytovene) • I.V. foscarnet (Foscavir)
Herpes simplex virus (HSV) infection	• Vesicular lesions around mucosal orifices of the face and genitals • Debilitation	• I.V. acyclovir (Zovirax) for HSV encephalitis • Oral acyclovir to suppress HSV • Topical acyclovir for a small outbreak of local lesions
Protozoal infections		
Pneumocystis jiroveci pneumonia	• Fever • Nonproductive cough • Progressive shortness of breath	• I.V. cotrimoxazole for treatment and prevention • I.V. or inhalation pentamidine for patients who can't tolerate or don't respond to co-trimoxazole
Toxoplasmosis	• Focal neurologic defects, such as seizures and hemiparesis • Encephalitis manifestations, such as headache, confusion, and lethargy	• Oral pyrimethamine (Daraprim) and sulfadiazine
Cryptosporidiosis	• Protracted watery stools • Severe vomiting • Fluid and electrolyte imbalances	• Oral antidiarrheals • Fluid replacement • Nutritional support
Bacterial infections		
Mycobacterium avium-intracellulare infection	• Fever • Weight loss • Weakness • Abdominal pain • Frequent watery stools • Anorexia	• Oral clarithromycin
M. tuberculosis infection	• Fever • Fatigue • Weight loss • Productive, purulent cough	• Combination oral therapy with isoniazid and rifampin plus either pyrazinamide or ethambutol
Fungal infections		
Candidiasis	• Painless mouth lesions • Pain with swallowing • Retrosternal chest pain • Nausea and vomiting	• Nystatin suspension for oral candidiasis • Topical antifungal creams, such as clotrimazole (Mycelex) or ketoconazole (Nizoral), for cutaneous candidiasis • Oral ketoconazole for esophageal candidiasis • Clotrimazole or miconazole creams, vaginal tablets, or suppositories for vaginal candidiasis • Ketoconazole, itraconazole, or fluconazole for systemic candidiasis
Cryptococcosis	• High fever, headache, and malaise (early) • Photophobia, stiff neck, nausea, vomiting, and mental changes (late)	• Systemic therapy with amphotericin B or fluconazole

(continued)

Box 17-3: **AIDS Indicator Diseases (continued)**

Disease	Clinical Signs and Symptoms	Treatments
Neoplasms **Kaposi's sarcoma**	• Pigmented, raised, nonblanching skin lesions • Pain when lesion impinges on organs or nerves	• Intralesional and systemic chemotherapy • Cryotherapy • Radiation therapy • Biological response modifiers and antiretrovirals
Non-Hodgkin's lymphoma	• Painless, enlarged lymph node, usually in the neck (early) • Fever, night sweats, and weight loss (late)	• Chemotherapy

Anaphylaxis

- Description
  - Anaphylaxis is an acute, potentially fatal, multisystem organ response to an allergen. After the initial exposure to an antigen, the immune system produces specific immunoglobulin (Ig) antibodies in the lymph nodes; helper T cells enhance the process
  - The IgE antibodies then bind to membrane receptors located on mast cells and basophils
  - After the body re-encounters the antigen, the IgE antibodies, or cross-linked IgE receptors, recognize the antigen as foreign; this activates the release of powerful chemical mediators, which cause an increase in vascular permeability, bronchoconstriction, urticaria, and hypotension
  - Substances that most commonly cause anaphylaxis include foods; certain medications, such as antibiotics, radiocontrast dyes, and anesthetic agents; insect stings; and latex
  - Some cases have no identifiable cause
- Signs and symptoms
  - Signs and symptoms range from mild to severe and usually affect the skin and/or mucous membranes, respiratory, cardiovascular, and GI systems
  - A mild reaction consists of peripheral tingling, a sensation of warmth, a feeling of fullness in the throat, pruritus, nasal congestion, and tearing; the reaction occurs within 2 hours of exposure
  - A moderate reaction includes more pronounced flushing, warmth, anxiety, and itching
  - A severe reaction typically occurs immediately after exposure
    - Signs and symptoms include complaints of a feeling of impending doom or fright, headache, and a display of apprehension and restlessness
    - Skin symptoms include flushing, urticaria, angioedema, pruritus, and edema
    - Respiratory symptoms include a feeling of a "lump" in their throat, difficulty swallowing, hoarseness, coughing, wheezing, dyspnea, and complains of chest tightness
    - Cardiovascular symptoms are dizziness, syncope, weakness, chest pain, and palpitations
    - Gastrointestinal symptoms are dysphagia, nausea, vomiting, diarrhea, and abdominal cramps
    - The reaction can progress to shock and cardiac arrest
- Diagnosis and treatment
  - Diagnosis is based on the patient's history and signs and symptoms
  - Skin testing can identify a specific allergen
  - Treatment aims to maintain the patient's airway, breathing, and circulation. Supplemental oxygen, endotracheal intubation, and ventilator support are used to maintain and support airway and breathing. IV fluids and vasopressors (dopamine) are using to maintain the cardiovascular system
  - The patient may require immediate administration of epinephrine 1:1,000 aqueous solution, 0.3 to 0.5 mL given subcutaneously every 20 to 30 minutes for up to three doses, or 5 mL of a 1:10,000 solution given by slow I.V. infusion every 5 to 10 minutes as needed; if I.V. administration isn't possible, endotracheal or intraosseous administration may be used
  - Drug treatment may also include corticosteroids (methylprednisolone, hydrocortisone, prednisone) and diphenhydramine (Benadryl) given I.V., I.M., or by mouth, bronchodilators (albuterol), H2 receptor antagonists cimetidine (Tagamet), ranitidine (Zantac), and famotidine (Pepcid)

- Nursing interventions
  - Provide supplemental oxygen, and prepare to assist with insertion of an endotracheal tube, if necessary
  - Insert a peripheral I.V. line and maintain patent I.V. access if necessary
  - Continually reassure the patient, and explain all tests and treatments
  - If the patient undergoes skin or scratch testing, monitor for signs of a serious allergic response; keep emergency resuscitation equipment readily available
  - Administer prescribed drugs; be aware that epinephrine is considered a first-line agent for treatment
  - Give inhaled beta-2 agonists (albuterol) as ordered, typically 10 mg/hour via continuous nebulization or 2.5 mg every 15 to 20 minutes via nebulization
  - Expect to administer oral antihistamines and steroids for 72 hours
  - Monitor the patient's vital signs and respiratory status, and note the response to treatment
  - If a specific allergen is identified, teach the patient and family about the type of allergy or allergen responsible for the patient's signs and symptoms
  - Teach the patient and family about the signs and symptoms of a reaction and the importance of carrying and becoming familiar with an anaphylaxis kit; make sure they learn how to use the kit before the need arises, and teach them about the need for medical identification jewelry to identify the allergy

Latex Allergy

- Description
  - Latex allergy is a type 1, IgE-mediated hypersensitivity reaction or type IV cell-mediated response to products that contain natural rubber latex
  - It can cause reactions that range from local dermatitis to life-threatening anaphylaxis
- Signs and symptoms
  - Hypotension due to vasodilation and increased vascular permeability, tachycardia, urticaria, and pruritus may occur
  - Other signs or symptoms include difficulty breathing and bronchospasm, wheezing, stridor, and angioedema
- Diagnosis and treatment
  - Diagnosis is based primarily on history and physical assessment of the patient
  - Radioallergosorbent test shows IgE antibodies specific to latex
  - Patch test causes hives along with itching and redness
  - The best treatment is prevention by avoiding exposure to airborne particles and use of latex-free products
  - Drug therapy may include corticosteroids, antihistamines, and histamine-2 receptor antagonists before and after latex exposure
  - For acute emergency, perform cardiopulmonary resuscitation, administer epinephrine, assist with tracheostomy, provide oxygen therapy, and administer volume expanders, I.V. vasopressors, and other drugs to reverse bronchospasm
- Nursing interventions
  - Make sure that products that aren't available free of latex are wrapped in cloth before they come in contact with the skin of a hypersensitive patient
  - Use powder-free, vinyl gloves
  - When adding medication to an I.V. bag, inject the drug through the spike port, and not the rubber latex port
  - Urge the patient to wear a tag identifying the latex allergy
  - Instruct the patient to avoid tomatoes, bananas, avocados, chestnuts, and kiwi fruits because they contain proteins similar to those present in rubber
  - Teach the patient to be aware of all latex-containing products and to use vinyl or silicone products instead

Rheumatoid Arthritis

- Description
  - Rheumatoid arthritis (RA) is an autoimmune disease that causes chronic inflammation of the small joints of the hands and wrists and the surrounding muscles, tendons, ligaments, and blood vessels. It may progress to other joints and body tissues, including the heart, lungs, kidneys, and skin
  - The joints are usually affected on both sides of the body in a symmetrical pattern

- Rheumatoid arthritis is characterized by periods of flares and remissions
- It can cause permanent joint damage and deformity
- The cause is unknown and there is no cure. It affects three times as many women as men between ages 30 and 50 and becomes more evident during the winter
- Signs and symptoms
  - Edema, redness, and stiffness causing pain and loss of function and ROM in the affected joints
  - Other signs and symptoms may include malaise; fever; anemia; rheumatoid nodules near joints; dull, aching joint pain; and joint deformity
  - Rheumatoid arthritis may be associated with pericarditis and pneumonitis
- Diagnosis and treatment
  - Diagnosis is based on patient history, physical examination, X-rays, and serologic blood tests, including rheumatoid factor, citrulline antibody, CBC, erythrocyte sedimentation rate (ESR), serum complement, and C-reactive protein (CRP)
  - Risk factors include genetics, smoking, silica inhalation, periodontal disease, and gut flora
  - 75% to 80% of patients with a positive rheumatoid factors test have the disease and 50% to 75% of people with RA have citrulline antibodies
  - Other diagnostic tests may include immunologic studies, synovial biopsy, X-rays, and magnetic resonance imaging
  - Treatments aim to educate patients and manage symptoms such as joint inflammation, pain, decreased ROM, and loss of use. Joint immobilization or splinting is used to decrease damage to the affected joint. Medications, physical therapy, and occasionally surgery are also used to manage symptoms from joint damage
  - Disease-modifying antirheumatic drugs (DMARDs) slow the progression of RA and decrease the risk of permanent damage to the joints and surrounding tissue; DMARDs include methotrexate, sulfasalazine (Azulfidine), and minocycline (Arestin)
  - Immunosuppressants act to suppress the immune system; they include azathioprine (Imuran), cyclophosphamide (Cytoxan), chlorambucil (Leukeran), and cyclosporine (Sandimmune)
  - Tumor necrosis factor alpha inhibitors are used to inhibit the inflammatory response. These include etanercept (Enbrel), infliximab (Remicade), and adalimumab (Humira)
  - Various anti-inflammatories are prescribed: acetylsalicylates (aspirin), low-dose steroids (prednisone), and nonsteroidal anti-inflammatory drugs (NSAIDs), including ibuprofen (Advil or Motrin), naproxen (Aleve), ketoprofen (Orudis and Oruvail), etodolac (Lodine), celecoxib (Celebrex), and diclofenac (Voltaren, Cataflam)
  - Misoprostol (Cytotec), sucralfate (Carafate), proton pump inhibitors (Prevacid) may be given to prevent NSAID-induced gastric ulcers
  - Gold salts such as gold thioglucose (Solganal), gold thiomalate (Myochrysine), and auranofin (Ridaura) may be prescribed to reduce inflammation; opioid analgesics may be used to relieve pain; antimalarials such as chloroquine (Aralen) and hydroxychloroquine (Plaquenil) are used for immunosuppression to prevent further joint destruction. Azathioprine (Imuran and Azasan) and cytotoxic agents such as methotrexate (Trexall and Rasuvo) may be used to decrease synovial inflammation; and sulfasalazine (Azulfidine) may be used to reduce inflammation in patients who have responded inadequately to salicylates or NSAIDs
  - Supplements that are frequently recommended for RA patients include omega-3 fatty acids, calcium + vitamin D for bone health, and folic acid to help with side effects of methotrexate
  - Corticosteroid injections into the affected joint and surrounding tissues for inflammation
  - Surgical interventions include joint repair or prosthetic replacement and synovectomy (removal of the synovium)
  - Lymphapheresis or plasmapheresis may be used for some patients
- Nursing interventions
  - Explain the treatment regimen and the involvement of each member of the health care team to the patient
  - Administer drugs as prescribed, and monitor for therapeutic and adverse reactions; drug therapy may need to be changed if adverse reactions are intolerable or therapeutic effects don't occur
  - Monitor the patient for relief of pain, stiffness, and soreness; patients have periods of remission and "flare" when symptoms increase
  - Help the patient with self-care, including ROM exercises, splint application, and ambulatory aid use
  - Provide modified utensils and equipment suggested by the occupational therapist to help conserve small joint and muscle function
  - Provide rest periods in the morning and evening, with the patient lying supine in bed to maintain strength while preventing flexion contractures; teach the patient not to overexert

- Provide a quiet environment for nighttime sleep; patients with acute RA require 8 to 10 hours of sleep
- Discuss home maintenance activities recommended by the occupational therapist to ensure that the patient understands needed changes
- Prepare the patient for surgery if indicated
- Provide postoperative care appropriate for the surgery
- Encourage compliance with treatments to achieve optimal results
- Encourage the patient to verbalize concerns about body image and changes in quality of life
- Provide information on available resources for assistance in the patient's home with meals and ADLs

Systemic Lupus Erythematosus

- Description
  - Systemic lupus erythematosus (SLE) is a chronic, systemic autoimmune disease that causes skin, heart, lung, and kidney inflammation with periods of exacerbations and remission
  - It varies in severity from mild to rapidly progressing with multiple organ involvement
  - Although its cause is unknown, SLE affects nine times as many women as men, primarily between ages 15 and 45; it's more common in Blacks and Asians than in Whites
  - Discoid lupus is a less severe form of SLE that chiefly affects the skin, producing raised, red, scaly lesions on the face, shoulders, and upper back as well as hair loss
- Signs and symptoms
  - Primary features include arthritis with synovitis, a characteristic butterfly rash over the nose and cheeks (develops in 50% of patients), and fever
  - Other effects may include diffuse and patchy hair loss, fatigue, weight loss, photosensitivity, renal failure (acute or chronic), seizures, psychosis, pleuritis, endocarditis, myocarditis, Raynaud's phenomenon, anemia, abdominal pain, menstrual irregularities, leukopenia, anemia, and lymph node enlargement throughout the body
- Diagnosis and treatment
  - Diagnosis may be based on patient history; physical examination; serologic studies, such as CBC with differential, ESR or CRP, antinuclear antibody tests, and lupus erythematosus cell test; electrocardiography; joint and chest X-rays; kidney function studies (urinalysis, BUN, and creatinine); lumbar puncture; arthrocentesis; and renal biopsies
  - The presence of 4 of the 11 American College of Rheumatology criteria for SLE is almost always indicative of a diagnosis of SLE. These include serositis, oral ulcers, arthritis, photosensitivity, blood disorders, renal involvement, antinuclear antibodies, immunologic phenomena (presence of antibodies), neurologic disorder, malar rash (butterfly rash on face), and discoid rash
  - Treatment typically calls for NSAIDs such as ibuprofen (Advil, Motrin), naproxen (Aleve), and diclofenac (Voltaren) and corticosteroids (prednisone) to decrease inflammation
  - Other drugs—immunosuppressants such as cyclophosphamide (Cytoxan), methotrexate, azathioprine (Imuran), cyclosporine (Sandimmune), belimumab (Benlysta), cardiotonics such as digoxin (Lanoxin), and antimalarials such as hydroxychloroquine (Plaquenil)—are prescribed based on the severity of the disease
- Nursing interventions
  - Monitor vital signs to evaluate the extent of inflammation
  - Observe the patient for rash to help differentiate SLE from discoid lupus
  - Monitor the patient for reports of arthritis, joint or chest pain, respiratory difficulties, and other symptoms; SLE symptoms vary among patients
  - Monitor the patient for seizures, headaches, and vision disturbances; neurologic problems may accompany the disease
  - Monitor the patient for numbness and tingling of the hands and feet; peripheral neuropathy may occur
  - Monitor the degree of fatigue, color of skin and conjunctivae, and color of stools; anemia is common in patients with SLE
  - Test urine and stool for occult bleeding, a possible adverse effect of prescribed medications
  - Provide for rest periods to avoid fatigue; promote independence in activities of daily living to improve self-esteem
  - Encourage the patient to express feelings about changes in body image and the chronic nature of the disease
  - Teach the patient about family planning, genetic counseling, medications, the treatment plan, avoidance of sun exposure, and wearing protective clothing and sunscreen when outdoors

Review Questions

Question 1. The nurse is preparing a female patient with SLE for discharge. Which instructions should the nurse include in the teaching plan?

A. Exposure to sunlight will help control skin rashes.
B. No activity limitations are necessary between flareups.
C. Report any changes in urination pattern.
D. Corticosteroids may be stopped when symptoms are relieved.

Correct answer: C SLE can cause damage to the glomeruli in the kidneys. Option A is incorrect because sunlight and other sources of ultraviolet light may exacerbate the disease. Option B is incorrect because fatigue can cause a flareup of SLE, and patients should be encouraged to pace activities and plan for rest periods. Corticosteroids, Option D, must be gradually tapered because they can suppress the function of the adrenal gland. Abruptly stopping corticosteroids can cause adrenal insufficiency, a potentially life-threatening situation.

Question 2. A patient with rheumatoid arthritis has a history of long-term NSAID use and, consequently, has developed peptic ulcer disease. To treat this condition, the nurse should expect to administer:

A. antibiotics.
B. ticlopidine.
C. prednisone.
D. misoprostol.

Correct answer: D NSAIDs decrease prostaglandin synthesis. Misoprostol, a synthetic analog of prostaglandin, is used to treat and prevent NSAID-induced gastric ulcers. (Option A) NSAID-induced peptic ulcer disease is not linked to *H. pylori*, and it does not require antibiotics. Ticlopidine (Option B) is an antiplatelet drug used to reduce the risk of stroke. Prednisone (Option C) is a glucocorticosteroid used to treat several inflammatory disorders and may promote gastric ulcer development.

Question 3. The nurse is providing care for a patient with AIDS and *Pneumocystis jiroveci* pneumonia. The patient is receiving trimethoprim/sulfamethoxazole (Bactrim). What's the best evidence that the therapy is working?

A. Patient is afebrile and SOB has resolved.
B. Whitening of lung fields on the chest X-ray.
C. Improved patient vitality and activity tolerance.
D. Development of leukocytosis.

Correct answer: A *P. jiroveci* pneumonia is a protozoal infection of the lungs. Bactrim is a first-line antibiotic used to treat this illness. Because a common manifestation of the infection is SOB and fever, improvements in these areas suggest success of the therapy. Sudden weight gain (Option A), whitening of the lung fields on chest X-ray (Option B), and development of leukocytosis (Option D) aren't evidence of therapeutic success.

Question 4. A patient with SLE who receives immunosuppressants develops a fever. The nurse should:

A. administer prescribed antipyretics.
B. place the patient in isolation.
C. apply cooling measures immediately.
D. notify physician.

Correct answer: D Immunosuppressants impair the patient's immunocompetence and predispose the patient to infection. Fever is a sign of infection; therefore, it's important to notify physician. Option A should be withheld until cultures have been obtained. Isolation (Option B) isn't indicated unless the absolute neutrophil count is less than 1,000/μL. Cooling measures (Option C) may be indicated, but they don't have priority over organism identification.

Question 5. Which finding distinguishes rheumatoid arthritis from osteoarthritis?

A. Crepitus with ROM
B. Symmetry of joint involvement
C. Elevated serum uric acid levels
D. Dominance in weight-bearing joints

Correct answer: B Rheumatoid arthritis is bilateral and symmetrical; by contrast, osteoarthritis and gouty arthritis are unilateral. Crepitus (Option A) is usually associated with osteoarthritis. Elevated serum uric acid levels (option C) are common in patients with gout. Dominance in weight bearing joints (options D) is seen in osteoarthritis.

Question 6. A patient is admitted with acute bronchitis. During the admission interview, the patient tells the nurse about an allergy to bananas. Based on this statement, the patient may also have an allergy to which drug or substance?

A. IV contrast dye
B. Cephalosporins
C. Penicillins
D. Latex

Correct answer: D Patients who are allergic to certain cross-reactive foods—including apricots, avocados, bananas, cherries, chestnuts, grapes, kiwis, passion fruit, peaches, and tomatoes—may also be allergic to latex. When exposed to latex, they may have an allergic response similar to the one these foods produce. Patients with allergies to shellfish may be allergic to IV contrast dye (Option A). Hypersensitivity reactions to cephalosporins (Option B) are more common in patients with penicillin allergy. There's no link between food allergies and penicillin (Option C).

Question 7. A patient with AIDS is prescribed zidovudine (Retrovir), 200 mg by mouth every 4 hours. When teaching the patient about this drug, the nurse should provide which instruction?

A. "Take zidovudine with meals."
B. "Take zidovudine on an empty stomach."
C. "Take zidovudine every 4 hours around the clock."
D. "It is ok to continue herbal supplements."

Correct answer: C To be effective, zidovudine must be taken every 4 hours around the clock. Food doesn't affect absorption of this drug, so the patient may take zidovudine either with food (Option A) or on an empty stomach (Option B). To avoid serious drug interactions, the patient should check with the physician before taking any supplements (Option D).

Question 8. In a patient who has HIV infection, the CD4+ level is measured to determine the:

A. presence of opportunistic infections.
B. level of the viral load.
C. if they are cured of the infection.
D. the ability of the immune system to fight infections.

Correct answer: D The CD4+ level in the blood of a patient with HIV infection is measured to determine the extent of damage to the immune system and how efficient it will be in fighting infections. Although the level does indicate the risk for developing an opportunistic infection, it doesn't identify specific infections (Option A). Different diagnostic tests are used to determine the viral load level (Option B). There is no cure for HIV (Option C).

Question 9. An 18-year-old patient complains of fatigue, weight loss, and a low-grade fever and symmetrical pain in the fingers, elbows, and ankles. Which condition is suspected?

A. Anemia
B. Leukemia
C. Rheumatic arthritis
D. SLE

Correct answer: C Fatigue, weight loss, and a low-grade fever are all early indications of many immune system diseases, including anemia (Option A), leukemia (Option B), and SLE (Option D). However, only rheumatic arthritis is associated with symmetrical pain in the fingers, elbows, wrists, ankles, and knees.

Question 10. Which antibody is involved in anaphylaxis?

A. IgE
B. IgA
C. IgG
D. IgM

Correct answer: A If you have an overreaction to an allergen, your body produces IgE, which can result in anaphylaxis. Option B is incorrect because IgA antibodies are produced by the mother and secreted in colostrum and breast milk. Option C is incorrect because it is the antibody involved in the humoral response of the immune system. Option D is incorrect because IgM is the primary antibody involved in fighting bacterial and viral infections.

Selected References

Campbell, R. L., & Kelso, J. M. (2017). Anaphylaxis: Emergency treatment. In R. M. Walls (Ed.), *UpToDate*. Wolters Kluwer. Retrieved from www.uptodate.com

Hamilton, R. G. (2017). Latex allergy: Management. In B. S. Bochner (Ed.), *UpToDate*. Wolters Kluwer. Retrieved from www.uptodate.com

Sax, P. E. (2017). Acute and early HIV infection: Clinical manifestations and diagnosis. In J. G. Bartlett (Ed.), *UpToDate*. Wolters Kluwer. Retrieved from www.uptodate.com

Smith, H. R., & Brown, A. (2017, May 26). *Rheumatoid arthritis*. Retrieved on March 27, 2017 from http://emedicine.medscape.com/article/331715-overview

Venables, P. J., & Maini, R. N. (2017). Diagnosis and differential diagnosis of rheumatoid arthritis. In J. R. O'Dell (Ed.), *UpToDate*. Wolters Kluwer. Retrieved from www.uptodate.com

Wallace, D. J. (2017). Diagnosis and differential diagnosis of systemic lupus erythematosus in adults. In D. S. Pisetsky (Ed.), *UpToDate*. Wolters Kluwer. Retrieved from www.uptodate.com

Chapter 18

Eye, Ear, and Nose Disorders

Introduction

- Disorders of the eye, ear, and nose can be particularly disruptive to activities of daily living (ADLs)
- Full visual function requires normal brain function, an intact retina, a clear lens, and normal intraocular pressure (IOP)
- Common vision disorders result from alterations in ocular function or anatomy due to disease, trauma, the aging process, or abnormal IOPs; patients with significantly impaired vision may be frightened, anxious, and require special nursing care
- Hearing loss is a common disability that affects millions of people and causes significant alterations in ADLs; sclerotic disorders and vestibular dysfunction can be especially upsetting. It is important that other means of communication such as writing, picture board, or even a sign language interpreter be available if necessary to ensure the accurate transmission of information between the patient and the health care team
- Although the nose is the primary organ of smell, nasal disorders can affect taste and the smooth passage of air during respirations
- Nursing history
  - The nurse asks the patient about their *chief complaint*
    - A patient with an eye disorder may report having diplopia, visual floaters, iridescent vision, vision loss, eye pain, or photophobia
    - The patient may also report decreased visual acuity or clarity, defects in color vision, and difficulty seeing at night
    - A patient with an ear disorder may experience hearing loss, tinnitus, pain, discharge, or dizziness
    - A patient with a nose disorder may experience nasal stuffiness, nasal discharge, or epistaxis
  - The nurse then questions the patient about their *present illness*
    - Ask the patient about their symptom(s), including when it started, associated symptoms, location, radiation, intensity, duration, frequency, and precipitating and alleviating factors
    - Ask about the use of glasses and contact lenses
    - Ask about the use of prescription and over-the-counter (OTC) drugs, herbal remedies, and vitamin and nutritional supplements
  - The nurse asks about the *medical history*
    - Question the patient about a history of allergies, hypertension, diabetes, cerebrovascular accident, multiple sclerosis, syphilis, human immunodeficiency virus, or sleep apnea
    - Ask about corrective eye surgery
    - Ask the patient about previous ear problems or injuries, frequent colds, allergens, headaches, nose or head trauma, and sinus complaints
  - The nurse then assesses the *family history*
    - Ask about a family history of eye disorders, such as cataracts, glaucoma, or blindness
    - Question the patient about a family history of diabetes and hypertension
    - Question the patient about a family history of eye, ear, and nose problems
  - The nurse obtains a *social history*
    - Ask about work, exercise, diet, use of recreational drugs and alcohol, and hobbies
    - Also ask about stress, support systems, and coping mechanisms

○ Question the patient about exposures to chemicals, flying debris, noise, fumes, or infectious agents; ask about the use of protective equipment for eyes (safety goggles), respiratory system (masks), and ears (ear plugs)

○ Ask the visually impaired patient how they manage ADLs

- Physical assessment
  - Nurse begins with *inspection*
    - ○ Observe the patient's eye movements and ability to focus
    - ○ Note the appearance of the eyelids, eyeballs, and lacrimal apparatus
    - ○ Examine the conjunctiva, sclera, iris, anterior chamber, and cornea
    - ○ Check both pupils for equality of size and shape, pupillary reaction to light, and accommodation
    - ○ Test visual acuity using a Snellen chart and near-vision chart
    - ○ Specialized optometric and ophthalmic tests may be ordered, such as optical coherence tomography (OCT), visual field testing, fundus photography, IOP measurements, etc.
    - ○ Test extraocular muscles by assessing the corneal light reflex and cardinal positions of gaze
    - ○ Examine intraocular structures using an ophthalmoscope (this may be challenging in the nondilated pupil)
    - ○ Observe the ears for position and symmetry; inspect the auricles for lesions, nodules, or redness; check the ear canal for drainage, foreign bodies, and cerumen
    - ○ Examine the auditory canal, tympanic membrane, and malleus with an otoscope
    - ○ Assess hearing using Weber's and Rinne's tests and pure tone audiometry
    - ○ Observe the nose for position, symmetry, swelling, deformity, and color; note any nasal discharge or flaring
    - ○ Inspect the nasal cavity for septal deviation or perforation; examine the vestibule and turbinates for redness, softness, and discharge
    - ○ Assess the patient's sense of smell
    - ○ Examine the nostrils using a nasal speculum; note color, patency, and the presence of exudate
  - Next, the nurse uses *palpation*
    - ○ Gently palpate the eyelids, noting any swelling or complaints of tenderness; eyeballs should feel equally firm, but not hard or rigid
    - ○ Palpate the lacrimal sac while observing the punctum for excessive tearing or drainage
    - ○ Palpate the mastoid area and ear for tenderness, redness, or warmth
    - ○ Palpate the nose for pain, tenderness, swelling, and deformity
    - ○ Palpate the sinuses for tenderness

Age-Related Macular Degeneration

- Description
  - Age-related macular degeneration (AMD) is characterized by small clusters of yellowish debris (called drusen) beneath the retina
  - When drusen are located in the macular area, they cause visual loss
  - Central vision is most often affected
  - Two types of AMD exist: dry type and wet type
    - ○ *Dry-type* AMD is atrophic and nonexudative and is responsible for 85% to 90% of cases; in this type of AMD, the outer layers of the retina slowly break down
    - ○ *Wet-type* AMD is neovascular and exudative and may have an abrupt onset; symptoms result from the proliferation of abnormal vessels under the retina. Early identification of the progression to wet type is essential for prompt treatment and improved outcomes
  - Although the cause of AMD is unknown, increasing age, ethnicity, and genetic factors are risk factors for development of the disease. Smoking is the main modifiable risk factor
  - AREDS or AREDS 2 antioxidant vitamin and mineral supplementation should be considered for patients with intermediate to advanced AMD
  - AMD is the most common cause of visual loss in people age 60 and older
- Signs and symptoms
  - In dry-type AMD, drusen can be seen beneath the retina; atrophy of the retinal pigment epithelium (RPE) also occurs

- In wet-type AMD, the patient has subretinal fluid accumulation or hemorrhage with a yellow-green discoloration that's sometimes surrounded by a pigment ring; in the advanced stage, exudates and fibrovascular scarring occur
- Grayness, haziness, or a blind spot may appear in the area of central vision; words may look blurred on a page, straight lines may appear to have kinks in them, and colors may seem dimmer
- The disorder may also cause difficulty with night vision and changing light conditions
- Diagnosis and treatment
  - Indirect ophthalmoscopy may show changes in the macular region of the fundus
  - The Amsler grid test may detect visual distortion. Have the patient check their monocular vision individually daily
  - Fluorescein angiography may show leaking vessels (choroidal neovascular membranes) in the subretinal neovascular net. Note: Fundus fluorescein angiography (FFA) is commonly nauseating for a short period. Prevent IV extravasation when administering the test. Counsel the patient on side effects and risk factors, including allergic reactions
  - Indocyanine green videoangiography identifies hidden or occult choroidal neovascular membranes
  - Optical coherence tomography may help identify choroidal neovascular membranes, subretinal fluid, and retinal thickening
  - Although no known cure exists for dry-type AMD, some evidence indicates that a diet high in beta-carotene, zinc, and vitamins A, C, and E may slow the progression of the disease (AREDS supplements)
  - For wet-type AMD, treatment targets the development and progression of angiogenesis; laser treatments may be used
  - Drug therapy may include a vascular endothelial growth factor (VEG-F) antagonist or the monoclonal antibody bevacizumab (Avastin). Anti-VEG-F is first line of treatment for neovascular (wet) AMD
  - Vitrectomy removes all or part of the vitreous humor. This may be done after a vitreous hemorrhage or if a posterior vitreous detachment is causing traction on the retina
  - Macular translocation shifts the macula away from the choroidal neovascular membranes
  - Photodynamic therapy (Visudyne) may also be helpful to seal the exudative neovascularization of wet AMD
- Nursing interventions
  - Teach the patient and family about the disorder, including treatment and follow-up care
  - Teach the patient to self- monitor for visual changes using monocular Amsler Grid testing and to promptly report any changes
  - Determine the extent of the patient's vision loss
  - Help the patient obtain optical aids such as magnifiers
  - Assist the patient with adaptations to accommodate his vision changes; promote safety
  - If the provider approves, suggest AREDs formulated vitamin supplements. Urge the patient to use eye protection such as glasses or sunglasses that block ultraviolet light to protect his eyes from ultraviolet light
  - Offer emotional support
  - Encourage the patient to express his fears and concerns, especially those related to vision loss and its impact on his ability to function
  - Refer the patient to local support organizations as appropriate

Box 18-1: Nursing Care for Intravitreal Injections

Intravitreal injection

- Prepare the patient for the procedure by verifying the order, informed consent is signed, the right patient, right drug, right dose, and right site.
- Perform visual acuity and IOP tests.
- Recline the patient. Administer preinjection drops (dilation, antibiotic, and/ or anesthetic) as ordered. Perform periocular cleansing per policy. Prepare intravitreal medication syringe and supplies. Assist provider with procedure as needed.
- Postinjection, administer eye drops as ordered and check visual acuity. Notify provider if visual acuity is worse than "count fingers."
- Review discharge instructions with patient. Educate patient to report increased pain or decreased vision.

- If Visudyne photodynamic therapy (with laser) is instituted, the patient must remain out of direct sunlight for (5) days to prevent significant photosensitivity reactions. The patient must be fully protected when leaving the office, with hat, gloves, longs sleeves, and pants
- If fluorescein dye test is performed, the patient should be aware of the appearance of a jaundiced skin color that may last for a day
- The patient undergoing any ophthalmic treatment should have a designated driver

Cataracts

- Description
  - Cataracts come in several forms (see *Types of Cataracts*, page 305) and are caused by a gradual degradation of the optical quality of the crystalline lens
  - It is a common cause of gradual vision loss that usually affects both eyes
- Signs and symptoms
  - Gradual painless blurring eventually leads to poor reading vision, reduced vision at night and in bright sunlight, and vision loss
  - Other effects may include halos around lights, milky pupils, and unpleasant glares
  - Cataracts naturally progress over time with no chance of recovery outside of surgical intervention
- Diagnosis and treatment
  - Indirect ophthalmoscopy or slit-lamp examination confirms the diagnosis
  - Cataracts can be surgically treated by extracapsular extraction, which removes the anterior capsule and its contents; intracapsular extraction, which removes the entire lens in the capsule; or phacoemulsification, which uses ultrasonic vibration to fragment the lens
    - In the United States, small incision phacoemulsification with foldable intraocular lens (IOL) implantation is the standard surgery for cataracts
  - Corrective lenses may be prescribed to improve vision
    - A plastic IOL implant may be inserted in the eye as part of the surgical procedure
    - Cataract glasses (glasses with magnifying lenses) or contact lenses may be prescribed 6 to 8 weeks after surgery
- Preoperative nursing interventions
  - Explain the importance of compliance in a preadmission interview
  - Make sure that someone can drive the patient to and from the day surgery center
  - Tell the patient to tilt his head backward when shampooing to prevent jarring the eye and increasing IOP
  - Administer a preoperative stool softener to prevent straining during defecation, which increases IOP
  - Explain preoperative and postoperative care to decrease the patient's anxiety
  - Answer questions and encourage the patient to discuss concerns
- Postoperative nursing interventions
  - Review postoperative instructions to improve compliance and prevent complications; the patient may have difficulty reading instructions because of impaired vision
  - Tell the patient not to bend, strain, lift, cough, sneeze, or rub the eye postoperatively; these actions can increase IOP, which can lead to complications, such as bleeding, vitreous herniation, vision loss, pain, and wound dehiscence; rubbing also increases the chance of infection
  - Tell the patient not to make quick movements or read, which could irritate the patched eye or dislodge an implanted lens
  - Teach the patient or family member how to administer eye medications properly; tell the patient to avoid using OTC eyedrops
  - Teach the patient how to clean the eye to prevent infection
  - Have the patient wear an eye shield and patch to protect the eye from injury; tell him to keep the eye patch dry and to wear an eye shield while sleeping
  - Tell the patient to call the practitioner if any of these signs or symptoms occur: eye pain that is increasing or that isn't relieved with analgesics, yellow or green discharge, temperature above 100°F (37.8°C), blurred vision, a significant reduction in vision, progressive redness, periocular swelling, nausea and vomiting, and seeing halos around lights
  - Explain postoperative activity restrictions
    - The patient may walk, climb stairs, watch television, and perform ADLs but should avoid engaging in strenuous physical activity and lifting more than 10 lb (4.5 kg)

> ### Box 18-2: **Types of Cataracts**
>
> There are several forms of cataracts. They occur at various points in the life cycle, but the treatment for each is the same.
>
> | Type of Cataract | Description |
> |---|---|
> | Complicated | Develop as secondary effects in patients with uveitis, glaucoma, retinitis pigmentosa, or retinal detachment or with systemic disease, such as diabetes, hypoparathyroidism, or atopic dermatitis; also develop after exposure to ionizing radiation or infrared rays. |
> | Congenital | Develop in utero at the anterior or posterior ocular pole; associated with heredity or maternal rubella infection in the first trimester. |
> | Senile | Occur after age 50 as part of aging; the nuclear portion of the lens becomes increasingly dense, transparency decreases, and light rays strike the opaque lens and scatter. |
> | Toxic | Result from drug or chemical toxicity with dinitrophenol, ergot, naphthalene, or phenothiazines. |
> | Traumatic | Can occur at any age and are caused by mechanical trauma or exposure to chemicals, radiation, or toxic substances; the capsule ruptures, swelling occurs, and opacity increases; usually unilateral. |

- ○ The patient may bathe or shower but should avoid getting water on the eye patch by tilting his head back when shampooing
- ○ The patient should avoid bending from the waist and hanging the head forward; a long-handled grabber may be used to pick up objects
- Make sure the patient is cared for by a family member or friend after surgery
- Advise the patient to refrain from sexual activity until he receives his practitioner's approval

Glaucoma

- Description
  - This group of disorders is often characterized by high IOP and optic nerve damage that affects peripheral vision
  - There are two main forms of glaucoma:
  - *Open-angle* (also known as *chronic, simple,* or *wide angle*) glaucoma begins insidiously and progresses slowly
    - ○ Up to 40% of primary open-angle glaucoma has a normotensive IOP. There is commonly evidence of optic nerve or retinal nerve fiber layer damage and evidence of visual field abnormalities
  - *Angle-closure* (also known as *acute* or *narrow angle*) glaucoma occurs suddenly and can cause permanent vision loss in 48 to 72 hours
- Signs and symptoms
  - Open-angle glaucoma may cause no symptoms, or it may cause a dull morning headache, mild aching in the eyes, loss of peripheral vision, halos around lights, and reduced visual acuity (especially at night) that's uncorrected by glasses
  - Acute angle-closure glaucoma causes the rapid onset of pain and pressure over the eye, blurred vision, decreased visual acuity, halos around lights, and nausea and vomiting
- Diagnosis and treatment
  - Tonometry measurements reveal increased IOP; visual field tests measure loss of peripheral vision
  - Ophthalmoscopy shows the effects of glaucoma on the optic disc (called cupping), whereas gonioscopy measures the angle of the anterior chamber of the eye
  - Other diagnostic tests may include slit-lamp examination and fundus photography
  - Drugs that may be used to treat glaucoma include topical adrenergic agonists, cholinergic agonists, beta-adrenergic blockers, and topical or oral carbonic anhydrase inhibitors that reduce IOP by decreasing the production of aqueous humor
  - Surgery or laser treatments may be performed for patients who are unresponsive to drug therapy (see *Procedures for Glaucoma,* page 306)

Box 18-3: Procedures for Glaucoma

Argon laser trabeculoplasty (ALT) is a first-line therapy for different types of glaucoma. It's used either instead of drug therapy or if drug therapy can't control the increased intraocular pressure (IOP). Performed as an outpatient procedure, ALT directs 40 to 80 laser beams into the trabecular network, creating holes through which the aqueous humor can return to the venous circulation.

For patients who are unresponsive to drug therapy or ALT, or aren't suitable candidates for these treatments, a trabeculectomy may be performed. In this glaucoma filtration procedure, a flap of sclera is dissected free to expose the trabecular meshwork. This discrete tissue block is then removed, and a surgical hole is made in the periphery of the iris. The opening allows aqueous humor to flow out under the conjunctiva by creating a filtering bleb. Often, drugs such as 5-fluorouracil are applied during or after the procedure to control scarring and reclosure of the hole.

Patients for whom trabeculectomy has failed to maintain lower IOP or who are at high risk for failure may need a tube shunt implanted to keep the drainage pathway artificially open. These shunts are surgically kept closed with an absorbable suture to allow healing time. Because of the time required before the shunt is operational and the difficulty of medically controlling IOP after surgery, the patient may undergo a trabeculectomy at the same time. Usually, this site fails about the same time as the shunt is healed, providing for continuous pressure reduction.

When other treatments have failed to control IOP, transscleral cyclophotocoagulation may be performed. Between 20 and 40 laser beams are directed into the ciliary body of the eye to decrease its production of aqueous fluid.

Laser peripheral iridotomy is used to correct the narrow angle between the iris and the trabecular meshwork that blocks appropriate drainage of aqueous humor in patients with angle-closure glaucoma. A laser beam creates a small hole in the peripheral iris, allowing the fluid to flow to the anterior chamber of the eye, which also results in opening of the angle of the eye.

- Bed rest is recommended for patients with acute angle-closure glaucoma
- Nursing interventions
  - Encourage patient compliance by teaching the patient about the disease process and treatment
  - Since glaucoma is a "silent disease," compliance is especially important. Open-angle glaucoma is a top cause of blindness worldwide
  - Postoperatively, give medications, as ordered to dilate the pupil and topical corticosteroids to rest the pupil and protect the affected eye
  - Administer pain medication, antiemetics, and stool softeners, as ordered
  - Encourage the patient to be ambulatory immediately after surgery
  - Teach the patient to avoid activities that can increase IOP such as straining during bowel movements

Deviated Nasal Septum

- Description
  - The nasal septum, which bisects the nasal cavity, is made up of cartilage and bone; deviations are common
  - Although septal deviation typically is asymptomatic, it can cause nasal obstruction and increase the risk of sinusitis and epistaxis
  - Deviated nasal septum may be congenital or caused by trauma
- Signs and symptoms
  - Signs and symptoms of deviated septum include drying, crusting nasal discharge and other mucosal changes, as well as bleeding that can block the sinus opening
  - The patient may report shortness of breath and difficulty breathing through the nose and may also report sinusitis and headache
  - Upper respiratory tract infection or nasal trauma can exacerbate symptoms
- Diagnosis and treatment
  - Diagnosis is based on visual inspection of the nasal mucosa with a bright light and nasal speculum
  - Short-term treatment consists of decongestants, antihistamines, and nasal saline rinses to open the nasal airway and analgesics to relieve headache
  - Long-term treatment may require septoplasty or submucous resection of the septum; in these procedures, the septum is surgically straightened and then stabilized with sutures and packing (consisting of petroleum jelly, iodoform, and soft gauze) for 24 to 48 hours

- Indications for surgery include nasal hemorrhage and an inability to pack the nose adequately because of deformity, recurrent sinusitis resulting from blocked sinus openings, and such signs and symptoms as snoring, breathing through the mouth, dry mouth, and shortness of breath
- Surgery is performed under local or general anesthesia and may require overnight hospitalization; its complications include septal hematoma, infection, hemorrhage, septal perforation, anosmia, and cosmetic deformity
- Preoperative nursing interventions
  - Determine the severity of the nasal airway obstruction; a patient with a blocked nasal airway needs humidification, oral hygiene, and other comfort measures
  - Teach the patient about postoperative care to reduce anxiety and promote compliance
- Postoperative nursing interventions
  - Keep the patient's head elevated 30 degrees to promote drainage, reduce edema, and maintain a patent airway
  - Check the patient's vital signs and airway frequently to ensure that the packing hasn't slipped posteriorly, which could block the oral airway; take rectal, ear, or axillary temperatures while the packing is in place because the patient's only airway is his oral airway
  - Watch for nasal bleeding and frequent swallowing; inspect the pharynx with a penlight if bleeding is suspected; keep emergency suction equipment at the patient's bedside
  - Encourage the patient to expectorate oral secretions; record the amount and describe the secretions
  - Change the 2″ × 3″ gauze dressing or drip pad, as needed, and record the frequency and amount of drainage
  - Urge the patient to avoid swallowing blood, which can lead to nausea and vomiting
  - Provide comfort measures, and administer analgesics, as needed, to decrease pain and promote participation in care
  - Use a face tent to provide humidified air, and frequently perform oral hygiene measures; because air breathed in through the mouth isn't humidified like air breathed in through the nose, the oral mucous membranes can become dry
  - Inform the patient of limitations and safety measures, such as not blowing his nose to prevent injury to the surgical site; if sneezing is necessary, the patient should open the mouth to release the pressure of the sneeze
  - Tell the patient to notify the practitioner if signs or symptoms of infection, hemorrhage, or hematoma occur, including bleeding, pain, swelling, redness, fever, headache, or foul-smelling drainage

Otitis Externa

- Description
  - Otitis externa is an acute or chronic inflammation of the external auditory canal. The pinna or tympanic membrane may also be involved
  - Risk factors include water in the ear canal (swimmer's ear), trauma to the skin of the ear (such as cotton swab, piercing site), use of objects in the canal that impact wax (earplugs, hearing aids), and endocrine disorders (such as diabetes mellitus) that can predispose a patient to infections
  - *Staphylococcus aureus* and *Pseudomonas* are the most common types of bacteria that cause otitis externa. Acute otitis externa (AOE) is caused by a bacteria in 98% of cases. A fungal cause is more likely in chronic otitis externa than AOE
- Signs and symptoms
  - AOE is a cellulitis of the ear skin and subdermis. A diagnosis requires evidence of diffuse inflammation of a rapid onset within 48 hours, occurring in the last 3 weeks
  - Symptoms of ear canal inflammation include one or more of the following: otalgia, ear itching, or fullness. Ear canal pain and temporal mandibular joint pain may be increased with jaw motion
  - Signs of ear canal inflammation include one or more of the following: tenderness of the tragus and/ or pinna, diffuse erythema, and/or edema of the canal. Otorrhea, regional lymphadenopathy, tympanic membrane erythema, or cellulitis of the pinna and adjacent skin may also be seen
  - Fungal otitis externa may not produce any symptoms
- Diagnosis and treatment
  - Microscopic examination, if performed, reveals the causative organism
  - Otoscopy shows a swollen external ear canal, debris, and erythema. Occasionally, regional cellulitis and periauricular lymphadenopathy are noted
  - Treatment includes cleaning debris from the ear canal under direct visualization

- With mild, chronic otitis externa, the patient may need specially fitted earplugs for showering or swimming
- Oral analgesics help control pain; topical anesthetics are not recommended
- Topical antimicrobial ear drops are first-line treatment. They commonly include acetic acid or an antibiotic, with or without a corticosteroid. Suspected or known nonintact TM should not receive ototoxic ear drops. An antifungal will be prescribed for otomycosis. Only severe bacterial infections require oral antibiotics
- Nursing interventions
  - Clean and dry the patient's ear gently and thoroughly
  - Give prescribed drugs. If the ear canal is severely swollen, a wick may be inserted to deliver medication throughout the canal. Tell the patient to not remove the wick until instructed to do so; however, it may fall out on its own as the edema subsides
  - To prevent recurrence, tell the patient to avoid potential irritants and to dry ears thoroughly. A few drops of a 50/50 mixture of 5% acetic acid solution (white household vinegar) in 70% rubbing alcohol after swimming can help dry the ear and adjust the pH to prevent AOE. Mild AOE can be often be self-treated with a 50/50 solution of 5% acetic acid solution (white household vinegar) and distilled water
  - Warn against cleaning the ears with cotton-tipped applicators or other objects

Otitis Media

- Description
  - Otitis media (OM) commonly results from poorly functioning eustachian tubes
  - There are various presentations of the disorder with different treatments
    - Acute otitis media (AOM) is a common childhood condition. It is characterized by a rapid onset of signs and symptoms of inflammation in the middle ear, commonly viral or bacterial in origin
    - Otitis media with effusion (OME) is the presence of middle-ear effusion (MEE) without signs or symptoms of an acute infection
    - OME may precede or predispose to AOM, occur after AOM, or occur as a result of eustachian tube dysfunction related to an upper respiratory tract infection. It is important to distinguish between the two because antibiotics are not indicated for OME, and many cases of AOM do not need antibiotics as well
    - MEE/OME may persist for several weeks or months
    - Chronic OME is the persistence of OME for 3 months or more. Persistent OME may lead to hearing loss, balance problems, behavior problems, recurrent AOM, and reduced school performance
  - The pathogens that most commonly cause AOM include *Streptococcus pneumoniae*, *Haemophilus influenzae*, and *Moraxella catarrhalis*
  - Complications of OM include rupture of the tympanic membrane, hearing loss, vertigo, meningitis, and septicemia
- Signs and symptoms
  - Preverbal children may display holding or tugging at the ear, excessive crying, fever, or altered sleep patterns. Older children and adults may report a rapid onset of otalgia, fever, fullness of the ear
  - The patient may also experience a sensation of fullness in the ear as well as popping or crackling sounds when swallowing or chewing
  - Other signs and symptoms may include purulent discharge from the ear (otorrhea), evidence of hearing loss, and, if tympanic membrane ruptures, pain that abruptly ceases
- Diagnosis and treatment
  - The patient's history may include upper respiratory infection or allergies
  - Otoscopic examination shows fluid MEE behind the tympanic membrane; in chronic OM, it reveals thickening or scarring of the tissue
    - The normal TM is translucent and pearly gray with the ability to visualize landmarks
    - OME will have MEE but typically no other signs
    - AOM typically shows MEE with a bulging erythematous TM. If the TM has perforated, there may be a hole seen and fluid in the external ear canal
    - Pneumatic otoscopy is the standard tool for diagnosis of the presence of MEE by reduced movement of the TM in AOM and OME
  - Culture and sensitivity testing of the exudate, if ordered
  - A complete blood count, if performed, may show leukocytosis (if AOM results from bacteria)
  - Radiographic studies, if performed, may demonstrate mastoid involvement

- Tympanometry may be performed
- An age-appropriate hearing test may be performed for persistent OME
- Treatment aims to eradicate the underlying cause, for instance, eliminating eustachian tube obstruction
- Medications for AOM include antibiotics; amoxicillin is generally first line unless the patient is allergic. Acetaminophen or ibuprofen is given as needed for pain
- Surgical procedures (for select cases of OME with documented hearing loss or recurrent AOM) include myringotomy and aspiration of middle-ear fluid, followed by insertion of a polyethylene tube into the tympanic membrane
  - Educate the parent's on the expected duration of tube function (months to years), recommended follow-up schedule, and detection of complications
  - Tympanostomy tube otorrhea (TTO) may occur and is treated with topical antibiotics
  - There are no routine water precautions needed for children with tympanostomy tubes, unless TTO is present
- Nursing interventions
  - Teach the patient and his family about the disorder, including treatment and follow-up care
  - Many cases of mild to moderate childhood AOM will resolve without antibiotics. The provider may take a "watch and wait" approach with appropriate follow-up (within 48 hours of onset for persistence of symptoms, or sooner for worsening) for:
    - Age 6 months to 23 months: nonsevere unilateral AOM
    - Age 24 months or older: nonsevere unilateral or bilateral AOM
  - Administer analgesics, antipyretics, and antibiotics as ordered
  - Watchful waiting with follow-up office testing and evaluation 3 months from diagnosis is appropriate for most OME not at high risk for complications
  - Chronic OME is reevaluated at 3 to 6 month intervals
  - Allow the patient and his family to verbalize their feelings and concerns; answer all questions and provide emotional support
  - Provide clear, concise explanations
  - Discourage over-the-counter antihistamines, intranasal steroids or decongestants as these are not proven to help and can cause side effects
  - Teach the patient or parent when to call for an evaluation of ear problems
  - Swallowing during take-off and landing of airplane flights can help even out pressure
  - If temporary mild to moderate hearing loss occurs, teach the patient/ family ways to manage impaired communication. Teach them to report worsening or persistence of hearing loss as appropriate
  - Prepare the patient and family for possible surgery; provide appropriate postoperative care

Otosclerosis

- Description
  - Otosclerosis (or hardening of the ear) is an overgrowth of bone that impedes normal ossicular motion and can fix the stapes to the oval window
  - Otosclerosis is the most common cause of progressive conductive hearing loss in adults with normal tympanic membranes
  - The disease has a familial tendency and usually occurs between ages 15 and 50; twice as many women are affected as men
  - Pregnancy may trigger the onset in women
- Signs and symptoms
  - Progressive hearing loss, which may be unilateral at first and may become bilateral, typically begins at an early age
  - Vertigo also can occur
  - The patient may report hearing his own voice better than the voices of others
- Diagnosis and treatment
  - Diagnostic tests may include audiometry; electronystagmography; caloric testing; magnetic resonance imaging or computed tomography; Weber's, Rinne's, and Romberg's tests; and facial nerve testing
  - Hearing aids are recommended to improve hearing
  - Stapedectomy (surgical removal of the stapes) may be done, and the stapes may be replaced by a

prosthesis; complications of this procedure, which is typically performed under local anesthesia, include continued hearing loss, granuloma, oval window rupture that causes perilymph fistula, inflammation, infection, prosthesis displacement, and temporary taste changes

- Preoperative nursing interventions
  - Use alternative communication methods as needed; a patient with severe hearing loss may need written instructions or a signing oral interpreter
  - Discuss preoperative tests and postoperative care to reduce anxiety and promote compliance
  - Encourage the patient to discuss anxieties and expectations; clarify misconceptions, and inform him that his hearing won't improve until 6 weeks after surgery because of edema and packing
- Postoperative nursing interventions
  - Elevate the head of the patient's bed 30 degrees; position him according to the practitioner's orders—on the unaffected side to prevent graft displacement or on the affected side to facilitate drainage
  - Monitor vital signs, and check dressings for bleeding; attempt to quantify bleeding
  - Check for headache, stiff neck, fever, and vertigo, which are signs and symptoms of complications
  - Observe the patient for edema, meningitis, labyrinthitis, and infection
  - Keep dressings intact; when removed, observe the site for bleeding, redness, drainage, and edema
  - Clean the suture line as directed; use aseptic technique to prevent infection, and watch for signs of infection
  - Keep packing intact; it's absorbable, and it shouldn't be removed
  - Assess facial nerve functioning twice daily to detect nerve compromise
  - Administer pain medications, as needed, to allow the patient to participate in care
  - Help the patient get out of bed to prevent falls
  - Remind the patient to avoid rapid head movements, which can cause the dizziness that commonly occurs after surgery
  - Tell the patient not to blow his nose and to keep his mouth wide open when coughing or sneezing
- Discharge nursing interventions
  - Provide written instructions to increase compliance
  - Tell the patient to avoid strenuous activity for 1 to 3 weeks but to return to work after 1 week as prescribed; strenuous activity can result in perilymph fistula and may dislodge the prosthesis
  - Instruct the patient to keep the ear dry for 6 weeks; he can shampoo his hair after 1 week; to avoid getting water in the affected ear while bathing, he should plug the ear with a cotton ball coated with petroleum jelly
  - Tell the patient not to travel by air for 2 to 3 weeks to prevent barotrauma
  - Tell the patient to avoid people with colds or upper respiratory tract infections for 4 to 6 weeks; these infections can spread to the middle ear by way of the eustachian tube
  - Instruct the patient to report drainage, fever, otalgia (ear pain), vertigo, redness, and tenderness of the incision site
  - Tell the patient to change the cotton ball covering the ear canal daily and as needed but not to disturb the packing in the ear canal
  - Show the patient how to perform daily incision care

Retinal Detachment

- Description
  - Retinal detachment is the accumulation of subretinal fluid that causes separation of the sensory layers of the retina from the underlying RPE; without treatment, the entire retina may detach, causing severe vision impairment and possible blindness
  - It may be caused by degenerative changes in the retina or vitreous gel which result in traction, intraocular inflammation, or mechanical trauma
  - Rhegmatogenous retinal detachment (RRD) is the most common type and occurs when a tear in the retina leads to subretinal fluid accumulation and separation from the RPE
  - Risk factors for premature posterior vitreous detachment (that may lead to RRD) include high myopia, prior intraocular surgery, family history, and RRD in the other eye. Some conditions are associated with higher incidence of RRD, including Marfan's syndrome, Ehlers-Danlos syndrome, Stickler syndrome, and homocysteinuria. Metabolic disease or vascular disease can also predispose to retinal detachment
- Signs and symptoms

- Signs and symptoms may occur slowly or suddenly
- Early symptoms may include flashes of light (photopsias) and a new floaters; left untreated, progressive loss of vision or shadow in one area may occur (some describe as if curtain is being pulled before the eye). Early detection and treatment are necessary for the best outcome
- An afferent pupillary defect may be seen if the detachment is clinically significant
- Asymptomatic detachments can occur
- Visual acuity and IOP should be checked
- Diagnosis and treatment
  - Diagnosis depends on ophthalmoscopy (both direct and indirect) after full pupil dilation; fundus photography, FFA, OCT, visual field examination, and ultrasonography may also be useful
  - Surgical treatment attempts to close the breaks in the layers by re-establishing contact between the retina and underlying RPE
  - Without intervention, the risk of blindness in a symptomatic retinal detachment is great
  - One or a combination of several types of surgery may be performed
    - *Diathermy* uses extreme heat to seal the edges of the torn RPE
    - *Laser photocoagulation* uses laser-generated heat to injure the tissue and cause scars, which create a fibrous adhesion to seal the hole
    - *Cryotherapy* uses nitrous oxide (also known as laughing gas) or carbon dioxide to injure the tissue by freezing it; the injury leaves a scar, which seals the retinal hole
    - *Scleral buckling* places a band around the globe of the eye to bring the choroid into contact with the retina and hold it in place until adhesion occurs
    - *Intraocular tamponade with a gas bubble can push the detached retina toward the eye wall*
    - *Vitrectomy may be needed*
- Preoperative nursing interventions
  - Pretreatment, the patient should be placed on reduced activity, and possibly bilateral eye patching
  - Place the patient on bed rest, patch the eye as prescribed, and position the patient's head so that the retinal tear or hole is at the lowest point of the eye (if the detachment is toward the outer side of the head, have the patient lie on the affected side with the bed flat); these interventions help prevent further detachment
  - Provide emotional support to the patient who may be distraught at the potential loss of vision
  - Prepare the patient for surgery by cleaning his face and giving him antibiotics and eyedrops, as ordered
  - Teach the patient about the role of the retina and why floaters, flashes of light, and decreased vision occur
  - Allow the patient and family to discuss their concerns
  - Explain the preoperative routines and the surgical procedure
  - The patient should be aware that intervention may produce an anatomically restored contact between the retina and RPE and is done to prevent further deterioration. Often, visual acuity is mostly restored, but this is not guaranteed
- Postoperative nursing interventions
  - Position the patient as directed; **the position varies according to the surgical procedure**
  - Tell the patient to avoid activities that increase IOP, such as sneezing, coughing, vomiting, lifting, straining during defecation, bending from the waist, and rapidly moving the head; increased IOP may cause more fluid to flow behind the retina before healing is complete
  - Administer eyedrops, antiemetics, analgesics, and antibiotics, as ordered; to reduce corneal edema and discomfort, apply ice packs as ordered
  - Tell the patient to notify the practitioner immediately if he experiences floaters, flashes of light, blurred vision, or pain that isn't relieved with analgesics; these symptoms indicate recurrence of detachment
  - Teach the patient to recognize and report the signs and symptoms of infection, such as temperature above 100°F (37.8°C), yellow or green discharge, increased redness or pulling of the eye or lid, and vision loss
  - Show the patient how to administer eye medications and change dressings using sterile technique to decrease the risk of infection
  - Tell the patient to wear the eye shield at night or when napping to prevent accidental injury to the eye
  - Discuss when the patient can return to work, resume ADLs, and drive or perform strenuous activities

Review Questions

Question 1. The nurse is caring for a patient who underwent stapedectomy. To prevent postoperative complications, the nurse should instruct the patient to:

A. sneeze with her mouth open.
B. frequently blow her nose.
C. clean her operated ear with a cotton-tipped applicator twice a day.
D. resume bending and straining when she's no longer experiencing ear pain.

Correct answer: A If sneezing can't be avoided, the patient should sneeze with her mouth open. This will prevent changes of air pressure in the middle ear, which can dislodge the prosthesis and graft. Option B is incorrect because blowing the nose and coughing should be avoided. Option C is incorrect because small objects, such as cotton-tipped applicators, shouldn't be inserted into the ear. Option D is incorrect because straining during a bowel movement and bending should be avoided for at least 2 to 3 weeks or as instructed by the practitioner.

Question 2. The nurse is assessing a 32-year-old patient with otosclerosis. The nurse should be aware that the patient's hearing loss:

A. will resolve in 4 to 6 weeks without intervention.
B. typically affects both ears.
C. occurred suddenly.
D. is associated with ear pain.

Correct answer: B The hearing loss associated with otosclerosis is typically bilateral, although one ear may show a greater impairment. Option A is incorrect because otosclerosis is a progressive disorder that is not self-limiting. Option C isn't correct because otosclerosis develops slowly over time. Because otosclerosis doesn't cause ear pain, Option D is incorrect.

Question 3. The nurse is teaching a patient with a detached retina who underwent scleral buckling on the left eye. The procedure included gas injection into the vitreous. Which of the following statements indicates that the patient understands the nurse's instructions?

A. "I should lie on my abdomen with my head turned to the right."
B. "I'll lie face down with my head turned to the left."
C. "I'll lie face up with my head turned to the right."
D. "I should lie on my back with my head turned to the left."

Correct answer: B In a scleral buckling, the sclera is flattened against the retina. A piece of silicone is attached to the sclera with a band that encircles the eye to keep the retina in contact with the choroid and sclera. Air or other gases may be injected into the vitreous to float up against the retina and promote retinal reattachment. When a gas is used, the patient is positioned on his abdomen with the head turned to the affected eye (in this situation, the left side) so that the gas will float up against the retina and aid in reattachment. The positions in Options A, C, and D don't allow the gas to float up against the retina.

Question 4. The nurse is providing care for a patient following right cataract removal surgery. In which position should the nurse place the patient?

A. Right-side lying
B. Prone
C. Supine
D. Trendelenburg's

Correct answer: C Positioning the patient on his back or inoperative side prevents pressure on the operative eye. Right side-lying (Option A) or prone position (Option B) may put external pressure on the affected eye. Trendelenburg's position (Option D) may increase intraocular pressure.

Question 5. Which position would be the most appropriate for a patient who has undergone stapedectomy?

A. On the affected side
B. On the unaffected side
C. Prone
D. Sims'

Correct answer: B The patient should be positioned on his unaffected side, with the operative ear up. He shouldn't be placed on the affected side (Option A) or prone (Option C). Although Sims' position (Option D) is a side-lying position, it doesn't take into consideration which side is best for after ear surgery.

Question 6. Which symptom would occur in a patient with a detached retina?

A. Flashing lights and floaters
B. Homonymous hemianopia
C. Loss of central vision
D. Ptosis

Correct answer: A Signs and symptoms of retinal detachment include abrupt flashing lights, floaters, loss of peripheral vision (not central vision, as in Option C), and a sudden shadow or curtain in the vision. Occasionally, vision loss is gradual. Homonymous hemianopia (Option B) can occur in stroke and traumatic brain injuries. Ptosis (Option D) can result from a stroke. Note that central vision loss CAN occur, if the macula is lifted off. The question may need to say, which is mostly likely to occur in a patient with a detached retina?

Question 7. A 72-year-old patient is being discharged from same-day surgery after having a cataract removed from his right eye. Which discharge instruction should the nurse give the patient?

A. "Sleep on the operative side."
B. "Resume all activities as before."
C. "Don't rub or place pressure on the eyes."
D. "Wear an eye shield all day and remove it at night."

Correct answer: C Rubbing or placing pressure on the eyes increases the risk of accidental injury to ocular structures. The nurse would caution against sleeping on the operative side—not on the operative side (Option A)—to reduce the risk of accidental injury to ocular structures. The nurse shouldn't tell the patient to resume all activities (Option B); activities such as lifting objects, straining, strenuous exercise, and sexual activity can increase IOP. An eye shield should be worn at night, not during the day (Option D); during waking hours, the patient should wear glasses or shaded lenses to protect the eye after the eye dressing has been removed.

Question 8. Which of the following increases a 40-year-old patient's risk of developing cataracts?

A. A history of frequent streptococcal throat infections
B. Maternal exposure to rubella during pregnancy
C. Increased IOP
D. Prolonged use of steroidal anti-inflammatory agents

Correct answer: D Prolonged use of steroidal anti-inflammatory agents increases the risk of developing cataracts. The other risk factors don't contribute to the development of cataracts.

Question 9. In caring for a patient after cataract surgery, the nurse should tell the patient to notify his physician of which of the following conditions?

A. Blurred vision
B. Eye pain
C. Glare
D. Itching

Correct answer: B The patient shouldn't experience pain after cataract surgery; pain may indicate hyphema, or clouding in the anterior chamber, and infection. The patient might normally experience the other symptoms after cataract surgery.

Question 10. An 89-year-old patient has eye pressures of 27 OD and 29 OS. When questioned, the patient has noticed seeing halos around lights for a year or 2, but denies pain, blurred vision, or headache. A visual field exam shows reduced peripheral vision. Which of the following is most likely?

A. Normal aging eyes
B. Open-angle glaucoma
C. Acute angle-closure glaucoma
D. Cataracts

Correct answer: B Loss of peripheral vision is not normal, although glaucoma incidence increases with age. Acute closed angle glaucoma is associated with elevated IOP and halos around lights, but this patient has had the halos for over a year and the predominant symptom of pain is missing. Cataracts may have decreased vision and halos around lights, but it is not associated with elevated IOP or peripheral vision loss.

- *A firm globe would only be present if the IOP is significantly elevated. You can have glaucoma and a normal IOP (once treated). You can have a soft globe with glaucoma and a firm globe in the absence of glaucoma.*

Question 11. The nurse is caring for a 7-year-old boy with unilateral ear pain since yesterday. The provider notes an inflamed ear canal with debris, and has diagnosed uncomplicated right external otitis. Which of the following instructions is correct?

A. You will need to have a tympanostomy tube placed to drain the fluid from your middle ear.
B. Use a cotton swab to clear out your ears once a week; this will help prevent future infections.
C. When you put in the antibiotic drops, lay down on your left side and leave the drops in for 3 to 5 minutes before getting up.
D. Pull the wick out in an hour.

Correct answer: C Rationale: Option A is incorrect because a tympanostomy tube is not indicated for an external otitis media. Option B is incorrect because cotton swabs increase the risk of trauma to the ear canal and predispose to otitis externa. Option D is incorrect because the patient should leave the wick in until it falls out on its own, or when directed, but an hour isn't long enough. Option C is correct.

Question 12. The provider diagnosed a patient, age 3, with left otitis media and recommended "watching and waiting." Which of the following statements is correct in educating the patient's mother?

A. If symptoms worsen or don't get better in 2 days, have the provider see the patient again for evaluation.
B. Give over-the-counter cough medicine as needed.
C. The child will need ear tubes or hearing will be lost.
D. If the ear begins draining, put some clove oil in it until you see the provider.

Correct answer: A Rationale: Watching and waiting is appropriate for many cases of nonsevere unilateral acute otitis media if reliable follow-up is possible in 48 to 72 hours, or sooner is worsening symptoms. Option B is incorrect because OTC cough medicine is not appropriate for young children. Acetaminophen or ibuprofen may be helpful for discomfort, though. Option C is incorrect because there is no indication that Mary needs ear tubes for AOM. Option D is incorrect because an acute onset of draining ear could indicate a ruptured TM, and nothing should be placed in the ear unless ordered by the provider.

Selected References

American Academy of Ophthalmology. (2015). American Academy of Ophthalmology Retina/ Vitreous Panel. Preferred Practice Panel Guidelines. Age-related macular degeneration. Retrieved from https://www.aao.org/preferred-practice-pattern/age-related-macular-degeneration-ppp-2015

American Academy of Ophthalmology. (2016). Cataract in the adult eye preferred practice pattern. Retrieved from http://dx.doi.org/10.1016/j.ophtha.2016.09.027

American Optometric Association. (2004). Optometric clinical practice guideline on care of the patient with retinal detachment and related peripheral vitreoretinal disease. Retrieved from https://www.aoa.org/documents/optometrists/CPG-13.pdf

American Society of Ophthalmic Registered Nurses. (2016). ASORN recommended practice: Intravitreal injections. Retrieved from http://www.asorn.org/client_data/files/2014/305_asornintravitrealinjections_final.pdf

Lieberthal, A. S., Carroll, A. E., Chonmaitree, T., Ganiats, T. G., Hoberman, A., Jackson, M. A., ... Tunkel, D. E. (2013, February 25). The diagnosis and management of acute otitis media. *Pediatrics, 131*, e964–e999. Retrieved from http://dx.doi.org/10.1542/peds.2012-3488

Prum, Jr, B. E., Rosenberg, L. F., Gedde, S. J., Mansberger, S. L., Stein, J. D., Moroi, S. E., ... Williams, R. D. (2015). Primary open-angle glaucoma preferred practice pattern® guidelines. *Ophthalmology.*2016;123(1):P41–P111. Retrieved from http://www.aaojournal.org/article/S0161-6420(15)01276-2/fulltext

Rosenfeld, R. M., Schwartz, S. R., Cannon, C. R., Roland, P. S., Simon, G. R., Kumar, K. A., ... Robertson, P. J. (2014). Clinical practice guideline: Acute otitis externa executive summary. *Otolaryngology-Head and Neck Surgery, 150*(2), 161–168. Retrieved from http://dx.doi.org/10.1177/0194599813517659

Rosenfeld, R. M., Schwartz, S. R., Pynnonen, M. A., Tunkel, D. E., Hussey, H. M., Fichera, J. S., ... Schellhase, K. G. (2013). Clinical practice guidelines: Tympanostomy tubes in children. *Otolaryngology-Head and Neck Surgery, 149*(1S), S1–S35. Retrieved from http://dx.doi.org/10.1177/0194599813487302

Rosenfeld, R. M., Shin, J. J., Schwartz, S. R., Coggins, R., Gagnon, L., Hackell, J. M., ... Corrigan, M. D. (2016). Clinical practice guideline: Otitis media with effusion (update). *Otolaryngology-Head and Neck Surgery, 154*(1S), S1–S41. Retrieved from http://dx.doi.org/10.1177/0194599815623467

Wu, L. (2017). Rhegmatogenous retinal detachment. Retrieved on June 1, 2017, from http://emedicine.medscape.com/article/1224737-overview

Chapter 19

Perioperative Nursing

Introduction

- Perioperative nursing includes three phases of the surgical experience: the preoperative, intraoperative, and postoperative phases
- It's a specialty that provides interprofessional continuity of care of the surgical patient
- It occurs in various inpatient and outpatient settings

Preoperative Phase

- Description
  - The preoperative period begins when the decision for surgery is made
  - It definitively ends when the patient is transferred to the operating room table, but it functionally ends when the patient is transferred to the holding area
- Psychosocial assessment
  - The preoperative psychosocial assessment aims to identify sources of the patient's concerns and anxiety; it includes assessing the patient's understanding of the surgery, previous surgical experiences, specific concerns or feelings about the surgery, and spiritual and/or cultural beliefs
  - Determine the patient's language, communication patterns, and presence of any cognitive or psychological impairments; arrange for assistance as needed
- Health history
  - Collect a thorough past medical history, making note of preexisting illnesses
  - Inquire about use of medications, herbal or over-the-counter remedies, tobacco, alcohol, or drugs. Make note of any that could interfere with anesthesia or contribute to postoperative complications, and check with the health care provider regarding how medications are to be taken prior to surgery
  - Ask about the patient's surgical history, including any reactions to anesthesia, or postoperative reactions such as unusual nausea or vomiting
  - Obtain a history of allergies, such as to drugs, adhesive tape, latex, Betadine, soap, and/or foods
  - Ask about implanted prosthetics, pacemakers, and body jewelry, which may affect the use of electrocautery equipment
  - Perform a baseline pain assessment. Ask about the patient's current level of pain or discomfort, and assess expectations about postoperative pain relief
- Physical assessment
  - Obtain baseline objective information by collecting vital signs, height, and weight; check for presence of dentures or dental caps; assess skin for lesions, rashes, or pressure injuries
  - Assess the cardiovascular, pulmonary, GI, GU, and neurologic systems for baseline functioning
  - Confirm that a chest X-ray has been performed, if ordered, to detect lung disease
  - If the patient is 40 years old or older or has a cardiac history, obtain an electrocardiogram to provide a baseline and detect any arrhythmias
  - Obtain a blood sample for baseline complete blood count and electrolyte levels; follow agency policy for drawing blood for typing and crossmatching

- Review the results of liver function tests, blood urea nitrogen, serum creatinine, and urinalysis to determine postoperative risk factors
- If the patient is a woman of childbearing age, determine her pregnancy status using urine or serum testing
- Notify operating room staff of any skin concerns; they may be able to position to prevent further compromise of tissue
- Preoperative teaching
  - Provide a description of and reasons for preoperative tests
  - Explain preoperative routines, time of surgery, expected length of surgery, and estimated amount of time in the postanesthesia care unit (PACU)
  - Advise the patient to refrain from smoking and consuming alcohol for 48 hours before surgery
  - Explain the recovery process, including the place where the patient will awaken, nursing care provided, monitoring of vital signs, equipment used, and the time he or she will return to the room
  - Cover the probable postoperative course: anticipated treatments, need to increase activity as soon as possible, need to cough and deep-breathe despite discomfort, method and timing of pain medication administration, and anticipated discharge needs
  - Inform that nothing by mouth is to be consumed 6 to 8 hours (per surgeon's instructions) before surgery; explain which of the patient's usual medications, if any, will be given prior to surgery
  - Explain any special procedures that must be performed before surgery, such as bowel preparation, cleaning with antimicrobial cleaners, and hair removal; hair should be removed with clippers—not by shaving—to reduce the risk of infection
  - Tell family members what time the patient will leave for surgery, where they can wait during surgery, when the health care provider will contact them about surgery results, and when they can visit with the patient
- Informed consent
  - Informed consent must be obtained by the health care provider and placed in the electronic health record before the patient receives any type of preanesthesia medication
  - The informed consent document indicates the specific procedure to be performed; includes a list of possible complications, disfigurement, disability, and removal of body parts; is clearly worded in simple terms; and contains the patient's or guardian's signature
- Preanesthesia medication
  - Preanesthesia medication is usually given while the patient is in the holding area. Depending on the types of medication given, effects are intended to decrease anxiety, provide sedation, induce amnesia, decrease pharyngeal secretions, slow hydrochloric acid production, and/or prevent allergic reactions to anesthetics
  - If ordered, prophylactic antibiotics are to be given within 1 hour of surgical incision
- Preoperative checklist
  - On the preoperative checklist, document actions, such as removing jewelry and dentures (and to whom they were given), checking patient identification, verifying the surgical site, asking the patient to void, ensuring that all needed documents are available, and administering medications as prescribed

Intraoperative Phase

- Description
  - The intraoperative phase begins when the patient is transferred to the operating table and ends when he or she is transferred to the PACU or recovery room
  - Universal protocol is required to prevent wrong site, wrong procedure, and wrong patient surgical errors
  - Various types of anesthesia and anesthetics may be used (see *Types of anesthesia*, page 317)

Postoperative Phase

- Description
  - The postoperative phase begins when the surgery is complete and the patient has been transferred to the PACU and ends with a follow-up evaluation in the clinical setting or at home

Box 19-1: **Types of Anesthesia**

A patient may receive general, regional, or local anesthesia.

Type of Anesthesia	Description
General	• Blocks awareness centers in the brain • Produces unconsciousness, body relaxation, and loss of sensation • Is administered by inhalation or I.V. infusion
Regional	• Inhibits excitatory processes in nerve endings or fibers • Provides analgesia within a specific body area • Doesn't produce unconsciousness • Is administered by nerve block, I.V. regional block with tourniquet, spinal (intrathecal) block, or epidural block
Local	• Blocks nerve impulse transmission at the site of action • Provides analgesia within a limited area • Doesn't produce unconsciousness • Is administered topically or by infiltration

- PACU nurses provide initial assessment, care, and treatments while the patient recovers from the anesthesia; when the patient's activity level, respirations, blood pressure, level of consciousness (LOC), and oxygen saturation are stable, per PACU discharge criteria, he or she is transferred to the regular medical-surgical unit
- Basic nursing actions
  - Verify the patient's identity, and obtain the report from the PACU nurse
  - Position the patient properly in bed. Obtain baseline vital signs, and apical and peripheral pulsations. Assess airway, respirations, and lung sounds, and continue to complete a head-to-toe general assessment (including LOC and neuromotor function) with focus on the operative organ system
  - Administer oxygen if ordered; a patient with a history of coronary artery disease should receive oxygen continuously until mobile. Be alert for signs of respiratory depression from anesthesia
  - Notify the health care provider if the patient can't maintain an arterial oxygen saturation greater than 90% or a partial pressure of arterial oxygen greater than 80 mm Hg
  - Inspect surgical site dressings for drainage and bleeding; reinforce dressings as ordered and needed
  - Check I.V. fluids, medications being given, and new orders; assess the I.V. site for patency
  - Check patency of drainage tubes and urinary catheters; document character of drainage; and start an intake and output record
  - Assess postoperative pain levels; provide comfort measures and prescribed drug therapies
  - Assess bowel sounds and maintain nasogastric suction, if present; continue nothing-by-mouth status until active peristalsis is present and the health care provider places a dietary order
  - Relieve postoperative discomforts, such as vomiting, abdominal distention, hiccups, and constipation (see *Managing postoperative discomforts*, page 318)
- Promoting recovery
  - Monitor fluid balance to ensure adequate tissue perfusion, maintain renal function, and prevent metabolic acidosis; be alert for tachycardia or hypotension, which may indicate a fluid volume deficit
  - Monitor electrolyte levels, and correct imbalances as ordered
  - Maintain nutrition by gradually increasing the patient's diet, as ordered and tolerated, and encourage foods high in protein and vitamin C
  - Increase activity daily as ordered; consult with the physical therapy staff as needed
  - Care for surgical wounds and drains, and provide urinary catheter care; remove the urinary catheter as soon as possible after surgery to decrease risk for CAUTI
  - Monitor for local and systemic signs and symptoms of infection and other complications
  - Teach the patient and family about the care being provided and how to continue postoperative recovery after discharge; obtain a home health referral if needed
  - Provide psychosocial support; refer to inpatient spiritual or social services assistance as needed; provide information about outpatient support groups or community services

Box 19-2: Managing Postoperative Discomforts

The following chart summarizes the causes of postoperative discomforts and associated nursing interventions.

Discomfort	Cause	Nursing Interventions
Vomiting	• **Fluid or air accumulation in the stomach • Stomach inflation • Food and fluid ingestion before peristalsis returns • Psychological factors • Adverse drug reactions • Pain • Electrolyte imbalances	• Encourage the patient to lie quietly in bed. • Administer antiemetics as prescribed. • Prevent aspiration of vomitus by positioning appropriately. • Maintain an accurate record of fluid intake and output. • Maintain adequate hydration. • Provide comfort measures. • Provide therapeutic listening if a psychological factor is identified
Abdominal distention	• Loss of normal peristalsis for 24 to 48 hours after surgery • Swallowing air during recovery from anesthesia	• Have the patient turn in bed, ambulate as tolerated, and perform leg exercises if able. • Withhold very hot or cold liquids when peristalsis is sluggish. • Insert a rectal tube as ordered to stimulate lower colonic peristalsis and gas passage. • Apply heat to the abdomen to expand gas and stimulate peristalsis. • Insert a nasogastric tube as ordered to aspirate fluid or gas. • Administer an enema as ordered to facilitate flatus and bowel movement.
Hiccups	• Intermittent spasms of the diaphragm that may result from direct, indirect, or reflexive irritation of the phrenic nerve	• Have the patient rebreathe carbon dioxide at 5-minute intervals by inhaling and exhaling into a paper bag. • Collaborate with the health care provider to determine is aspiration of the stomach should be performed, if hiccups are caused by gastric dilation. • Collaborate with the health care provider to request blockage of the phrenic nerve by using local infiltration. • Administer a phenothiazine as prescribed.
Constipation	• Local inflammation, peritonitis, or abscess • Weakness resulting from surgery	• Administer an enema as ordered to facilitate a bowel movement. • Administer a stool softener, as prescribed, in the early postoperative phase. • Assess for use of opioid medication, which can increase constipation. • Encourage early ambulation. • Increase fluids and dietary intake as prescribed.

Postoperative Complications

- Venous thromboembolism (VTE)
  - Description
    - VTE can occur in any surgical patient, especially those who may have impaired peripheral circulation.
    - It may result from positioning during surgery, pressure from a pillow or blanket roll placed under the knees after surgery, or concentration of blood caused by loss of fluid or dehydration (see *Chapter 7, Cardiovascular disorders*, for details)
- Hemorrhage
  - Description
    - Hemorrhage after an operation may occur after anesthesia induction or as a result of internal bleeding due to surgical manipulation

- Classified as primary, intermediary, or secondary
  - Primary hemorrhage occurs at the time of the operation
  - Intermediary (or reactive) hemorrhage occurs within the first few hours after the operation as a result of the return of normal blood pressure and its effect on clots in untied vessels, or from a slipped ligature
  - Secondary hemorrhage occurs some time after the operation as a result of insecure taping or erosion of a vessel by a drainage tube
- Signs and symptoms
  - A patient with hemorrhage may experience apprehensiveness, restlessness, agitation, thirst, tinnitus, and progressive weakness followed by cold, moist, pale skin and pallid lips and conjunctivae; increased pulse rate; reduced blood pressure; decreased temperature; rapid, deep respirations; and a rapid decrease in hemoglobin level
- Nursing interventions
  - Assess for location of bleeding; apply pressure to the area, if accessible
  - Provide supplemental oxygen, and maintain a patent airway
  - Monitor the patient's vital signs frequently
  - Give blood transfusions, I.V. fluids, and drugs as ordered to hemodynamically stabilize the patient's condition
  - Prepare the patient for surgery, if necessary
- Paralytic ileus
  - Description
    - Paralytic ileus is a physiologic form of intestinal obstruction that can develop after abdominal surgery, after anesthesia, after manipulation of the GI tract, or because of the stress response; it usually resolves spontaneously in 2 to 3 days
  - Signs and symptoms
    - A patient with paralytic ileus may have severe abdominal distention, extreme distress and, possibly, vomiting with diminished or absent bowel sounds
    - The patient may be severely constipated or may pass flatus and very small, liquid stools
  - Nursing interventions
    - Maintain nothing-by-mouth status until bowel sounds return
    - Administer I.V. fluids as ordered
    - Encourage frequent position changes and ambulation
    - Decreasing opioid use and chewing gum may help resolve ileus
    - If paralytic ileus doesn't resolve, insert a nasogastric tube as ordered
- Pulmonary embolism
  - Description
    - An embolus is a foreign body, gas bubble, blood clot, or piece of tissue that travels in the bloodstream
    - A pulmonary embolism occurs when an embolus is dislodged from its original site and is carried in the blood to the main pulmonary artery or one of the pulmonary branches (see *Chapter 9, Respiratory disorders*, for details)
    - It's common in patients who have experienced trauma, immobilized patients and elderly patients, and is considered a serious complication
- Respiratory complications
  - Description
    - The most common postoperative problem, respiratory complications are serious; their incidence is higher in patients undergoing abdominal surgery
    - The most common respiratory complications are atelectasis, bronchitis, bronchopneumonia, lobar pneumonia, and pleurisy
  - Signs and symptoms
    - Signs and symptoms vary according to the cause of the respiratory complication but may include adventitious breath sounds, chest pain, cough, sputum production, hemoptysis, cyanosis, nasal flaring, shortness of breath, dyspnea, tachypnea, orthopnea, retractions, accessory muscle use, and decreased respiratory excursion
    - Other findings include changes in cognition, anxiety, diaphoresis, fatigue, tachycardia, and fever
  - Nursing interventions
    - Closely monitor respiratory status, breath sounds, pulse oximetry, respiratory rate and depth, skin color, use of accessory muscles, vital signs, and LOC

- ○ Provide supplemental oxygen as ordered, and initiate continuous monitoring of oxygen saturation levels by pulse oximetry
- ○ Obtain a chest X-ray, as ordered
- ○ Provide chest physiotherapy, and encourage coughing, deep breathing, and regular use of incentive spirometry to mobilize and facilitate removal of secretions
- ○ Reposition frequently, and assist with ambulation
- ○ Administer drugs, such as antibiotics and bronchodilators, as prescribed
- ● Shock
  - ● Shock is the most serious postoperative complication
  - ● Classified as hypovolemic, cardiogenic, neurogenic, or septic (see *Chapter 6, Disruptions in homeostasis,* for details)
- ● Wound dehiscence and evisceration
  - ● Description
    - ○ Dehiscence may occur when the edges of the wound fail to join properly, or separate after they seem to be healing normally
    - ○ Evisceration may occur if a portion of the viscera protrudes through the incision
    - ○ Dehiscence and evisceration are most likely to occur 6 to 7 days after surgery
    - ○ Factors that may contribute to dehiscence and evisceration include poor nutrition, diabetes, chronic pulmonary or cardiac disease, localized wound infection, and stress on the incision
    - ○ Stress on the incision from coughing or vomiting may cause abdominal distention or severe stretching, leading to dehiscence
  - ● Nursing interventions
    - ○ If dehiscence or evisceration occurs, take the following steps:
      - ○ Place sterile dressings soaked in normal saline over exposed viscera or dehiscence
      - ○ Monitor vital signs and report any signs of shock
      - ○ Place the patient on bed rest, and notify the surgeon immediately
      - ○ Don't allow the patient to have anything by mouth; he may need to have surgery
- ● Wound infection
  - ● Description
    - ○ Infections of the surgical wound account for many postoperative infections (see *Chapter 5, Principles of wound care,* for details)

Review Questions

Question 1. A patient undergoes a surgical procedure that requires the use of general anesthesia. For which condition does the nurse monitor the patient?

A. anemia
B. atelectasis.
C. dehydration.
D. peripheral edema.

Correct answer: B Atelectasis occurs when the postoperative patient fails to move, cough, and breath deeply. With good nursing care, this is an avoidable complication. Anemia (Option A) is a rare complication that usually occurs in patients who lose a significant amount of blood or continue bleeding postoperatively. Fluid shifts that occur postoperatively may result in dehydration (Option C) and peripheral edema (Option D), but the patient is at higher risk for atelectasis.

Question 2. The nurse has just administered preoperative medication to a patient will have surgery in 30 minutes. What is the appropriate nursing action after medication administration?

A. Obtain vital signs
B. direct the patient to the bathroom down the hall.
C. place the bed in low position with the side rails up.
D. confirm that the medication will immediately induce sleep.

Correct answer: C The focus of nursing actions should always remain on patient safety. Vital signs (Option A) should be taken before the preoperative medication is given. The patient should void before the preoperative medication is given—not after (Option B). When the preoperative medication is given, the bed should be placed in low position, with the side rails raised, and a call light in reach (Option C). The patient may not be asleep (Option D), but drowsiness will occur.

Question 3. The nurse is caring for a patient who was given pain medication before leaving the PACU. Upon returning to the medical-surgical room, the patient reports experiencing pain and requests more pain medication. Which is the appropriate nursing action?

A. Document the pain level only.
B. Give a half dose of the as-needed ordered medication.
C. Notify the practitioner that the patient is continuing to experience pain.
D. Tell the patient that it will be 4 hours before more pain medication can be given.

Correct answer: C The practitioner should be notified of the patient's concern so that new medication orders can be established. The patient's pain should be documented (Option A); however, the nurse also needs to provide assessment and interventions. The nurse cannot independently alter a dose without first consulting the practitioner (Option B). A patient who's experiencing pain after surgery shouldn't have to wait 4 hours for pain relief (Option D).

Question 4. The nurse is evaluating a patient postoperatively for infection. Which assessment finding requires further immediate nursing intervention?

A. A rectal temperature of 100°F (37.8°C)
B. The presence of an indwelling urinary catheter
C. A white blood cell (WBC) count of 9,000/μL
D. Redness, warmth, and tenderness in the incision area

Correct answer: D Redness, warmth, and tenderness in the incision area may indicate a postoperative infection; this requires immediate nursing intervention. A rectal temperature of 100°F (Option A) is normal in a postoperative patient because of the inflammatory process. The presence of any invasive device (Option B) predisposes a patient to infection but alone doesn't indicate infection; this does not require immediate nursing intervention. Because a normal WBC count ranges from 4,000 to 10,000/μL, Option C is incorrect.

Question 5. The nurse is caring for a patient with a postoperative wound evisceration. What is the priority nursing action?

A. Place the patient on nothing-by-mouth status.
B. Explain to the patient what is happening, and provide support.
C. Avoid pushing the protruding organs back into the abdominal cavity.
D. Cover the protruding organs with sterile gauze moistened with sterile saline solution.

Correct answer: D Immediately covering the wound with moistened gauze prevents the organs from drying. Options A and C can be undertaken after Option D. Both the gauze and the saline solution must be sterile to reduce the risk of infection. Explaining what is happening and providing support (Option B) may reduce the patient's anxiety but this isn't the priority action.

Question 6. A patient in the postoperative phase of abdominal surgery has orders to advance the diet as tolerated. The patient has tolerated ice chips and a clear liquid diet. As the next step, the nurse would expects advancement to which type of diet?

A. soft
B. general
C. full liquid
D. sodium-restricted

Correct answer: C After a clear liquid diet, which is nutritionally inadequate but minimally irritating to the stomach, a patient advances to a full-liquid diet next, which adds bland and protein foods. A soft diet (Option A) comes after that, which omits foods that are hard to chew or digest. A regular or general diet (Option B) has no limitations. A sodium-restricted diet (Option D) is ordered when the health care provider wishes to control the amount of sodium intake for health purposes.

Question 7. The patient's intake and output record contains the following information: milk, 180 mL; orange juice, 60 mL; one serving scrambled eggs; one slice toast; one can Ensure oral nutritional supplement, 240 mL; I.V. dextrose 5% in water at 100 mL/hour; 50 mL water after twice daily medications. Medications are given at 9:00 a.m. and 9:00 p.m. How will the nurse document the patient's total intake for the 7 a.m. to 3 p.m. shift?

A. 1,000 mL
B. 1,250 mL
C. 1,330 mL
D. 1,380 mL

Correct answer: C The patient's total intake is 1,330 mL, based on the following equation: $180 + 60 + 240 + 800$ (which is 100 mL/hour × 8 hours) $+ 50 = 1,330$.

Question 8. Which action will the nurse undertake to follow principles of asepsis?

A. Maintaining a sterile environment
B. Keeping the environment as clean as possible
C. Testing for microorganisms in the environment
D. Cleaning an environment until it is free from germs

Correct answer: B Asepsis is the process of avoiding contamination from outside sources by keeping the environment clean. A clean environment has a reduced number of microorganisms, but isn't necessarily sterile (the absence of all microorganisms) (Option A). Testing for microorganisms or culturing (Option C) isn't indicated for asepsis. Cleaning an environment until it is free from germs (Option D) would result in a sterile environment.

Question 9. On the first day after thoracotomy, the nurse's assessment of the patient reveals a temperature of 100°F (37.8°C), a heart rate of 96 beats/minute, blood pressure of 136/86 mm Hg, and shallow respirations of 24 breaths/minute, with rhonchi heard at the lung bases. The patient reports incisional pain at a level of 6 out of 10. What is the priority nursing intervention?

A. Providing pain medication as ordered
B. Assisting the patient out of bed to ambulate
C. Administering ibuprofen (Motrin) as ordered to reduce fever
D. Encouraging the patient to cough and deep-breathe

Correct answer: A Although all the interventions are incorporated within the plan of care, relieving pain and making the patient comfortable take priority. Medication for temperature (Option B) can take place after addressing pain, although this temperature is not unexpected in the early post-operative period. Addressing pain gives the patient the ability to achieve the other objectives (Options C and D).

Question 10. Which nursing intervention will the nurse include in the plan of care for a patient with atelectasis?

A. Administer oxygen continuously at 2 L/minute.
B. Encourage cough and deep-breathing every 4 hours.
C. Have the patient use an incentive spirometer every hour.
D. Assist the patient with ambulation up to a chair every day.

Correct answer: C Incentive spirometry is used to prevent or treat atelectasis. Performed every hour, it produces deep inhalations that help open the collapsed alveoli. Giving oxygen (Option A) doesn't encourage deep inhalation. Coughing and deep breathing (Option B) is a good intervention but rarely results in as deep an inspiratory effort as incentive spirometry; it should also be performed more frequently than every 4 hours. Getting the patient out of bed to a chair (Option D) helps expand the lungs and stimulate deep breathing, but it's not as important as regular incentive spirometry.

Selected References

American Society of PeriAnesthesia Nurses. (2015a). *2015-2017 Peri-anesthesia nursing standards, practice recommendations and interpretive statements*. Retrieved from https://www.aspan.org/Clinical-Practice/ASPAN-Standards.

Association of periOperative Registered Nurses (AORN). (2015b). Correct site surgery tool kit. Retrieved from https://www.aorn.org/guidelines/clinical-resources/tool-kits/correct-site-surgery-tool-kit.

Association of periOperative Registered Nurses (AORN). (2016a). *Guideline for preoperative patient skin antisepsis. 2016 guidelines for perioperative practice*. Denver, CO: Author.

Association of periOperative Registered Nurses (AORN). (2016b). *Guideline for transfer of patient care information. 2016 guidelines for perioperative practice*. Denver, CO: Author.

Association of periOperative Registered Nurses (AORN). (2016c). *Guidelines for perioperative practice* (2016 ed.). Denver, CO: Author.

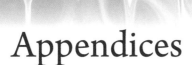

Appendices

NANDA-I Taxonomy II by Domain

The following is a list of the NANDA International 2015–2017 taxonomy II according to their domain (area of activity, investigation, or interest).

Domain: Health Promotion

- Deficient diversional activity
- Deficient community health
- Frail elderly syndrome
- Ineffective health maintenance
- Ineffective family health management
- Ineffective health management
- Ineffective protection
- Noncompliance
- Readiness for enhanced health management
- Risk for frail elderly syndrome
- Risk-prone health behavior
- Sedentary lifestyle

Domain: Nutrition

- Deficient fluid volume
- Excess fluid volume
- Imbalanced nutrition: Less than body requirements
- Ineffective breast-feeding
- Impaired swallowing
- Ineffective infant feeding pattern
- Insufficient breast milk

- Interrupted breast-feeding
- Neonatal jaundice
- Obesity
- Overweight
- Readiness for enhanced breast-feeding
- Readiness for enhanced fluid balance
- Readiness for enhanced nutrition
- Risk for deficient fluid volume
- Risk for electrolyte imbalance
- Risk for imbalanced fluid volume
- Risk for impaired liver function
- Risk for neonatal jaundice
- Risk for overweight
- Risk for unstable blood glucose level

Domain: Elimination and Exchange

- Bowel incontinence
- Constipation
- Chronic functional constipation
- Diarrhea
- Dysfunctional gastrointestinal motility
- Functional urinary incontinence
- Impaired gas exchange
- Impaired urinary elimination
- Overflow urinary incontinence
- Perceived constipation
- Readiness for enhanced urinary elimination
- Reflex urinary incontinence
- Risk for chronic functional constipation
- Risk for constipation
- Risk for dysfunctional gastrointestinal motility
- Risk for urge urinary incontinence
- Stress urinary incontinence
- Urge urinary incontinence
- Urinary retention

Domain: Activity/Rest

- Activity intolerance
- Bathing self-care deficit
- Decreased cardiac output
- Disturbed sleep pattern
- Dressing self-care deficit
- Dysfunctional ventilatory weaning response
- Fatigue
- Feeding self-care deficit
- Impaired bed mobility
- Impaired home maintenance
- Impaired physical mobility
- Impaired sitting
- Impaired spontaneous ventilation
- Impaired standing
- Impaired transfer ability
- Impaired walking
- Impaired wheelchair mobility
- Ineffective breathing pattern
- Ineffective peripheral tissue perfusion

- Insomnia
- Readiness for enhanced self-care
- Readiness for enhanced sleep
- Risk for activity intolerance
- Risk for decreased cardiac output
- Risk for decreased cardiac tissue perfusion
- Risk for disuse syndrome
- Risk for impaired cardiovascular function
- Risk for ineffective cerebral tissue perfusion
- Risk for ineffective gastrointestinal perfusion
- Risk for ineffective peripheral tissue perfusion
- Risk for ineffective renal perfusion
- Self-neglect
- Sleep deprivation
- Toileting self-care deficit
- Wandering

Domain: Perception/Cognition

- Acute confusion
- Chronic confusion
- Deficient knowledge
- Ineffective impulse control
- Impaired memory
- Impaired verbal communication
- Labile emotional control
- Readiness for enhanced communication
- Readiness for enhanced knowledge
- Risk for acute confusion
- Unilateral neglect

Domain: Self-Perception

- Chronic low self-esteem
- Disturbed body image
- Disturbed personal identity
- Hopelessness
- Readiness for enhanced self-concept
- Risk for chronic low self-esteem
- Risk for compromised human dignity
- Risk for disturbed personal identity
- Readiness for enhanced hope
- Risk for situational low self-esteem
- Situational low self-esteem

Domain: Role Relationships

- Caregiver role strain
- Dysfunctional family processes
- Impaired parenting
- Impaired social interaction
- Ineffective relationship
- Ineffective role performance
- Interrupted family processes
- Parental role conflict
- Readiness for enhanced family processes
- Readiness for enhanced parenting
- Readiness for enhanced relationship

- Risk for caregiver role strain
- Risk for ineffective relationship
- Risk for impaired attachment
- Risk for impaired parenting

Domain: Sexuality

- Ineffective sexuality pattern
- Ineffective childbearing process
- Readiness for enhanced childbearing process
- Risk for disturbed maternal-fetal dyad
- Risk for ineffective childbearing process
- Sexual dysfunction

Domain: Coping/Stress Tolerance

- Anxiety
- Autonomic dysreflexia
- Chronic sorrow
- Complicated grieving
- Compromised family coping
- Death anxiety
- Decreased intracranial adaptive capacity
- Defensive coping
- Disabled family coping
- Disorganized infant behavior
- Fear
- Grieving
- Impaired individual resilience
- Impaired mood regulation
- Ineffective activity planning
- Ineffective coping
- Ineffective denial
- Posttrauma syndrome
- Powerlessness
- Rape-trauma syndrome
- Readiness for enhanced coping
- Readiness for enhanced family coping
- Readiness for enhanced organized infant behavior
- Readiness for enhanced power
- Readiness for impaired resilience
- Relocation stress syndrome
- Risk for autonomic dysreflexia
- Risk for complicated grieving
- Risk for compromised resilience
- Risk for disorganized infant behavior
- Risk for ineffective activity planning
- Risk for posttrauma syndrome
- Risk for powerlessness
- Risk for relocation stress syndrome
- Stress overload

Domain: Life Principles

- Decisional conflict
- Impaired emancipated decision-making
- Impaired religiosity

- Moral distress
- Readiness for enhanced decision-making
- Readiness for enhanced emancipated decision-making
- Readiness for enhanced religiosity
- Readiness for enhanced spiritual well-being
- Risk for impaired emancipated decision-making
- Risk for impaired religiosity
- Risk for spiritual distress
- Spiritual distress

Domain: Safety/Protection

- Contamination
- Delayed surgical recovery
- Hyperthermia
- Hypothermia
- Impaired dentition
- Impaired oral mucous membrane
- Impaired skin integrity
- Impaired tissue integrity
- Ineffective airway clearance
- Ineffective thermoregulation
- Latex allergy response
- Risk for adverse reaction to iodinated contrast media
- Risk for allergy response
- Risk for aspiration
- Risk for contamination
- Risk for bleeding
- Risk for corneal injury
- Risk for delayed surgical recovery
- Risk for dry eye
- Risk for falls
- Risk for hypothermia
- Risk for imbalanced body temperature
- Risk for impaired skin integrity
- Risk for impaired tissue integrity
- Risk for infection
- Risk for injury
- Risk for latex allergy response
- Risk for other-directed violence
- Risk for perioperative hypothermia
- Risk for perioperative positioning injury
- Risk for peripheral neurovascular dysfunction
- Risk for impaired oral mucous membrane
- Risk for poisoning
- Risk for pressure ulcer
- Risk for self-directed violence
- Risk for self-mutilation
- Risk for shock
- Risk for sudden infant death syndrome
- Risk for suffocation
- Risk for suicide
- Risk for thermal injury
- Risk for trauma
- Risk for urinary tract injury
- Risk for vascular trauma
- Self-mutilation

Domain: Comfort

- Acute pain
- Chronic pain
- Chronic pain syndrome
- Impaired comfort
- Labor pain
- Nausea
- Readiness for enhanced comfort
- Risk for loneliness
- Social isolation

Domain: Growth/Development

- Risk for delayed development
- Risk for disproportionate growth

Nursing Implications of Diagnostic Tests

To provide appropriate care for a patient undergoing a diagnostic test, the nurse must understand the test and its uses, prepare the patient properly (including verifying that informed consent has been obtained and explaining the procedure), and monitor the patient carefully before and after the test.

Test and Description	Uses of Test	Patient Preparation	Nursing Implications
Radiologic (X-ray) Tests			
Abdominal Flat Plate of Abdomen or Kidneys, Ureters, and Bladder (KUB)			
X-ray of the abdomen or kidneys, ureters, and bladder	• Detecting abdominal masses, bowel obstructions, ileus, or perforation • Detecting renal and bladder masses and some renal calculi	• Have the patient remove clothing and metal objects. • Instruct the patient to take a deep breath and hold it while the X-ray is taken.	• Cover the patient's reproductive organs with a lead shield. • Don't perform this test on a pregnant patient.
Angiography			
X-ray of arterial blood vessels using contrast media (dye)	• Identifying femoral artery occlusion • Detecting arterial peripheral vascular disease • Checking for aneurysms, tumors, or vascular anomalies • Determining status of cerebral circulation • Determining condition of coronary arteries • Identifying blood flow dynamics	• Instruct the patient to fast for 3 to 8 hours before the test. • Mark peripheral pulses with a pen. • Tell the patient to expect a warm, flushing sensation when the dye is injected.	• Check for allergies to shellfish or iodine and for a prior reaction to dye before the X-ray. • Observe the patient for signs of hemorrhage or hematoma at the insertion site. • Monitor vital signs. • Document the type of vascular closure device used and status of the dressing. • Ambulate the patient per the standards for the type of closure device used. • Check the peripheral pulses bilaterally. • Compare color and temperature in extremities. • Monitor the patient for allergic reactions to the dye, such as diaphoresis, hypotension, wheezing, angioedema, and laryngospasm. • Monitor the patient for signs of cerebral emboli, such as slurred speech, confusion, and hemiparesis (one-sided weakness). • Encourage the patient to drink adequate fluids.

(continued)

Test and Description	Uses of Test	Patient Preparation	Nursing Implications
Radiologic (X-ray) Tests (continued)			
Arthrography/Arthogram			
Visualization of the shape and integrity of a joint capsule following the injection of contrast media, air, or both	• Determining the cause of joint pain and swelling • Determining the progression of joint disease • Diagnosing joint disorders and synovial cysts	• Tell the patient that crackling noises may be heard in the joint after the procedure due to the injection of air during the procedure. • Explain that a local anesthetic will be used.	• Assess the patient for allergies to contrast media or local anesthesia. • After the test, assess the joint for swelling, and apply ice if needed. • Administer an analgesic for pain and discomfort. • Don't perform this test on a pregnant patient.
Bone Densitometry			
Measures bone mineral density	• Diagnosing osteoporosis and monitoring its progression	• Tell the patient to wear clothing that's easily removed from the hip area and without zippers or metal fasteners. • Make sure the patient avoids calcium products for 24 hours before the test.	• Tell the patient to remain still during the test. • Contraindicated in pregnancy
Cardiac Catheterization and Coronary Angiography			
X-ray examination of coronary vessels using dye injected through a catheter in the femoral or antecubital vein (for right-sided cardiac catheterization) or in the femoral or brachial artery (for left-sided cardiac catheterization)	• Determining size and structure of cardiac chambers • Measuring pressures and volumes in cardiac chambers • Determining valve structure and function • Determining pressure in pulmonary vessels • Determining extent of damage from heart disease • Determining condition of coronary vessels • Facilitating infusion of thrombolytic agents into occluded coronary arteries • Performing angioplasty, atherectomy, and stent insertion	• Have the patient fast for 3 to 8 hours before the test. • Prepare the patient for a warm, flushing sensation when the dye is injected. • Scrub and clip hair around the catheter insertion site. • If prescribed, administer pretest medications, such as an antihistamine, a steroid, a sedative, or a tranquilizer. • Have the patient void before receiving the pretest medication or before going to the cardiac catheterization laboratory. • Mark peripheral pulses. • If the patient is on metformin (Glucophage), this medication should not be taken on the day of the test and held for 48 hours posttest.	• Check for allergies to shellfish or iodine and for a prior reaction to dye before the test. • Have the patient remove dentures and jewelry before the test. • Start an I.V. infusion before the test and maintain it during and after the test. • Obtain baseline vital signs, and monitor them continuously during the test and frequently after the test. • Monitor peripheral pulses below the insertion site each time vital signs are taken. • After the test, maintain pressure to the insertion site, and keep the extremity flat and immobilized with a sandbag. • Maintain bed rest for 4 to 6 hours and then ambulate the patient. • Tell the patient to avoid heavy lifting and vigorous activity for several days unless the practitioner orders further restrictions. • Check the catheter insertion site for hemorrhage or hematoma; apply ice if needed. • Document the type of vascular closure device used and status of the dressing. • Have emergency equipment available to treat complications, such as arrhythmias, anaphylaxis, pneumothorax, and hemopericardium. • Encourage the patient to drink fluids after the test.

(continued)

Test and Description	Uses of Test	Patient Preparation	Nursing Implications
Radiologic (X-ray) Tests (continued)			
Chest X-ray			
Visualization of the lungs, heart, and bony structures	• Detecting lung diseases or tumors • Diagnosing chronic obstructive pulmonary disease • Identifying infections • Diagnosing abnormal rib conditions • Detecting cardiomegaly • Identifying location of central lines and endotracheal tubes • Identifying fluid or air accumulation	• Have the patient remove metal objects. • Instruct the patient to take a deep breath and hold it while the X-ray is taken.	• Cover the patient's reproductive organs with a lead shield. • Don't perform this test on a pregnant patient.
Computed Tomography (CT) Scan, Computed Axial Tomography Scan, and Spiral CT Scan			
Multidimensional visualization of a body part using a computer-controlled, focused X-ray beam of various speeds; contrast media may be used to enhance visualization	• Visualizing brain lesions, tumors, edema, and other conditions (cerebral CT scan) • Identifying herniated disks, tumors, and other abnormalities (spinal CT scan) • Visualizing tumors and chest lesions (thoracic CT scan) • Visualizing liver, pancreas, spleen, gallbladder, reproductive tract, and abdominal cavity for abnormalities (abdominal CT scan) • Detecting kidney abnormalities, such as tumors and calculi (renal CT scan)	• If dye is used, maintain nothing-by-mouth (NPO) status 3 to 8 hours before the test. • If the patient is undergoing a cerebral CT scan, remove hairpins and jewelry, and administer a sedative, as prescribed. • Explain that flushing or nausea may occur after injection of contrast media. • Patients taking metformin (Glucophage) should be instructed to withhold medication for 48 hours prior to the test and for a period of time after the test.	• Check for allergies to shellfish or iodine and for a prior reaction to dye before the test. • Tell the patient to remain still during the test and breathe steadily. • Prepare the patient for the large and confining machinery; assess the patient for claustrophobia. • If dye was used, check for signs of iodine reaction and acute renal failure after the test. If an allergic reaction occurs, administer an antihistamine as prescribed. • Monitor for hypoglycemia or acidosis in patients who withheld metformin prior to the test. • Encourage the patient to drink fluids after the test.
Excretory Urography (IVP)			
X-ray visualization of the urinary tract using I.V. injected, iodine-based contrast media that concentrates in the urinary tract; also known as intravenous pyelography	• Determining the size, shape, and function of the kidneys, ureters, and bladder • Detecting tumors, cysts, or renal calculi • Detecting other renal diseases • Detecting urinary outlet obstruction	• Maintain NPO status 8 to 12 hours before the test. • Administer a laxative the evening before the test. • Check to make sure no barium studies have been performed within 4 days of the IVP. • If the patient is on metformin (Glucophage), this medication should not be taken on the day of the test and should be held for 48 hours posttest.	• Check for allergies to shellfish or iodine and for a prior reaction to dye. • Check urine output and blood urea nitrogen (BUN) level; the test usually isn't performed on oliguric patients or on those with a BUN level > 40 mg/dL. • Observe for an allergic reaction to the dye. If an allergic reaction occurs, administer a steroid or antihistamine as prescribed. • Monitor urine output. • Encourage the patient to drink fluids after the test.

(continued)

Test and Description	Uses of Test	Patient Preparation	Nursing Implications
Radiologic (X-ray) Tests (continued)			
GI Series			
Upper: X-ray examination of the esophagus, stomach, and small bowel after the patient swallows contrast media, such as barium or diatrizoate meglumine (Gastrografin) *Lower:* X-ray examination of the large intestine by inserting barium by way of an enema	• Examining the stomach for ulcerations, cancer, or other diseases • Diagnosing hiatal hernia • Detecting esophageal varices, pyloric stenosis, or foreign bodies • Detecting diverticula • Checking for tumors or obstructions • Detecting inflammatory bowel disease	• Maintain NPO status after midnight. • Tell the patient that the test may take 1 to 2 hours. • Make sure the patient receives a clear liquid diet the day before the test. • Instruct the patient on the bowel cleansing preparation ordered. • Maintain NPO status for 3 to 8 hours before the test. • If the patient is on metformin (Glucophage), this medication should not be taken on the day of the test and should be held for 48 hours posttest	• Don't allow the patient to eat until the test is completed. • Give a laxative, as prescribed, after an X-ray series using barium. • Increase fluid intake posttest unless contraindicated • Note stool color and consistency to ensure that the barium has been passed. • Advise the patient who has received diatrizoate meglumine (Gastrografin) that diarrhea may occur. • Administer enemas, bisacodyl suppositories, or saline enemas at 6 a.m. the morning of the test; make sure the drainage is clear. • Encourage increased fluid intake on the day before the test. • Administer a laxative or an enema, as prescribed, to expel the barium. • Advise the patient that the barium may make stools appear a light color for several days after the test. • Tell the patient to report lack of bowel movements to the physician; retained barium can cause bowel obstruction and fecal impaction. • Contraindicated in pregnancy
Hysterosalpingography			
X-ray that visualizes the uterine cavity, fallopian tubes, and peritubal area; Fluoroscopic radiographs obtained as contrast medium flows through the uterus and fallopian tubes	• Detecting tubal abnormalities • Detecting uterine abnormalities such as congenital malformations • Confirming the presence of fistulas or peritubal adhesions • Evaluating the cause of repeated miscarriage • Diagnosing infertility	• Check the patient's history for recent pelvic infection and notify practitioner. • Tell the patient that antibiotics may be given before or after the test. • Explain that the test should take place 2 to 5 days after menstruation ends. • Warn the patient that she might experience moderate cramping during the test. • Tell the patient to perform bowel preparation the night before the test, as ordered. • If the patient is on metformin (Glucophage), this medication should not be taken on the day of the test and held for 48 hours posttest	• Teach the patient that she can return to pretest activities gradually. • Monitor the patient for signs and symptoms of infection, uterine perforation, bleeding, and adverse reaction to the contrast medium. • Premedicate the patient for cramping as ordered.

(continued)

Test and Description	Uses of Test	Patient Preparation	Nursing Implications
Radiologic (X-ray) Tests (continued)			
Mammography			
X-ray examination of the breast's soft tissue structures Fluid-field digital mammography (FFDM) Computer-aided detection (CAD) and three-dimensional (3D) breast imagery	• Detecting benign breast cysts, mastitis, or abscess • Screening for malignant breast tumors	• Have the patient remove clothing and jewelry from the waist up and put on a gown. • Prepare the patient for pinching and discomfort as the breast tissue is compressed. • Tell the patient not to use powder or deodorant the day of the test because both may leave residue that could be mistaken for areas of calcification. • The American Cancer Society recommends yearly mammograms for women between the ages of 45 to 54 years old and every other year for women 55 and older if they are in good health and expected to live 10 years or longer	• Tell the patient to remain still during the test. • Tell the patient that breast augmentation may be an interfering factor.
Myelography			
X-ray examination of the spinal column using contrast media	• Detecting tumors or other obstructions of the spinal tract • Locating herniated intervertebral disks	• Tell the patient to increase fluid intake the day before the test; fasting for 2 to 6 hours before the test may be required. • Tell the patient to remain still on the X-ray table, which will be tilted downward. • Inform the patient that a lumbar puncture is performed to instill the dye. • Notify the radiologist if there is history of seizures or asthma, or use of an antidepressant, phenothiazine, blood thinner, or diabetic drugs like metformin, as these drugs may be stopped 1 to 2 days before the test.	• Check for allergies to shellfish or iodine and for a prior reaction to dye. Maintain the patient's position, as prescribed, after the test; maintain bed rest for 3 to 4 hours, and then tell the patient to avoid bending over or strenuous activities for 1 to 2 days. • Keep the patient's head elevated at 30 to 45 degrees to prevent seizures. • Encourage fluid intake to eliminate the contrast media and prevent headache. • Observe the patient for signs of dye reactions. • Observe the patient for signs of meningeal irritation. • Monitor the patient's ability to void after the test. • Monitor vital signs after the test.

(continued)

Test and Description	Uses of Test	Patient Preparation	Nursing Implications
Radiologic (X-ray) Tests (continued)			
Percutaneous Transhepatic Cholangiography			
Visualization of the biliary system using contrast media injected I.V. or through a T tube	• Identifying calculi or obstructions in the biliary system • Detecting calculi or other obstructions in the common bile duct after surgery (T-tube cholangiography)	• Maintain NPO status for 3 to 8 hours before the test. • Obtain written consent • An I.V. antibiotic may be administered prior to the test via a T tube. • Tell the patient that an anesthesia will be injected into the abdominal skin site and will sting. • If the patient is on metformin (Glucophage), this medication should not be taken on the day of the test and should be held for 48 hours posttest.	• Check for allergies to shellfish or iodine and for a prior reaction to dye before the test. • Observe the patient for allergic reactions, inflammation, and sepsis. • Monitor vital signs frequently until patient is stable. • Watch for nausea and vomiting after the test. • Contraindicated in pregnancy
Venography			
X-ray examination of the peripheral venous system using contrast media	• Detecting deep vein thrombosis • Evaluating varicose veins	• Explain the test to the patient. • Maintain NPO status for 3 to 4 hours before the test.	• Check for allergies to shellfish or iodine and for a prior reaction to dye before the test. • Check the examination site for signs of inflammation or infection. • Observe the patient for systemic signs of infection. • Monitor vital signs and pulses in the affected area.
Endoscopic Tests			
Arthroscopy			
Visualization of the internal joint structures, through a fiberoptic endoscope	• Detecting torn cartilage or ligaments • Assessing arthritic changes • Performing corrective surgery through arthroscope	• Perform standard preoperative preparations. • If the patient will receive general anesthesia, maintain NPO status for at least 8 hours before the test. • Clip hair from and scrub the affected area.	• Check the incision site for infection. • Assess neurovascular status of the affected extremity. • Keep the joint elevated and extended. • Apply ice to decrease edema, and administer an analgesic, as prescribed, to relieve pain. • Instruct the patient to avoid using the joint for several days and strenuous activity; if necessary, teach crutch walking. • Tell the patient that sutures are usually removed in 7 days.

(continued)

Test and Description	Uses of Test	Patient Preparation	Nursing Implications
Endoscopic Tests (continued)			
Bronchoscopy			
Visualization of the trachea and bronchi through a fiberoptic bronchoscope	• Detecting tumors or inflammation • Obtaining sputum culture • Biopsying accessible lesions • Removing foreign bodies and excessive secretions • Locating bleeding sites in the tracheobronchial tree	• Maintain NPO status for 6 to 12 hours before the test. • Have the patient remove dentures and contact lenses. • Administer pretest medications, such as atropine, to decrease secretions and a sedative or tranquilizer to relax the patient. • Spray lidocaine in the back of the throat to decrease discomfort from the tube	• Maintain NPO status until the gag reflex returns. • Monitor vital signs frequently until the patient is stable. • Monitor respiratory status; this test poses a risk of laryngospasm. • Have emergency resuscitation equipment available. • Note any hemoptysis. • Provide gargling solutions or lozenges to relieve sore throat.
Colonoscopy			
Visualization of the colon using a flexible endoscope	• Detecting tumors • Detecting and removing polyps • Identifying sites of bleeding • Detecting ulceration and bowel inflammation	• Confirm that the patient hasn't undergone a barium test in the past 14 days. • Have the patient maintain a clear fluid diet for up to 3 days before the test. • Discontinue anticoagulants and aspirin as directed by the health care provider prior to the procedure. • Make sure the patient performs the bowel cleansing preparation ordered. • Maintain NPO status for 8 hours before the test. • Administer an analgesic and a sedative, as prescribed.	• Maintain NPO status after the test until the patient is alert. • Observe the patient for bleeding and abdominal pain; the patient is at risk for bowel perforation and hemorrhage, especially if a biopsy was performed or polyps were removed. • Monitor vital signs until the patient is stable. • Explain that flatus and gas pain are common after the test. • Encourage fluid intake.
Cystoscopy			
Visualization of the urethra and bladder cavity; may include retrograde pyelography (X-ray visualization of the ureters after dye is injected)	• Detecting tumors and calculi • Establishing cause of hematuria • Determining cause of infection • Biopsying prostate (bladder) or urethra • Resecting bladder tumors	• If the patient will receive general anesthesia, maintain NPO status for 8 hours before test. • Discontinue aspirin and anticoagulants as directed by health care provider prior to the procedure • Encourage fluid intake the day before the test. • Administer a pretest analgesic, if prescribed, 1 hour before the test. • Prepare the patient for the lithotomy position and the use of an irrigation system. • Tell the patient that an anesthetic gel may be inserted into the urethra before the test.	• Monitor urine output and vital signs. • Remember that urine may be pink and contain clots. • Report any hemorrhage or difficulty voiding. • Monitor the patient for signs of gram-negative sepsis, such as chills, fever, tachycardia, and hypotension; administer a prophylactic antibiotic if prescribed. • Monitor vital signs and I & O frequently until the patient is stable. • Encourage increased fluid intake for at least 24 hours postprocedure. • If bladder spasms occur, give warm sitz baths and an antispasmodic, as prescribed.

(continued)

Test and Description	Uses of Test	Patient Preparation	Nursing Implications

Endoscopic Tests (continued)

Endoscopic Retrograde Cholangiopancreatography (ERCP)

Test and Description	Uses of Test	Patient Preparation	Nursing Implications
Visualization of the bile and pancreatic ducts using an endoscope and contrast media	• Detecting obstructions, such as tumors, cysts, and calculi • Detecting cirrhosis and pancreatic disease	• Maintain NPO status for 8 hours before the test. • Administer a pretest medication, such as an opioid analgesic or sedative, as prescribed. • If the patient is on metformin (Glucophage), this medication should not be taken on the day of the test and should be held for 48 hours posttest • Discontinue anticoagulants and aspirin as directed by health care provider prior to the procedure	• Check for allergies to shellfish or iodine and for a reaction to previous tests using dye. • Maintain NPO status until the gag reflex returns. • Check vital signs frequently, and observe the patient for signs of inflammation and sepsis. • Monitor the patient for signs of pancreatitis, such as abdominal pain, nausea, and vomiting. • Monitor the patient for signs of respiratory distress. • Provide gargling solutions or lozenges to relieve sore throat. • Contraindicated in pregnancy

Esophagogastroduodenoscopy (EGD)

Test and Description	Uses of Test	Patient Preparation	Nursing Implications
Direct visualization of the esophagus, stomach, and duodenum	• Detecting gastric ulcers or esophagitis • Detecting tumors • Determining site of bleeding • Detecting hiatal hernia	• Maintain NPO status for 8 to 12 hours before the test. • Have the patient remove dentures. • Administer medications, such as atropine, a sedative or tranquilizer, or an opioid analgesic, 1 hour before the test, as prescribed.	• Maintain NPO status until the gag reflex returns. • Place the patient on his side to prevent aspiration. • Monitor vital signs frequently until the patient is stable. • Check for complications, such as fever, hemorrhage, abdominal pain, and dyspnea. • Inform the patient that retained air may cause bloating, belching, and flatus and he may have a sore throat or hoarseness.

Sigmoidoscopy

Test and Description	Uses of Test	Patient Preparation	Nursing Implications
Visualization of the rectum and sigmoid colon using a flexible endoscope	• Screening for polyps and colorectal cancer • Inspecting for inflammatory disease • Detecting hemorrhoids and other perirectal conditions	• Administer two saline enemas the morning of the test. • Maintain NPO status for 8 hours before the test. • Confirm that the patient hasn't undergone a barium test in the past 14 days.	• Observe the patient for signs of bleeding or perforation. • Explain that the test may cause gas pain and flatus and may cause slight rectal bleeding if biopsies were obtained.

Nuclear (Radioisotope) Scans

Bone Scan

Test and Description	Uses of Test	Patient Preparation	Nursing Implications
I.V. administration of a radioisotope followed by a bone scan 2 to 3 hours later	• Determining condition of bone • Detecting bone disease and degeneration • Detecting metastasis	• Don't limit oral intake. • Force fluids (four to six glasses of water between isotope administration and scanning). • Have the patient void before the scan.	• Tell the patient to remain still during the test. • Remember that no radiation precautions are needed after the test. • Encourage increased fluid intake to hasten isotope elimination, which occurs in 6 to 24 hours. • No breast-feeding for up to 3 days posttest.

(continued)

Test and Description	Uses of Test	Patient Preparation	Nursing Implications

Nuclear (Radioisotope) Scans (continued)

Brain Scan

I.V. administration of a radioisotope followed by a brain scan 30 minutes to 3 hours later	• Detecting intracranial lesions • Evaluating cerebral perfusion	• Don't limit oral intake. • Explain the test to the patient.	• Tell the patient to remain still during the test with the hands at the sides. • Remember that no radiation precautions are needed after the test. • Encourage fluid intake.

Cardiac Perfusion Scan, Thallium Scan, Myocardial Perfusion Heart Scan

I.V. administration of a radioisotope followed by imaging in 10 to 60 minutes. If part of a stress test, thallium is given before exercise and then reimaging is done at peak exercise.	• Screening for ischemic heart disease • Determining coronary perfusion after a myocardial infarction (MI) • Assessing cardiac chambers • Assessing for coronary artery disease (CAD)	• Have the patient fast per facility procedure. • Restrict smoking before a thallium stress test. • Tell the patient to avoid drugs for erectile dysfunction (ED) such as sildenafil (Viagra) for 48 hours before the test.	• Remember that no special radiation precautions are needed for this test. • If a stress test is performed, monitor vital signs after the test. • Encourage the patient to drink increased fluids for 24 to 48 hours after the test. • ED drugs can cause severe hypotension when mixed with nitroglycerin, which may be required during the test. • If a stress test is performed also, instruct the patient to wear walking shoes. • Contraindicated in pregnancy

Gallbladder Scan, HIDA Scan, Hepatobiliary Scan

I.V. administration of a radioisotope followed by imaging	• Determining gallbladder function • Identifying gallstones or other obstruction • Detecting infection of the gallbladder	• Tell the patient not to eat for 4 hours before the scan. • Explain that images will be taken at 10- to 15-minute intervals over 1 to 2 hours. • Tell the patient with acute pain that a positive test may result in further medical treatment or surgery.	• Don't perform the test on a pregnant or nursing patient. • Encourage fluid intake to hasten radioisotope elimination over 1 to 2 days. • Do not breast-feed for up to 3 days posttest.

Leukocyte Scan

Injection of indium-tagged leukocytes to detect infection location	• Locating sources of infection that are difficult to detect, such as those in bone, the abdomen, or the kidneys	• Make sure the patient's blood is drawn, tagged with indium, and reinjected before imaging.	• No special follow-up care is required.

Liver and Spleen Scan

I.V. administration of a radioisotope followed by imaging within 30 minutes	• Determining size, shape, and position of liver and spleen • Identifying liver pathology • Assessing condition of liver after abdominal trauma	• Check with the radiology department about oral intake limitations. • Explain the test to the patient, especially the positions used.	• Tell the patient to remain still during the test. • Remember that no radiation precautions are needed after the test. • Encourage increased fluids for 24 to 48 hours posttest. • Watch the patient for anaphylactic or pyrogenic reaction. • Contraindicated in pregnancy • Do not breast-feed for up to 3 days posttest

(continued)

Test and Description	Uses of Test	Patient Preparation	Nursing Implications
Nuclear (Radioisotope) Scans (continued)			
Lung Scan			
I.V., inhalation, or ventilation administration of a radioisotope followed by imaging; time varies with route of administration	• Determining lung function • Assessing pulmonary vascular perfusion • Determining presence of pulmonary embolism ($\dot{V}/\dot{Q}$ scan)	• Don't limit oral intake. • Explain the test to the patient.	• Tell the patient to remain still during the test. • Inform the patient undergoing a xenon ventilation scan that he or she must hold the breath on request during the test. • Monitor vital signs frequently. • Remember that no radiation precautions are needed after the test. • Increase fluid intake for up to 24 to 48 hours posttest • Contraindicated in pregnancy
Lymphoscintigraphy			
Following subcutaneous administration of a radioisotope, a scanner detects the gamma rays emitted by affected lymph nodes.	• Diagnosing lymphedema • Locating sentinel lymph nodes in breast cancer and malignant melanoma	• Explain that the skin around the tumor site or in the distal extremity will be injected with a very tiny needle.	• Don't perform the test on a pregnant patient. • Tell the patient that the length of time after injection until scanning varies and may include postexercise testing in patients with lymphedema. • Remember that no radiation precautions are needed after the test.
Positron Emission Tomography (PET) Scan			
Inhalation or infusion of high-energy radioactive tracers (attached to glucose, water, or ammonia) and use of computer-based nuclear imaging to measure blood flow, tissue composition, and metabolism	• Detecting coronary artery disease (CAD) and assessing ischemic tissue and myocardial viability with or without exercise testing • Detecting tumor, stroke, and epilepsy • Charting progress of CAD, collateral coronary artery circulation, head injury, stroke, Alzheimer's disease, Parkinson's disease, and certain biochemical abnormalities associated with psychiatric disorders • Providing measurements of $\dot{V}/\dot{Q}$ relationship and lung perfusion	• Tell the patient not to eat for 4 hours before the scan, but to drink plenty of water. • If the patient is diabetic, tell the patient to follow the practitioner's instructions on which diabetic drugs to take before the test. • Patients who are confused or agitated may require sedation. • Urinary catheterization may be necessary for colon or kidney studies. • Tell the patient to abstain from caffeine, alcohol, and tobacco 24 hours before the test.	• Check blood glucose level; diabetic patients will receive special instructions before the test. • Prepare the patient for the length of the test and any sensations the patient may hear or feel (light-headedness, dizziness, and headache are common). • Don't perform this test on a pregnant patient. • Document the patient's weight for use in determining the dose of radioactive material. • Encourage the patient to increase fluids after the test. • Contraindicated in pregnancy • No breast-feeding for up to 3 days posttest
Renal Scan			
I.V. administration of a radioisotope followed immediately or within 30 minutes by imaging	• Determining renal function • Identifying kidney position, size, and shape	• Don't limit oral intake. • Encourage fluid intake (two to three glasses of water about 30 minutes before the test). • Have the patient void before the scan.	• Make sure the test isn't scheduled within 24 hours of excretory urography because the patient should be well hydrated. • Remember that no radiation precautions are needed after the test. • Encourage fluid intake to hasten radioisotope elimination.

(continued)

Test and Description	Uses of Test	Patient Preparation	Nursing Implications

Nuclear (Radioisotope) Scans (continued)

Single-Photon Emission Computed Tomography (SPECT)

Following injection of radionuclide, the scanner detects the radiation emitted as it rotates around to obtain a 3D image of the target	• Detecting specific types of cancer such as neuroendocrine tumors • Detecting cancer that has metastasized to the bone • Confirming diagnosis of Alzheimer's disease • Detecting location of an infection, stress fractures, spondylosis, brain abnormalities, cardiac dysfunction, thyroid tumors, or plus flow of blood	• Maintain NPO status 4 hours before the scan. • Tell the patient the test takes about 1 hour.	• Prepare the patient for the length of the test and any sensations the patient may hear or feel (light-headedness, dizziness, and headache are common). • Encourage the patient to drink fluids after the test.

Thyroid Scan

Oral administration of radioactive iodine followed by scanning within 2 to 24 hours	• Determining thyroid size, shape, and function • Identifying pathologic conditions, especially adenomas	• Check on drug restrictions; thyroid drugs, cough syrup, multiple vitamins, and some oral contraceptives may be restricted from 1 to several weeks before the test. • NPO for 8 hours prior to test or per protocol	• Check for iodine allergies. • Make sure the test isn't administered to a pregnant patient because it can damage the fetus. • Remember that no radiation precautions are needed after the test. • Increase fluid intake posttest • No breast-feeding for up to 3 days posttest

Magnetic and Ultrasound Studies

Endoscopic Ultrasonography

Combines ultrasonography and endoscopy to visualize the GI wall and adjacent structures and allows ultrasound imaging with high resolution	• Evaluating or staging lesions of the esophagus, stomach, duodenum, pancreas, ampulla, biliary ducts, and rectum • Evaluating submucosal tumors	• Instruct the patient to fast for 6 to 8 hours before the test. • Administer an I.V. sedative to help the patient relax before the test. • Some procedures may require prior bowel cleansing.	• Make sure the patient is scheduled for abdominal ultrasonography before a barium test is done; retained barium interferes with ultrasound readings. • Obesity and excess gas in the bowel can interfere with the accuracy of the results.

Magnetic Resonance Imaging (MRI)

Visualization of body parts by exposing body cells to small magnets and tracking the cells' reaction (can be done with or without contrast)	• Detecting abnormalities in all body parts, including bones and joints • Studying bone structure	• Have the patient remove metal objects, such as jewelry and hairpins. • Identify surgeries or wounds with metal implants, rods, or pacemakers, which would be a contraindication to MRI. • Have the patient take preprocedure anxiolytic for claustrophobia, if ordered.	• Prepare the patient for being placed inside the large, doughnut-shaped electromagnet. (Open MRIs are available in some areas.) • Tell the patient to remain still during the test; assess for claustrophobia. • Tell the patient to expect loud clicking sounds during the test. • Encourage the patient to relax during the test. • Contraindicated in pregnancy

(continued)

Test and Description	Uses of Test	Patient Preparation	Nursing Implications
Magnetic and Ultrasound Studies (continued)			
Transesophageal Echocardiography (TEE)			
Invasive procedure using an esophageal scope to place a probe behind the heart to better visualize the heart and its structures	• Assessing left atrial anatomy and function and prosthetic valve function • Diagnosing cardiac masses and aneurysms • Assessing cardiac tamponade, endocarditis, and intracardiac thrombi	• Maintain NPO status for 6 hours before the test. • Attach electrocardiogram (ECG) leads and blood pressure cuff. • Position the patient on the table to allow for esophageal intubation. • Administer sedatives as ordered. • Remove the patient's dentures.	• Prepare the patient for the procedure and use of sedation and local anesthetic. • Closely monitor ECG, blood pressure, and oxygen saturation during and after the test. • Have suctioning equipment readily available in case of vomiting. • Keep the patient NPO until fully awake and gag reflex has returned.
Ultrasonography (Ultrasound of the Abdomen)			
Visualization of underlying soft tissues and body structures using high-frequency sound waves that echo from the underlying body parts, producing scans, waveforms, or sounds	• Identifying gallstones • Differentiating between liver masses and other causes of jaundice • Diagnosing renal masses • Determining fetal presence and growth; visualizing uterus, ovaries, and fallopian tubes • Assessing blood flow (Doppler) and detecting occlusion or aneurysm • Assessing heart valve movement and heart size, position, and shape (echogram) • Evaluating thyroid gland size and structure • Detecting abdominal aneurysms	• Explain the test to the patient based on the body site being evaluated. • For a transabdominal scan, which requires a full bladder, instruct the patient to drink several glasses of water and not to void. For a kidney, gallbladder, spleen, or abdominal scan, instruct the patient to fast for 8 to 12 hours before the test.	• Tell the patient he or she can resume activity and diet as ordered. • Monitor the patient for signs and symptoms of perforation or bleeding. • Tell the patient to avoid alcohol and driving for 24 hours after the test if I.V. sedation was used.
Biopsies			
Liver Biopsy			
Removal of hepatic tissue by way of needle aspiration for microscopic examination	• Detecting tumors • Diagnosing hepatocellular disease, especially cirrhosis	• Check the patient's platelet count and coagulation studies; this test is contraindicated in a patient with a platelet count <100,000/µL and in patients with bleeding disorders. • Maintain NPO status for 6 to 8 hours before the test. • Give vitamin K, if prescribed, before and after the test. • Administer a sedative as prescribed. • Tell the patient to report use of aspirin, nonsteroidal anti-inflammatory drugs (NSAIDs), or anticoagulants to the practitioner before the test.	• Report abnormal prothrombin times to the practitioner. • Tell the patient that the test requires supine positioning and placement of the right hand under the head. • Have the patient practice exhaling and holding the breath in that position. • Place the patient on the right side for 2 hours after the test to apply pressure on the liver and prevent hemorrhage. • Monitor vital signs and assess for pain in the chest or shoulder; give an analgesic as prescribed. • Observe the patient for signs of hemorrhage and pneumothorax. • Monitor vital signs frequently until the patient is stable.

(continued)

Test and Description	Uses of Test	Patient Preparation	Nursing Implications
Biopsies (continued)			
Other Tissue Biopsies			
Removal of organ tissue for microscopic examination	• Detecting malignant tumors • Identifying pathologic cellular changes	• Preparation for a patient undergoing other tissue biopsy is similar to that for a liver biopsy.	• Nursing care for the patient undergoing other tissue biopsy is similar to that for a liver biopsy.
Electrodiagnostic Tests			
Electrocardiography (EKG, ECG, Electrocardiogram)			
Noninvasive test that gives a graphic representation of the heart's electrical activity; ambulatory or Holter monitoring records the ECG over a 24-hour period; stress testing records the ECG during increasing levels of exercise.	• Detecting ischemia, injury, and necrosis • Identifying conduction delays, bundle blocks, fascicular blocks, and arrhythmias • Identifying chamber enlargement • Determining cardiac status after MI • Assessing the effectiveness of cardiac drugs and treatments • Determining pacemaker activity • Determining safe limits of exercise	• Tell the patient that the skin may be prepared with alcohol or sandpaper or shaved so the electrodes hold. • For a stress test, instruct the patient to withhold food and fluids for 3 hours before the test. • Instruct the patient to wear loose-fitting clothing and supportive shoes. • Tell the patient to immediately report chest discomfort, shortness of breath, fatigue, leg cramps, or dizziness. • Show the patient how to record activity and symptoms in a diary for Holter monitoring. • Tell the patient that there's no risk of electrical shock.	• Withhold medications, as ordered, before the stress test. • Have emergency equipment available during stress testing. • Obtain a resting ECG and baseline vital signs before the stress test. • Monitor vital signs, and assess the patient for signs and symptoms of cardiovascular instability during and after the stress test. • Help the patient remove electrodes after the test and clean skin.
Electroencephalography			
Noninvasive test that records the electrical activity of the brain via scalp electrodes	• Identifying seizure activity • Assessing and locating cerebral lesions and injury • Evaluating trauma and drug intoxication • Determining brain death • Evaluating sleep disorders	• Explain to the patient that he or she will be subjected to stimuli, such as lights and sounds. • Tell the patient to lie still during the test. • Reassure the patient that electrical shock won't occur. • Tell the patient to wash the hair the night before the test but not to apply any conditioners, sprays, or gels. • Tell the patient he may need to avoid sleep the night before the test if his study requires sleep testing.	• Withhold alcohol, stimulants, caffeine-containing beverages and chocolate and refrain from smoking 8 hours before the test. • Withhold medications such as sedatives and anticonvulsants, as directed, for 24 to 48 hours before the test. • Help the patient remove any electrode gel from the hair and scalp after the test.

(continued)

Test and Description	Uses of Test	Patient Preparation	Nursing Implications
Biopsies (continued)			
Electromyography (EMG)			
Needle insertion into selected muscles at rest and during voluntary contraction picks up nerve impulses and measures nerve conduction time.	• Determining the severity and location of nerve entrapment to diagnose conditions, such as carpal tunnel syndrome or herniated disk • Diagnosing peripheral nervous system disorders such as polyneuropathies • Evaluating disorders of the muscles and motor neurons, such as amyotrophic lateral sclerosis and myasthenia gravis	• Explain to the patient that he or she will experience discomfort during needle insertion. • Tell the patient that he or she will be asked to flex and relax muscles during the procedure.	• Withhold medications, such as NSAIDs or pyridostigmine bromide before the test, as ordered. • Administer analgesics, as prescribed, after the test. • Check the needle insertion sites for bleeding and inflammation.
Evoked Potential Studies			
Electrodes on the skin and scalp to record electrical activity in the brain in response to sensory (visual, auditory, or somatosensory) stimulation	• Diagnosing multiple sclerosis • Assessing hearing and vision, optic nerve disorders, and acoustic neuromas • Detecting abnormalities affecting the brain and spinal cord such as neuropathies • Determining brain death	• Have the patient wash the hair the night before the test but not to apply any conditioners, sprays, or gels. • Tell the patient what to expect, based on the type of stimulus being used.	• Help the patient remove any electrode gel from the hair after the test.

Nursing Implications in Oncology Care

Cancer is a group of diseases characterized by uncontrolled growth and spread of abnormal cells. In the United States, it's the second leading health problem and the cause of one of every four deaths.

Various risk factors for cancer have been identified:

- Tobacco is associated with cancers of the lung, mouth, tongue, upper airway, bladder, kidney, pancreas, and esophagus
- Alcohol is associated with cancers of the mouth, pharynx, larynx, esophagus, and liver
- Occupational exposure to carcinogens is associated with leukemia and cancers of the lung, skin, liver, bladder, nose, kidney, esophagus, and pancreas
- Viruses are associated with cancers of the liver and cervix, Burkitt's lymphoma, Kaposi's sarcoma, and lymphoma
- Radiation exposure is associated with leukemia, melanoma, and cancers of the lip, thyroid, lungs, breast, and digestive organs
- Hormones are associated with endometrial and breast cancer
- A high-fat, low-fiber diet is associated with cancers of the colon, prostate, breast, esophagus, and stomach

In patients with cancer, normal cells go through a multistage process of change. During initiation, they're exposed to factors that damage them, causing mutation of their genetic codes. There are at least four types of genes that, when damaged, cause a normal cell to behave abnormally. These are oncogenes, tumor supressor genes, suicide genes, and deoxyribonucleic acid (DNA)-repair genes. During promotion, the mutated cells respond to additional factors that promote their growth. During invasion, continuous cellular division causes pressure and destruction of surrounding tissues by enzymes released from the cancer cells to promote the spread of disease. During metastasis, the cancer cells spread to other sites in the body that are far from the primary tumor site.

Tumors are classified as benign or malignant. In benign tumors, cells grow abnormally but don't metastasize or invade surrounding tissue. In malignant tumors, abnormal cells can spread, resulting in death for the host cells.

Cancers are anatomically staged using the TNM (tumor, node, metastasis) classification, which stages disease based on the size, penetration, and invasion of the primary tumor; the presence, extent, and location of regional node involvement; and the presence or absence of metastasis. Cancer also can be histologically graded as grade 1 (highly differentiated cells that resemble the tissue of origin most closely), 2 (intermediate differentiation), 3 (essentially undifferentiated cells), and 4 (highly undifferentiated, anaplastic cells). Patients with grade 4 disease have the poorest prognosis.

Cancer treatment has four goals:

- Cure by eradicating the cancer to ensure long-term survival
- Control by arresting tumor growth
- Palliation by alleviating symptoms when the disease is beyond control
- Prophylaxis by providing treatment when the patient is at increased risk for tumor development, spread, or recurrence
- Treatment may include surgery, radiation therapy, chemotherapy, bone marrow transplantation, biotherapy, or any combination of these options

Surgery

For a patient with cancer, different types of surgery may be performed for different reasons.

Diagnostic surgery is used to diagnose specific types of cancer. Examples include laparotomy and incisional, excisional, aspiration, or needle biopsies.

Staging surgery determines the extent of the disease and the need for additional therapy. Examples include exploratory surgery, tumor delineation, and multiple biopsies.

Definitive and curative surgery removes as much of the tumor as possible. Examples include local excision of cancer in situ, cryosurgery, laser surgery, electrosurgery, and en bloc (in one piece) dissection.

Preventive and prophylactic surgery is performed on tissues or organs at high risk for developing subsequent cancer because of family history, congenital disposition, or underlying conditions. Examples include colectomy, orchiopexy, and oophorectomy.

Reconstructive surgery is used to repair anatomic defects and improve function and appearance after cancer surgery. Examples include ostomies, breast reconstruction, and prosthesis placement.

Palliative surgery promotes patient comfort and quality of life by relieving the symptoms of advanced disease. Examples include neurosurgical management of pain, removal of obstructive metastasis, and treatment of oncologic emergencies.

Surgery to insert a mechanical device is performed to facilitate treatment or patient comfort. Devices may be inserted to facilitate drug administration, collect blood samples, or implant radioactive substances.

Preoperative and postoperative care related to these types of surgery is similar to that for other types of surgery.

Radiation Therapy

Radiation therapy is the use of high-energy radiation in doses large enough to eradicate disease but small enough to minimize adverse effects. Radiation rays cause one or both strands of the DNA molecule to break, thereby preventing cellular division or replication. Rapidly dividing, well-oxygenated, poorly differentiated cancer cells are most sensitive to the effects of radiation.

Various types of radiation therapy may be used. With external beam therapy, the radiation source is outside the body. With internal therapy (brachytherapy), the radiation source is placed directly on the body surface or near the body area to be irradiated. With interstitial therapy, the radiation source is implanted into the involved tissues. With systemic therapy, the radiation source is absorbed into the circulation and travels throughout the body.

For internal, interstitial, or systemic radiation, safety guidelines include following safety procedures based on the type, dose, method, and half-life of the radioisotope and minimizing exposure to radiation by maintaining a safe distance and placing shields between people and radioisotope devices.

Follow additional safety guidelines for interstitial radiation therapy with sealed (contained in seals, wires, or ribbons) or unsealed sources:

- Assign the patient to a private room, and mark the door with a radiation therapy safety sign
- Assess the patient's self-care ability
- Protect staff and the patient's family members from exposure to radiation by implementing time and distance restrictions, using shielding devices, and safely handling body fluids, depending on the sealed or unsealed status of the radiation source. Keep a safety container in the patient's room
- Prevent dislodgment of implanted radiation devices. Check linens, bedpans, and other equipment for signs of a dislodged implant
- If the implant becomes dislodged, contact the radiation therapy department
- Provide reassurance that when the radiation source is gone, the patient is no longer radioactive

Also follow additional safety guidelines for systemic radiation therapy:

- Wear protective gloves when handling the patient's radioactive body fluids or items that come in contact with the patient's body fluids
- Use disposable food trays and eating utensils
- Keep nondisposable items, linens, and other equipment in plastic bags in the patient's room to be scanned for radioactivity before removal

Chemotherapy

Chemotherapy is the use of antineoplastics to destroy or retard cancer cell growth. Chemotherapeutic drugs affect normal and cancer cells by interfering with DNA synthesis or cellular function during the cell cycle. They have the greatest effect on rapidly dividing cells, such as those found in bone marrow, mucous membranes, and hair follicles. The guiding principle of chemotherapy is to administer agents in doses large enough to eradicate disease but small enough to minimize adverse effects and the damage to the normal cells.

Chemotherapeutic drugs are used as adjuvant therapy with either surgery or radiotherapy. Many classes of antineoplastics are used for chemotherapy. Alkylating agents are cell cycle nonspecific drugs that cross-link and break DNA strands, causing cell death. They're used to treat leukemias, lymphomas, and myelomas. Examples include cyclophosphamide (Cytoxan), pentostatin (Nipent), cladribine (Leustatin), chlorambucil (Leukeran), lomustine (CeeNU), carmustine (Gliadel), carboplatin, and cisplatin (Platinol), which is also classified as a heavy metal with alkylating properties.

Antimetabolite agents are cell cycle specific for the S phase. They block or interfere with normal DNA or ribonucleic acid synthesis by competing for placement as a metabolite needed by the cell. They're used to treat leukemias, testicular and ovarian tumors, lymphomas, sarcomas, and lung and breast cancers. Examples include methotrexate (Trexall), fludarabine (Fludara), and 5-fluorouracil.

Antibiotics are cell cycle nonspecific drugs that interfere with DNA synthesis by inserting a compound between the DNA helix strands. They're used to treat Wilms' tumor, neuroblastoma, lymphomas, ovarian and testicular cancers, and breast cancer. Examples include doxorubicin, bleomycin, and daunorubicin (Cerubidine).

Vinca or plant alkaloids are cell cycle specific for the M phase. They block cell division by inhibiting spindle formation during mitosis. They're used to treat leukemia, Hodgkin's disease, non-Hodgkin's lymphoma, neuroblastoma, Wilms' tumor, and cancers of the lung, breast, and testes. Examples include vincristine, vinblastine, and docetaxel (Taxotere).

Topoisomerase I inhibitors cause DNA damage during DNA synthesis. They're used to treat colorectal cancer, metastatic ovarian cancer, and small-cell lung cancer. Examples include irinotecan (Camptosar) and topotecan (Hycamtin).

Steroids and hormones, which are used in combination with other drugs, alter the environment that bathes the cell. They're used to treat leukemias, lymphomas, and reproductive organ tumors. Examples include prednisone, estrogen, progestin, flutamide, and the antiestrogen tamoxifen.

Miscellaneous antineoplastics are also available; paclitaxel, for example, inhibits microtubular function and is used to treat metastatic breast and ovarian cancer.

Follow these safety guidelines when preparing, administering, or disposing of chemotherapeutic drugs:

- Prepare drugs under a laminar hood to prevent air from flowing into your face (usually prepared by a pharmacist)
- Wear two pair of disposable gloves and a cuffed gown when mixing drugs
- Perform hand hygiene before putting gloves on and after removing gloves
- Don't eat, drink, smoke, or chew gum in the drug preparation area
- If a chemotherapeutic drug touches the skin, wash the area thoroughly with nonabrasive soap and water as soon as possible
- If a chemotherapeutic drug touches the eye, flood the eye immediately with clear water or eyewash and seek medical attention
- Use spill kits for large spills on work areas or the floor
- Don't store food or drink with chemotherapeutic drugs
- Perform hand hygiene before and after administering drugs, and wear gloves
- Don't dispose of materials by clipping needles, breaking syringes, or removing needles from syringes
- Use needles, syringes, tubing, and connectors with Luer lock attachments
- Use gauze pads when removing chemotherapy syringes and needles from injection ports or spikes from I.V. bags
- Use an absorbent pad under the injection site to contain spillage
- Avoid hand-to-eye and hand-to-mouth contact when handling chemotherapeutic drugs or contaminated body fluids
- Dispose of equipment used to administer chemotherapeutic drugs in accordance with the regulations governing disposal of toxic and chemical wastes

Bone Marrow Transplantation

Although bone marrow transplantation is a complex treatment with a high potential for severe complications, it has become a viable option for many patients with various malignant disorders. Bone marrow transplantation may be considered for patients with various disorders, such as leukemia, lymphoma, multiple myeloma, neuroblastoma, metastatic breast cancer, ovarian cancer, and small-cell lung cancer.

Before transplantation, the patient receives high and potentially lethal doses of radiation and chemotherapy that produce an immunosuppressed state and damage and destroy the patient's bone marrow, creating space for replacement with healthy donor marrow. There are three types of donor marrow:

1. Autologous donor marrow, the most commonly transplanted type, is harvested from the recipient during disease remission, processed, and kept in frozen storage to be reinfused at a later date. Peripheral blood stem cells can be similarly harvested by leukapheresis and are then processed and stored for later use
2. Allogenic donor marrow is harvested from a relative or a person with similar human leukocyte antigen tissue type
3. Synergic donor marrow is harvested from an identical twin

The donor marrow is usually infused 48 to 72 hours after the last dose of radiation or chemotherapy. Potential immediate adverse reactions include allergic response (urticaria, chills, fever), fluid overload, and pulmonary system response to fat emboli. Potential complications include infection, hemorrhage, liver veno-occlusive disease, renal insufficiency, GI disturbances, multiple organ dysfunction syndrome, and graft-versus-host disease.

Nursing implications for care are based on the care plan for any severely immunosuppressed patient and include:

- Prevention of exposure to nosocomial infections posttransplantation (strict aseptic techniques must be maintained)
- Recognition of early signs of posttransplantation complications and graft rejection (early treatment may reverse the rejection process)
- Provision of extensive patient and family teaching before and after transplantation
- Recognition of the patient's and family's need for emotional support during the transplantation process

Biotherapy

Biotherapy stimulates and enhances the body's immune response against tumor cells. Biotherapeutic drugs include bacillus Calmette-Guérin vaccine, human tumor antigens, monoclocal antibodies such as rituximab (Rituxan), interferon, and growth factors.

Many biological response modifiers (BRMs) have been approved by the Food and Drug Administration since the mid-1980s.

The following BRMs have had success in treating select cancers:

- Interferon is a protein that regulates the immune response and has antiviral and antiproliferative characteristics at the cellular level. Interferon is used to treat hairy cell leukemia and chronic myelogenous leukemia. Interferon also treats hairy cell leukemia plus malignant melanoma and follicular lymphoma
- Interleukins are produced by leukocytes to promote hematopoiesis. Interleukin-2 (Proleukin) treats metastatic melanomas and renal cell cancers. Interleukin-11 (Neumega) prevents or treats thrombocytopenia in nonmyeloid cancers
- Monoclonal antibodies may be tagged with radioisotopes for diagnostic testing or to kill target cancer cells; tositumomab (Bexxar) is used to treat B-cell lymphoma. Other monoclonal antibodies suppress autoimmune destruction of transplants or inhibit malignant cells (without radioactivity), such as rituximab (Rituxan) for non-Hodgkin's lymphoma, cetuximab (Erbitux) for metastatic colorectal cancer, and trastuzumab (Herceptin) for breast cancer
- Colony-stimulating factors occur naturally in the body and mediate hematopoiesis. Filgrastim (Neupogen) and sargramostim (Leukine) are commonly used to stimulate white blood cell production; epoetin alfa (Epogen) is used to stimulate red blood cell production

Many adverse effects are associated with these treatments. Nursing implications include

- Familiarity with potential adverse effects and complications of BRMs
- Careful monitoring and documentation of patient response to treatment
- Extensive patient and family teaching

Cancer-Related Problems

Various problems can result from cancer treatment or from the disease itself. To provide quality care, see the chart below for common cancer-related problems and their nursing implications.

Cancer-Related Problem	Nursing Implications
Alopecia	
To the patient, alopecia may be the most distressing adverse reaction. If caused by chemotherapy, alopecia is temporary. Radiation-induced alopecia, however, may be permanent.	• Prepare the patient for alopecia. Inform the patient that hair loss is usually gradual and may be reversible after treatment ends. • Inform the patient that alopecia may be partial or complete and that it affects men and women. • Inform the patient that alopecia may affect the scalp, eyebrows, eyelashes, and body hair. • Discuss ways to improve self-image—for example, by using wigs, hats, cosmetics, and scarves.
Anemia	
Anemia can develop slowly over several courses of treatment or may be due to the disease.	• Assess the patient for dizziness, fatigue, pallor, and shortness of breath on minimal exertion. • Monitor the patient's hematocrit, hemoglobin level, and red blood cell count. Remember that a patient dehydrated from nausea, vomiting, or anorexia may exhibit a false-normal hematocrit. After this patient is rehydrated, the hematocrit will decrease. • Be prepared to administer a blood transfusion to a symptomatic patient, as prescribed. • Instruct the patient to rest frequently and to increase dietary intake of iron-rich foods. Advise the patient to take a multivitamin with iron as prescribed.

(continued)

Cancer-Related Problem	Nursing Implications
Bone Marrow Suppression	
Bone marrow suppression is the most common and potentially serious adverse reaction to antineoplastics.	• Watch for the blood count nadir because that's when the patient is at greatest risk for the complications of leukopenia, thrombocytopenia, and anemia. • Plan a patient-teaching program about bone marrow suppression, including information about blood counts, potential infection sites, personal hygiene, and measures to take to prevent unnecessary exposure. • Place the patient on neutropenic precautions according to institutional policy.
Constipation	
Constipation is common in patients with colon cancer; it may indicate neurotoxicity caused by chemotherapy, or it may be caused by narcotic pain control.	• Assess the patient for bowel sounds, abdominal distention or pain, and fecal impaction. • Encourage fluid intake of 3 qt (2.8 L) daily unless contraindicated. • Modify the diet to include more fiber. • Administer a laxative, stool softener, enema, or suppository, as prescribed. • Monitor amount and number of stools.
Depression	
Depression is described as a persistent sad or dysphoric mood.	• Assess the patient's psychosocial status. • Encourage the patient to verbalize concerns and needs. • Offer to refer the patient to a cancer care counselor. • Administer antidepressants, as prescribed.
Diarrhea	
A common reaction to chemotherapy and radiation therapy, diarrhea can cause fluid and electrolyte imbalances if severe.	• Monitor fluid intake and output. • Assess the patient for signs of dehydration and electrolyte imbalances. • Assess the patient for bowel sounds, abdominal cramps, and rectal irritation. • Obtain stool cultures as prescribed. • Administer an antidiarrheal as prescribed. • Provide good perianal hygiene. • Encourage fluid intake, and modify the diet as needed.
Dyspnea	
Dyspnea may result from lung cancer and is typically described as shortness of breath but also refers to difficult or uncomfortable breathing.	• Assess the patient's breath sounds and pulse oximetry and watch for peripheral edema. • Provide oxygen therapy if saturation levels fall below 92%, as ordered. • Encourage the patient to pace activities with rest periods, and assist with daily activities as needed. • Administer respiratory therapy as prescribed.
Fatigue	
Fatigue is a general feeling of physical or emotional exhaustion and lack of energy that may result from anemia, decreased nutritional intake, or increased cell destruction by treatment.	• Assess the patient's ability to sleep or rest and level of fatigue. • Assess the patient for signs of increased metabolic processes, such as fever and disease progression. • Assist the patient with daily activities. • Minimize physical fatigue by pacing activities and allowing adequate time for sleep and rest. • Help the patient examine coping strategies.
Leukopenia	
Leukopenia increases the patient's risk of infection, especially if the granulocyte count is under 1,000/mm^3.	• Provide information about good hygiene, and assess the patient frequently for signs and symptoms of infection. • Teach the patient to recognize and report the signs and symptoms of infection, such as fever, cough, sore throat, or a burning sensation on urination. • Teach the patient how and when to take his temperature. • Caution the patient to avoid crowds and people with colds or the flu during the nadir. • Remember that the inflammatory response may be decreased and the complications of leukopenia more difficult to detect if the patient is receiving a corticosteroid. • Administer colony-stimulating factors, as prescribed.

(continued)

Cancer-Related Problem	Nursing Implications
Nausea and Vomiting	
Nausea and vomiting can result from gastric mucosal irritation, chemical irritation of the central nervous system, or psychogenic factors that may be activated by sensations, suggestions, or anxiety related to chemotherapy.	• Control the chemical irritation by administering combinations of antiemetics as prescribed. • Monitor the patient for signs and symptoms of aspiration because most antiemetics sedate. • Control psychogenic factors by helping the patient perform relaxation techniques before chemotherapy to minimize feelings of isolation and anxiety. • Encourage the patient to express feelings of anxiety. • Encourage the patient to listen to music or to engage in relaxation exercises, meditation, or hypnosis to promote feelings of control and well-being. • Adjust the drug administration time to meet the patient's needs. Some patients prefer treatments in the evening when they find sedation comfortable. Patients who are employed may prefer their treatments on their days off.
Sexual Dysfunction	
Sexual dysfunction is a physical or emotional inability to express oneself sexually that can result from treatment or the disease.	• Assess the patient for sexual concerns related to fatigue, anemia, nausea, vomiting, or body image. • If the patient is male, assess him for impotence; if the patient is female, assess her for menstrual problems. • Give the patient information about the disease's effects and treatment. • Discuss specific measures to help the patient adapt to sexuality changes, such as using different positions and lubrication. • Advise the patient that contraception is advisable during chemotherapy (or radiation therapy) to prevent birth defects from chromosomal damage. • Allow the partner to visit the patient in private. • Refer the patient to counselors or support groups, as needed.
Stomatitis	
Although epithelial tissue damage can affect any mucous membrane, the most common site is the oral mucosa. Stomatitis is temporary and can range from mild and barely noticeable to severe and debilitating. (Debilitation may result from poor nutrition during acute stomatitis.)	• Initiate preventive mouth care before chemotherapy to provide comfort and decrease the severity of the stomatitis. • Provide therapeutic mouth care, including topical antibiotics, if prescribed, and cessation of mouthwash use. • Encourage use of oral anesthetics before meals, pain medication, or both, if prescribed. • Assess the need for diet change or alternate form of nutrition (tube feedings, total parenteral nutrition).
Thrombocytopenia	
Thrombocytopenia may occur with leukopenia. When the platelet count is under 50,000/mm^3, the patient is at risk for bleeding. When it's under 20,000/mm^3, the patient is at severe risk and may require a platelet transfusion.	• Assess the patient for bleeding gums, increased bruising or petechiae, hypermenorrhea, tarry stools, hematuria, and coffee-ground vomitus. • Advise the patient to avoid cuts and bruises and to use a soft toothbrush and an electric razor. • Instruct the patient to report sudden headaches, which could indicate potentially fatal intracranial bleeding. • Instruct the patient to use a stool softener, as prescribed, to prevent colonic irritation and bleeding. • Instruct the patient to avoid using a rectal thermometer and receiving I.M. injections to prevent bleeding.

Nursing Implications in Clinical Pharmacology

The following chart identifies drugs by class and summarizes their indications, contraindications, adverse reactions patients can experience, and nursing implications.

Common Drugs	Indications	Contraindications	Adverse Reactions	Nursing Implications
Drugs that Affect the Autonomic Nervous System				
Cholinergics (Parasympathomimetics)				
ambenonium (Mytelase); bethanechol (Duvoid), carbachol, edrophonium (Tensilon), neostigmine (Prostigmin), pilocarpine (Carpine), pyridostigmine (Mestinon, Regonol)	• Glaucoma (carbachol, pilocarpine) • Nonobstructive urine retention (bethanechol) • Neurogenic bladder (bethanechol) • Abdominal distention and ileus (bethanechol) • Myasthenia gravis (ambenonium, edrophonium, neostigmine, pyridostigmine)	• Potential GI or urinary obstruction • Enlarged prostate	• Nausea, vomiting, and diarrhea • Headache • Hypotension • Muscle weakness • Increased bronchial secretions, salivation, and sweating • Bradycardia • Abdominal cramping • Respiratory depression	• Monitor the patient's GI and urinary status. • Monitor vital signs. • Administer atropine as an antidote. • Determine what other drugs the patient is taking. Use of another cholinergic increases the risk of cholinergic crisis; use of an anticholinergic may inhibit the effects of the cholinergic.
Anticholinergics (Parasympatholytics, Cholinergic Blockers)				
atropine, benztropine mesylate (Cogentin), dicyclomine (Bentyl), glycopyrrolate (Robinul), meclizine (Antivert), propantheline, scopolamine (Transderm Scōp), trihexyphenidyl	• Bradycardia (atropine) • Decrease saliva and bronchial secretions preoperatively (atropine, scopolamine, glycopyrrolate) • Parkinsonism (benztropine, trihexyphenidyl) • Motion sickness (scopolamine) • Peptic ulcer or bowel spasm (propantheline, dicyclomine) • Produce mydriasis (atropine)	• Angle-closure glaucoma • Hemorrhage, tachycardia, and GI or urinary obstruction	• Dry mouth and difficulty swallowing • Photophobia, blurred vision, and dizziness • Constipation • Urinary retention	• Assess mucous membranes for dryness. • Tell the patient to report blurred vision and dizziness; if these symptoms are present, help the patient with daily activities to prevent injury. • Report sudden eye pain to the physician, and withhold next dose. • Assess vital signs
Adrenergics (Sympathomimetics)				
albuterol, dobutamine, dopamine (Intropin), ephedrine, epinephrine (Adrenalin, EpiPen Auto-Injector), isoetharine, isoproterenol (Isuprel), metaproterenol, norepinephrine (Levophed), phenylephrine (Neo-Synephrine), pseudoephedrine (Sudafed), salmeterol	• Bronchodilation (albuterol, isoproterenol) • Cardiac stimulation (epinephrine, dobutamine) • Hypotension (dopamine, norepinephrine) • Enhance renal perfusion (dopamine) • Allergic reactions (epinephrine) • Nasal congestion (ephedrine)	• Angle-closure glaucoma • Tachyarrhythmias	• Arrhythmias, tachycardia, and hypertension • Nervousness and restlessness • Hypotension	• Monitor vital signs, breath sounds, and electrocardiogram (ECG) results. • Measure output to detect adequate renal perfusion.

(continued)

Common Drugs	Indications	Contraindications	Adverse Reactions	Nursing Implications
Drugs that Affect the Autonomic Nervous System (*continued*)				
Adrenergic Blockers (Sympatholytics)				
Alpha-adrenergic blockers: ergotamine (Cafergot), phentolamine (Regitine) *Beta-adrenergic blockers:* atenolol, metoprolol (Lopressor), nadolol (Corgard), propranolol (Inderal), timolol	• *Alpha-adrenergic blockers:* hypertension from pheochromocytoma (phentolamine), vascular headaches (ergotamine) • *Beta-adrenergic blockers:* hypertension (atenolol, propranolol, timolol), angina (atenolol, propranolol), arrhythmias (propranolol), vascular headache (propranolol), glaucoma (timolol)	• *Alpha-adrenergic blockers:* myocardial infarction (MI) and pregnancy • *Beta-adrenergic blockers:* heart failure (with caution), heart block, and bronchospasm	• *Alpha-adrenergic blockers:* cardiac arrhythmias, hypotension, and tachycardia • *Beta-adrenergic blockers:* bradycardia, dizziness, vertigo, and bronchospasm	• Monitor vital signs, especially blood pressure and pulse. • Monitor circulatory status. • Don't discontinue the drug abruptly.
Neuromuscular Blockers				
atracurium, pancuronium, succinylcholine (Anectine), tubocurarine, vecuronium	• Relax skeletal muscles during surgery (succinylcholine) • Reduce muscle spasm during induced seizures (tubocurarine) • Manage ventilator-dependent patients (pancuronium) • Facilitate intubation (atracurium)	• Hypersensitivity • Malignant hypertension	• Excessive bronchial secretions, respiratory depression, and bronchospasm • Malignant hyperthermia	• Protect the patient's airway. • Assess the patient's level of pain. • Monitor vital signs.
Analgesics and Opioids				
Opioid Analgesics				
buprenorphine (Buprenex), codeine, fentanyl (Duragesic, Sublimaze), hydromorphone (Dilaudid), meperidine (Demerol), morphine (Duramorph, MS Contin), oxycodone (Percodan, Percocet), pentazocine (Talwin)	• Moderate to severe pain • Anesthesia adjunct (meperidine, morphine) • Acute pulmonary edema (morphine) • Cough (codeine) • Acute MI (morphine)	• Central nervous system (CNS) depression • Respiratory depression • Acute alcohol withdrawal • Liver disease, respiratory problems, and renal disease (use with caution)	• Respiratory depression • Orthostatic hypotension • Dizziness, ataxia, drowsiness, and euphoria • Tolerance • Physical and psychological dependence	• Assess the patient's level of pain and the effectiveness of pain relief measures. • Administer the drug before pain is severe. • Monitor respiratory status and blood pressure. • Assess bowel function; continued use of opioid agents can cause severe constipation. • For an overdose, naloxone (Narcan) is the antidote.
Opioid Antagonists				
nalmefene, naloxone, naltrexone (Revia)	• CNS depression in opioid overdose • Respiratory depression in opioid overdose • Opioid detoxification in a former addict	• Opioid dependence (use with caution). Acute withdrawal symptoms may develop. • Cardiac irritability (use with caution)	• Hypotension and hypertension	• Monitor vital signs, respiratory status, and level of consciousness until the effects of the opioid have worn off. • Assess the patient's level of pain. • Protect the patient's airway.

(*continued*)

Common Drugs	Indications	Contraindications	Adverse Reactions	Nursing Implications
Analgesics and Opioids (*continued*)				
Nonopioid Analgesics and Antipyretics				
acetaminophen (Tylenol), acetylsalicylic acid (aspirin), phenazopyridine	• Mild to moderate musculoskeletal or nerve pain (acetaminophen, aspirin) • Fever (acetaminophen, aspirin) • Inflammation (aspirin) • Arthritis (aspirin) • Urinary tract pain (phenazopyridine)	• Pregnancy (except acetaminophen) • Bleeding disorders and ulcers (aspirin) • Chickenpox (danger of Reye's syndrome with aspirin)	• GI upset and heartburn • Prolonged bleeding time (aspirin)	• Assess the patient's level of pain and the effectiveness of pain relief measures. • Administer the drug before meals for optimal effect or with meals to alleviate GI symptoms.
Nonsteroidal Anti-Inflammatory Drugs (NSAIDs)				
celecoxib (Celebrex), diclofenac (Voltaren), fenoprofen (Nalfon), ibuprofen (Advil, Motrin), ketorolac (Toradol), meclofenamate, naproxen (Aleve, Naprosyn), piroxicam (Feldene), sulindac (Clinoril), tolmetin	• Inflammation associated with arthritis, gout, bursitis, and other inflammatory disorders • Pain associated with general aches • Fever	• Bleeding disorders (use with caution) • Ulcers and GI problems (use with caution) • Hypersensitivity to sulfonamides (celecoxib) • Use cautiously in patients with severe liver disease or chronic alcohol abuse	• GI bleeding, nausea, and vomiting • Prolonged bleeding time	• Assess the patient's level of pain and the effectiveness of pain relief measures. • Assess the patient for GI symptoms.
Drugs that Affect the Central Nervous System				
CNS Stimulants				
amphetamine (Adderall), caffeine, dextroamphetamine (Dexedrine), methamphetamine (Desoxyn), methylphenidate (Ritalin), pemoline	• Narcolepsy (amphetamine, methylphenidate, pemoline) • Attention deficit hyperactivity disorder (methamphetamine, methylphenidate, pemoline) • Appetite control (amphetamine, caffeine, dextroamphetamine, methamphetamine)	• Hypertension, angina, or cardiovascular disease • Glaucoma • Hyperthyroidism • History of drug abuse	• Insomnia, restlessness, and irritability • Hypotension and tachycardia • Drug dependence and tolerance	• Tell the patient to avoid caffeine-containing drinks. • Monitor blood pressure and pulse. • Monitor weight.
Anticonvulsants				
Barbiturates: primidone (Mysoline) *Benzodiazepines*: clonazepam (Klonopin), diazepam (Valium), lorazepam (Ativan) *Hydantoins*: fosphenytoin, mephenytoin, phenytoin (Dilantin)	• Generalized tonic-clonic seizures (barbiturates, hydantoins, carbamazepine) • Partial seizures (barbiturates, hydantoins, carbamazepine, lamotrigine, levetiracetam, oxcarbazepine)	• Hypersensitivity • Bone marrow suppression • Blood dyscrasias	• Drowsiness, ataxia, sedation, and dizziness • Leukopenia • Gingival hyperplasia (hydantoins)	• Assess seizure activity. • Administer the drug with food to decrease GI upset. • Don't administer the drug with milk or antacids, which can interfere with absorption. • Tell the patient not to take the drug with alcohol or other CNS depressants.

(continued)

Common Drugs	Indications	Contraindications	Adverse Reactions	Nursing Implications
Drugs that Affect the Central Nervous System *(continued)*				
Anticonvulsants *(continued)*				
Succinimides: ethosuximide (Zarontin), methsuximide (Celontin) *Other:* carbamazepine (Tegretol), lamotrigine (Lamictal), levetiracetam (Keppra), oxcarbazepine (Trileptal), valproic acid (Depakene)	• Absence seizures (benzodiazepines, succinimides, valproic acid) • Status epilepticus (benzodiazepines) • For sedation and as anxiolytics (benzodiazepines, barbiturates)			• Assess oral mucous membranes, particularly noting gum hyperplasia. • Monitor serum levels. • Don't discontinue the drug abruptly.
Antiparkinsonians				
amantadine, bromocriptine mesylate (Parlodel), carbidopa-levodopa (Sinemet), levodopa, pergolide, ropinirole (Requip), selegiline (Eldepryl)	• Parkinson's disease (increase levels of dopamine) • Drug-induced extrapyramidal symptoms (amantadine) • Antiviral (amantadine)	• Angle-closure glaucoma • Cardiac disease and pyloric obstruction (use with caution)	• Nausea and vomiting • Orthostatic hypotension • Involuntary body movements	• Supervise the patient's activity when drug therapy is started. • Tell the patient to get up slowly to prevent orthostatic hypotension. • Be aware that some anticholinergics, such as trihexyphenidyl and benztropine, may also be used to treat Parkinson's disease.
Sedatives, Hypnotics, and Anxiolytics				
Antihistamines: diphenhydramine (Benadryl), hydroxyzine (Vistaril), promethazine *Barbiturates:* pentobarbital, secobarbital (Seconal) *Benzodiazepines:* clonazepam (Klonopin), diazepam (Valium), lorazepam (Ativan)	• Anxiety (hydroxyzine and benzodiazepines) • Insomnia (diphenhydramine, barbiturates) • Sedation (promethazine, barbiturates)	• Preexisting CNS depression • Respiratory depression • History of drug abuse	• Drowsiness, dizziness, and confusion • Decreased blood pressure and pulse rate	• Assess the patient's mental status. • Be aware that the effects of these drugs are potentiated by alcohol and other sedatives, hypnotics, or anxiolytics. • Keep in mind that barbiturates decrease the effectiveness of warfarin (Coumadin) and oral contraceptives.
Antidepressants				
Selective serotonin-reuptake inhibitors (SSRIs): citalopram (Celexa), escitalopram (Lexapro), fluoxetine (Prozac), paroxetine (Paxil), sertraline (Zoloft) *Tricyclics:* amitriptyline, imipramine (Tofranil), nortriptyline (Pamelor) *Other:* venlafaxine (Effexor)	• Clinical depression • Obsessive-compulsive disorder (fluoxetine, paroxetine, sertraline) • Panic disorder (SSRIs, venlafaxine)	• Hypotension (tricyclics) • Cardiovascular disease (tricyclics) • Use of monoamine oxidase inhibitors (SSRIs) in combination or within 14 days of use	• Cardiac adverse effects (tricyclics) • Anticholinergic effects (tricyclics) • GI irritation (SSRIs) • Nervousness and insomnia (SSRIs) • Hypertension (venlafaxine)	• Monitor the patient carefully for adverse reactions, which may occur before therapeutic effect, which takes 2 to 4 weeks. • Monitor the patient taking SSRIs for nervousness and insomnia.

(continued)

Common Drugs	Indications	Contraindications	Adverse Reactions	Nursing Implications
Drugs that Affect the Cardiovascular System				
Antianginals				
Beta-adrenergic blockers (see page 349) *Calcium channel blockers:* amlodipine (Norvasc), diltiazem (Cardizem), nicardipine (Cardene), nifedipine (Procardia), verapamil *Nitrates:* isosorbide dinitrate (Isordil), isosorbide mononitrate, nitroglycerin (Nitro-Dur) Ranolazine (Ranexa)	• Chest pain caused by ischemia of the coronary arteries • Decrease the heart's workload and reduce the need for oxygen	• Uncontrolled hypotension or hypertension • Heart failure or heart block	• Headache • Hypotension • Flushing	• Assess anginal pain before, during, and after administration of nitroglycerin. • Be aware that the patient should avoid using these agents during the night to prevent drug tolerance. • Monitor pulse rate and blood pressure before administering antianginals. • Treat headache (a common adverse reaction) with mild analgesics.
Antiarrhythmics				
Class IA (sodium channel blockers): disopyramide (Norpace), moricizine, procainamide, quinidine gluconate *Class IB (sodium channel blockers):* lidocaine (Xylocaine), mexiletine, phenytoin (Dilantin), tocainide *Class IC (sodium channel blockers):* flecainide (Tambocor), propafenone (Rythmol) *Class II (beta-adrenergic blockers):* atenolol (Tenormin), metoprolol (Lopressor), propranolol (Inderal) *Class III:* amiodarone (Cordarone), dofetilide (Tikosyn), dronedarone (Multaq), ibutilide (Corvert) *Class IV (calcium channel blockers):* diltiazem (Cardizem), verapamil (Calan) *Miscellaneous or unclassified:* adenosine (Adenocard), atropine, digoxin (Lanoxin), magnesium sulfate	• Cardiac arrhythmias, specifically, atrial fibrillation, premature ventricular contractions, ventricular tachycardia and fibrillation, and supraventricular tachycardia • Promote normal sinus rhythm with regular ventricular response	• Heart block • Heart failure • Sinus bradycardia	• Nausea • Hypotension • Dyspnea • Heart failure, heart block, and new arrhythmias	• Monitor vital signs and ECG results. • Monitor oxygenation status. • Educate the patient about the importance of taking these medications at regularly scheduled times. • Teach the patient and family how to monitor pulse rate and blood pressure.

(continued)

Common Drugs	Indications	Contraindications	Adverse Reactions	Nursing Implications
Drugs that Affect the Cardiovascular System (*continued*)				
Antihypertensives				
Angiotensin-converting enzyme (ACE) inhibitors: captopril (Capoten), enalapril (Vasotec), lisinopril (Zestril), benazepril (Lotensin), quinapril (Accupril), ramipril (Altace) *Angiotensin II receptor blockers:* candesartan (Atacand), irbesartan (Avapro), losartan (Cozaar), olmesartan (Benicar), telmisartan (Micardis), valsartan (Diovan) *Beta-adrenergic blockers:* atenolol (Tenormin), metoprolol (Lopressor), nadolol (Corgard), propranolol (Inderal) *Calcium channel blockers:* diltiazem (Cardizem), nicardipine (Cardene), nifedipine (Procardia), verapamil *Central-acting adrenergic inhibitors:* clonidine (Catapres), methyldopa *Diuretics: Peripheral-acting adrenergic inhibitors:* guanethidine sulfate, reserpine *Peripheral vasodilators:* diazoxide, hydralazine, nitroprusside sodium, prazosin (Minipress), terazosin (Hytrin)	• Hypertension	• Heart failure • Bradycardia • Hypotension	*Life-threatening* • Hemolytic anemia • Hepatic necrosis • Leukopenia *Commonly seen* • Dry mouth • Drowsiness • Dizziness • Impotence • Nasal congestion • Nausea • Orthostatic hypotension • Skin rash • Dry, hacking cough (with ACE inhibitors)	• Assess blood pressure before administering the drug. • Monitor pulse rate and blood pressure. • Assess the patient for orthostatic hypotension; supervise ambulation if orthostatic hypotension occurs. • Monitor daily weight and intake and output.
Antilipemics				
atorvastatin (Lipitor), cholestyramine, colestipol (Colestid), ezetimibe (Zetia), fluvastatin (Lescol), lovastatin (Mevacor), niacin, pravastatin (Pravachol), rosuvastatin (Crestor), simvastatin (Zocor)	• Reduce serum lipid levels when dietary measures haven't been successful. • Primary prevention of cardiac events (atorvastatin, fluvastatin, lovastatin, pravastatin, rosuvastatin, simvastatin)	• Fat-soluble vitamin deficiency • Severe constipation or bowel obstruction • History of GI disorders and impaired liver function (use with caution)	• Abdominal discomfort • Diarrhea • Nausea and vomiting (cholestyramine, colestipol) • Muscle pain • Increased liver enzyme levels (atorvastatin, ezetimibe, fluvastatin, lovastatin, pravastatin, rosuvastatin, simvastatin) • Constipation (cholestyramine)	• Assess the patient's dietary habits. • Monitor bowel elimination patterns, and document changes. • Report changes in GI status. • Monitor liver function tests. • Teach the patient and family how to reduce other risks of cardiac disease.

(continued)

Common Drugs	Indications	Contraindications	Adverse Reactions	Nursing Implications
Drugs that Affect the Cardiovascular System (*continued*)				
Cardiac Glycoside				
digoxin (Lanoxin)	• Heart failure • Atrial tachyarrhythmias (to control ventricular rate)	• Uncontrolled ventricular arrhythmias • Complete heart block • MI, cardiac myopathy, and renal impairment (use with caution)	• Nausea and vomiting • Bradycardia • Hypotension • Weakness and fatigue	• Monitor the apical pulse before administering the drug and hold if pulse is <60 beats/minute. • Check for signs and symptoms of toxic reaction (anorexia, nausea, vomiting, fatigue, weakness, and bradycardia). • Monitor electrolyte levels (imbalances increase the potential for toxic reaction, especially hypokalemia).
Diuretics				
Carbonic anhydrase inhibitors: acetazolamide (Diamox) *Loop diuretics:* bumetanide (Bumex), ethacrynic acid (Edecrin), furosemide (Lasix) *Osmotic diuretics:* mannitol (Osmitrol), urea *Potassium-sparing diuretics:* spironolactone (Aldactone), triamterene (Dyrenium) *Thiazide diuretics:* chlorothiazide (Diuril), chlorthalidone, hydrochlorothiazide (Oretic), indapamide	• Heart failure, edema, and hypertension • Cerebral edema (mannitol) • Glaucoma (acetazolamide, mannitol)	• Hypotension • Kidney failure (anuria) • Hypovolemia • Hypokalemia (for non–potassium-sparing diuretics)	• Dehydration • Hypotension and orthostatic hypotension • Electrolyte imbalances • Hypokalemia • Arrhythmias • Muscle cramps • Photosensitivity	• Monitor weight, fluid balance, blood pressure, and electrolyte levels. • Assess the patient for signs of fluid overload. • Administer diuretics at times that don't disturb the patient's sleep. • Review drug interactions, especially those involving digoxin and lithium. • Be aware that hypokalemia can lead to arrhythmias, muscle cramps, and digoxin toxicity. • Keep in mind that lithium excretion is decreased with concomitant use of loop, potassium-sparing, or thiazide diuretics; this can cause lithium toxicity. • Teach the patient about diet restrictions.
Anticoagulants and Thrombolytics				
Anticoagulants: dalteparin (Fragmin), enoxaparin (Lovenox), heparin, warfarin (Coumadin), dabigatran (Pradaxa), rivaroxaban (Xarelto) *Thrombolytics:* alteplase (Activase), streptokinase (Streptase)	• Treat and prevent clotting disorders, such as deep vein thrombosis, phlebitis, pulmonary embolus, peripheral vascular disease, and disorders arising from prolonged bed rest (anticoagulants) • Used in emergent situations, such as dissolving clots in coronary arteries, pulmonary arteries, and deep veins and preventing the extension of MI (thrombolytics)	• Bleeding or coagulation disorders • Active bleeding and blood dyscrasias • Active ulcer disease • Cancer	• Bleeding and thrombocytopenia • Potentially severe allergic responses (thrombolytics)	• Monitor partial thromboplastin time (heparin) and prothrombin time (warfarin). • Monitor the patient for signs and symptoms of bleeding (such as bleeding gums or presence of blood in stool). • Reduce the number of punctures; apply pressure to puncture sites. Make sure thrombolytics are administered only in settings in which the patient can be closely monitored.

(continued)

Common Drugs	Indications	Contraindications	Adverse Reactions	Nursing Implications
Drugs that Affect the Cardiovascular System *(continued)*				
Anticoagulants and Thrombolytics (continued)				
				• If the patient is taking dalteparin and enoxaparin, educate him about subcutaneous drug administration. • Educate the patient and family about necessary precautions when taking anticoagulants, such as using a soft toothbrush and an electric razor, returning for routine laboratory tests, avoiding aspirin and ibuprofen, and informing other physicians and dentists about anticoagulant therapy. • Teach patients about decreasing foods high in vitamin K when taking warfarin (Coumadin)
Antianemics				
Iron products: ferrous gluconate, ferrous sulfate, iron dextran (DexFerrum, InFeD) *Vitamins:* cyanocobalamin (vitamin B_{12}), folic acid *Other:* darbepoetin alfa (Aranesp), epoetin alfa (Epogen, Procrit)	• Iron deficiency anemia (iron products) • Pernicious anemia and vitamin B_{12} deficiency (cyanocobalamin) • Folic acid deficiency (folic acid) • Anemia of chronic disease (epoetin alfa, darbepoetin alfa)	• Don't administer until type of anemia has been diagnosed • GI disturbances • Hypersensitivity to the drug	• Constipation, diarrhea, dark stools, GI upset, and staining at the injection site of I.M. preparations (iron products) • Allergic reactions and peripheral vascular thrombosis with cyanocobalamin • Hyperkalemia, hypertension, arthralgia, edema (epoetin alfa, darbepoetin alfa)	• Assess the patient's nutritional status. • Assess hemoglobin level and hematocrit and total body stores of iron. • Teach the patient and family the importance of a balanced diet. • Tell the patient and family that oral preparations are best absorbed on an empty stomach. • Tell the patient and family that iron products turn the stools black or dark green. • Teach the patient and family how to administer subcutaneous injections (epoetin alfa, darbepoetin alfa).
Drugs that Affect the Respiratory System				
Bronchodilators				
Beta-adrenergic agonists albuterol, epinephrine, isoetharine, isoproterenol (Isuprel), metaproterenol, salmeterol, terbutaline, *Phosphodiesterase inhibitors* Theophylline aminophylline	• Bronchospasm associated with asthma, bronchitis, and other chronic obstructive pulmonary diseases • Acute bronchospasm	• Untreated cardiac arrhythmias • Coronary artery disease	• Tachycardia and arrhythmias • Nervousness • Headache	• Assess breath sounds, respiratory status, sputum production, and vital signs. • Teach the patient and family how to administer inhaled medications. • Monitor serum levels (theophylline).

(continued)

Common Drugs	Indications	Contraindications	Adverse Reactions	Nursing Implications
Drugs that Affect the Respiratory System (*continued*)				
Antitussives, Expectorants, and Mucolytics				
Antitussives: codeine, dextromethorphan, diphenhydramine (Benadryl) *Expectorants:* guaifenesin *Mucolytics:* acetylcysteine, potassium iodide– saturated solution	• Unproductive or excessive cough • Promote rest	• Hypersensitivity • Chronic obstructive pulmonary disease	• Nausea • Drowsiness	• Assess respiratory status, cough, and sputum production. • Encourage increased fluid intake to reduce mucous viscosity.
Drugs that Affect the GI System				
Antacids				
aluminum hydroxide; aluminum hydroxide and magnesium hydroxide; aluminum hydroxide, magnesium hydroxide, and simethicone (Mylanta); calcium carbonate (Rolaids, Tums); magaldrate and simethicone	• Hyperacidity • Gastroesophageal reflux • Peptic ulcer disease	• Undiagnosed abdominal pain • Renal failure (antacids with magnesium, which can't be excreted and may produce hypermagnesemia and toxic drug levels) • Impaired GI motility	• Stomach cramps • Diarrhea (magnesium) • Constipation (aluminum)	• Assess bowel elimination patterns. • If the patient is on a sodium-restricted diet, instruct the patient and family to check the sodium content of antacids. • Don't administer antacids within 1 to 2 hours of other medications because they may delay absorption.
Antidiarrheals				
attapulgite (Kaopectate), bismuth subsalicylate (Pepto-Bismol), diphenoxylate with atropine (Lomotil), loperamide (Imodium)	• Acute diarrhea • Chronic diarrhea	• Undiagnosed abdominal pain • Hypersensitivity reactions • Infectious diarrhea	• Constipation • Drowsiness (atropine, loperamide)	• Assess bowel elimination patterns. • Assess fluid and electrolyte balance.
Antiemetics				
dimenhydrinate (Dramamine), granisetron (Kytril), meclizine (Antivert), metoclopramide (Reglan), ondansetron (Zofran), prochlorperazine, promethazine, scopolamine (Transderm Scōp), trimethobenzamide (Tigan)	• Depress the vomiting center in the medulla by acting on the chemoreceptor trigger zone (metoclopramide, prochlorperazine, promethazine, trimethobenzamide, granisetron ondansetron) • Decrease the effects of motion on the vomiting center (dimenhydrinate, meclizine, scopolamine)	• Intestinal obstruction • Sedative use (use with caution)	• Drowsiness • Hypotension • Extrapyramidal reactions (metoclopramide, prochlorperazine, promethazine)	• Assess the patient for symptoms of nausea and vomiting. • Assess GI status, including bowel sounds and presence of abdominal pain. • Monitor intake and output. • Ensure adequate hydration.

(continued)

Common Drugs	Indications	Contraindications	Adverse Reactions	Nursing Implications
Drugs that Affect the GI System (*continued*)				
Antiulceratives				
Histamine-2 (H₂) antagonists: cimetidine (Tagamet), famotidine (Pepcid), nizatidine (Axid), ranitidine (Zantac) *Prostaglandin-like:* misoprostol (Cytotec)	• *H₂-antagonists:* treat and prevent gastric and duodenal ulcers, treat gastric hypersecretion • *Prostaglandin-like:* inhibit gastric acid secretion in patients taking high doses of nonsteroidal anti-inflammatory drugs by synthetically mimicking prostaglandin	• *H₂-antagonists:* impaired liver or kidney function (use with caution), hypersensitivity reactions • *Prostaglandin-like:* pregnancy (has an oxytocic action)	• *H₂-antagonists:* confusion, dizziness, headache • *Prostaglandin-like:* diarrhea and abdominal pain	• Assess the patient for changes in mental status (H₂-antagonists). • Don't administer antiulceratives with antacids; antacids can interfere with the absorption of H₂-antagonists. • Instruct the patient to take misoprostol with meals and at bedtime to help decrease diarrhea.
Proton Pump Inhibitor				
lansoprazole (Prevacid), omeprazole (Prilosec), pantoprazole (Protonix)	• Peptic ulcer disease • Gastroesophageal reflux disease • Erosive esophagitis	• Lactation	• Nausea • Diarrhea • Headache	• Treatment course is about 8 weeks. The long-term effects of this amount of acid suppression are unknown at this time.
Pepsin Inhibitor				
sucralfate (Carafate)	• Peptic ulcer disease (forms a protective coating over the ulcer)	• Safe use in pregnancy or lactation not established	• Constipation • Impaired absorption of other drugs	• Give on an empty stomach about 1 hour before meals and at bedtime.
Laxatives				
Bulk-forming agents: methylcellulose (Citrucel), psyllium (Metamucil) *Lubricants:* hyperosmolar agents, lactulose, magnesium citrate, magnesium hydroxide, magnesium sulfate (Epsom salts), mineral oil, phosphates and biphosphates *Stimulants:* bisacodyl, castor oil *Stool softeners:* docusate calcium, docusate sodium (Colace)	• Constipation associated with many conditions and medications • Straining during defecation (stool softeners)	• GI conditions, such as abdominal pain, nausea, and vomiting • Diarrhea	• Cramping • Nausea and vomiting • Damage to the bowel or rectum with chronic use • Electrolyte imbalance and dehydration	• Assess bowel elimination patterns. • Assess the patient for previous use of laxatives. • Monitor stools. • Teach the patient and family that a high-fiber diet, fluids, and exercise promote regular patterns of elimination.

(continued)

Common Drugs	Indications	Contraindications	Adverse Reactions	Nursing Implications
Drugs that Affect the Endocrine System				
Antidiabetics				
Insulins: rapid-acting (Novolog), Humalog short-acting (Humulin R, Novolin R), intermediate-acting (NPH insulin, Humulin N), mixed (Humulin 70/30), basal or long-acting (insulin detemir [Levemir], insulin glargine [Lantus]) *Oral antidiabetics:* acetohexamide, chlorpropamide (Diabinese), glimepiride (Amaryl), glipizide (Glucotrol), glyburide (Diabeta), tolazamide, tolbutamide *Biguanide:* metformin (Glucophage) *Alpha glucosidase inhibitors:* acarbose (Precose), miglitol (Glyset) *Meglitinide:* repaglinide (Prandin) *Thiazolidinedione: pioglitazone* (Actos) *Dipeptidyl-peptidase 4 (DPP-4) inhibitor* Sitagliptin (Januvia) *Glucagon-like peptide-1 receptor agonist* exenatide (Byetta)	• *Insulin:* type 1 and type 2 diabetes mellitus when oral antidiabetics, diet, and weight control are ineffective • *Oral antidiabetic:* type 2 diabetes mellitus • *Biguanide:* type 2 diabetes (used to decrease hepatic production of glucose) • *Alpha glucosidase inhibitor:* type 2 diabetes (blocks absorption of carbohydrate) • *Meglitinide:* type 2 diabetes (stimulates release of insulin from pancreas) • *Thiazolidinedione:* type 2 diabetes (reduces cellular insulin resistance)	• Hypersensitivity to a specific insulin • Hypoglycemia • Renal impairment, hepatic dysfunction, alcohol abuse (metformin) • Concomitant administration of other drugs with renal tubular excretion such as cimetidine (metformin) • Impaired liver function (acarbose) • Type 1 diabetes (repaglinide) • New York Heart Association (NYHA) class III or IV cardiac status pioglitazone	• Hypoglycemia • Lipodystrophy (insulin) • Weight gain, GI upset, anorexia, nausea, and diarrhea (metformin) • Vitamin B_{12} malabsorption (metformin) • Risk of lactic acidosis with kidney disease (metformin) • Flatulence, abdominal distention, and diarrhea (acarbose) • May increase liver function test results (acarbose)	• Monitor blood glucose levels. • Assess the patient for signs and symptoms of hypoglycemia and hyperglycemia. • Assess dietary habits and the patient's knowledge of diet restrictions. • Monitor actual dietary intake. • Make sure the patient and family are taught about diabetes and its treatment, including medications, diet, insulin monitoring, hypoglycemia and hyperglycemia, and the effects of illness and stress.
Antithyroids				
methimazole (Tapazole), potassium iodide, propylthiouracil, sodium iodide	• Hyperthyroidism • Graves' disease	• Pregnancy and lactation • Hypersensitivity to iodine or iodide preparations	• Rash • Nausea and vomiting • Anorexia • Hypothyroidism	• Assess the patient's nutritional status. • Monitor T_3 and T_4 levels. • Monitor weight weekly. • Tell the patient to take the medication at the same time every day.
Thyroid Hormones				
levothyroxine (Synthroid), thyroid	• Supplement or replace natural thyroid hormone • Hypothyroidism, myxedema, goiter, postthyroidectomy	• Hyperthyroidism • Thyrotoxicosis • Untreated adrenal insufficiency • Acute MI	• Tachycardia • Nervousness • Insomnia • Increased appetite • Weight loss	• Assess the patient's nutritional status. • Monitor T3 and T4 levels. • Administer the drug in the morning on an empty stomach to prevent insomnia and increase absorption. • Assess the patient for symptoms of cardiovascular disease.

(continued)

Common Drugs	Indications	Contraindications	Adverse Reactions	Nursing Implications
Drugs Used to Treat Inflammation, Allergy, and Organ Rejection				
Adrenocorticosteroids				
cortisone acetate, dexamethasone, hydrocortisone sodium succinate (Solu-Cortef), methylprednisolone (Medrol), methylprednisolone sodium succinate (Solu-Medrol), prednisolone (Prelone), prednisone, triamcinolone	• Replacement therapy in patients with adrenal insufficiency • Shock (to increase cardiac output and blood pressure) • Inflammatory disorders, such as joint diseases, GI disorders, and skin allergies • Cerebral edema	• Peptic ulcer disease • Tuberculosis • Severe infections • Autoimmune disorders, heart failure, diabetes, and glaucoma (use with caution)	• Water and sodium retention • Mood swings • Hyperglycemia • Acne and facial hair growth • GI distress • Masked signs of infection • Hypokalemia	• Monitor weight, blood pressure, and blood counts. • Administer oral doses with milk or food to decrease the risk of GI distress. • Assess the patient for signs and symptoms of fluid retention, hypokalemia, hyperglycemia, and mental changes. • Wean the patient from steroid therapy. • Tell the patient to avoid infected people, immunizations, vaccinations, and skin testing.
Antihistamines				
brompheniramine, cetirizine (Zyrtec), chlorpheniramine, desloratadine (Clarinex), diphenhydramine (Benadryl), fexofenadine (Allegra), loratadine, promethazine	• Allergic symptoms from common allergies, drug allergies, and severe allergic reactions • Nausea and vomiting • Motion sickness • Increase effect of analgesics and promote sedation	• Drug hypersensitivity • Glaucoma • Emphysema • CNS depression and seizure disorders (use with caution)	• Sedation and drowsiness • Dry mouth • Hypotension • GI upset	• Assess the patient for known allergies. • Protect a sedated patient from injury. • Provide adequate hydration. • Tell the patient to avoid activities that require mental alertness, to avoid alcohol, to take the drug with food to prevent GI distress, and to maintain adequate fluid intake.
Immunosuppressants				
azathioprine (Imuran), cyclosporine (Neoral, Sandimmune)	• Prevent rejection of organ transplants • Severe rheumatoid arthritis	• Bone marrow suppression • Severe infections • Kidney and liver disease (use with caution)	• Anorexia • Nausea and vomiting • Chills and fever • Anaphylactic reactions • Oral inflammation	• Assess the patient for signs and symptoms of infection. • Protect the patient from exposure to infectious agents. • Educate the patient and family about the signs and symptoms of infection. • Warn the patient not to use cyclosporine products interchangeably without physician supervision. • Tell the patient to avoid people with infections and to practice strict oral hygiene.

(continued)

Common Drugs	Indications	Contraindications	Adverse Reactions	Nursing Implications
Drugs Used to Treat Infection				
Antibacterials				
Aminoglycosides: amikacin (Amikin), gentamicin (Garamycin), kanamycin, neomycin, streptomycin, tobramycin (Tobrex) *Cephalosporins (1st, 2nd, 3rd, & 4th generations):* cefaclor, cefazolin, cefixime (Suprax), cefoxitin, ceftazidime (Fortaz), ceftriaxone (Rocephin), cefuroxime sodium (Zinacef), cephalexin (Keflex), cefdinir (Omnicef), cefepime (Maxipime) *Fluoroquinolones:* ciprofloxacin (Cipro), levofloxacin (Levaquin), ofloxacin *Penicillins:* amoxicillin, ampicillin (Principen), oxacillin, ticarcillin *Macrolides:* azithromycin (Zithromax), clarithromycin (Biaxin), erythromycin (Erythrocin) *Sulfonamides:* cotrimoxazole (Bactrim), sulfamethoxazole, sulfisoxazole *Tetracyclines:* demeclocycline (Declomycin), doxycycline (Vibramycin), oxytetracycline, tetracycline, minocycline HCL (Minocin) *Other:* chloramphenicol, clindamycin (Cleocin), methenamine hippurate (hiprex), nitrofurantoin (Macrodantin), vancomycin (Vancocin)	• Bacterial infections • Infections caused by spirochetes, rickettsiae, and other organisms • Urinary tract infections (sulfonamides, cephalosporins, methenamine mandelate, nitrofurantoin)	• Hypersensitivity • Liver or renal failure	• Superinfections, especially with broad-spectrum agents • Allergic reactions • GI distress	• Assess the patient for signs and symptoms of infection. • Check for a history of allergy. • Withhold the medication if an allergic response occurs.

(continued)

Common Drugs	Indications	Contraindications	Adverse Reactions	Nursing Implications
Drugs Used to Treat Infection (*continued*)				
Antifungals				
amphotericin B, amphotericin B lipid products (ABELCET, AmBisome, Amphotec), clotrimazole, fluconazole (Diflucan), miconazole, nystatin (Mycostatin)	• Systemic and local fungal infections • Candida infections • Ringworm infections	• Hypersensitivity • Renal failure	• Nausea and vomiting • Blood dyscrasias • Headache, fever, and chills • Skin irritation • Hypersensitivity reactions	• Assess the patient for signs and symptoms of infection. • Assess the infected areas. • Wear gloves when applying topical preparations. • Be aware of proper dosing. Doses of amphotericin B lipid products aren't interchangeable with conventional amphotericin B.
Anthelmintics				
lindane, mebendazole, metronidazole (Flagyl), quinine sulfate	• Malaria • Roundworm, pinworm, whipworm, hookworm, tapeworm, lice, and other parasitic infections	• Myasthenia gravis (quinine) • Pregnancy and lactation	• GI disturbances • Dizziness • Eczema (lindane)	• Teach the patient how to take the medication properly. • Emphasize basic hygiene, such as regular hand hygiene and not sharing personal items with others. • If the patient is receiving metronidazole, assess him for signs of candidal overgrowth. • Advise the patient that all sexual partners should be treated with metronidazole. • Administer quinine with food to prevent GI irritation.
Antituberculotics				
ethambutol (Myambutol), isoniazid (INH), rifampin (Rifadin), rifapentine (Priftin), streptomycin	• Tuberculosis (TB) prevention in those who are exposed to it • Active TB	• Hypersensitivity • Liver disease	• Nausea and vomiting • Risk of damage to the liver, kidneys, and optic nerve	• Assess the patient's pulmonary status. • Keep in mind that antacids can delay the absorption of isoniazid and that isoniazid inhibits phenytoin metabolism. • Tell the patient that rifampin may cause the saliva, sputum, sweat, urine, and stools to appear reddish brown or reddish orange. • Educate the patient and family about the importance of continuing long-term multidose therapy even after symptoms have subsided.

(*continued*)

Common Drugs	Indications	Contraindications	Adverse Reactions	Nursing Implications
Drugs Used to Treat Infection (*continued*)				
Antivirals				
acyclovir (Zovirax), amantadine, didanosine (Videx), famciclovir (Famvir), foscarnet (Foscavir), ganciclovir (Cytovene), indinavir (Crixivan), oseltamivir (Tamiflu), valacyclovir (Valtrex), zalcitabine, zidovudine (Retrovir)	• Viral infections • Genital, encephalic, and ophthalmic herpes simplex • Influenza A and influenza B virus prevention • Human immunodeficiency virus	• Hypersensitivity • Pregnancy	• Dizziness • Headache • Nausea and vomiting • Diarrhea • Hypotension • Renal failure • Peripheral neuropathy • Pancreatitis	• Assess the patient for signs and symptoms of infection. • Maintain adequate fluid intake. • Wear gloves when applying topical preparations.
Antihyperuricemics				
Anti-inflammatory: colchicine *Uric acid synthesis inhibitor:* allopurinol (Zyloprim) *Uricosurics:* probenecid	• Uric acid buildup prevention (probenecid, allopurinol) • Decrease acute joint inflammation from increased uric acid (colchicine)	• History of renal calculi (probenecid) • Hypersensitivity • Impaired liver or kidney function • Peptic ulcer disease	• GI irritation • Skin reactions • Bone marrow depression	• Encourage the patient to drink at least 2 qt (2 L) of fluid per day. • Administer after meals to decrease GI distress. • Tell the patient that he should discontinue allopurinol and call the physician if a rash develops.

Common Infectious Disorders

Disorder	Characteristics
Bacterial Infections	
Anthrax	Bacterial infection characterized as cutaneous, inhalational, or intestinal • Diagnosis confirmed by isolation of *Bacillus anthracis* from cultures of blood, skin, lesions, or sputum • Signs and symptoms directly related to the location of infection. Cutaneous anthrax is characterized by a small, elevated, itchy lesion, which develops into a vesicle and then a painless ulcer, along with enlarged lymph glands. Inhalational anthrax is characterized by flulike symptoms initially, followed by severe respiratory difficulty and shock. With intestinal anthrax, fever, nausea, vomiting, and decreased appetite occur, which progress to abdominal pain, hematemesis, and severe diarrhea.
Chlamydia	Sexually transmitted infection caused by *Chlamydia trachomatis* • Can cause urethritis and pelvic inflammatory disease
Conjunctivitis	Bacterial or viral infection of the conjunctiva of the eye • Culture from the conjunctiva identifies the causative organism. • Associated with hyperemia of the eye, discharge, tearing, pain, and photophobia
Gonorrhea	Sexually transmitted infection caused by *Neisseria gonorrhoeae*, a gram-negative, oxidase-positive *Diplococcus* • After exposure, epithelial cells at infection site become infected and the disease begins to spread locally. • Disease pattern depends on the individual infected and the site of infection.
Listeriosis	Infection caused by weakly hemolytic, gram-positive bacillus *Listeria monocytogenes* • Primary method of person-to-person transmission is neonatal infection in utero or during passage through an infected birth canal. • Disease may cause abortion, premature delivery, stillbirth, or organ abscesses in fetuses. • Neonates may have tense fontanelles due to meningitis, be irritable or lethargic, have seizures, or be comatose.

(continued)

Disorder	Characteristics
Bacterial Infections *(continued)*	
Lyme disease	Infection caused by *Borrelia burgdorferi* spirochetes. • Transmitted by ixodid tick, which injects spirochete-laden saliva into the bloodstream or deposits fecal matter on the skin • After 3 to 32 days, spirochetes migrate outward, typically causing a ringlike rash, called *erythema chronicum migrans.* • Spirochetes disseminate to other skin sites or organs through the bloodstream or lymphatic system. • Spirochetes may survive for years in joints, or they may die after triggering an inflammatory response in the host. • As infection progresses through three stages, neurologic symptoms and impairment worsen.
Meningitis	Meningeal inflammation caused by bacteria, viruses, protozoa, or fungi. The most common types are bacterial and viral. • Disease occurs when infecting organisms enter the subarachnoid space and cause an inflammatory response. The organisms gain access to the cerebrospinal fluid, where they cause irritation of the tissues bathed by the fluid. • Characteristic signs include fever, chills, headache, nuchal rigidity, vomiting, photophobia, lethargy, coma, positive Brudzinski's and Kernig's signs, increased deep tendon reflexes, widened pulse pressure, bradycardia, and rash.
Otitis media	Inflammation of the middle ear caused by a bacterial infection • Disease is commonly accompanied by a viral upper respiratory infection. • Viral symptoms occur, generally followed by ear pain.
Peritonitis	Acute or chronic inflammation of the peritoneum caused by bacterial invasion • Onset commonly sudden, with severe and diffuse abdominal pain • Pain intensifies and localizes in the region of infection.
Pertussis (whooping cough)	Highly contagious respiratory infection usually caused by the nonmotile, gram-negative coccobacillus *Bordetella pertussis* and, occasionally, by the related similar bacteria *B. parapertussis* or *B. bronchiseptica* • Transmitted by direct inhalation of contaminated droplets from a patient in an acute stage. It may also spread indirectly through soiled linen and other articles contaminated by respiratory secretions. • After approximately 7 to 10 days, *B. pertussis* enters the tracheobronchial mucosa, where it produces progressively tenacious mucus. • Known for its associated spasmodic cough, characteristically ending in a loud, crowing inspiratory whoop. Complications include apnea, hypoxia, seizures, pneumonia, encephalopathy, and death.
Pneumonia	Infection of the lung parenchyma that's bacterial, fungal, viral, or protozoal in origin • The lower respiratory tract can be exposed to pathogens by inhalation, aspiration, vascular dissemination, or direct contact with contaminated equipment. When inside, the pathogen begins to colonize and infection develops. • Bacterial infection initially triggers alveolar inflammation and edema, which produces an area of low ventilation with normal perfusion. Capillaries become engorged with blood, causing stasis. As alveolocapillary membranes break down, alveoli fill with blood and exudates, causing atelectasis, or lung collapse.
Salmonellosis	Disease caused by a serotype of the genus *Salmonella*, a member of the *Enterobacteriaceae* family • Most common species of *Salmonella* include *S. typhi*, which causes typhoid fever; *S. enteritidis*, which causes enterocolitis; and *S. choleraesuis*, which causes bacteremia. • Nontyphoidal salmonellosis usually follows ingestion of contaminated dry milk, chocolate bars, pharmaceuticals of animal origin, or contaminated or inadequately processed foods, especially eggs and poultry. • Characteristic symptoms include fever, abdominal pain or cramps, and severe diarrhea with enterocolitis.
Shigellosis	Acute intestinal infection caused by the bacteria *Shigella*, a member of the *Enterobacteriaceae* family. It's a short, nonmotile, gram-negative rod. • Transmission occurs primarily through the fecal-oral route. • After an incubation period of 1 to 4 days, *Shigella* organisms invade the intestinal mucosa and cause inflammation. • Symptoms can range from watery stools to fever, cramps, and stools with pus, mucus, or blood.

(continued)

Disorder	Characteristics
Bacterial Infections (continued)	
Tetanus	Acute exotoxin-mediated infection caused by the anaerobic, spore-forming, gram-positive bacillus *Clostridium tetani* • Transmission occurs through a puncture wound that's contaminated by soil, dust, or animal excreta containing *C. tetani* or by way of burns and minor wounds. • After *C. tetani* enters the body, it causes local infection and tissue necrosis. It also produces toxins that then enter the bloodstream and lymphatics and eventually spread to central nervous system (CNS) tissue. • Disease is characterized by marked muscle hypertonicity, hyperactive deep tendon reflexes, and painful, involuntary muscle contractions. Severe muscle spasms can last up to 7 days.
Toxic shock syndrome (TSS)	Acute bacterial infection caused by toxin-producing, penicillin-resistant strains of *Staphylococcus aureus*, such as TSS toxin-1 or staphylococcal enterotoxins B and C. It can also be caused by *Streptococcus pyogenes*. • Menstrual TSS is associated with tampon use. • Nonmenstrual TSS is associated with infections, such as abscesses, osteomyelitis, pneumonia, endocarditis, bacteremia, and postsurgical infections. • Signs and symptoms include fever, hypotension, renal failure, and multisystem involvement.
Tuberculosis	Infectious disease transmitted by inhaling *Mycobacterium tuberculosis*, an acid-fast bacillus, from an infected person • Bacilli are deposited in the lungs, the immune system responds by sending leukocytes, and inflammation results. After a few days, leukocytes are replaced by macrophages. Bacilli are then ingested by the macrophages and carried off by the lymphatics to the lymph nodes. Macrophages that ingest the bacilli fuse to form epithelioid cell tubercles, tiny nodules surrounded by lymphocytes. • Caseous necrosis develops in the lesion, and scar tissue encapsulates the tubercle. The organism may be killed in the process or exist in a dormant state. • Dormant organisms may reactivate and cause local disease in the presence of immunosuppression.
Urinary tract infection	Infection most commonly caused by enteric gram-negative bacilli • Results from microorganisms entering the urethra and then ascending into the bladder • Commonly causes urgency, frequency, and dysuria
Viral Infections	
Cytomegalovirus infection	A deoxyribonucleic acid (DNA) virus that's a member of the herpes virus group • Transmission can occur horizontally (person-to-person contact with secretions), vertically (mother to neonate), or through blood transfusions. • The virus spreads through the body in lymphocytes or mononuclear cells to the lungs, liver, GI tract, eyes, and CNS, where it commonly produces inflammatory reactions, particularly in immunocompromised hosts.
Ebola	Ebola is an infection caused by a virus in the family of Filoviridae. • The Ebola virus is found in several African countries. • Ebola is spread through blood or body fluids such as urine, saliva, sweat, feces, emesis, breast milk, and semen. It can also be spread by direct contact of bodily fluids with objects such as needles and syringes contaminated with the Ebola virus. • Signs and symptoms generally occur between 2 and 21 days after exposure. Primary clinical manifestations include muscle pain, weakness, diarrhea, fatigue, diarrhea, vomiting, abdominal pain, and unexplained bleeding. • Currently, there is no vaccine or medicine approved to treat Ebola. • (Retrieved from CDC.gov/vhf/ebola/about.html)
Herpes simplex virus (HSV)	HSV is an enveloped, double-stranded DNA virus that causes both herpes simplex type 1 and type 2. • Type 1 HSV is transmitted via oral and respiratory secretions; type 2 HSV is transmitted via sexual contact. • During exposure, the virus fuses to the host cell membrane and releases proteins, turning off the host cell's protein production or synthesis. The virus then replicates and synthesizes structural proteins. The virus pushes its nucleocapsid (protein coat and nucleic acid) into the cytoplasm of the host cell and releases the viral DNA. • Complete virus particles capable of surviving and infecting a living cell are transported to the cell's surface. • Characteristic painful, vesicular lesions are usually observed at the site of initial infection.

(continued)

Disorder	Characteristics
Viral Infections (continued)	
Herpes zoster	Caused by a reactivation of varicella-zoster virus that has been lying dormant in the cerebral ganglia or the ganglia of posterior nerve roots. • Small, painful, red, nodular skin lesions develop on areas along nerve paths. • Lesions change to vesicles filled with pus or fluid.
Human immunodeficiency virus (HIV) infection	A ribonucleic acid (RNA) retrovirus that causes acquired immunodeficiency syndrome (AIDS). • Virus passes from one person to another through blood-to-blood and sexual contact. In addition, an infected pregnant woman can pass HIV to her baby during pregnancy or delivery as well as through breast-feeding. • Most people with HIV infection develop AIDS; however, current combination drug therapy in conjunction with treatment and prophylaxis of common opportunistic infections can delay the natural progression and prolong survival.
Infectious mononucleosis	Viral illness caused by the Epstein-Barr virus, a B-lymphotropic herpes virus. • Most cases spread by the oropharyngeal route, but transmission by blood transfusion or during cardiac surgery is also possible. • The virus invades the B cells of the oropharyngeal lymphoid tissues and then replicates. • Dying B cells release the virus into the blood, causing fever and other symptoms. During this period, antiviral antibodies appear and the virus disappears from the blood, lodging mainly in the parotid gland.
Influenza	A contagious respiratory illness caused by influenza viruses. • Symptoms include fever, cough, sore throat, and muscle aches. • Virus could progress to eye infections, pneumonia, and acute respiratory distress.
Monkeypox	Rare disease caused by the monkeypox virus, which belongs to the Orthopoxvirus group. • In humans, monkeypox causes swollen lymph nodes, fever, headache, muscle aches, backache, exhaustion, and a papular rash with lesions that eventually crust and fall off.
Mumps	Acute viral disease caused by an RNA virus classified as *Rubulavirus* in the *Paramyxoviridae* family • Virus is transmitted by droplets or by direct contact. • Characterized by enlargement and tenderness of parotid gland and swelling of other salivary glands
Rabies	Rapidly progressive infection of the CNS caused by an RNA virus in the *Rhabdoviridae* family • Transmitted by the bite of an infected animal through the skin or mucous membranes or, occasionally, in airborne droplets or infected tissue • The rabies virus begins replicating in the striated muscle cells at the bite site and then spreads along the nerve pathways to the spinal cord and brain, where it replicates again and causes a fatal encephalitis.
Respiratory syncytial virus	Infection of the respiratory tract caused by an enveloped RNA paramyxovirus • The organism is transmitted from person to person by respiratory secretions or by touching contaminated surfaces. • Bronchiolitis or pneumonia ensues and, in severe cases, may damage the bronchiolar epithelium. • Interalveolar thickening and filling of alveolar spaces with fluid may occur. • The virus is more common in winter and early spring.
Rubella	An enveloped positive-stranded RNA virus classified as a Rubivirus in the *Togaviridae* family • Transmitted through contact with the blood, urine, stool, or nasopharyngeal secretions of an infected person. It can also be transmitted transplacentally. • The virus replicates first in the respiratory tract and then spreads through the bloodstream. • Characteristic maculopapular rash usually begins on the face and then spreads rapidly.
Rubeola (measles)	Acute, highly contagious paramyxovirus infection that's spread by direct contact or by contaminated airborne respiratory droplets • Portal of entry is the upper respiratory tract. • Characterized by Koplik's spots (lesions on the buccal mucosa) and a pruritic macular rash that becomes papular and erythematous • Can be associated with encephalitis and pneumonia

(continued)

Disorder	Characteristics
Viral Infections (continued)	
Smallpox	Acute contagious virus caused by the variola virus, a member of the _Orthopoxvirus_ family • Transmitted from person to person by infected aerosols and air droplets. • The incubation period, which is usually 12 to 14 days, is followed by the sudden onset of influenza-like symptoms including fever, malaise, headache, and severe back pain. • Between 2 and 3 days later, the patient may feel better; however, the characteristic rash appears, first on the face, hands, and forearms and then after a few days progressing to the trunk. Lesions also develop in the mucous membranes of the nose and mouth and then ulcerate and release large amounts of virus into the mouth and throat.
Varicella (chickenpox)	Common, highly contagious exanthem caused by the varicella-zoster virus, a member of the herpes virus family • Transmitted by respiratory droplets or contact with vesicles. In utero infection is also possible • Characterized by a pruritic rash of small, erythematous macules that progress to papules and then to clear vesicles on an erythematous base
Viral pneumonia	Lung infection caused by any one of a variety of viruses, transmitted through contact with an infected individual • The virus first attacks bronchiolar epithelial cells, causing interstitial inflammation and desquamation. • Virus invades bronchial mucous glands and goblet cells and then spreads to the alveoli, which fill with blood and fluid. In advanced infection, a hyaline membrane may form.
Zika	A viral infection that is spread primarily from the bite of an _Aedes_ species mosquito • Transmission and spread can also occur from a pregnant woman to her unborn fetus; pregnant women should avoid travel where the Zika virus is prevalent. • Primary symptoms include fever, rash, headache, joint pain, red eyes, and muscle pain. • There is currently no vaccine or medicine approved to treat Zika. (Retrieved from www.cdc.gov/zika)
Fungal Infections	
Histoplasmosis	Fungal infection caused by _Histoplasma capsulatum_, a dimorphic fungus • Transmitted through inhalation of _H. capsulatum_ spores or invasion of spores after minor skin trauma • Initially, infected person may be asymptomatic or have symptoms of mild respiratory illness, sometimes progressing into more severe illness affecting several organ systems.
Protozoal Infections	
Toxoplasmosis	Infection caused by the intracellular parasite _Toxoplasma gondii_, which affects both birds and mammals • Transmitted to humans by ingestion of tissue cysts in raw or undercooked meat or by fecal-oral contamination from infected cats. Direct transmission can also occur during blood transfusions, organ transplants, or bone marrow transplants. • When tissue cysts are ingested, parasites are released, which quickly invade and multiply within the GI tract. The parasitic cells rupture the invaded host cell and then disseminate to the CNS, lymphatic tissue, skeletal muscle, myocardium, retina, and placenta. • As the parasites replicate and invade adjoining cells, cell death and focal necrosis occur, surrounded by an acute inflammatory response, which are the hallmarks of this infection. • After the cysts reach maturity, the inflammatory process is undetectable and the cysts remain latent within the brain until they rupture. • In the normal host, the immune response checks the infection, but this isn't so with immunocompromised or fetal hosts. In these patients, focal destruction results in necrotizing encephalitis, pneumonia, myocarditis, and organ failure.
Trichinosis	Infection caused by the parasite _Trichinella spiralis_ and transmitted through ingestion of uncooked or undercooked meat that contains encysted larvae • After gastric juices free the larva from the cyst capsule, it reaches sexual maturity in a few days. The female roundworm burrows into the intestinal mucosa and reproduces. • Larvae then travel through the lymphatic system and the bloodstream. They become embedded as cysts in striated muscle, especially in the diaphragm, chest, arms, and legs.

CDC Hand Hygiene Guidelines Fact Sheet

The Centers for Disease Control and Prevention (CDC) has released these guidelines to improve adherence to hand hygiene in health care settings.

- Improved adherence to hand hygiene (i.e., hand washing or use of alcohol-based hand rubs) has been shown to terminate infection outbreaks in health care facilities; reduce transmission of antimicrobial-resistant organisms, such as methicillin-resistant *Staphylococcus aureus* (MRSA); and reduce overall infection rates.
- In addition to traditional handwashing with soap and water, the CDC recommends the use of alcohol-based hand rubs by health care personnel for patient care because these products address some of the obstacles that health care professionals face when caring for patients.
- Handwashing with soap and water remains a sensible strategy for hand hygiene in non–health care settings and is recommended by the CDC and other experts.
- Health care personnel should wash with soap and water when their hands are visibly soiled.
- The use of gloves does not eliminate the need for hand hygiene. Likewise, the use of hand hygiene does not eliminate the need for gloves. Gloves reduce hand contamination by 70% to 80%, prevent cross-contamination, and protect patients and health care personnel from infection. Hand rubs should be used before and after contact with each patient just as gloves should be changed before and after contact with each patient.
- When using an alcohol-based hand rub, the product should be applied to the palm of one hand. The hands and fingers should then be rubbed together, covering all surfaces, until hands are dry. Note that the volume needed to reduce the number of bacteria on hands varies by product.
- Alcohol-based hand rubs significantly reduce the number of microorganisms on the skin, are fast acting, and are less likely to cause skin irritation.
- Health care personnel who care for patients who are at high risk of acquiring infections, such as those in intensive care units (ICU) or in transplant units, should avoid wearing artificial nails and keep natural nails less than a quarter-inch long. When evaluating hand hygiene products for potential use in health care facilities, administrators or product selection committees should consider the relative efficacy of antiseptic agents against various pathogens and the acceptability of hand hygiene products by personnel. Characteristics of a product that can affect acceptance and therefore usage include its smell, consistency, and color as well as its effect on the skin, particularly skin dryness.
- As part of its recommendations, the CDC is asking health care facilities to develop and implement a system for measuring improvements in adherence to these hand hygiene guidelines. Some of the suggested performance indicators include periodic monitoring of hand hygiene adherence and providing feedback to personnel regarding their performance, monitoring the volume of alcohol-based hand rub used per 1,000 patient-days, monitoring adherence to policies dealing with wearing artificial nails, and diligently assessing the adequacy of health care personnel hand hygiene when outbreaks of infection occur.
- Allergic contact dermatitis due to alcohol hand rubs is very uncommon. However, with increasing use of such products by health care personnel, it is likely that true allergic reactions will occasionally be encountered.
- Cleansing with alcohol-based hand rubs takes less time than traditional handwashing. In an 8-hour shift, an estimated 1 hour of an ICU nurse's time will be saved by using an alcohol-based hand rub.
- The guidelines should not be construed to legalize product claims that are not allowed by a Food and Drug Administration (FDA) product approval according to the FDA's *Over-the-Counter Drug Review*, nor are they intended to apply to consumer use of the products discussed.

Source: Centers for Disease Control and Prevention. (2002, October 25). *Hand hygiene fact sheet*. Office of Communication, Division of Media Relations. Retrieved from http://cdc.gov/media/pressrel/fs021025.htm

CDC Isolation Precautions

Standard precautions are generally always used unless otherwise indicated, or they are used in conjunction with other precaution measures. The length of time for isolation precautions will vary depending on the nature and seriousness of the patient's infection or disease. Check with the facility's infection control department, local and state health departments, and the Centers for Disease Control and Prevention (CDC), because recommendations can change for individual diseases or for new and emerging infections.

Precautions	Equipment Needed	Indications
Standard precautions: Used for all patients regardless of diagnosis or presumed infection	• Gloves are indicated for use with all patients when touching blood and body fluids, mucous membranes, or broken skin, when handling items or touching surfaces soiled with blood or body fluids, and when performing venipuncture and other vascular access procedures. • Masks and protective eyewear or a face shield are needed to protect mucous membranes of the mouth, nose, and eyes during procedures that may generate drops of blood or other body fluids. • A gown or apron is indicated during procedures that are likely to generate splashing of blood or other body fluids.	Used when coming in contact with any of the following: • Blood • All body fluids, secretions, and excretions, except sweat, regardless of whether they contain visible blood • Skin that is not intact • Mucous membranes
Airborne precautions (used in addition to standard precautions): Used when microorganisms may be carried through air and dispersed widely by air currents, resulting in inhalation or deposition on a susceptible host	• Special air handling and ventilation procedures are needed to prevent the spread of infection. • Use of an N95 particulate respirator is indicated when entering an infected patient's room.	Used for patients known to have or suspected of having a serious illness transmitted by airborne droplet nuclei, such as: • Herpes zoster virus • Influenza virus (H1N1 strain) • Monkeypox virus • Rubeola (measles) • Severe acute respiratory syndrome • Smallpox (variola) • Tuberculosis, mycobacterial infection • Varicella-zoster virus
Droplet precautions (used in addition to standard precautions): Used when infectious agents may be transmitted through large-particle droplets (>5 μm) traveling short distances of 3′ or less and/or when those droplets may come in contact with the conjunctivae or nasal or oral mucous membranes of a susceptible person	• A mask is indicated to protect the mucous membranes.	Used for patients known to have or suspected of having a serious illness transmitted by large-particle droplets, such as: • Epiglottiditis (due to *Haemophilus influenzae* type b) • Diphtheria (pharyngeal) • Influenza virus (human seasonal, pandemic) • Meningitis (*H. influenzae* type b) • Meningococcal disease (sepsis, meningitis, pneumonia) • Mumps (infectious parotitis) • *Mycoplasma pneumoniae* • Parvovirus B19 (*erythema infectiosum*) • Pertussis (whooping cough) • Pneumonic plague (Yersinia pestis) • Pneumonia (adenovirus; *H. influenzae* type b in infants and children; meningococcal; group A *Streptococcus*) • Rhinovirus

(continued)

Precautions	Equipment Needed	Indications
		• Rubella (German measles) • Rubeola • Severe acute respiratory syndrome • Streptococcal disease (group A major skin disease, wound, or burn; pharyngitis or scarlet fever in infants and young children; pneumonia; serious invasive disease) • Viral hemorrhagic fever viruses (Lassa, Ebola, Marburg, Crimean-Congo)
Contact precautions (used in addition to standard precautions): Used to reduce the risk of transmitting infectious agents by direct or indirect contact (direct contact transmission can occur through patient care activities that require physical contact; indirect contact transmission involves a susceptible host coming in contact with a contaminated, usually inanimate, object in the patient's environment)	• A gown and gloves are indicated, and dedicated equipment (thermometer, stethoscope, and blood pressure cuff) is used for each patient.	Used for patients known to have or suspected of having a serious illness easily transmitted by direct patient contact or by contact with items in the patient's environment, such as: • Bronchiolitis • *Clostridium difficile* gastroenteritis • Congenital rubella • Conjunctivitis (acute viral/acute hemorrhagic) • Cutaneous diphtheria • Ebola virus • Furunculosis, staphylococcal infection (infants and young children) • Hepatitis A virus (diapered or incontinent patients) • Herpes simplex virus (herpesvirus hominis): mucocutaneous (disseminated or primary severe) or neonatal • Herpes zoster virus • Human metapneumovirus • Impetigo • Influenza, avian virus (H5N1, H7, and H9 strains) • Pediculosis (head lice) • Monkeypox • Multidrug-resistant organisms, infection, or colonization (MRSA, vancomycin-resistant *Enterococcus*, vancomycin-intermediate and vancomycin-resistant *S. aureus*, extended-spectrum beta-lactamase–resistant *S. pneumoniae*) • Parainfluenza virus infection, respiratory infection in infants and young children • Pneumonia (adenovirus, *Burkholderia cepacia*) • Poliomyelitis • Pressure ulcer (major, infected) • Respiratory infectious disease (acute in infants and children) • Respiratory syncytial virus (infants, young children, and immunocompromised adults) • Rotavirus (gastroenteritis) • Scabies • Severe acute respiratory syndrome • Shigellosis • Smallpox (variola) • Staphylococcal disease (major) • Streptococcal disease (group A major skin, wound, or burn) • Vaccinia virus (vaccination site infection with eczema vaccinatum; fetal, generalized, or progressive vaccinia) • Varicella-zoster virus • Viral hemorrhagic fever viruses (Lassa, Ebola, Marburg, Crimean-Congo) • Wound infections (major)

Data from Siegel, J. D., Rhinehart, E., Jackson, M., Chiarello, L., & the Healthcare Infection Control Practices Advisory Committee. (2007). *2007 guideline for isolation precautions: Preventing transmission of infectious agents in healthcare settings.* Retrieved from http://www.cdc.gov/hicpac/pdf/isolation/Isolation2007.pdf

Guide to Laboratory Test Results

This chart provides normal values for common laboratory tests, including chemistry, hematology, and coagulation tests. Where indicated, conventional and SI units are given.

Laboratory Test	Conventional	SI Units
Comprehensive Metabolic Panel		
Alanine aminotransferase	Male: 10 to 40 U/L Female: 7 to 35 U/L	0.17 to 0.68 µkat/L 0.12 to 0.60 µkat/L
Albumin	3.5 to 5 g/dL	35 to 50 g/L
Alkaline phosphatase	45 to 115 U/L	45 to 115 U/L
Aspartate aminotransferase	10 to 36 U/L	0.17 to 0.60 µkat/L
Bilirubin, total	0.3 to 1 mg/dL	5 to 17 µmol/L
Blood urea nitrogen	6 to 20 mg/dL	2.1 to 7.5 mmol/L
Calcium	8.8 to 10.4 mg/dL	2.2 to 2.6 mmol/L
Carbon dioxide	22 to 26 mEq/L	22 to 26 mmol/L
Chloride	100 to 108 mEq/L	100 to 108 mmol/L
Creatinine	Male: 0.8 to 1.3 mg/dL Female: 0.6 to 0.9 mg/dL	62 to 115 µmol/L 53 to 97 µmol/L
Glucose	70 to 100 mg/dL	3.9 to 6.1 mmol/L
Potassium	3.5 to 5.2 mEq/L	3.5 to 5.2 mmol/L
Protein, total	6.3 to 8.3 g/dL	64 to 83 g/L
Sodium	136 to 145 mEq/L	136 to 145 mmol/L
Lipid Panel		
Total cholesterol	<200 mg/dL	<5.05 mmol/L
High-density lipoprotein cholesterol	>60 mg/dL	>1.55 mmol/L
Low-density lipoprotein cholesterol	<130 mg/dL	<3.36 mmol/L
Very-low–density lipoprotein cholesterol	<130 mg/dL	<3.4 mmol/L
Triglycerides	<150 mg/dL	<1.7 mmol/L
Thyroid Panel		
Thyroid-stimulating hormone	0.4 to 4.2 mIU/L	0.4 to 4.2 mIU/L
Thyroxine, free	0.9 to 2.3 ng/dL	10 to 30 nmol/L
Thyroxine, total	5 to 13.5 mcg/dL	60 to 165 mmol/L
Triiodothyronine	80 to 200 ng/dL	1.2 to 3 nmol/L
Other Chemistry Tests		
Albumin, globulin ratio	3.4 to 4.8 g/dL	34 to 38 g/dL
Ammonia	<50 ng/dL	<36 µmol/L
Amylase	25 to 125 U/L	0.4 to 2.1 µkat/L

(continued)

Laboratory Test	Conventional	SI Units
Other Chemistry Tests (continued)		
Anion gap	8 to 14 mEq/L	8 to 14 mmol/L
Bilirubin, direct	<0.5 mg/dL	<6.8 μmol/L
Calcitonin	Male: <16 pg/mL Female: <8 pg/mL	<16 ng/L <8 ng/L
Calcium, ionized	4.65 to 5.28 mg/dL	1.1 to 1.25 mmol/L
Cortisol	a.m.: 7 to 25 mcg/dL p.m.: 2 to 14 mcg/dL	0.2 to 0.7 μmol/L 0.06 to 0.39 μmol/L
C-reactive protein	<0.8 mg/dL	<0.8 mg/L
Ferritin	Male: 20 to 300 ng/mL Female: 20 to 120 ng/mL	20 to 300 mcg/L 20 to 120 mcg/L
Folate	1.8 to 20 ng/mL	4.5 to 45.3 nmol/L
Gamma glutamyltransferase	Male: 7 to 47 U/L Female: 5 to 25 U/L	0.12 to 1.80 μkat/L 0.08 to 0.42 μkat/L
Glycosylated hemoglobin	4% to 7%	0.04 to 0.07
Homocysteine	<12 μmol/L	<12 μmol/L
Iron	Male: 65 to 175 mcg/dL Female: 50 to 170 mcg/dL	11.6 to 31.3 μmol/L 9 to 30.4 μmol/L
Iron-binding capacity	250 to 400 mcg/dL	45 to 72 μmol/L
Lactic acid	0.5 to 2.2 mEq/L	0.5 to 2.2 mmol/L
Lipase	Adults over 60: 10 to 140 U/L Adults under 60: 18 to 180 U/L	0.17 to 2.3 μkat/L 0.30 to 3 μkat/L
Magnesium	1.8 to 2.6 mg/dL	0.74 to 1.07 mmol/L
Osmolality	275 to 295 mOsm/kg	275 to 295 mOsm/kg
Phosphate	2.7 to 4.5 mg/dL	0.87 to 1.45 mmol/L
Prealbumin	19 to 38 mg/dL	190 to 380 mg/L
Uric acid	Male: 3.4 to 7 mg/dL Female: 2.3 to 6 mg/dL	202 to 416 μmol/L 143 to 357 μmol/L
Hematology Tests		
Hematocrit	Male: 42% to 52% Female: 36% to 48%	0.42 to 0.52 0.36 to 0.48
Hemoglobin	Male: 14 to 17.4 g/dL Female: 12 to 16 g/dL	140 to 174 g/L 120 to 160 g/L

Leukocytes
• Bands
• Basophils
• Eosinophils
• Lymphocytes
  ○ B lymphocytes
  ○ T lymphocytes
• Monocytes
• Neutrophils
	4,000 to 10,000/mm³
	0% to 5%
	0% to 1%
	1% to 3%
	25% to 40%
	270 to 640/mm³
	1,400 to 2,700/mm³
	2% to 7%
	54% to 75%
		4 to 10 × 10⁹/L
		0.03 to 0.08
		0 to 0.01
		0.01 to 0.03
		0.25 to 0.40
		—
		—
		0.02 to 0.07
		0.54 to 0.75

(continued)

Laboratory Test	Conventional	SI Units
Hematology Tests *(continued)*		
Platelets	140,000 to 400,000/mm³	140 to 400 × 10⁹/L
Red blood cell	Male: 4.2 to 5.4 million/mm³ Female: 3.6 to 5 million/mm³	4.2 to 5.4 × 10¹²/L 3.6 to 5 × 10¹²/L
Coagulation Tests		
Activated clotting time	107 ± 13 seconds	107 ± 13 seconds
Bleeding time	3 to 6 minutes	3 to 6 minutes
D-Dimer	<250 mcg/L	<1.37 nmol/L
Fibrinogen	200 to 400 mg/dL	2 to 4 g/L
International normalized ratio (therapeutic target)	2.0 to 3.0	2.0 to 3.0
Partial thromboplastin time	21 to 35 seconds	21 to 35 seconds
Prothrombin time	10 to 13 seconds	10 to 13 seconds

Posttest

Instructions

This posttest has been designed to evaluate your readiness to take the certification examination for medical-surgical nursing. Similar in form and content to the actual examination, the posttest consists of 150 questions based on brief clinical situations. The questions will help sharpen your test-taking skills while assessing your knowledge of medical-surgical nursing theory and practice.

To improve your chances for performing well, consider these suggestions:

1. Read each clinical situation and question closely. Weigh the four options carefully and then select the option that best answers the question. (*Note:* In this posttest, options are lettered A, B, C, and D to aid in later identification of correct answers and rationales. These letters won't appear on the certification examination.)
2. Completely darken the circle in front of the answer that you select using a #2 pencil. (You must use a #2 pencil when taking the certification examination if you take a paper and pencil test.) Don't use check marks, Xs, or lines.
3. If you decide to change your answer, erase the old answer completely. (The certification examination is scored electronically; an incomplete erasure may cause both answers to be scored, in which case you won't receive credit for answering the question.)
4. If you have difficulty understanding a question or are unsure of the answer, place a small mark next to the question number and, if time permits, return to it later. If you have no idea of the correct answer, make an educated guess. (Only correct answers are counted in scoring the certification examination, so guessing is preferable to leaving a question unanswered.)
5. After you complete the posttest, check your responses against the correct answers and rationales provided on pages 392 to 405.
6. Now, select a quiet room where you'll be undisturbed and begin.

Questions

Question 1. Prevention and early treatment of Lyme's disease are crucial because late complications of this disease include:

A. arthritis.
B. lung abscess.
C. renal failure.
D. sterility.

Question 2. A patient, age 28, is admitted with a suspected malignant melanoma on his left shoulder. When performing the physical assessment, the nurse would expect to find

A. a brown birthmark that has lightened in color.
B. a brown or black mole with red, white, or blue areas.
C. a red birthmark that has recently become darker.
D. an area of diffuse petechiae.

Question 3. A patient, age 32, is admitted with a tentative diagnosis of acquired immunodeficiency syndrome (AIDS). The practitioner orders a biopsy of his facial lesions; the preliminary biopsy report indicates Kaposi's sarcoma. The nurse's *best* approach would be to

A. explore the patient's feelings about his facial disfigurement.
B. inform the patient of the biopsy results, and support him emotionally.
C. pretend not to notice the lesions on the patient's face.
D. tell the patient that Kaposi's sarcoma is common in people with AIDS.

Question 4. A patient who is human immunodeficiency virus (HIV) positive begins zidovudine therapy. Which statement *best* describes the action of this drug?

A. It clears up skin lesions.
B. It eliminates the virus that causes AIDS.
C. It interferes with viral replication.
D. It stimulates the immune system.

Question 5. During routine hygiene care for a patient with AIDS, a nurse following standard precautions would take which action?

A. Place the patient in a private room.
B. Put on a mask, gloves, and a gown.
C. Use reverse isolation.
D. Wear gloves when giving mouth care.

Question 6. When assessing the skin of a patient with deep partial-thickness burns, what would the nurse expect to find?

A. Blisters of varying sizes, with areas of charred tissue
B. Cherry-red areas with weeping blisters
C. Dry, pale areas with no blister formation
D. Pearly-white areas with charred tissue

Question 7. A patient, age 23, underwent a rhinoplasty 6 hours ago. After administering his pain medication, the nurse notes that he is swallowing frequently. What is the most likely cause of the swallowing?

A. A normal response to the analgesic
B. An adverse reaction to the analgesic
C. Bleeding posterior to the nasal packing
D. Oral dryness caused by nasal packing

Question 8. A patient, age 72, has otosclerosis and is scheduled for a stapedectomy. During preoperative teaching, which instruction should the nurse give?

A. "Cough and sneeze with your mouth closed."
B. "Lie on the bed with your operative ear facing up."
C. "Try to get up and walk around as soon as you return from the operating room."
D. "Turn your head rapidly to prevent dizziness."

Question 9. During an eye assessment, a patient complains that "a curtain seems to be coming down in front of my eye." This complaint suggests which condition?

A. Blepharitis
B. Cataract
C. Glaucoma
D. Retinal detachment

Question 10. A patient, age 64, is receiving treatment for heart failure. The nurse should plan to teach about which drugs?

A. Antibiotics, vasopressors, and steroids
B. Digoxin, vasodilating agents, and diuretics
C. Vasoconstricting agents, beta-adrenergic blockers, and digoxin
D. Vasodilating agents, digoxin, and anti-inflammatory agents

Question 11. When assessing the patient with an acute dissecting thoracic aortic aneurysm, which finding would the nurse expect?

A. Decreased hemoglobin level and hematocrit
B. Hypertension
C. Severe chest pain
D. Slow respiratory rate

Question 12. A patient, age 72, has vascular disease. Which nursing intervention would be appropriate?

A. Advise him to wear knee-length stockings.
B. Caution him not to exercise daily.
C. Encourage him to avoid caffeine and nicotine.
D. Instruct him to soak both feet in cool water.

Question 13. A patient, age 38, has acute bronchitis. The nurse formulates a nursing diagnosis of *Ineffective airway clearance*. After implementing the care plan, the nurse would expect which outcome? The patient

A. exhibits increased anxiety.
B. maintains a respiratory rate of 24 breaths/minute.
C. maintains an arterial oxygen saturation of 90%.
D. maintains clear breath sounds.

Question 14. A patient, age 27, is admitted with complaints of severe fatigue, muscle weakness, and anorexia. He states he is recovering from the flu and has had severe nausea, frequent vomiting, and diarrhea. Blood is drawn for serum electrolyte measurements. Based on the patient's symptoms, the nurse should expect to find below normal levels of

A. bicarbonate.
B. calcium.
C. potassium.
D. sodium.

Question 15. The nurse who elicits a positive Chvostek's sign would suspect that the patient has which condition?

A. Hypercalcemia
B. Hyperkalemia
C. Hypocalcemia
D. Hypernatremia

Question 16. A patient, age 18, develops diabetes insipidus after a severe closed head injury. Which assessment findings would indicate that he also has hypernatremia?

A. Anorexia, muscle cramps, and a serum sodium level greater than 135 mEq/L
B. Cardiac arrhythmias, muscle weakness, nausea, and vomiting
C. Numbness, muscle cramps, and a positive Trousseau's sign
D. Thirst, dry and swollen tongue, and disorientation

Question 17. A patient, age 63, is resuscitated successfully after cardiac arrest. Blood studies show he is acidotic—a common finding in patients who have suffered cardiac arrest. What is the most likely explanation for the acidic serum pH?

A. Decreased tissue perfusion causes lactic acid production.
B. High doses of sodium bicarbonate administered affected the pH.
C. Irregular cardiac rhythms decrease cardiac output.
D. Fat-forming ketoacids are broken down.

Question 18. A patient, age 52, is admitted with a diagnosis of Cushing's syndrome. When analyzing the patient's laboratory data, the nurse expect to find

A. a decreased WBC count, hyponatremia, metabolic acidosis, and hyperglycemia.
B. decreased cortisol levels, an elevated serum glucose level, hypocalcemia, and hyponatremia.
C. glycosuria, hyperkalemia, a decreased cortisol level, and metabolic alkalosis.
D. hyperglycemia, an increased white blood cell (WBC) count, and elevated cortisol levels.

Question 19. A patient, age 68, has benign prostatic hyperplasia. He is admitted for cystoscopy and transurethral resection of the prostate (TURP). During preoperative teaching, the nurse notes that the patient seems very anxious. Exploring the patient's anxiety, the nurse learns he is sexually active and is worried about becoming impotent. How should the nurse deal with his concerns?

A. Advise him that TURP seldom causes impotence.
B. Advise him to speak with the surgeon.
C. Refer him to the psychiatric clinical nurse specialist.
D. Tell him not to worry because he will not become impotent after surgery.

Question 20. Six hours after undergoing TURP, a patient complains of severe bladder spasms. The nurse notes that his urinary drainage is burgundy colored and contains large clots, his skin feels cool to the touch, and a rounded swelling is palpable above his symphysis pubis. Which action should the nurse implement first?

A. Administer ordered antispasmodic agents.
B. Assess the patency of the continuous irrigation system.
C. Assess the patient for indications of shock.
D. Notify the attending practitioner.

Question 21. A patient, age 34, is scheduled for discharge after undergoing a modified retroperitoneal lymph node dissection for testicular cancer. He seems quiet and depressed, and the nurse asks if he has anything on his mind. "Now that I'm ready to go home," he says, "I keep thinking about the practitioner telling me I'll be sterile. I'm worried about how my wife will react, even though we didn't plan to have children." What would be the nurse's best response?

A. "Don't worry about being sterile if you didn't plan on having children anyway."
B. "I think you should ask the surgeon to talk with you and your wife about your concerns."
C. "Sterility is an expected result of the treatment. You can feel comforted by the fact that this disease has a high cure rate."
D. "Would you like to talk about your concerns?"

Question 22. During an assessment of a 32-year-old patient with endometriosis, the nurse is most likely to find

A. changes in body image, self-concept, and sexuality.
B. chronic, severe pain related to menstruation.
C. high anxiety with a need for perfection and control.
D. loss and grieving associated with infertility problems.

Question 23. A patient, age 49, returns from the postanesthesia care unit after a total abdominal hysterectomy and bilateral salpingo-oophorectomy to treat cervical cancer. Which nursing intervention has the highest priority at this time?

A. Assess the patient's pain level and response to analgesics.
B. Encourage the patient to do deep breathing and leg exercises.
C. Monitor the patient for indications of hemorrhage.
D. Provide emotional support to the patient.

Question 24. A patient, age 64, is found on the floor of his bathroom in his apartment after apparently falling and hitting his head on the bathtub. On admission to the neurologic unit, he has a decreased level of consciousness (LOC). The practitioner's orders are to elevate the head of the bed; keep the patient's head in neutral alignment, without neck flexion or head rotation; avoid sharp hip flexion; give an acetaminophen suppository, 300 mg, every 6 hours if the patient's temperature exceeds 99.8°F (37.7°C); and give dextrose 5% in water (D_5W) at 20 mL/hour. Which statement best describes the rationale for the positioning order?

A. It decreases cerebral arterial pressure.
B. It does not impede venous outflow.
C. It prevents aspiration of stomach contents.
D. It prevents flexion contractures.

Question 25. A patient with a head injury and reduced LOC is placed on a hypothermia blanket and given antipyretic medication. Which statement best describes the therapeutic value of these interventions?

A. They prevent hypoxia associated with diaphoresis.
B. They promote equalization of osmotic pressures.
C. They promote the integrity of intracerebral neurons.
D. They reduce brain metabolism and limit hypoxia.

Question 26. A patient, age 76, is transferred to the medical-surgical unit from the emergency department (ED) with a diagnosis of left-sided stroke in evolution. On admission to the unit, he has a blood pressure of 150/90 mm Hg, an apical pulse of 78 beats/minute and regular, a respiratory rate of 20 breaths/minute, and a rectal temperature of 100°F (37.8°C). The practitioner orders oxygen by nasal cannula at 2 L/minute; vital sign assessment every hour for the first 4 hours, every 2 hours for the next 4 hours, and then every 4 hours; I.V. D_5W in half-normal saline solution at a rate of 100 mL/hour; and no oral intake. When helping to transfer the patient to his bed, the nurse notices a snoring quality to his respirations. Which nursing action is the highest priority at this time?

A. Assess the patient's ability to communicate his needs.
B. Place items the patient may need to the right side of the bed.
C. Place the patient in Fowler's position.
D. Position the patient on his side, with the head of the bed elevated slightly.

Question 27. Two hours after a patient with left-sided stroke in evolution was admitted to the unit, the nurse measures his blood pressure at 170/80 mm Hg, apical pulse at 58 beats/minute and regular, respiratory rate at 14 breaths/minute, and axillary temperature at 101°F (38.3°C). What is the first action the nurse should take at this time?

A. Assess the patient for a distended bladder.
B. Assess the patient for signs of overhydration.
C. Assess the patient's vital signs more frequently.
D. Report the patient's vital signs to the practitioner.

Question 28. A patient, age 68, has a primary brain tumor. During the past 18 months, he has been admitted to the neurologic unit several times for surgery, radiation therapy, and chemotherapy. Today, he is admitted to investigate a recent onset of seizures. The nurse notes that the patient has become listless and sleepy. Which action should the nurse take first?

A. Ask the patient how he is feeling.
B. Assess the patient's verbal and motor responses and ability to open his eyes.
C. Call the practitioner and report the findings.
D. Continue observing the patient's behavior, which may be an adverse effect of phenytoin.

Question 29. A patient, age 16, has type 1 diabetes mellitus and is in the hospital for regulation of his disease. He tells the nurse he feels hungry, thirsty, tired, and weak, and he frequently asks to use the bathroom. What should the nurse do first?

A. Administer the patient's prescribed insulin.
B. Determine the patient's blood glucose level.
C. Give an additional snack with the patient's next meal.
D. Notify the practitioner immediately.

Question 30. A patient, age 39, has type 1 diabetes mellitus. When he arrives at the ED complaining of dizziness, the nurse notes that he seems weak, confused, and disoriented. His wife states that he took his usual morning dose of 6 units of regular insulin and 15 units of NPH insulin but ate little of his breakfast. What is the most likely cause of the patient's signs and symptoms?

A. Hyperglycemia
B. Hyperlipidemia
C. Hypoglycemia
D. Ketoacidosis

Question 31. A patient, age 19, is HIV positive. A diagnosis of AIDS would be confirmed when

A. malignant (non-Hodgkin's) lymphoma is diagnosed.
B. seroconversion takes place.
C. the enzyme-linked immunosorbent assay (ELISA) test is positive.
D. the Western blot test is positive.

Question 32. A patient, age 60, is admitted to the hospital with a diagnosis of pneumonia in the left lower lobe. His arterial blood gas (ABG) findings include pH 7.35, Pao_2 60 mm Hg, $Paco_2$ 40 mm Hg, and HCO_3^- 34 mEq/L. Based on these results, which nursing diagnosis has the highest priority?

A. Impaired gas exchange
B. Ineffective airway clearance
C. Ineffective breathing pattern
D. Risk for infection

Question 33. A patient, age 54, seeks medical attention for low-grade afternoon fevers, night sweats, loss of appetite, and a productive cough. The practitioner suspects pulmonary tuberculosis (TB), especially after the patient remarks that his wife recently was diagnosed with TB. A positive acid-fast bacillus sputum culture confirms that the patient has TB. Which nursing diagnosis has the highest priority?

A. Anxiety related to hearing the diagnosis
B. Deficient knowledge related to spread of the infection
C. Imbalanced nutrition: Less than body requirements related to not eating
D. Risk for injury related to infection

Question 34. A patient is taking isoniazid to treat TB. Which instruction should the nurse give him about this drug?

A. Drinking alcohol daily can cause drug-induced hepatitis.
B. Taking isoniazid with aluminum hydroxide minimizes GI upset.
C. Isoniazid is best absorbed when taken on an empty stomach.
D. Prolonged use of isoniazid causes dark, concentrated urine.

Question 35. A patient, age 41, undergoes a mitral valve replacement. Postoperatively, he has a chest tube connected to an underwater seal with suction. Three days after surgery, the nurse detects no bubbling in the underwater seal compartment. What would be the best nursing action at this time?

A. Assure the patient he is progressing and that the system is working properly.
B. Check the practitioner's order for amount of suction and increase the water seal by 10 cm.
C. Milk the chest tube, using slow, even strokes.
D. Speak with the practitioner to increase the amount of suction ordered.

Question 36. A patient, age 63, is admitted with acute bronchopneumonia. The nurse notes that he is in moderate respiratory distress. The patient has a history of emphysema-type chronic obstructive pulmonary disease (COPD). The practitioner orders strict bed rest. Which position would help the patient feel most comfortable?

A. High Fowler's position, using the bedside table as an armrest
B. Side-lying position with the head elevated 45 degrees
C. Semi-Fowler's position with legs elevated
D. Sims' position with the head elevated 90 degrees

Question 37. A patient, age 58, is brought to the ED complaining of chest pain and light-headedness. He has a history of stable angina pectoris. Blood is drawn for analysis, and an electrocardiogram (ECG) is done. A change in which component of the ECG tracing would alert the nurse that the patient is having a myocardial infarction (MI)?

A. P wave
B. R wave
C. QRS complex
D. ST segment

Question 38. The practitioner orders I.V. streptokinase for a patient with an evolving MI. During streptokinase therapy, the most important nursing assessment is for

A. cardiac arrhythmias.
B. increased chest pain.
C. signs of bleeding.
D. signs of pulmonary edema.

Question 39. A patient develops left ventricular dysfunction secondary to an MI. During the physical assessment, the nurse would expect to find:

A. bilateral basilar crackles.
B. elevated central venous pressure.
C. hepatojugular reflux.
D. pitting sacral edema.

Question 40. While monitoring a patient's cardiac rhythm, the nurse observes seven multifocal premature ventricular contractions (PVCs) on a 1-minute rhythm strip. What should the nurse do first?

A. Administer lidocaine as prescribed.
B. Change the ECG leads.
C. Continue to monitor the patient.
D. Have the patient change position.

Question 41. A patient, age 48, is recovering from an MI. When preparing him for discharge, the nurse should include all of the following instructions except:

A. "Avoid extremes of heat and cold."
B. "Eat several small meals each day."
C. "Lift weights daily to strengthen your arms."
D. "Monitor your pulse during physical activity."

Question 42. A patient is admitted with a diagnosis of hepatitis B. To prevent the spread of this infection, which measure is appropriate?

A. Blood and body fluid precautions
B. Contact precautions
C. Enteric precautions
D. Respiratory precautions

Question 43. For a patient with hepatitis B, which nursing intervention is not appropriate?

A. Assess the skin for excoriation.
B. Encourage frequent, small meals.
C. Provide rest periods after meals.
D. Provide a low-protein diet.

Question 44. A patient, age 53, comes to the ED short of breath. His respiratory rate is 45 breaths/minute; he cannot speak because of severe dyspnea. The patient's history reveals an MI and several episodes of heart failure. When auscultating his chest, what would the nurse expect to hear?

A. A friction rub and clear breath sounds
B. A friction rub and crackles
C. A murmur and crackles
D. An S_3 gallop and crackles

Question 45. A patient, age 55, is admitted with cor pulmonale secondary to advanced COPD. He has been a coal miner for 35 years. When performing the physical assessment, what would the nurse expect to find?

A. Distended neck veins, cyanosis, and reduced expiratory phase
B. Distended neck veins, right upper quadrant tenderness, and dependent edema
C. Dyspnea, cyanosis, and increased respiratory excursion
D. Dyspnea, cyanosis, and reduced respiratory rate

Question 46. Which nursing intervention would be most effective in improving the breathing of a patient with COPD?

A. Administering oxygen as prescribed
B. Alternating rest and activity
C. Implementing postural drainage and percussion
D. Teaching pursed-lip breathing

Question 47. A patient, age 64, is ready for discharge after hospitalization for an exacerbation of COPD. Which statement by the patient would indicate that he understands his discharge instructions?

A. "I'll eat several small meals during the day."
B. "I should do my most difficult activities when I first get up in the morning."
C. "I should plan to do my exercises after I eat."
D. "I should take my medicine at bedtime to prevent insomnia."

Question 48. A patient, age 65, is admitted with thyrotoxicosis. His history reveals hyperthyroidism. Laboratory results show that he has elevated T_3 and T_4 levels. The nurse would expect to administer which drugs?

A. Aminophylline, ephedrine, and theophylline
B. Dexamethasone, cortisol, and levothyroxine
C. Epinephrine, dopamine, and norepinephrine
D. Iodine, propylthiouracil, and propranolol

Question 49. A patient undergoes a subtotal thyroidectomy. Which interventions should the nurse implement for him immediately after surgery?

A. Assess vital signs every 15 minutes until stable; maintain the patient in semi-Fowler's position; give fluids as tolerated; keep a tracheostomy set at the bedside.
B. Assess vital signs every hour until stable; provide a liquid diet; maintain the patient in Trendelenburg's position; use mist inhalation.
C. Assess vital signs every 2 hours; keep the patient in a lateral recumbent position; provide the house diet; maintain strict intake and output.
D. Assess vital signs every 4 hours; maintain the patient in a supine position; withhold all oral intake; maintain strict intake and output; keep a tracheostomy set at the bedside.

Question 50. A patient, age 58, is admitted with complaints of anorexia, weight loss, and general body wasting. After a diagnostic workup, he is diagnosed with Addison's disease. Which statement best describes the pathophysiology of Addison's disease?

A. A tumor develops in the adrenal gland.
B. Release of adrenal medullary hormones is decreased.
C. Release of adrenocortical hormones is decreased.
D. Release of adrenocortical hormones is increased.

Question 51. A nurse on a telemetry unit teaches a student nurse the primary way coronary arteries receive blood flow. The nurse should emphasize that most of the blood flow to coronary arteries is supplied during which of the following?

A. Diastole
B. Expiration
C. Inspiration
D. Systole

Question 52. Which action is the first priority when caring for a patient exhibiting signs and symptoms of coronary artery disease?

A. Administering sublingual nitroglycerin
B. Decreasing anxiety
C. Educating the patient about his signs and symptoms
D. Enhancing myocardial oxygenation

Question 53. A patient with acute asthma showing inspiratory and expiratory wheezes and a decreased forced expiratory volume should be treated with which class of medication right away?

A. Beta-adrenergic blockers
B. Bronchodilators
C. Inhaled steroids
D. Oral steroids

Question 54. Which measure can reduce or prevent the incidence of atelectasis in a postoperative patient?

A. Chest physiotherapy
B. Incentive spirometry
C. Mechanical ventilation
D. Reducing oxygen requirements

Question 55. The heart rhythm of a patient in cardiac arrest undergoing cardiopulmonary resuscitation (CPR) deteriorates to ventricular fibrillation. Which action should the nurse take first?

A. Administer 0.5 mg of atropine I.V.
B. Administer 1 mg of epinephrine I.V.
C. Continue cardiopulmonary resuscitation.
D. Defibrillate with a monophasic defibrillator at 360 joules.

Question 56. Which sign or symptom typically signifies rapid expansion and impending rupture of an abdominal aortic aneurysm?

A. Abdominal pain
B. Absent pedal pulses
C. Angina
D. Lower back pain

Question 57. During discharge teaching, which instruction should the nurse give to a patient diagnosed with pancreatitis?

A. Avoid caffeinated foods and beverages.
B. Consume high-fat meals.
C. Consume low-calorie meals.
D. Limit daily alcohol intake.

Question 58. For a patient with peritonitis, which aspect of nursing care takes priority?

A. Fluid and electrolyte balance
B. Gastric irrigation
C. Pain management
D. Psychosocial care

Question 59. Which sign or symptom would a patient in the early stages of peritonitis exhibit?

A. Abdominal distention
B. Abdominal pain and rigidity
C. Hyperactive bowel sounds
D. Right upper quadrant pain

Question 60. While assessing a patient's heart sounds, the nurse hears a murmur at the second left intercostal space along the left sternal border. Which valve is most likely involved?

A. Aortic
B. Mitral
C. Pulmonic
D. Tricuspid

Question 61. Which blood test is the best indicator of myocardial injury?

A. Brain natriuretic peptide (BNP)
B. Creatine kinase (CK)
C. Lactate dehydrogenase (LD)
D. Troponin I

Question 62. A patient's ABG results are as follows: pH 7.16, partial pressure of arterial carbon dioxide ($Paco_2$) 80 mm Hg, partial pressure of arterial oxygen (Pao_2) 46 mm Hg, bicarbonate (HCO_3^-) 24 mEq/L, and arterial oxygen saturation (Sao_2), 81%. These ABG values indicate which condition?

A. Metabolic acidosis
B. Metabolic alkalosis
C. Respiratory acidosis
D. Respiratory alkalosis

Question 63. When giving emergency treatment to a patient with impending anaphylaxis secondary to a drug hypersensitivity, which action should the nurse take first?

A. Administer oxygen.
B. Insert an I.V. catheter.
C. Obtain a CBC.
D. Take vital signs.

Question 64. A hospitalized patient needs a central I.V. catheter inserted. The physician places the catheter in the subclavian vein. Shortly afterward, the patient develops shortness of breath and appears restless. Which action should the nurse perform first?

A. Administer a sedative.
B. Advise the patient to calm down.
C. Auscultate for breath sounds.
D. Check to see if the patient can have medication.

Question 65. Which class of medications protects the ischemic myocardium by blocking catecholamines and sympathetic nerve stimulation?

A. Beta-adrenergic blockers
B. Calcium channel blockers
C. Opioids
D. Nitrates

Question 66. Jugular vein distention is most prominent in which disorder?

A. Abdominal aortic aneurysm
B. Heart failure
C. Myocardial infarction
D. Pneumothorax

Question 67. Preoperative teaching for the patient about to have surgery should focus on which area?

A. Deciding if the patient should have the surgery
B. Giving emotional support to the patient and family
C. Giving minute details of the surgery to the patient and family
D. Providing general information to reduce patient and family anxiety

Question 68. A 165-lb (75-kg) patient with a pulmonary embolus is ordered to receive 20 units/kg/hour of heparin by I.V. infusion. How many units of heparin should he receive each hour?

A. 1,000
B. 1,200
C. 1,500
D. 1,700

Question 69. A patient complains that he sees a yellow halo around lights. Upon reviewing the patient's medication list, the nurse determines that this is most likely caused by a high level of which medication?

A. Digoxin
B. Enalapril
C. Furosemide
D. Metoprolol

Question 70. What information should the nurse include when teaching a patient about gout?

A. Good foot care will reduce complications.
B. The patient should be on a high-purine diet.
C. Uric acid crystals cause inflammatory destruction of the joint.
D. Uric acid production in the kidneys affects joints.

Question 71. Which sign or symptom typically occurs early in the development of multiple sclerosis (MS)?

A. Dementia
B. Diplopia
C. Joint swelling
D. Paralysis

Question 72. A patient recalls smelling an unpleasant odor before his seizure. Which term describes this symptom?

A. Atonic seizure
B. Aura
C. Ictus
D. Postictal experience

Question 73. A patient with a C6 spinal injury would most likely have which sign or symptom?

A. Aphasia
B. Hemiparesis
C. Paraplegia
D. Quadriplegia

Question 74. Medications used to treat peptic ulcer disease such as ranitidine (Zantac) work by:

A. neutralizing acid.
B. protecting the mucosal barrier.
C. reducing acid secretion.
D. stimulating gastrin release.

Question 75. During an assessment of a patient with a duodenal ulcer, the nurse finds that the patient experiences:

A. dull upper epigastric pain.
B. early satiety.
C. pain when he eats.
D. pain when he has an empty stomach.

Question 76. To reduce occurrences of dumping syndrome, the nurse should instruct the patient to do which of the following?

A. Eat three meals daily.
B. Follow a high-carbohydrate, low-fat, low-protein diet.
C. Rest after meals for 30 minutes.
D. Sip fluids with meals.

Question 77. What nursing action takes priority when caring for a patient hospitalized for acute cholecystitis?

A. Administering antibiotics
B. Assessing the patient for complications
C. Preparing the patient for lithotripsy
D. Preparing the patient for surgery

Question 78. After a right lower lobectomy for lung cancer, a patient returns to her room with a chest tube in place. The nurse formulates a care plan with a primary nursing diagnosis of Impaired gas exchange related to lung surgery. The expected outcome appropriate for this diagnosis is the patient will

A. maintain a pulse oximetry level above 93%.
B. perform incentive spirometry every 2 hours while awake.
C. request pain medication as needed.
D. sit upright, leaning slightly forward.

Question 79. A patient with cancer develops bilateral pleural effusions. During chest auscultation, which breath sounds should the nurse expect to hear?

A. Crackles
B. Diminished
C. Rhonchi
D. Wheezes

Question 80. After teaching a patient about rheumatoid arthritis, which statement indicates that the patient understands the disease process?

A. "I will definitely have to have surgery for this."
B. "It can get better and then worse again."
C. "It will never get any better than it is right now."
D. "Once it clears up, it will never come back."

Question 81. When teaching a patient about cardiomyopathy, which statement by the patient indicates that further teaching is needed about the causes of cardiomyopathy? "It's caused by

A. a virus."
B. bacteria."
C. certain drugs."
D. plaque in the arteries."

Question 82. While assessing a patient with dilated cardiomyopathy, the nurse notices that the ECG no longer has any P waves, only a fine wavy line. The ventricular rhythm is irregular, with a QRS duration of 0.08 second, and the heart rate is 110 beats/minute. The nurse interprets this rhythm as:

A. atrial fibrillation.
B. atrial flutter.
C. sinus tachycardia.
D. ventricular fibrillation.

Question 83. Which sign is one of the earliest indications of cardiogenic shock?

A. Altered LOC
B. Cyanosis
C. Decreased urine output
D. Presence of a fourth heart sound (S_4)

Question 84. According to the Seventh Report of the Joint National Committee on the Prevention, Detection, Evaluation, and Treatment of High Blood Pressure (JNC 7), what stage does a patient who has a continuous blood pressure reading of 142/90 mm Hg fall into?

A. Normal
B. Prehypertension
C. Stage 1 hypertension
D. Stage 2 hypertension

Question 85. A nurse knows that the kidneys play an important role in regulating blood pressure. When hypertension occurs, which kidney responses help normalize blood pressure?

A. Excreting sodium and retaining water
B. Excreting sodium and water
C. Retaining sodium and excreting water
D. Retaining sodium and water

Question 86. Which treatment is recommended for postoperative management of a patient who has undergone ligation and stripping?

A. Bed rest
B. Elastic leg compression
C. Ice packs
D. Sitting

Question 87. While assessing a patient with disseminated intravascular coagulation (DIC), the nurse suspects the patient has developed internal bleeding. Which sign indicates this condition?

A. Bradycardia
B. Hypertension
C. Increasing abdominal girth
D. Petechiae

Question 88. A patient with thrombocytopenia secondary to leukemia develops epistaxis. What should the nurse instruct the patient to do?

A. Blow his nose and then put lateral pressure on it.
B. Hold his nose while bending forward at the waist.
C. Lie supine with his neck extended.
D. Sit upright, leaning slightly forward.

Question 89. Instructions for a patient with systemic lupus erythematosus (SLE) should include information about which blood dyscrasia?

A. Dressler's syndrome
B. Essential thrombocytopenia
C. Polycythemia
D. von Willebrand's disease

Question 90. Which laboratory test results support the diagnosis SLE?

A. Elevated serum complement level and decreased C-reactive protein
B. Leukocytosis and elevated blood urea nitrogen (BUN) and creatinine levels
C. Pancytopenia and elevated antinuclear antibody (ANA) titer
D. Thrombocytosis and elevated sedimentation rate

Question 91. Which patient is most at risk for developing deep vein thrombosis (DVT)?

A. A 33-year-old male runner with Achilles tendonitis
B. A 35-year-old female 2 days postpartum
C. A 62-year-old female recovering from a total hip replacement
D. An ambulatory 70-year-old male who is recovering from pneumonia

Question 92. Which treatment would be most appropriate to relieve the pain of a patient admitted with DVT?

A. Applying heat
B. Bed rest
C. Exercise
D. Leg elevation

Question 93. A patient admitted with Parkinson's disease has an expressionless face and monotone speech. Which conclusion by the nurse is most accurate?

A. The patient is most likely depressed and should be left alone.
B. The patient probably has dementia.
C. The patient's antipsychotic medication may need adjustment.
D. These are common signs of Parkinson's disease.

Question 94. The nurse is assessing a patient's response to skeletal traction applied to the lower extremity. Which finding would be considered normal?

A. Coolness and pallor below the fracture level
B. Erythema and swelling immediately around the pin insertion site
C. Moderate to severe muscle spasms around the fracture area
D. Serous drainage and crust formation at the pin insertion site

Question 95. A patient has just returned from the postanesthesia care unit after undergoing internal fixation of a left femoral neck fracture. The nurse should place the patient in which position?

A. On his back with two pillows between his legs
B. On his left side with his right knee bent
C. On his right side with his left knee bent
D. Sitting at a 90-degree angle

Question 96. After surgical repair of a hip, which position is best for a patient's legs and hips?

A. Abducted
B. Adducted
C. Prone
D. Subluxated

Question 97. The nurse is auscultating the lungs of a patient following chest tube insertion. Which finding indicates correct chest tube placement?

A. Bronchial sounds heard at both bases
B. Bronchovesicular sounds heard over both lung fields
C. Crackles heard on the affected side
D. Vesicular sounds heard over upper lung fields

Question 98. Which physiologic effects of a pulmonary embolism would initially affect oxygenation?

A. A blood clot blocks perfusion and ventilation, producing profound hypoxia.
B. A blood clot blocks perfusion, producing hypoxia despite normal or supernormal ventilation.
C. A blood clot blocks ventilation, but perfusion is unaffected.
D. A blood clot blocks ventilation, producing hypoxia despite normal perfusion.

Question 99. A patient with a pulmonary embolism may have an umbrella filter placed in the vena cava for which reason?

A. To break up clots into insignificantly small pieces
B. To collect clots so that they do not reach the lungs
C. To prevent further clot formation
D. To slowly release an anticoagulant that dissolves any clots

Question 100. The nurse is caring for a patient with a pleural effusion. The patient asks, "What is a pleural effusion?" Which response would be appropriate for the nurse to make?

A. "It is the accumulation of fluid between the linings of the pleural space."
B. "It is the collapse of a bronchiole."
C. "It is the collapse of alveoli."
D. "It is the fluid in the alveolar space."

Question 101. Which oral medication is administered to prevent further thrombus formation?

A. Heparin
B. Furosemide
C. Metoprolol
D. Warfarin

Question 102. An hour after I.V. furosemide (Lasix) is administered to a patient with heart failure, a short burst of ventricular tachycardia appears on the cardiac monitor. Which electrolyte imbalance should the nurse suspect?

A. Hypocalcemia
B. Hypokalemia
C. Hypermagnesemia
D. Hypernatremia

Question 103. What signs and symptoms of pneumonia might an elderly patient first have that a younger patient is unlikely to have?

A. Altered mental status and dehydration
B. Fever and chills
C. Hemoptysis and dyspnea
D. Pleuritic chest pain and cough

Question 104. A patient with pneumonia develops dyspnea with a respiratory rate of 32 breaths/minute and difficulty expelling his secretions. The nurse auscultates his lung fields and hears bronchial sounds in the left lower lobe. The nurse determines that the patient requires which treatment first?

A. Antibiotics
B. Bed rest
C. Oxygen
D. Nutritional intake

Question 105. A patient was given morphine for pain. He is sleeping and has a respiratory rate of 4 breaths/minute. If action is not taken quickly, what reaction might he have?

A. An asthma attack
B. Respiratory arrest
C. Seizure
D. Waking up on his own

Question 106. After a patient undergoes a gastric resection, what postoperative care need should take priority?

A. Body image
B. Nutritional needs
C. Skin care
D. Spiritual needs

Question 107. During the first few days of recovery from ostomy surgery for ulcerative colitis, which aspect of patient care should take priority?

A. Body image
B. Ostomy care
C. Sexual concerns
D. Skin care

Question 108. A patient with Crohn's disease is experiencing an exacerbation. Which instruction should take priority when the nurse plans his care?

A. Controlling rectal bleeding
B. Encouraging ambulation
C. Increasing his current weight
D. Promoting bowel rest

Question 109. Which patient has the highest risk of developing anemia?

A. A patient who has had a gastrectomy
B. A patient with a colostomy following colon resection
C. A patient with frequent bouts of dumping syndrome
D. A patient with gastroesophageal reflux disease (GERD)

Question 110. The nurse is reviewing a 52-year-old patient's laboratory values. The platelet count is 75,000/μL. This value indicates which of the following?

A. A normal platelet count
B. Thrombocytopathy
C. Thrombocytopenia
D. Thrombocytosis

Question 111. The nurse is assessing a patient with ankylosing spondylitis. Which initial sign(s) or symptom(s) would the nurse most likely find in this patient?

A. Fatigue and night sweats
B. Low back pain
C. Neck pain and stiffness
D. Red, painful, swollen joints

Question 112. When reviewing the laboratory values of a patient recently diagnosed with chronic lymphocytic leukemia, which finding(s) might the nurse expect to find?

A. Elevated aspartate aminotransferase and alanine aminotransferase levels
B. Elevated sedimentation rate
C. Thrombocytopenia and increased lymphocytes
D. Uncontrolled proliferation of granulocytes

Question 113. When teaching a patient about multiple myeloma, which intervention should the nurse stress?

A. Drink at least 3 qt (3 L) of fluid daily.
B. Keep the lower extremities elevated.
C. Maintain bed rest.
D. Restrict fluid intake.

Question 114. An elderly patient has a wound that is not healing normally. Interventions should be based on which principle or test results?

A. Diminished immune functioning that interferes with the ability to fight infection
B. Kidney function test results
C. Laboratory test results
D. Poor wound healing, which is expected as part of the aging process

Question 115. During discharge teaching about corticosteroids, the patient asks the nurse what the drugs suppress. Which response by the nurse would be the most accurate?

A. Neural transmission
B. Pain receptors
C. The sympathetic response
D. The inflammatory response

Question 116. Which precautions should the nurse include in the care plan for a neutropenic patient with lymphoma?

A. Eliminate fresh fruits and vegetables, avoid enemas, and practice frequent hand hygiene.
B. Have the patient use a soft toothbrush and electric razor, avoid enemas, and watch for signs of bleeding.
C. Provide a clear liquid, low sodium diet.
D. Put on a mask, gown, and gloves when entering the patient's room.

Question 117. Objectives for treating diabetic ketoacidosis (DKA) include administering which of the following?

A. Blood products
B. Glucagon
C. Glucocorticoids
D. Insulin and I.V. fluids

Question 118. Which disease process releases enough insulin to prevent ketosis but not enough to prevent hyperglycemia?

A. Diabetes insipidus
B. Diabetic ketoacidosis
C. Hyperosmolar hyperglycemic nonketotic syndrome (HHNS)
D. Type 1 diabetes mellitus

Question 119. A patient with insulin-dependent diabetes mellitus may require which change to his daily routine during periods of infection?

A. Less insulin
B. More insulin
C. No changes
D. Oral antidiabetic agents

Question 120. A patient learns from the physician that he has Hodgkin's disease. After the physician leaves the room, the patient tells the nurse he is afraid of dying. Which response by the nurse is appropriate?

A. "Don't worry; many people survive this disease."
B. "Hodgkin's disease is very treatable."
C. "You should speak with your minister."
D. "You're afraid of dying?"

Question 121. A patient with a gunshot wound requires an emergency blood transfusion. His blood type is AB Rh negative. Which blood type would be the safest for him to receive?

A. AB Rh positive
B. A Rh positive
C. A Rh negative
D. O Rh positive

Question 122. The physician prescribes an enema for a patient with suspected appendicitis. Which action should the nurse take?

A. Assist the patient to the left lateral Sims' position.
B. Prepare 750 mL of irrigating solution warmed to 100°F (37.8°C).
C. Provide privacy and explain the procedure to the patient.
D. Question the physician about the order.

Question 123. A patient develops a small-bowel obstruction 5 days after undergoing surgery. A Miller-Abbott tube is inserted for bowel decompression. Which nursing diagnosis takes priority?

A. Acute pain
B. Deficient fluid volume
C. Excess fluid volume
D. Imbalanced nutrition: Less than body requirements

Question 124. A patient with irritable bowel syndrome is being prepared for discharge. Which meal plan should the nurse give the patient?

A. High-fiber, high-fat
B. High-fiber, low-fat
C. Low-fiber, high-fat
D. Low-fiber, low-fat

Question 125. Which laboratory values will a nurse interpret as confirming a patient's diagnosis of pancreatitis?

A. Decreased amylase, decreased lipase, decreased serum glucose, and increased serum calcium levels
B. Decreased amylase, decreased lipase, elevated serum glucose, and increased serum calcium levels
C. Elevated amylase, elevated lipase, elevated serum glucose, and decreased serum calcium levels
D. Elevated amylase, elevated lipase, decreased serum glucose, and decreased serum calcium levels

Question 126. A patient is being evaluated for hepatitis A. Which activity places him at the highest risk for contracting hepatitis A?

A. Eating a shrimp platter at a local restaurant
B. Having sexual intercourse with his fiancée
C. Helping his roommate with an epistaxis episode
D. Receiving an elective blood transfusion after surgery

Question 127. Which nursing measure takes priority for a patient with esophageal varices?

A. Controlling blood pressure
B. Recognizing hemorrhage
C. Teaching the patient about varices
D. Teaching the patient what foods to avoid

Question 128. When examining the laboratory values for a patient diagnosed with cirrhosis, the nurse would expect to find:

A. a prolonged prothrombin time.
B. an increased carbon dioxide level.
C. an increased pH.
D. an increased WBC count.

Question 129. A patient with cirrhosis complains that his skin always feels itchy. The nurse recognizes that the itching results from which abnormality associated with cirrhosis?

A. Decreased protein level
B. Increased aspartate aminotransferase level
C. Increased bilirubin level
D. Prolonged prothrombin time

Question 130. For gastric ulcer perforation, patient management should include:

A. administration of a histamine-2 (H_2)-receptor antagonist.
B. antacid administration.
C. fluid and electrolyte replacement.
D. removal of the nasogastric (NG) tube.

Question 131. Which discharge instruction should the nurse give to a patient after a prostatectomy?

A. Avoid straining at stool.
B. Report clots in the urine right away.
C. Return to your usual activities in 3 weeks.
D. Soak in a warm tub daily for comfort.

Question 132. Which discharge instructions should the nurse give to a patient undergoing treatment for acute pyelonephritis?

A. Avoid consuming any dairy products.
B. Recurrence is unlikely because you have been treated with antibiotics.
C. Return for follow-up urine cultures.
D. Stop taking the prescribed antibiotics when your signs and symptoms subside.

Question 133. A patient has undergone a radical cystectomy and has an ileal conduit for the treatment of bladder cancer. Which postoperative assessment finding should the nurse report to the physician immediately?

A. A dusky stoma
B. A red, moist stoma
C. Slight bleeding from the stoma when changing the appliance
D. Urine output of more than 30 mL/hour

Question 134. The nurse is caring for a patient with urine retention. The physician has ordered the patient to be catheterized. Which catheter would be the most appropriate for the nurse to select to perform the procedure?

A. Coudé
B. Indwelling urinary
C. Straight
D. Three-way

Question 135. A patient is injected with a radiographic contrast medium and immediately shows signs of dyspnea, flushing, and pruritus. Which intervention should take priority?

A. Applying a cold pack to the I.V. site
B. Calling the physician
C. Checking his vital signs
D. Making sure his airway is patent

Question 136. When caring for a patient following surgical ablation of the pituitary gland, the nurse should be alert for what condition?

A. Addison's disease
B. Cushing's syndrome
C. Diabetes insipidus
D. Hyperthyroidism

Question 137. A nurse can expect to see which signs and symptoms when a patient overproduces adrenocortical hormone?

A. Changes in skin texture and low body temperature
B. Hirsutism and obesity
C. Polyuria and dehydration
D. Weight loss and heat intolerance

Question 138. Sodium and water retention in a patient with Cushing's syndrome contribute to which commonly seen disorders?

A. Hypertension and heart failure
B. Hypoglycemia and dehydration
C. Hypotension and hyperglycemia
D. Pulmonary edema and dehydration

Question 139. Which disease process results from an absence or inadequate amount of insulin, leading to hyperglycemia and a series of biochemical disorders?

A. Diabetic ketoacidosis
B. Diabetes insipidus
C. HHNS
D. Hyperaldosteronism

Question 140. A patient is admitted with Graves' disease. Which laboratory test should the nurse expect to be ordered?

A. Lipid panel
B. Serum glucose
C. Serum calcium
D. Thyroid panel

Question 141. For a patient whose ICP fluctuates between 20 and 25 mm Hg, which nursing intervention would be most appropriate?

A. Encourage family member visitation.
B. Ensure that the patient's mean arterial pressure (MAP) is less than 60 mm Hg.
C. Lower the head of the bed to less than 15 degrees.
D. Reassess the patient's ABCs (airway, breathing, and circulation).

Question 142. A 33-year-old patient undergoes an L4 to L5 laminectomy. Which of the following would work best to prevent postoperative complications?

A. Encouraging the patient to be out of bed the first postoperative day
B. Limiting movement in bed and repositioning only when necessary
C. Maximizing bracing while in bed
D. Using a soft mattress

Question 143. An hour after receiving pyridostigmine bromide, a patient reports difficulty swallowing and excessive respiratory secretions. The nurse notifies the physician and prepares to administer which medication?

A. Acyclovir
B. Additional pyridostigmine bromide
C. Atropine
D. Edrophonium

Question 144. When assessing a patient with glaucoma, the nurse should expect which finding?

A. A soft globe on palpation
B. An intraocular pressure (IOP) of 15 mm Hg
C. Complaints of double vision
D. Complaints of halos around lights

Question 145. A patient with an above-the-knee amputation visits the orthopedic surgeon for a follow-up. Which comment to the nurse would indicate the patient is properly caring for the stump and prosthetic leg?

A. "I inspect the stump weekly to look for signs of redness, blistering, or abrasions."
B. "I put my prosthesis on before I get out of bed."
C. "I wash the stump every day with an antiseptic soap."
D. "I wipe out the socket of my prosthesis with a damp, soapy cloth weekly."

Question 146. Which type of shock should the nurse expect to observe in a patient experiencing tamponade?

A. Anaphylactic
B. Cardiogenic
C. Hypovolemic
D. Septic

Question 147. Which parameter should the nurse monitor frequently while a patient receives pentamidine isethionate (Pentam)?

A. Blood sugar levels
B. CBC
C. Coag studies
D. Heart rate

Question 148. A patient is ordered to receive 1,000 mL of 0.45% normal saline with 20 mEq of potassium chloride over 6 hours. The infusion set administers 15 gtt/mL. At how many gtt/minute should the nurse set the flow rate?

A. 36
B. 40
C. 42
D. 45

Question 149. An 82-year-old male patient with Parkinson's disease experiences frequent urinary incontinence. The nurse should perform which intervention first?

A. Apply a condom catheter.
B. Diaper the patient.
C. Insert an indwelling urinary catheter.
D. Provide skin care every 4 hours.

Question 150. A patient with a spinal cord injury says he has difficulty recognizing the signs and symptoms of urinary tract infection (UTI) before it becomes too late. Which of the following is an early indication of UTI?

A. Burning on urination
B. Fever and change in the clarity of urine
C. Frequency of urination
D. Lower back pain

Answers and Rationales

Question 1. Correct answer: A. If Lyme disease goes untreated, arthritis, neurologic problems, and cardiac abnormalities may arise as late complications. The first sign of Lyme disease is typically a skin lesion that enlarges and has a characteristic red border. However, not all patients develop this lesion. Options B, C, and D are incorrect because they aren't complications of Lyme disease.

Question 2. Correct answer: B. Melanomas have an irregular shape and lack uniformity in color. They may appear brown or black with red, white, or blue areas. Options A, C, and D contain inaccurate information.

Question 3. Correct answer: A. Facial lesions can contribute to situational low self-esteem and a disturbed body image. Kaposi's sarcoma is among the many psychosocial and physical traumas that may confront the patient with AIDS; anxiety, anger, grief, and depression are common emotional responses. The nurse who works with patients who have AIDS must develop excellent listening skills. The patient may be especially concerned that others will realize he has Kaposi's sarcoma. Option B is incorrect because the practitioner should inform the patient of the biopsy results, not the nurse. Option C ignores the patient's concerns. Option D doesn't provide emotional support to the patient.

Question 4.   Correct answer: C. Zidovudine inhibits deoxyribonucleic acid synthesis within the virus that causes AIDS, interfering with viral replication. Options A, B, and D inaccurately describe the drug's action.

Question 5.   Correct answer: D. Standard precautions stipulate that a health care worker who anticipates coming into contact with a patient's blood or body fluids must wear gloves; this protects the health care worker. Option A is incorrect because a private room doesn't provide a method of barrier protection, which is needed for standard precautions. Option B is incorrect because a mask is needed only for anticipated contact with airborne droplets of blood or body fluids; a gown and gloves are needed only for anticipated contact with splashes of blood or body fluids. Option C is incorrect because reverse isolation is used to protect the patient from the health care worker.

Question 6.   Correct answer: B. In partial-thickness burns, skin color varies from pink to cherry-red. Deep second-degree burns appear cherry-red and may have blisters that ooze fluid. Option A is incorrect because it describes superficial partial-thickness burns. Options C and D are incorrect because they describe full-thickness burns.

Question 7.   Correct answer: C. In a patient who has nasal packing in place, frequent swallowing may indicate bleeding in the posterior pharynx. Options A and B are incorrect because frequent swallowing isn't a response to analgesics. Option D is incorrect because mouth dryness causes thirst, not frequent swallowing.

Question 8.   Correct answer: B. To prevent pressure on the graft site, which may cause graft displacement, the nurse should instruct the patient to lie on the nonoperative side. Option A is incorrect because the patient should cough or sneeze with mouth open, not closed, to prevent increased pressure through the eustachian tube into the middle ear (which could displace the graft). Option C is incorrect because the patient should remain in bed for 24 hours after surgery to prevent graft displacement. Option D is incorrect because rapid head movement could cause vertigo.

Question 9.   Correct answer: D. With extensive, rapidly developing retinal detachment, a patient may report the sensation of a curtain dropping down in front of his or her eye. Options A, B, and C are incorrect because glaucoma, cataracts, and blepharitis don't cause this sensation.

Question 10.   Correct answer: B. The practitioner may prescribe digoxin for the patient with heart failure to increase contractility and slow the heart rate (and thus improve cardiac function); a vasodilating agent to decrease preload, afterload, and systemic vascular resistance; and a diuretic to reduce blood volume and venous pressure. None of the drugs listed in Option A are prescribed for the patient with heart failure. Option C inaccurately suggests that vasoconstricting agents are used. Option D inaccurately suggests that anti-inflammatory agents are used to treat heart failure.

Question 11.   Correct answer: C. When the dissecting aneurysm begins, severe chest pain (described as a tearing in the chest) develops; typically, the patient also has signs and symptoms of respiratory distress and ischemia of the central nervous system, limbs, kidneys, and mesenteric arterial system. Option B describes a possible cause—not a symptom—of the dissecting aneurysm. Options A and D aren't associated with this disorder.

Question 12.   Correct answer: C. The nurse should encourage the patient to avoid caffeine and nicotine because they constrict vessels and would further impair his circulation; this includes encouraging the patient to quit smoking or chewing tobacco, avoid drinking caffeine-containing beverages, and avoid ingesting such drugs as amphetamines. Option A is incorrect because it would impair circulation. The patient should exercise daily, unless pain is experienced, not avoid daily exercise, as Option B suggests. Option D is incorrect because the patient with peripheral vascular disease should keep the extremities warm and dry.

Question 13.   Correct answer: D. Maintaining clear breath sounds would indicate that the patient has effective airway clearance. Option A is incorrect because increased airway clearance would help decrease—not increase—the patient's anxiety. The respiratory rate in Option B is too high for an adult. The pulse oximetry reading in Option C is too low.

Question 14.   Correct answer: C. Lack of potassium intake (related to anorexia and nausea) plus potassium loss by way of gastric secretions (from vomiting) and intestinal fluids (from diarrhea) puts this patient at high risk for a below-normal serum potassium level. Option A is incorrect because vomiting would lead to metabolic alkalosis, and therefore, the serum bicarbonate level would be high—not low. Option B is incorrect because vomiting and diarrhea don't alter the body's calcium level; calcium is stored in bones. Option D is incorrect because vomiting may increase the serum sodium level.

Question 15. **Correct answer: C.** A positive Chvostek's sign (contraction of facial muscles when the facial nerve is tapped) indicates neuromuscular irritability, a sign of hypocalcemia. Options A, B, and D are incorrect because a positive Chvostek's sign doesn't appear with those conditions.

Question 16. **Correct answer: D.** Diabetes insipidus results from lack of antidiuretic hormone, which causes significant urine losses. Such losses, in turn, lead to hypernatremia (an elevated serum sodium level), which causes dry and sticky mucous membranes, thirst, swollen tongue, and disorientation. Option A is incorrect because a serum sodium level of 135 mEq/L falls within the normal range and muscle cramps are a sign of hyponatremia. Option B is incorrect because muscle irritability—not weakness—is characteristic of hypernatremia. Option C is incorrect because numbness and a positive Trousseau's sign indicate hypocalcemia.

Question 17. **Correct answer: A.** Cardiac arrest leads to ischemia (resulting from decreased tissue perfusion) and to subsequent cardiac insufficiency; cardiac insufficiency causes anaerobic metabolism (metabolism occurring without oxygen), leading to lactic acid production. Ischemia of any organ or body part can cause an increase in the lactic acid level. Option B is incorrect because sodium bicarbonate treatment causes alkalosis. Option C is incorrect because an irregular heartbeat doesn't necessarily cause acidosis. Option D is incorrect because this type of acidosis occurs in diabetes mellitus (diabetic ketoacidosis).

Question 18. **Correct answer: D.** In patients with Cushing's syndrome (hyperadrenalism), laboratory findings typically include sustained hyperglycemia, elevated cortisol levels, elevated WBC count, hypernatremia, and hypokalemia. Option A is incorrect because a decreased WBC count, hyponatremia, and metabolic acidosis aren't seen in Cushing's syndrome. Cushing's syndrome doesn't cause hyponatremia and hypocalcemia (Option B) or decreased cortisol level and hyperkalemia (Option C).

Question 19. **Correct answer: A.** The nurse should tell the patient that only 5% of patients experience impotence after TURP. If the patient continues to seem worried, however, the nurse should advise him to speak with his surgeon. Options B and D wouldn't give the patient a chance to express his concerns. Option C is incorrect because the nurse should help the patient express his concerns initially as well as give him appropriate information; this doesn't require a referral to a psychiatric clinical nurse specialist.

Question 20. **Correct answer: C.** The nurse first should check for indications of shock by taking the patient's vital signs. Clots in the urinary drainage indicate bleeding, which is common after TURP (especially during the first 2 postoperative hours). After making sure the patient isn't in shock, the nurse should check the irrigation system (Option B), notify the practitioner (Option D), and administer ordered antispasmodic agents (Option A) because spasms can precipitate bleeding.

Question 21. **Correct answer: D.** The nurse should elicit the patient's concerns and listen actively as he expresses these concerns. Option A is incorrect because although the patient didn't plan to have children, he may view his sterility as yet another threat to his masculinity. The testicular cancer probably already has threatened his self-concept. Option B isn't the best response because the nurse can and should help the patient explore his feelings. At a later time, the nurse may suggest that the patient talk with his practitioner. Option C is incorrect because it invalidates the patient's feelings.

Question 22. **Correct answer: B.** Pain is the most common symptom of endometriosis. Option D is incorrect because infertility is a possible consequence of endometriosis. Options A and C don't refer to the most likely assessment finding for a patient with endometriosis.

Question 23. **Correct answer: C.** Although all of the options are important nursing interventions, monitoring for hemorrhage is the highest priority. Hemorrhage can lead to a life-threatening situation for the patient. The nurse should assess for signs and symptoms of hemorrhage every 15 minutes for the first 1 hour, every 30 minutes × 2 hours, hourly × 2, and then q4h × 24 hours. Some institutions may require less frequently taken vital signs, but the nurse's awareness of this potential complication is paramount.

Question 24. **Correct answer: B.** Any activity or position that impedes venous outflow from the patient's head may increase blood volume inside the skull, possibly raising intracranial pressure (ICP). Increased ICP can cause brain damage and impair vital physiologic functions. Option A is incorrect because cerebral arterial pressure is affected by the balance between the arterial oxygen level and the arterial carbon dioxide level—not by the position ordered. Hypoxia or hypercapnia causes an increase in cerebral blood flow, thereby raising the ICP. Option C is incorrect because the ordered position doesn't prevent aspiration of stomach contents. Option D is incorrect because preventing flexion contractures isn't a priority at this time.

Question 25. Correct answer: D. The hypothermia blanket and antipyretic medication can induce hypothermia, which in turn decreases brain metabolism and makes the brain less vulnerable to hypoxia by decreasing the need for oxygen. Option A is incorrect because diaphoresis doesn't cause hypoxia; antipyretic medication may cause diaphoresis as vasodilation occurs. The osmotic pressure equalization (Option B) and integrity of intracerebral neurons (Option C) depend on an adequate supply of oxygen, carbon dioxide, and glucose and may occur as a result of decreased cerebral metabolism and hypoxia.

Question 26. Correct answer: D. A stroke in evolution refers to continuing neurologic changes over 24 to 48 hours. The patient should be placed on his side because leaving a patient on his back may cause the tongue to fall backward as well as the aspiration of secretions, resulting in airway obstruction that in turn may induce atelectasis and pneumonia. Option B is inappropriate for this patient because of weakness on the right side (resulting from his left-sided brain lesion). Options A and C aren't priorities.

Question 27. Correct answer: D. A brain injury, such as the one this patient has suffered, can cause increased ICP. Slow respirations, a slow pulse, and elevated pulse pressure are associated with compromised cerebral circulation. These changes signal increasing ICP—a condition that calls for practitioner notification so that prompt medical intervention can help prevent additional damage. Although Options A, B, and C also are important, the nurse should take these actions only *after* notifying the practitioner.

Question 28. Correct answer: B. Listlessness and sleepiness suggest the patient has a decreased LOC—the earliest sign that his condition is deteriorating. Option B describes the components of the Glasgow Coma Scale, which the nurse should use to obtain an objective determination of the patient's LOC. Options A, C, and D are appropriate, but don't take precedence over objective determination of the patient's LOC.

Question 29. Correct answer: B. Polyphagia (increased appetite), polydipsia (increased thirst), lethargy, and polyuria (increased urination) signal hyperglycemia and indicate a need to determine the patient's glucose level. Option A is incorrect because although giving insulin will affect the blood glucose level, changes in the insulin regimen may need to be made based on the patient's clinical manifestations and the current blood glucose level. Option C would worsen the patient's hyperglycemia. Option D is incorrect because the practitioner should be notified of the patient's symptoms, current insulin regimen, etc., *after* determining the patient's actual glucose level for optimal glucose management.

Question 30. Correct answer: C. Dizziness, weakness, confusion, and disorientation signal an insulin reaction and severe hypoglycemia—a common finding in diabetic patients who take insulin but miss a meal. Hyperglycemia (Option A) and ketoacidosis (Option D) are rare in a patient with diabetes who takes insulin and decreases his nutritional intake. Option B is incorrect because hyperlipidemia (an excessive blood fat level) doesn't cause hypoglycemia.

Question 31. Correct answer: A. AIDS isn't diagnosed until an AIDS-indicator condition occurs. Option B is incorrect because seroconversion is the basis for establishing that a patient is HIV positive, not for diagnosing AIDS. Options C and D are incorrect because the ELISA test and the Western blot test identify HIV antibodies in the blood; a patient who is HIV positive has already tested positive for HIV antibodies. Being HIV positive isn't synonymous with a diagnosis of AIDS.

Question 32. Correct answer: A. Because the patient's ABG measurements reveal hypoxemia, impaired gas exchange has the highest priority. Option B is incorrect because the data don't indicate a problem with the patient's airway. Option C isn't relevant because the patient has a normal $Paco_2$ level, which means that his breathing pattern isn't a problem. Option D is incorrect because the patient with pneumonia already has an infection.

Question 33. Correct answer: B. Because the patient isn't in acute distress, the highest-priority nursing diagnosis is *Deficient knowledge related to spread of the infection*. Options A, C, and D must be addressed but aren't priorities at this time; as the nurse gives the patient information about TB, these other nursing diagnoses may diminish in importance.

Question 34. Correct answer: A. Drinking alcohol daily during isoniazid therapy can induce drug-related hepatitis. Option B is incorrect because the patient should avoid concomitant use of aluminum-containing antacids with isoniazid because they impair isoniazid absorption. Option C is incorrect because the patient should take isoniazid with meals for maximal absorption and to decrease GI upset. Option D gives false information.

Question 35. Correct answer: A. Lack of bubbling in the water seal chamber denotes the air has been removed from the pleural cavity; progress has been made toward chest tube removal. There is no need to increase the level of the water seal (Option B). Option C is inappropriate, and the suction would be decreased or removed in this situation—not increased (Option D).

Question 36. Correct answer: A. High Fowler's position elevates the clavicles and helps the lungs to expand, thereby easing respirations. The other options wouldn't promote more comfortable breathing.

Question 37. Correct answer: D. An active ischemic injury in the myocardium causes displacement of the ST segment. Options A, B, and C aren't associated with an MI.

Question 38. Correct answer: C. Bleeding is a major complication associated with streptokinase therapy because streptokinase promotes systemic thrombolysis by activating plasminogen to form the proteolytic enzyme plasmin, which degrades fibrin clots. Another complication to streptokinase is an allergic response. Although streptokinase may cause reperfusion arrhythmias, Option A is incorrect because these arrhythmias usually require no treatment. Streptokinase isn't associated with chest pain (Option B) or pulmonary edema (Option D).

Question 39. Correct answer: A. Signs and symptoms of acute left ventricular dysfunction are associated primarily with pulmonary congestion, which is characterized by bilateral bibasilar crackles. Options B, C, and D are signs of right-sided heart failure.

Question 40. Correct answer: A. Various protocols are available for managing ventricular arrhythmias. Typically, the patient with more than five or six PVCs per minute is treated, especially if the PVCs are multifocal; lidocaine is the most commonly used agent. Options B, C, and D don't address the patient's immediate needs.

Question 41. Correct answer: C. Exercising the upper extremities—especially with heavy lifting—can strain the myocardium. Options A, B, and D are appropriate discharge instructions for a patient recovering from an MI.

Question 42. Correct answer: A. Blood and body fluid precautions are needed because hepatitis B is transmitted through the serum and body fluids. Options B, C, and D are inappropriate for a patient with this disease.

Question 43. Correct answer: D. The patient with hepatitis B needs a high-protein—not low-protein—diet to enhance the recovery of injured liver cells. Options A, B, and C are appropriate for a patient with hepatitis B.

Question 44. Correct answer: D. An S_3 gallop is characteristic of heart failure; crackles indicate the presence of intra-alveolar fluid, which may result from left-sided heart failure. Option A is incorrect because this patient wouldn't have clear breath sounds. Option B is incorrect because pleurisy, not heart failure, causes a friction rub. Option C is incorrect because heart failure doesn't cause a murmur.

Question 45. Correct answer: B. Cor pulmonale is a form of right-sided heart failure caused by pulmonary disease; only Option B lists signs of right-sided heart failure. Option A is incorrect because the patient with diagnosed COPD will have a prolonged expiratory phase. Option C is incorrect because respiratory excursion is reduced with COPD. Option D is incorrect because the patient with COPD and cor pulmonale will have an increased respiratory rate.

Question 46. Correct answer: D. Pursed-lip and diaphragmatic breathing, which increase carbon dioxide elimination, are the most effective ways to improve this patient's breathing. Option A must be done cautiously in patients with COPD because their breathing stimulus depends on a low arterial oxygen content. Option B would improve the patient's activity tolerance but not his ventilation. In conjunction with breathing exercises, Option C is used to remove retained secretions and thus improve gas exchange.

Question 47. Correct answer: A. Because this patient may feel full after even a small meal, he should eat smaller, more frequent, high-calorie meals to obtain the energy he needs for breathing. Option B is incorrect because most patients with COPD tolerate activity better if it's spaced throughout the day with frequent rest periods. Option C is incorrect because the patient should exercise before eating to conserve the energy and blood flow for digestion. Option D is incorrect because taking a bronchodilator at bedtime may contribute to insomnia.

Question 48. Correct answer: D. Iodine reduces thyroid vascularity and prevents release of thyroid hormone into the circulation. Propylthiouracil, which blocks thyroid hormone synthesis, is the drug most commonly used to treat hyperthyroidism; methimazole has similar effects and can be used in patients allergic to propylthiouracil. Propranolol, a beta-adrenergic blocker, is used to decrease patient anxiety and the cardiac effects of hyperthyroidism. The drugs listed in Option A are used primarily to treat asthma and may lead to increased excitability and tachycardia in a patient with hyperthyroidism. Option B is incorrect because levothyroxine is used to treat hypothyroidism, not hyperthyroidism. The adrenergic agents listed in Option C are inappropriate for the hyperthyroid patient because they would further stimulate the cardiovascular system, which is already under stress from hypermetabolism.

Question 49. Correct answer: A. Because hemorrhage and respiratory obstruction can develop after a subtotal thyroidectomy, the nurse must monitor vital signs every 15 minutes until the patient is stable and then every 30 minutes to 1 hour for the next several hours. Semi-Fowler's position promotes comfort and breathing and allows immobilization, which is needed to prevent strain on the suture line. Fluids should be given unless the patient experiences nausea and vomiting or has difficulty swallowing. A tracheostomy set is needed because airway obstruction may result from edema. Option B is incorrect because Trendelenburg's position would cause a decreased number of respirations and edema at the surgical site. Options C and D are incorrect because vital signs should be monitored more frequently, and the patient should be in semi-Fowler's position.

Question 50. Correct answer: C. In Addison's disease (adrenocortical insufficiency), the release of adrenocortical hormones diminishes. Option A is incorrect because Addison's disease is thought to have an autoimmune etiology. Option B is incorrect because Addison's disease doesn't affect hormones produced by the adrenal medulla. Option D is incorrect because adrenocortical hormone release decreases rather than increases.

Question 51. Correct answer: A. Most of the blood flow to coronary arteries is supplied during diastole. Breathing patterns (Options B and C) don't affect blood flow. Coronary arteries receive only a minute portion of blood during systole (Option D).

Question 52. Correct answer: D. Enhancing myocardial oxygenation is always the first priority when a patient exhibits signs or symptoms of cardiac compromise. Without adequate oxygen, the myocardium suffers damage. Administering sublingual nitroglycerin to treat acute angina (Option A), decreasing the patient's anxiety (Option B), and educating the patient (Option C) are important aspects of care delivery but don't take first priority.

Question 53. Correct answer: B. Bronchodilators are the first line of treatment for asthma because bronchoconstriction is the cause of reduced airflow. Beta-adrenergic blockers (Option A) aren't used to treat asthma and can cause bronchoconstriction. Inhaled or oral steroids (Options C and D) may be given to reduce the inflammation but aren't used for emergency relief.

Question 54. Correct answer: B. Incentive spirometry requires the patient to take deep breaths and promotes lung expansion. Chest physiotherapy (Option A) helps mobilize secretions but won't prevent atelectasis. Placing the patient on mechanical ventilation (Option C) or reducing the patient's oxygen requirements (Option D) won't affect the development of atelectasis.

Question 55. Correct answer: D. To attempt to convert the rhythm, the nurse should first defibrillate the patient with a monophasic defibrillator at 360 joules. If this fails, then the nurse should continue CPR (Option C) for 2 minutes and attempt to defibrillate again. Epinephrine (Option B) may be given, but not until after the first two defibrillation attempts. Atropine (Option A) is given for symptomatic bradycardia.

Question 56. Correct answer: D. Lower back pain results from expansion of the aneurysm. The expansion causes pressure in the abdominal cavity, and the pain is referred to the lower back. Abdominal pain (Option A) is the most common symptom resulting from impaired circulation. Absent pedal pulses (Option B) are a sign of no circulation and occur after a ruptured aneurysm or in peripheral vascular disease. Angina (Option C) is associated with atherosclerosis of the coronary arteries.

Question 57. Correct answer: A. A patient with pancreatitis should avoid foods and beverages that can cause a relapse of the disease, including caffeine, which is a stimulant that will further irritate the pancreas. The patient should maintain a diet low in fats and high in calories, especially carbohydrates, not high in fats (Option B) or low in calories (Option C). The patient should avoid all alcohol, not just limit his intake (Option D), because chronic alcohol use is one of the causes of pancreatitis.

Question 58. Correct answer: A. Because peritonitis can advance to shock and circulatory failure, fluid and electrolyte balance takes priority to maintain hemodynamic stability. Although the patient may periodically need gastric irrigation (Option B) to ensure patency of the nasogastric tube, pain management (Option C) for comfort, and psychosocial care (Option D) to address concerns such as anxiety, these don't take priority.

Question 59. Correct answer: B. Peritonitis is characterized by abdominal pain that causes rigidity of the abdominal muscles. Abdominal distention (Option A) may occur as a late sign but doesn't occur early on. Bowel sounds may be normal or decreased, not increased (Option C). Right upper quadrant pain (Option D) is characteristic of cholecystitis or hepatitis.

Question 60. Correct answer: C. Abnormalities of the pulmonic valve are auscultated at the second left intercostal space along the left sternal border. Abnormalities of the aortic valve (Option A) are heard at the second intercostal space to the right of the sternum; of the mitral valve (Option B), at the fifth intercostal space at the left midclavicular line; and of the tricuspid valve (Option D), at the third and fourth intercostal spaces along the left sternal border.

Question 61.   Correct answer: D. Troponin I levels rise rapidly and are detectable within 1 hour of myocardial injury; they aren't detectable in people without cardiac injury. BNP levels (Option A) are used to screen for and determine the progress of heart failure. Because CK (Option B) is widely distributed in tissues, elevations in total serum CK lack specificity for cardiac damage. LD (Option C) is present in almost all body tissues and not specific to heart muscle, although LD isoenzymes may be useful in diagnosing cardiac injury.

Question 62.   Correct answer: C. Because the patient's $Paco_2$ is high at 80 mm Hg and his metabolic measure (HCO_3^-) is normal, he has respiratory acidosis. If he had an HCO_3^- below 22 mEq/L, he would have metabolic acidosis (Option A). His pH is less than 7.35, indicating acidosis, which eliminates metabolic and respiratory alkalosis (Options B and D) as possibilities.

Question 63.   Correct answer: A. The first action the nurse should take is administering oxygen. The nurse can then take vital signs (Option D) and immediately notify the physician. If the patient doesn't already have an I.V. catheter in place, the nurse can insert one (Option B) if anaphylactic shock is developing. Obtaining a CBC (Option C) wouldn't help resolve the emergency situation.

Question 64.   Correct answer: C. Because this is an acute episode, the nurse should listen to the patient's lungs to see if anything has changed (e.g., the development of a pneumothorax). The nurse shouldn't check to see if the patient can have medication (Option D), nor should she give this patient medication, especially a sedative (Option A), if he's having difficulty breathing. This patient is having an acute episode, and giving him support rather than advising him to calm down (Option B) is more appropriate.

Question 65.   Correct answer: A. Beta-adrenergic blockers work by blocking beta receptors in the myocardium, reducing the response to catecholamines and sympathetic nerve stimulation. They protect the myocardium, helping to reduce the risk of another infarction by decreasing the workload of the heart and decreasing myocardial oxygen demand. Calcium channel blockers (Option B) reduce the workload of the heart by decreasing the heart rate. Opioids (Option C) reduce myocardial oxygen demand, promote vasodilation, and decrease anxiety. Nitrates (Option D) reduce myocardial oxygen consumption by decreasing left ventricular end-diastolic pressure (preload) and systemic vascular resistance (afterload).

Question 66.   Correct answer: B. Jugular vein distension results from elevated venous pressure and indicates a failure of the heart to pump. Jugular vein distention isn't a symptom of abdominal aortic aneurysm (Option A) or pneumothorax (Option D). Although a severe MI (Option C) can progress to heart failure, the MI itself doesn't cause jugular vein distention.

Question 67.   Correct answer: D. The nurse's role is to provide general information about the surgery and what to expect before and after surgery and to give emotional support during this time. The nurse's role isn't to decide if the patient should have surgery (Option A) or to give minute details of the surgery (Option C). If the patient or family requests extremely detailed information, the surgeon should answer their questions. Emotional support alone (Option B) during this time isn't sufficient.

Question 68.   Correct answer: C. A 165-lb patient weighs 75 kg (2.2 lb = 1 kg). 20 units × 75 kg × 1 hour = 1,500 units/hour.

Question 69.   Correct answer: A. One of the most common signs of digoxin toxicity is the visual disturbance known as the yellow halo sign. The other medications aren't associated with such a side effect.

Question 70.   Correct answer: C. The patient needs to know that uric acid crystals collect in the joint of the great toe and cause inflammation. Good foot care (Option A) doesn't affect the development of complications. The patient should be on a low-purine diet, not a high-purine diet (Option B). The kidneys excrete uric acid, an end product of purine metabolism; they don't produce uric acid (Option D).

Question 71.   Correct answer: B. Early indications of MS include slurred speech and diplopia. Although depression and a short attention span may occur, dementia (Option A) is rarely associated with MS. Muscle spasms and joint stiffness are manifestations of MS, but not joint swelling (Option C). Paralysis (Option D) is a late symptom of MS.

Question 72.   Correct answer: B. An aura occurs in some patients as a warning before a seizure. The patient may experience a certain smell, a vision such as flashing lights, or a sensation. Atonic seizure (Option A) or drop attack refers to an abrupt loss of muscle tone. Ictus (Option C) is the seizure itself. During a postictal experience (Option D), which occurs after a seizure, the patient may be confused, somnolent, and fatigued.

Question 73.   Correct answer: D. Quadriplegia occurs as a result of cervical spine injuries. Aphasia (Option A) refers to difficulty expressing or understanding spoken words as in stroke patients. Hemiparesis (Option B) describes weakness of one side of the body. Paraplegia (Option C) occurs as a result of injury at or below the thoracic area of the spinal cord.

Question 74. Correct answer: C. Histamine-2 receptor antagonists such as ranitidine reduce acid secretion; they work by inhibiting, not stimulating, gastrin secretion (Option D). Antacids neutralize acid (Option A), and mucosal barrier fortifiers protect the mucosal barrier (Option B).

Question 75. Correct answer: D. A patient with a duodenal ulcer feels pain when his stomach is empty; eating food or taking antacids relieves the pain. The other symptoms result from gastric ulcer.

Question 76. Correct answer: C. To reduce the occurrences of dumping syndrome, the patient should be taught to lie down after eating for 30 minutes; eat smaller, more frequent meals in a semirecumbent position, not three meals a day (Option A); avoid sweets and follow a low-carbohydrate, high-protein, moderate-fat diet, not a high-carbohydrate, low-fat, low-protein diet (Option B); and drink fluids 30 to 45 minutes before or after meals—not with meals (Option D).

Question 77. Correct answer: B. The nurse should first assess this patient for such complications as perforation, fever, abscess, fistula, and sepsis; only after that should the nurse administer antibiotics (Option A) to reduce the infection. Surgery (Option D) is performed after the acute infection has subsided. Only a small percentage of these patients undergo lithotripsy (Option C).

Question 78. Correct answer: A. A pulse oximetry level above 93% and a normal respiratory rate demonstrate probable lung expansion and normal chest tube functioning. Using an incentive spirometer (Option B) would be an intervention used to achieve the expected outcome. Requesting pain medication as needed (Option C) is an expected action for a nursing diagnosis of *Acute pain*. Sitting upright, leaning slightly forward (Option D), suggests that the patient still has impaired gas exchange because this position increases lung expansion.

Question 79. Correct answer: B. In pleural effusion, fluid accumulates in the pleural space, impairing transmission of normal breath sounds. Because of the acoustic mismatch, breath sounds are diminished. Crackles (short explosive or popping sounds) (Option A) commonly accompany atelectasis, interstitial fibrosis, and left-sided heart failure. Rhonchi (low-pitched sounds with a snoring quality) (Option C) suggest secretions in the large airways. Wheezes (high-pitched, hissing sounds) (Option D) result from narrowed airways, as in asthma, COPD, and bronchitis.

Question 80. Correct answer: B. The patient with rheumatoid arthritis needs to understand that the disease is somewhat unpredictable characterized by periods of exacerbation and remission. Although there's no cure (Option D), symptoms can be managed at times (Option C). Surgery (Option A) may be indicated in some cases, but not always.

Question 81. Correct answer: D. Cardiomyopathy isn't usually caused by plaque in the arteries or atherosclerosis. The etiology in most cases is a viral (Option A) or bacterial (Option B) infection or cardiotoxic effects of drugs (Option C) or alcohol.

Question 82. Correct answer: A. Atrial fibrillation is defined as chaotic, asynchronous, electrical activity in the atrial tissue. On an ECG, uneven baseline fibrillating waves appear rather than distinguishable P waves. Atrial flutter (Option B) results in sawtooth flutter waves. P waves are present in sinus tachycardia (Option C). Ventricular fibrillation (Option D) results in a chaotic rhythm with no QRS complexes.

Question 83. Correct answer: A. Initially, the decrease in cardiac output results in a decrease in cerebral blood flow that causes restlessness, agitation, or confusion. Cyanosis (Option B), decreased urine output (Option C), and presence of a fourth heart sound (Option D) are all later signs of shock.

Question 84. Correct answer: C. According to JNC 7, a systolic blood pressure of 140 to 159 mm Hg or a diastolic pressure of 90 to 99 mm Hg represents stage 1 hypertension. A systolic pressure less than 120 mm Hg and diastolic pressure less than 80 mm Hg are considered normal (Option A). A systolic pressure of 120 to 139 mm Hg or diastolic pressure of 80 to 89 mm Hg represents prehypertension (Option B). A systolic pressure greater than or equal to 160 mm Hg or diastolic pressure greater than or equal to 100 mm Hg represents stage 2 hypertension (Option D).

Question 85. Correct answer: B. The kidneys respond to a rise in blood pressure by excreting sodium and excess water. This response ultimately affects systolic blood pressure by regulating blood volume. Retaining sodium and water (Option D) would only further increase blood pressure. Sodium and water travel together across the membrane in the kidneys; one can't travel without the other (Options A and C).

Question 86. Correct answer: B. Elastic leg compression helps venous return to the heart, thereby decreasing venous stasis. Bed rest (Option A) and sitting (Option D) are contraindicated because both promote decreased blood return to the heart and venous stasis. Although ice packs (Option C) help reduce edema, they also cause vasoconstriction and impede blood flow.

Question 87.   Correct answer: C. As blood collects in the peritoneal cavity, dilation and distention of the abdomen occur, causing an increase in abdominal girth. The patient with DIC would have hypotension and tachycardia, not bradycardia (Option A) and hypertension (Option B). Petechiae (Option D) result when blood from tiny blood vessels leaks into the skin.

Question 88.   Correct answer: D. The upright position, leaning slightly forward, avoids increasing vascular pressure in the nose and helps the patient avoid aspirating blood. Nose blowing (Option A) can dislodge any clotting that has occurred. Bending at the waist (Option B) increases vascular pressure and promotes bleeding rather than stopping it. Lying supine (Option C) won't prevent aspiration of blood.

Question 89.   Correct answer: B. Essential thrombocytopenia is linked with immunologic disorders, such as SLE and HIV. Dressler's syndrome (Option A) is pericarditis that occurs after an MI and isn't linked to SLE. Moderate to severe anemia is associated with SLE, not polycythemia (Option C). A type of hemophilia, von Willebrand's disease (Option D) isn't linked to SLE.

Question 90.   Correct answer: C. Laboratory findings for patients with SLE usually show pancytopenia, elevated ANA titer; decreased serum complement levels, not elevated serum complement levels; and an elevated C-reactive protein level, not decreased level (Option A). Thrombocytosis and elevated sedimentation rate (Option D) are not diagnostic for SLE. Patients may have elevated BUN and creatinine levels (Option B) from nephritis, but the increase doesn't indicate SLE.

Question 91.   Correct answer: A. DVT is more common in immobilized patients who have had surgical procedures such as total hip replacement. Pregnancy (Option B) can cause varicose veins, which can lead to venous stasis, but it isn't a primary cause of DVT. A patient recovering from an injury (Option C) or pneumonia (Option D) may have decreased mobility but isn't at the highest risk for developing DVT.

Question 92.   Correct answer: D. Leg elevation alleviates the pressure caused by thrombosis and occlusion by assisting venous return. Applying heat (Option A) would dilate the vessels and pool blood in the area of the thrombus, increasing the risk of further thrombus formation. Bed rest (Option B) adds to venous stasis by increasing the risk of thrombosis formation. When DVT is diagnosed, ambulation is encouraged to improve circulation to the extremity, but exercise (Option C) isn't recommended for the first 10 to 14 days after an acute DVT attack until the clot is more firmly attached and the patient is on anticoagulants.

Question 93.   Correct answer: D. The nurse should recognize that these are common signs of Parkinson's disease, which results from degeneration of the substantia nigra in the basal ganglia of the brain where dopamine is produced and stored. This degeneration results in motor dysfunction. These aren't the typical signs of depression (Option A) or dementia (Option B). The effects of antipsychotic medication (Option C) can mimic the extrapyramidal signs of Parkinson's disease, but these drugs aren't indicated for treating Parkinson's disease.

Question 94.   Correct answer: D. Serous drainage around the pin insertion site is a normal finding; some institutions don't recommend crust removal because of its protective nature. A pale, cool extremity (Option A) may indicate arterial compromise. Erythema and swelling (Option B) signal infection. Severe muscle spasms (Option C) may indicate improper alignment of the body or traction.

Question 95.   Correct answer: A. The operative leg must be kept abducted to prevent dislocation of the hip. Placing the patient on the left or right side with knee bent (Options B and C) doesn't promote abduction, and acute flexion of the operated hip may cause dislocation. The head of the bed may be raised 35 to 49 degrees, not 90 degrees (Option D).

Question 96.   Correct answer: A. After surgical repair of the hip, the legs and hips should be in the abducted position. The adducted, prone, and subluxated positions (Options B, C, and D) don't keep the prosthesis within the acetabulum.

Question 97.   Correct answer: B. If the chest tube is inserted correctly, the nurse will hear normal bronchovesicular breath sounds in that area, and the patient's oxygenation status will improve; the patient should undergo a chest X-ray to ensure reexpansion. Options A, C, and D are abnormal breath sounds.

Question 98.   Correct answer: B. The blood clot blocks blood flow to a region of the lung tissue. That area remains ventilated, but because blood flow is blocked, no gas exchange can occur in that region, and a ventilation-perfusion mismatch occurs. Ventilation (Options A, C, and D) isn't initially affected by a blood clot because air can still move normally through the bronchial tree.

Question 99.   Correct answer: B. The umbrella filter is placed in a patient in whom anticoagulation is contraindicated to prevent further clots from entering the lungs. Filters may remain permanently or be retrieved after the danger of emboli has passed. The filter doesn't break up the clots (Option A), prevent further clot formation (Option C), or release anticoagulants (Option D).

Question 100. Correct answer: A. Pleural fluid normally seeps continually into the pleural space from the capillaries lining the parietal pleura and is reabsorbed by the visceral pleural capillaries and lymphatics. Any condition that interferes with either the secretion or drainage of this fluid can lead to a pleural effusion. The collapse of alveoli (Option C) or a bronchiole (Option B) has no particular name. Fluid within the alveolar space (Option D) isn't in the pleural space; such fluid accumulation can result from heart failure or adult respiratory distress syndrome.

Question 101. Correct answer: D. Warfarin prevents vitamin K from synthesizing certain clotting factors. This oral anticoagulant can be given over the long term. Heparin (Option A) is a parenteral anticoagulant that interferes with coagulation by readily combining with antithrombin; it can't be given by mouth. Neither furosemide (Option B) nor metoprolol (Option C) affects anticoagulation.

Question 102. Correct answer: B. Furosemide is a potassium-depleting diuretic that can cause hypokalemia. In turn, hypokalemia increases myocardial excitability, leading to ventricular tachycardia. Hypocalcemia (Option A), which slows conduction through the atrioventricular junction, can cause such bradyarrhythmias as atrioventricular block. Hypermagnesemia (Option C) may lead to bradycardia, not tachycardia. Hypernatremia (Option D) may cause sinus tachycardia as a result of water loss.

Question 103. Correct answer: A. Although fever, chills, hemoptysis, dyspnea, cough, and pleuritic chest pain (Options B, C, and D) are the common signs and symptoms of pneumonia, an elderly patient may first appear with only an altered mental status and dehydration resulting from a blunted immune response.

Question 104. Correct answer: C. The patient is having difficulty breathing and is probably becoming hypoxic. As an emergency measure, the nurse can provide oxygen without waiting for a physician's order. Antibiotics (Option A) may be warranted, but this isn't a nursing decision. The patient should be maintained on bed rest (Option B) if he's dyspneic to minimize his oxygen demands, but providing additional oxygen will deal more immediately with his problem. The patient will need nutritional support (Option D), but while dyspneic, he may be unable to spare the energy needed to eat and at the same time maintain adequate oxygenation.

Question 105. Correct answer: B. Opioids such as morphine can cause respiratory arrest if given in large quantities. It's unlikely the patient will have an asthma attack (Option A), a seizure (Option C), or wake up on his own (Option D).

Question 106. Correct answer: B. After gastric resection, a patient may require total parenteral nutrition or jejunostomy tube feedings to maintain adequate nutritional status, which promotes healing. Body image (Option A) isn't the major concern for the patient at this point because clothing can cover the incision site. Although the patient needs wound care at the incision site to prevent infection, he doesn't need additional skin care measures (Option C). If spiritual needs (Option D) arise, they should be addressed when the patient demonstrates a readiness to share those needs.

Question 107. Correct answer: B. Although all the nurse should address body image (Option A), sexual concerns (Option C), and skin care (Option D) as needed, ostomy care–including the crucial task of helping the patient learn to safely manage the ostomy before discharge–takes priority.

Question 108. Correct answer: D. Promoting bowel rest takes priority during an acute exacerbation of Crohn's disease. The nurse accomplishes this by decreasing activity, not encouraging ambulation (Option B), and initially putting the patient on nothing-by-mouth status, not taking steps to increase his weight (Option C); although weight loss may occur, bowel rest still takes priority. Rectal bleeding (Option A) doesn't typically occur in Crohn's disease.

Question 109. Correct answer: A. Lack of intrinsic factor following gastrectomy could cause pernicious anemia as the result of the patient's inability to absorb vitamin B_{12}. The presence of a colostomy (Option B), dumping syndrome (Option C), or GERD (Option D) wouldn't place a patient at risk for developing anemia.

Question 110. Correct answer: C. Thrombocytopenia is a decreased number of platelets. In adults, this would be less than 100,000/µL. A normal platelet count (Option A) ranges from 150,000/µL to 450,000/µL. Thrombocytopathy (Option B) is platelet dysfunction, and thrombocytosis (Option D) is an excess number of platelets.

Question 111. Correct answer: B. Typically, intermittent low back pain is the first indication of ankylosing spondylitis. Although ankylosing spondylitis may cause fatigue, it rarely produces night sweats (Option A). Neck pain and stiffness (Option C) from involvement of the cervical spine are relatively late manifestations. Red, painful, swollen joints (Option D) occur with rheumatoid arthritis.

Question 112. **Correct answer: C.** Chronic lymphocytic leukemia causes a proliferation of small, abnormal, mature B lymphocytes and decreased antibodies; it can also cause thrombocytopenia. Uncontrolled proliferation of granulocytes (Option D) occurs in myelogenous leukemia. Erythrocyte sedimentation rate (Option B) and aspartate aminotransferase and alanine aminotransferase (Option A) levels aren't affected.

Question 113. **Correct answer: A.** The patient needs to drink 3 to 5 qt (3 to 5 L) of fluid each day—not restrict fluid intake (Option D)—to dilute calcium and uric acid, reducing the risk of renal dysfunction. The lower extremities don't need to be elevated (Option B). Walking, not bed rest (Option C), is encouraged to prevent further bone demineralization.

Question 114. **Correct answer: A.** Immune function is important in the healing process, and diminished functioning may slow or prevent the healing process from taking place. Laboratory and kidney function test results (Options B and C) are important but aren't the main factors in determining interventions. Although wound healing declines with age (Option D), healthy behaviors (such as proper nutrition and exercise) can enhance the older patient's response to tissue trauma.

Question 115. **Correct answer: D.** Corticosteroids suppress eosinophils, lymphocytes, natural killer cells, and other microorganisms, inhibiting the natural inflammatory process in an infected or injured part of the body. This promotes resolution of inflammation, stabilizes lysosomal membranes, decreases capillary permeability, and depresses phagocytosis of tissues by WBCs, thus blocking the release of more inflammatory materials. Corticosteroids don't affect the neural transmission (Option A), pain receptors (Option B), or sympathetic response (Option C).

Question 116. **Correct answer: A.** Neutropenia occurs when the absolute neutrophil count falls below 1,000/mm^3, reflecting a severe risk for infection. The nurse should provide a low-bacterial diet, which means eliminating fresh fruits and vegetables; avoid invasive procedures such as enemas because they increase the infection risk; and practice frequent hand hygiene to lower the infection risk. Using a soft toothbrush and electric razor, avoiding enemas, and monitoring for bleeding (Option B) are thrombocytopenia precautions. A neutropenic patient doesn't need a clear liquid diet or sodium restrictions (Option C). Putting on a mask, gown, and gloves when entering the patient's room (Option D) is reverse isolation.

Question 117. **Correct answer: D.** A patient with DKA would receive insulin to lower glucose and I.V. fluids to correct hypotension. Glucagon (Option B) is given to treat hypoglycemia; DKA involves hyperglycemia. Blood products (Option A) aren't needed to correct DKA. Glucocorticoids (Option C) aren't needed because the adrenal glands aren't involved.

Question 118. **Correct answer: C.** In HHNS, enough insulin is released to prevent ketosis but not enough to prevent hyperglycemia. Diabetes insipidus (Option A) doesn't involve hyperglycemia. Diabetic ketoacidosis (Option B) involves hyperglycemia and ketosis. In type 1 diabetes mellitus (Option D), the body does not produce insulin.

Question 119. **Correct answer: B.** During periods of infection or illness, an insulin-dependent patient may need even more insulin—not less insulin (Option A) or no change (Option C)—to compensate for increased blood glucose levels. Because the patient has insulin-dependent diabetes, oral antidiabetic agents (Option D) wouldn't be indicated.

Question 120. **Correct answer: D.** Repeating what the patient has said (or describing his feelings) encourages the patient to elaborate on his thoughts and feelings. Telling him not to worry (Option A) or saying that Hodgkin's disease is very treatable (Option B) ignores his feelings and offers false reassurance. Telling a patient what to do, such as calling his minister (Option C), also ignores his feelings.

Question 121. **Correct answer: C.** Human blood can contain an inherited D antigen. People with the D antigen have Rh-positive blood type; those lacking the antigen have Rh-negative blood. A person with Rh-negative blood must receive Rh-negative blood, not Rh-positive blood (Options A, B, and D). If an Rh-negative person receives Rh-positive blood, he develops anti-Rh agglutinins, and subsequent transfusions with Rh-positive blood may cause serious reactions, including clumping and hemolysis of red blood cells.

Question 122. **Correct answer: D.** Enemas are contraindicated in an acute abdominal condition of unknown origin (such as suspected appendicitis) as well as after recent colon or rectal surgery or MI, so the nurse should question the physician about the order. Options A, B, and C are correct only when enema administration is appropriate.

Question 123. **Correct answer: B.** Fluid shifts to the site of the bowel obstruction, causing a fluid deficit—not excess fluid (Option C)—in the intravascular spaces. If the obstruction isn't resolved immediately, the patient may experience *Imbalanced nutrition: Less than body requirements* (Option D); however, *Deficient fluid volume* takes priority. The patient also may experience pain (Option A), but that nursing diagnosis also takes lower priority.

Question 124.   Correct answer: B. The patient with irritable bowel syndrome needs to be on a diet that is high in fiber (at least 25 g/day) but doesn't contain fatty foods, which may precipitate symptoms. The other options provide too little fiber or too much fat.

Question 125.   Correct answer: C. Inflammation of the pancreas causes it to excrete pancreatic enzymes. The inflammation also causes a blockage of the ducts from the pancreas to the GI tract; therefore, the pancreatic enzymes are released into the blood, resulting in an elevation of amylase and lipase levels. Carbohydrate metabolism is impaired secondary to damage to pancreatic beta cells. This impairment causes the patient to become hyperglycemic. As in many other disease processes, the serum calcium level decreases because of the saponification of calcium by fatty acids in the area of the inflamed pancreas.

Question 126.   Correct answer: A. Hepatitis A can result from contact with contaminated feces and may be transmitted through infected water, milk, or food, especially shellfish from contaminated waters. Hepatitis B results from blood or sexual contact (Options B and C). Hepatitis C is usually caused by contact with infected blood, including blood transfusions (Option D).

Question 127.   Correct answer: B. Recognizing the rupture of esophageal varices, or hemorrhage, takes priority because the patient could succumb to this quickly. Although not as important, the nurse should also focus on controlling blood pressure (Option A) because doing so helps reduce the risk of variceal rupture. Lower priority measures include teaching the patient what foods he should avoid (such as spicy foods) (Option D) and explaining what varices are (Option C).

Question 128.   Correct answer: A. Clotting factors may not be produced normally when a patient has cirrhosis, indicating an increased potential for bleeding and resulting in a prolonged prothrombin time. There's no associated change in carbon dioxide level (Option B) or pH (Option C) unless the patient is developing other comorbidities, such as metabolic alkalosis. In acute cirrhosis, the WBC count can be, but isn't always, elevated (Option D).

Question 129.   Correct answer: C. High bilirubin levels irritate peripheral nerves, causing an intense itching sensation. Itching isn't a symptom of decreased protein levels (Option A), increased aspartate aminotransferase levels (Option B), or prolonged prothrombin time (Option D).

Question 130.   Correct answer: C. The patient should receive fluid and electrolyte replacement as well as antibiotics and blood replacement. He should undergo NG tube suctioning to prevent further spillage of stomach contents into the perineal cavity, not have an NG tube removed (Option D). H_2-receptor antagonists (Option A) and antacids (Option B) aren't helpful in this situation.

Question 131.   Correct answer: A. Straining at stool after prostatectomy can cause bleeding. Small blood clots or pieces of tissue commonly are passed in the urine for up to 2 weeks postoperatively (Option B). Other activities are resumed based on the guidance of the physician (Option C). Sexual intercourse and driving are usually prohibited for about 3 weeks; exercising and returning to work are usually prohibited for about 6 weeks. Tub baths (Option D) are prohibited because they cause dilation of pelvic blood vessels.

Question 132.   Correct answer: C. The patient needs to return for follow-up urine cultures because he may have asymptomatic bacteriuria. Consuming dairy products (Option A) won't contribute to pyelonephritis. The patient must take the full course of antibiotics, regardless of his signs and symptoms (Option D). Pyelonephritis can recur as a relapse or new infection, frequently within 2 weeks of completing therapy (Option B).

Question 133.   Correct answer: A. A dusky or cyanotic stoma indicates insufficient blood supply, an emergency that needs prompt intervention. The stoma should be red and moist (Option B), indicating adequate blood flow. Slight bleeding from the stoma when changing the appliance (Option C) may occur because the intestinal mucosa is fragile. A urine output of less than 30 mL/hour or no urine output for more than 15 minutes should be reported; a urine output of more than 30 mL/hour is normal (Option D).

Question 134.   Correct answer: C. Urine retention is usually a temporary problem that requires insertion of a straight catheter. A coudé catheter (Option A) is used only when it's difficult to insert a standard catheter, usually because of an enlarged prostate. An indwelling urinary catheter (Option B) is used for longer-term bladder problems. A three-way catheter (Option D) is used for patients who need bladder irrigation such as after a prostate resection.

Question 135.   Correct answer: D. The patient is showing signs of an allergy to the iodine in the contrast medium. The first action is to make sure the patient's airway is patent. If it's compromised, the nurse should call a cardiac arrest code. Checking the patient's vital signs (Option C) and calling the physician (Option B), although important nursing actions, should take place after making sure the patient's airway is patent. Applying a cold pack to the I.V. site (Option A) isn't indicated.

Question 136.   Correct answer: C. Although the cause of diabetes insipidus is unknown, it may occur secondary to head trauma, brain tumors, or surgical ablation of the pituitary gland. Addison's disease (Option A) is caused by a deficiency of cortical hormones, whereas Cushing's syndrome (Option B) results from an excess of cortical hormones. Hyperthyroidism (Option D) occurs when the thyroid gland secretes high levels of thyroid hormone.

Question 137.   Correct answer: A. Overproduction of adrenocortical hormone results in hirsutism and obesity. Changes in skin texture and low body temperature (Option B) indicate thyroid hormone underproduction. Polyuria and dehydration (Option C) indicate diabetic ketoacidosis. Weight loss and heat intolerance (Option D) indicate thyroid hormone overproduction.

Question 138.   Correct answer: A. In a patient with Cushing's syndrome, increased mineralocorticoid activity, which results in sodium and water retention, commonly contributes to hypertension and heart failure. Hypoglycemia and dehydration (Option B) are uncommon in a patient with Cushing's syndrome. Diabetes mellitus and hyperglycemia may develop, but hypotension (Option C) isn't part of the disease process. Pulmonary edema and dehydration (Option D) also aren't complications of Cushing's syndrome.

Question 139.   Correct answer: A. Diabetic ketoacidosis stems from an absence or inadequate amount of insulin and leads to a series of biochemical disorders. Diabetes insipidus (Option B) is caused by a deficiency of vasopressin. HHNS (Option C) is a coma state characterized by hyperglycemia and hyperosmolarity. Hyperaldosteronism (Option D) is an excess of aldosterone production, causing sodium and fluid excesses and hypertension.

Question 140.   Correct answer: D. Graves' disease is another name for hyperthyroidism, which would require a thyroid panel. A patient with Graves' disease wouldn't typically need serum glucose or calcium levels (Options B and C) or a lipid panel (Option A) because Graves' disease involves the thyroid.

Question 141.   Correct answer: D. The nurse should always reassess the patient's ABCs when his ICP is elevated (normal ICP ranges from 0 to 15 mm Hg). External stimulation, such as visitors (Option A), should be limited because it could increase the patient's ICP. The patient's MAP should be maintained at or above 60 mm Hg, not below 60 mm Hg (Option B). The head of the bed should be elevated between 15 and 30 degrees to promote venous drainage, not lowered to less than 15 degrees (Option C).

Question 142.   Correct answer: A. In most cases, patients should be out of bed the first postoperative day. Frequent repositioning rather than limiting movement (Option B), using a chairlike brace for the lower back when out of bed rather than maximizing bracing while in bed (Option C), and using a firm rather than soft mattress (Option D) help to minimize complications.

Question 143.   Correct answer: C. These symptoms suggest cholinergic crisis or excessive acetylcholinesterase medication and typically appear 45 to 60 minutes after the last dose of acetylcholinesterase inhibitor. Atropine, an anticholinergic drug, is used to antagonize acetylcholinesterase inhibitors. The other drugs are acetylcholinesterase inhibitors. Edrophonium (Option D) is used to diagnose and pyridostigmine bromide (Option B) is used to treat myasthenia gravis and would worsen these symptoms. Acyclovir (Option A) is an antiviral and wouldn't be used to treat these symptoms.

Question 144.   Correct answer: D. Complaints of halos around lights is a common finding in a patient with glaucoma. Other signs and symptoms include IOP—not an IOP of 15 mm Hg (Option B), which falls within the normal range of 10 to 21 mm Hg—loss of peripheral vision or blind spots, reddened sclera, a firm globe (not a soft globe, as in Option A), decreased accommodation, and occasional eye pain; patients may also be asymptomatic. Glaucoma doesn't cause double vision (Option C).

Question 145.   Correct answer: B. The prosthesis should be applied upon rising in the morning. The stump and prosthesis should be inspected and cleaned daily with a mild soap, not an antiseptic soap (Option C) and not weekly (Options A and D). The prosthesis should be kept clean to prevent irritation or pressure areas from dirt or bacteria.

Question 146.   Correct answer: B. In tamponade, fluid accumulates in the pericardial sac, hindering motion of the heart muscle and causing it to pump inefficiently, which results in signs of cardiogenic shock. Anaphylactic and septic shock (Options A and D) are types of distributive shock in which fluid is displaced from the capillaries and leaks into surrounding tissues. Hypovolemic shock (Option C) involves the actual loss of fluid.

Question 147.   Correct answer: A. Pentamidine isethionate can cause hyperglycemia or hypoglycemia. The patient's electrolyte levels, heart rate, and CBC (Options B, C, and D) can be monitored less frequently.

Question 148. **Correct answer: C.** The flow rate is determined by the rate of infusion and the number of drops per milliliter of fluid being administered: gtt/mL × amount to be infused divided by the number of minutes = the I.V. flow rate.

15 gtt/mL × 1,000 mL = 15,000

15,000 mL divided by 360 minutes = 41.6 gtt/minute, which rounds up to a flow rate of 42 gtt/minute.

Question 149. **Correct answer: A.** A condom catheter uses a condom-type device to drain urine away from the patient. Diapering the patient (Option B) will not keep urine away from the body and the patient (if alert) or the family may object because they feel it's demeaning to the patient. Because the patient with Parkinson's disease is already prone to infections of the urinary tract, he shouldn't have an indwelling urinary catheter inserted (Option C). The nurse should provide skin care as soon as the patient is incontinent to prevent skin maceration and breakdown, not just every 4 hours (Option D).

Question 150. **Correct answer: B.** The patient with a spinal cord injury should recognize fever and change in the clarity of urine as early indications of a UTI. Lower back pain (Option D) is a late sign. The patient with a spinal cord injury may not have burning or frequency of urination (Options A and C).

Analyzing the Posttest

Total the number of *incorrect* responses to the posttest. A score of 1 to 14 indicates that you have an excellent knowledge base and that you're well prepared for the certification examination; a score of 15 to 29 indicates adequate preparation, although more study or improvement in test-taking skills is recommended; a score of 30 or more indicates the need for intensive study before taking the certification examination.

For a more detailed analysis of your performance, complete the self-diagnostic profile worksheet.

Self-Diagnostic Profile for Posttest

In the top row of boxes, record the number of each question you answered incorrectly. Then beneath each question number, check the box that corresponds to the reason you answered the question incorrectly. Finally, tabulate the number of check marks on each line in the right-hand column marked "Totals." You now have an individualized profile of weak areas that require further study or improvement in test-taking ability before you take the Medical-Surgical Nursing Certification Examination.

Question Number   **Totals**

Test-Taking Skills

1. Misread question

2. Missed important point

3. Forgot fact or concept

4. Applied wrong fact or concept

5. Drew wrong conclusion

6. Incorrectly evaluated distractors

7. Mistakenly filled in wrong circle

8. Read into question

9. Guessed wrong

10. Misunderstood question

Selected References

ACC atlas of pathophysiology (3rd ed.). (2009). Philadelphia, PA: Lippincott Williams & Wilkins.

American Heart Association. (2010). 2010 American Heart Association guidelines for cardiopulmonary resuscitation and emergency cardiovascular care science. *Circulation, 122*(18), S3.

American Pain Society. (2008). *Principles of analgesic use in the treatment of acute pain and cancer pain* (6th ed.). Glenview, IL: Author.

Baranoski, S., & Ayello, S. E. (2011). *Wound care essentials: Practice principles* (3rd ed.). Philadelphia, PA: Lippincott Williams & Wilkins.

Bickley, L. (2008). *Bates' guide to physical examination and history taking* (11th ed.). Philadelphia, PA: Lippincott Williams & Wilkins.

Fauci, A. S., Kasper, D., Hauser, S., Longo, D., Jameson, J. L., & Loscalzo, J. (2008). *Harrison's principles of internal medicine* (17th ed.). New York, NY: McGraw-Hill.

Ignatavicius, D., & Workman, L. (2009). *Medical-surgical nursing: Patient-centered collaborative care.* Philadelphia, PA: W.B. Saunders.

Lippincott's guide to infectious diseases. (2010). Philadelphia, PA: Lippincott Williams & Wilkins.

Medical-surgical nursing made incredibly easy! (3rd ed.). (2011). Philadelphia, PA: Lippincott Williams & Wilkins.

Melnyk, B., & Fineout-Overholt, E. (2010). *Evidence-based practice in nursing & healthcare: A guide to best practice.* Philadelphia, PA: Lippincott Williams & Wilkins.

Nettina, S. (2009). *Lippincott manual of nursing practice* (9th ed.). Philadelphia, PA: Lippincott Williams & Wilkins.

Nursing 2012 drug handbook (32nd ed.). (2011). Philadelphia, PA: Lippincott Williams & Wilkins.

Pillitteri, A. (2009). *Maternal and child health nursing: Care of the childbearing and childrearing family* (6th ed.). Philadelphia, PA: Lippincott Williams & Wilkins.

Porth, C. M. (2010). *Essentials of pathophysiology* (3rd ed.). Philadelphia, PA: Lippincott Williams & Wilkins.

Smeltzer, S. C., Bare, B. G., Hinkle, J. L., & Cheever, K. H. (2009). *Brunner and Suddarth's textbook of medical-surgical nursing* (12th ed.). Philadelphia, PA: Lippincott Williams & Wilkins.

Suadoni, M. T. (2009). Raised intracranial pressure: Nursing observations and interventions. *Nursing Standard, 23*(43), 35–40.

Taylor, C., Lillis, C., & Lynn, P. (2010). *Fundamentals of nursing: The art and science of nursing care* (7th ed.). Philadelphia, PA: Lippincott Williams & Wilkins.

Ward, S., & Hisley, S. (2009). *Maternal-child nursing care: Optimizing outcomes for mothers, children, and families.* Philadelphia, PA: F.A. Davis Company.

Woods, S. L., Froelicher, E. S., Motzer, S., & Bridges, E. (Eds.). (2009). *Cardiac nursing* (6th ed.). Philadelphia, PA: Lippincott Williams & Wilkins.

Yarbro, C. H., Wujcik, D., & Gobel, B. H. (2010). *Cancer nursing: Principles and practice* (7th ed.). Sudbury, MA: Jones & Bartlett Learning.